Fundamentals of

Pharmacology

For Nursing and Healthcare Students

Fundamentals of

Pharmacology

For Nursing and Healthcare Students

Edited by

IAN PEATE, EN(G), RGN, DipN (Lond) RNT, BEd (Hons), MA (Lond) LLM, OBE, FRCN, JP

Principal
School of Health Studies
Gibraltar Health Authority
St Bernard's Hospital
Gibraltar, UK

BARRY HILL, MSc ANP, PGCAP, PGCE, BSc (Hons), DipHE, O.A. Dip, Fellow (FHEA)

Senior Lecturer and Director of Education
(Employability) Faculty of Health and Life Sciences
Department of Nursing, Midwifery and Health
Northumbria University
Newcastle upon Tyne, UK

WILEY Blackwell

Registered Office(s)
John Wiley & Sons, Inc., 111 River Street, Hoboken, NJ 07030, USA
John Wiley & Sons Ltd, The Atrium, Southern Gate, Chichester, West Sussex, PO19 8SQ, UK

Editorial Office
9600 Garsington Road, Oxford, OX4 2DQ, UK

For details of our global editorial offices, customer services and more information about Wiley products visit us at www.wiley.com.

Wiley also publishes its books in a variety of electronic formats and by print-on-demand. Some content that appears in standard print versions of this book may not be available in other formats.

Limit of Liability/Disclaimer of Warranty
The contents of this work are intended to further general scientific research, understanding and discussion only and are not intended and should not be relied upon as recommending or promoting scientific method, diagnosis or treatment by physicians for any particular patient. In view of ongoing research, equipment modifications, changes in governmental regulations and the constant flow of information relating to the use of medicines, equipment and devices, the reader is urged to review and evaluate the information provided in the package insert or instructions for each medicine, equipment or device for, among other things, any changes in the instructions or indication of usage and for added warnings and precautions. While the publisher and authors have used their best efforts in preparing this work, they make no representations or warranties with respect to the accuracy or completeness of the contents of this work and specifically disclaim all warranties, including without limitation any implied warranties of merchantability or fitness for a particular purpose. No warranty may be created or extended by sales representatives, written sales materials or promotional statements for this work. The fact that an organisation, website or product is referred to in this work as a citation and/or potential source of further information does not mean that the publisher and authors endorse the information or services the organisation, website or product may provide or recommendations it may make. This work is sold with the understanding that the publisher is not engaged in rendering professional services. The advice and strategies contained herein may not be suitable for your situation. You should consult with a specialist where appropriate. Further, readers should be aware that websites listed in this work may have changed or disappeared between when this work was written and when it is read. Neither the publisher nor authors shall be liable for any loss of profit or any other commercial damages, including but not limited to special, incidental, consequential or other damages.

Library of Congress Cataloging-in-Publication Data

Names: Peate, Ian, editor. | Hill, Barry (Lecturer in nursing), editor.
Title: Fundamentals of pharmacology for nursing & healthcare students /
    edited by Ian Peate and Barry Hill.
Other titles: Fundamentals of pharmacology for nursing and healthcare students
Description: Hoboken, NJ : Wiley-Blackwell, 2021. | Includes
    bibliographical references and index.
Identifiers: LCCN 2020028463 (print) | LCCN 2020028464 (ebook) | ISBN
    9781119594666 (paperback) | ISBN 9781119594628 (adobe pdf) | ISBN
    9781119594673 (epub)
Subjects: MESH: Pharmacological Phenomena | Pharmaceutical Preparations |
    Drug Therapy
Classification: LCC RM301.25 (print) | LCC RM301.25 (ebook) | NLM QV 4 |
    DDC 615.1/9–dc23
LC record available at https://lccn.loc.gov/2020028463
LC ebook record available at https://lccn.loc.gov/2020028464

Cover Design: Wiley
Cover Image: © apomares/Getty Images

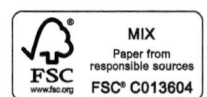

MIX
Paper from
responsible sources
FSC
www.fsc.org   FSC® C013604

Contents

Contents

Contents

Contributors

Jaden Allan
MSc, PG Dip, BSc (Hons), RN, SFHEA. Director of International Development and Recruitment. Senior Lecturer, Learning Laeadership Lead (Peer support), Department of Nursing, Midwifery and Health.

Jaden joined Northumbria University having spent several years working in a partnership hospital post as a practice placement facilitator (PPF) organising a range of health professional student placements and providing support to students and mentors during their clinical rotations. Jaden's clinical nursing experience is in critical care (respiratory, neurological and plastics) at the Newcastle upon Tyne NHS Foundation Trust, and earlier in acute surgery (GI and general) at Northumbria NHS Trust. Since joining the university, Jaden has held a number of complex module lead roles and he has been instrumental in developing the use of simulation within the nursing curriculum. Having many years of senior lecturer experience in teaching and leadership gives Jaden a sound foundation for his strategic and departmental work.

Over the past four years Jaden's roles have include Director of Programs and Director of Learning and Teaching (DLT) with responsibility for curricula revalidation, quality teaching and assessment monitoring, departmental development and university vision delivery. He has also led on departmental timetabling, and faculty integration of timetabling systems.

Jaden is currently working as Director of International Development and Recruitment for the faculty of Health and Life Sciences, liaising with international partners and universities to develop the university's portfolio of Transnational Education (TNE) and international students both on campus and globally.

Jaden has developed, and been implementation lead, for a number of complex practice modules in Northumbria University's UK BSc (Hons) Nursing program. He is a lead on the implementation for a BSc (Hons) Nursing curricula in Malta.

He has led the development, and the successful implementation, of the 'Learning Leadership scheme' within Northumbria's Nursing programs. This peer support scheme prepares and develops students on nursing programs to support newer students as they make the transition into higher education and the world of nursing.

Jaden's learning and teaching interests are developing clinical skills, simulation (all levels), leadership, peer support and compassion in nursing. Jaden also has a particular interest in the use of technology to enhance and share learning.

Nicola Clipperton
BSc (Hons) in Evidence Based Nursing Practice – Adult. Registered Nurse (RN).

Nicola began her nursing career in 2006, working as a Healthcare Assistant. In 2007, she attended the University of York, where she obtained her Adult Nursing degree. In 2010, Nicola moved to London to pursue a career in critical care. She worked for Imperial College Healthcare NHS Trust in the critical care department from 2010 to 2016, working her way up from newly qualified nurse to Senior Charge Nurse. While working in critical care, Nicola featured in the BBC2 documentary series; 'Hospital', providing an insight into the running of a busy London teaching hospital. In 2016, Nicola changed her focus toward oncology, where she became a Clinical Nurse Specialist, supporting those affected by bowel cancer. In 2018, Nicola relocated back to North Yorkshire and currently works as a Specialist Screening Practitioner for the National Bowel Cancer Screening Program for Public Health England.

Julie Derbyshire

Professional Doctorate (Education), MSc Practice Education and Development, BA (Hons) Education, DipHE Nursing, Certificate in Health Education, Registered General Nurse (RGN), Nursing Lecturer (NMC status), Fellow (FHEA).

Julie qualified as a Registered General Nurse in 1992 and specialised in neurosurgical/trauma nursing, working within a regional neurosciences unit at Newcastle General Hospital for eight years. Julie moved into a specialist practice development role in 2000 before taking on the role of a Lecturer in Health and Social Care at an FE college. In 2003, after one year at the college and completing a BA (Hons) in Education, Julie moved to a Senior Lecturer role in Adult Nursing at Northumbria University. During this time, she completed masters and doctoral level study. Julie teaches predominantly undergraduate nursing students and is current program lead for the registered degree nursing apprenticeship. Julie also teaches her specialist subject of neurology to postgraduate students from different healthcare professions. Her other key areas of interest are interprofessional learning (IPL), study skills, critical care, service improvement and practice learning.

Sadie Diamond-Fox

Masters of Clinical Practice in Advanced Critical Care Practice (ACCP), BSc (Hons) Adult Nursing, PGC Autonomous Healthcare Practice (AHP), Non-Medical Prescriber (V300). Registered Nurse. ACCP member of the Faculty of Intensive Care Medicine.

Sadie qualified as an Adult Nurse in 2008 and has since worked in various critical care departments including hepatobiliary, cardiothoracic, burns and general medical and surgical units. During this time she has progressed from Registered Nurse to her current specialist roles as Advanced Critical Care Practitioner (ACCP) and Senior Lecturer and PFNA content expert for Northumbria University's ACCP training programs.

Sadie has various national links and responsibilities within the critical care field. She is current Co-Lead for the Northern Region of ACCPs (ACCPNR), a regional group whose aim is to increase collaborative working of ACCPs to advance practice within critical care, while enhancing and supporting training and educational development. Sadie also sits on the North East Intensive Care Society (NEICS) Committee, which involves regular networking and engagement with international experts within the field, and collaboration with local critical care leads and practitioners.

Deborah Flynn

Doctor of Nursing, MA Medical Education, PGC Academic Practice, BSc (Hons) Health and Social Care, DipHE General Nursing, Registered Nurse (RN), Registered Teacher (NMC), Fellow (FHEA). Senior Lecturer Adult Nursing, Northumbria University.

Deborah became a student nurse in 1986 at BG Alexander Nursing College and Johannesburg General hospital (now Charlotte Maxeke Johannesburg Academic Hospital) in Johannesburg, South Africa, completing her studies as a Registered Nurse (general, community health and psychiatry) and Midwife in 1990. Deborah worked across the South African public and private sector in general surgical and neuro medical wards. From 1993 to 2002, she worked as a Staff Nurse rising to a Charge Nurse in Germany and Switzerland in a variety of disciplines. In 2002, she returned to Britain to work as a Staff Nurse on an acute stroke unit.

Entering the educational sector in 2005, Deborah progressed from Practice Educator to Senior Lecturer and has taught on both undergraduate and postgraduate programs. In 2018, she completed her doctorate exploring student nurses' experience of humour use in the clinical setting. Her key interests are clinical skills, humour in clinical care, stroke care, pharmacology and practice supervisor/assessor preparation.

Claire Ford

Fellow of Higher Education Academy (FHEA), PG Diploma Midwifery, BSc (Hons) Adult Nursing, Registered Nurse (RN). Lecturer Adult Nursing, Northumbria University.

Claire joined the teaching team at Northumbria University in 2013, having spent time working within perioperative care and completing a Postgraduate Diploma in Midwifery. She studied for her BSc (Hons) and PG Dip at Northumbria University, and won academic awards for both, as well as the Heath Award in 2009. As a Lecturer, she teaches a range of modules across pre-registration healthcare programs, both nationally and internationally, and has a passion for pain management, clinical skills, women's health, gynaecology, perioperative care and simulation. She also has an interest in using other forms of media and technology to facilitate and enhance deep learning and is the co-founder of the 'Skills for Practice' website, which acts as a central repository for videos, posters and podcasts focusing on a range of clinical nursing procedures. In 2016, the website was shortlisted for the Student Nursing Times Awards – Teaching Innovation of the Year. In addition to teaching, Claire is involved in several research projects. Her PhD study examines preoperative pain planning using both qualitative and quantitative data collection methods and is underpinned by a critical ethnographic methodology. She is also involved in another research project, exploring the use of technology-enhanced learning and virtual reality to augment undergraduate students' learning.

Alexandra Gatehouse

Alexandra Gatehouse graduated from Nottingham University in 2000 with a BSc (Hons) Physiotherapy, following Junior Rotations in the Newcastle Trust. She is specialised in Respiratory Physiotherapy in Adult Critical Care, also working within New Zealand. In 2012, Alex trained as an Advanced Critical Care Practitioner, completing a Masters in Clinical Practice in Critical Care and qualifying in 2014. Alex subsequently completed her non-medical prescribing qualification and continues to rotate within all of the Critical Care Units in Newcastle Upon Tyne, also enjoying teaching on the regional transfer course. She is a co-founder of the Advanced Critical Care Practitioner Northern Region Group and is a committee member of the North East Intensive Care Society. Alex has presented abstracts at the European Society of Intensive Care Medicine and the North East Intensive Care Society conferences.

Jan Guerin

Dip General Nursing (RSA), BSc Nursing Education (RSA), PGD ANP(UK), Diploma General Adult Critical Care(RSA), Diploma Trauma and Emergency Nursing Science (RSA), Cert LSM/BSLM(UK).

Jan qualified as a General Registered Nurse in South Africa in 1992. She gained 12 years of accumulative experience working in acute care settings within the field of adult emergency and critical care including 4 years as a lead lecturer for Trauma and Emergency Nursing. Jan moved to the UK in 2006 and joined Hammersmith Hospitals NHS Trust as a Senior Staff Nurse in adult General ITU, which included a year of secondment experience in Critical Care Outreach at Charing Cross Hospital. In 2017, Jan worked for the Hillingdon Hospitals NHS Trust and in the roles as an ITU Nurse Educator and Practice Nurse Educator as lead for Clinical skills. Jan, moved over to adult social care nursing in 2020, and is currently in a role as a Quality Business Partner with Sunrise Senior Living. Jan, has a special interest in health promotion and prevention of chronic disease and has been certified in Lifestyle Medicine with the British Society of Lifestyle Medicine (BSLM).

Annette Hand

Nursing MA, PG Dip CR, Dip HE, RGN. Nurse, Consultant/Associate, Professor/Clinical Lead – Nursing, Northumbria Healthcare NHS Trust/Northumbria University/Parkinson's Excellence Network.

Annette has a clinical academic position and divides her time between three roles; Nurse Consultant, Associate Professor and UK Clinical Lead for Nursing (Parkinson's).

Annette has worked in the field of Parkinson's for many years and as a Nurse Consultant has an active clinical, research, and educational role within this area. She qualified as a non-medical prescriber over 15 years ago and continues to use this skill in day-to-day clinical practice. She was the non-medical prescribing lead for Northumbria Healthcare NHS Foundation Trust for many years supporting and developing other non-medical prescribers. Annette, an Associate Professor with Northumbria University, has lectured on the Non-Medical Prescribing Program (V300) for over five years, supporting prescribing students and the continual development of the V300 Program. Annette was appointed to the national role of Clinical Lead for Nursing within the Parkinson's UK Excellence Network as part of the clinical leadership team. This role was developed to support service improvements through education, knowledge exchange and evidence-based practice and support the role of the Parkinson's Nurse across the UK.

Barry Hill

MSc Advanced Practice, PGC Academic Practice, BSc (Hons) Intensive Care Nursing, DipHE Adult Nursing, OA Dip Counseling Skills, Registered Nurse (RN). Registered Teacher (NMC RNT/TCH). Senior Fellow (SFHEA), Program Leader (Senior Lecturer) Adult Nursing, Northumbria University. Clinical Editor *British Journal of Nursing*.

Barry completed his Registered Nurse training at Northumbria University and Buckinghamshire Chilterns University College (BCUC). Barry's clinical experience has been gained at Imperial College NHS Trust, London, UK. Barry has worked as a Staff Nurse and Senior Staff Nurse in cardiac and general intensive care at the Milne ICU unit at St Mary's Hospital, London (Paddington). He worked in neuro trauma and general intensive care as a Charge Nurse at Charing Cross Hospital, London.

   Following this role, he worked as a Senior Charge Nurse at general intensive care (GICU) at Hammersmith Hospital, London. Finally, he worked as a Matron within the surgical division for Plastics, Orthopaedics, ENT and Major trauma (POEM) at Charing Cross Hospital, London. Barry is ICU qualified, has a clinical master's in advanced practice, is an NMC RN, independent prescriber (V300), and Registered Teacher. Barry is currently the Director of Education (Employability), Programme Leader BSc Adult Nursing, and Senior Lecturer at Northumbria University. He teaches undergraduate and postgraduate students from all disciplines. His key areas of interest are clinical educations, acute and critical care, clinical skills, independent prescribing, and pharmacology, and advanced level practice. Barry has published widely in journals and books and is a Fellow with the Higher Education Academy (FHEA).

Claire Leader

MA, PGCAP, BSc (Hons), RN, RM. Senior Lecturer in Adult Nursing at Northumbria University.

Claire began her career in 1995 studying Adult Nursing at the University of York before taking up a Staff Nurse post at the Leeds Teaching Hospital's Trust, initially within cardiothoracic surgery and later in the emergency department where she worked between 1998 and 2002. Following this, Claire spent time as a Nursing Officer in the Merchant Navy before returning to the UK to undertake her Midwifery Education at Huddersfield University. Following a move to the North East of England where Claire practised as a Midwife, she moved into the area of clinical research gaining valuable experience as a Research Nurse and Midwife, going on to lead teams within a number of speciality areas coordinating research studies for the National Institute of Health Research (NIHR). Within this role, Claire undertook the NIHR Advanced Leadership Program and has been involved in the development and delivery of the NIHR National Strategy for Clinical Research Nurses as well as contributing to the development of clinical–academic careers for Nurses, Midwives and Allied Health Professionals in the North East region. In 2018, Claire moved to Northumbria University and in addition to contributing to the development and delivery of a high-quality undergraduate curriculum, has continued to work collaboratively with the NIHR as well as the Royal College of Nursing in developing resources and initiatives which contribute to Nurse research careers.

Cecilia Mihaila

Cecilia, qualified as a Medical Doctor in Romania in 2006. Her medical training and experience was achieved working in the largest university hospital in Bucharest, which provided emergency and trauma healthcare services. Cecilia, moved to UK in 2010 and has been working in the NHS in Anaesthesia and Adult Intensive Care. She is passionate about cardiac care and has contributed by creating an "Out of Hospital Arrest Protocol" in 2014 following an in hospital audit result. She has also been involved in teaching sessions for the ICU Nursing Staff on airway management and cardiac arrest protocols following cardiac surgery. Cecilia is passionate about preventing chronic disease by supporting people to achieve optimal health through nutrition and lifestyle choices as a certified Health Coach.

Michelle Mitchell

Advanced Diploma in Adult Nursing, .BSc (Hons) in Practice Development, Registered Nurse (RN), Graduate Tutor, Learning Leadership Lead at Department of Nursing, Midwifery and Health, Northumbria University.

Michelle studied for both her Advanced Diploma in Adult Nursing and BSc (Hons) in Practice Development at Northumbria University. She was awarded the Heath Medal in 2013 for both academic and clinical excellence and was short listed nationally in 2014 in the category of 'Most Inspiration Student' in the Nursing Times awards. The majority of Michelle's clinical background is in primary care, where she worked for many years in varies areas including, community nursing, GP practice, palliative care, sexual health and with a focus on public health she was a stop smoking advisor. Entering the education sector at Northumbria University in 2014 Michelle teaches predominantly undergraduate nursing students across all subjects and is lead for an international public health module in Malta. Her PhD study examines the relationship between student nurses and their community assessors utilising a hermeneutic phenomenological methodology. Michelle is well published in books and journals and is a Fellow of the Higher Education Academy (FHEA).

Aby Mitchell

MSc Advanced Practice, PGCAP, TCH, BSc (Hons), RGN, FHEA. Senior Lecturer in Adult Nursing (Cohort Lead) at The University of West London.

Aby began her career in 1995 studying Adult Nursing at the Thames Valley University (now The University of West London) before taking up a Staff Nurse post at Wexham Park Hospital in the burns and plastics unit. In 1999, Aby took her first Community Staff Nurse post in Berkshire where she progressed to District Nursing Sister and then Team Leader for the District Nursing Service and Out of Hours Service. During that time, Aby developed her wound care practice and set up clinical services to treat and manage leg ulcers in the community. Aby left the community after 18 years in 2015 to start her career in lecturing with the University of West London. She currently works clinically one day a week as a Senior Clinical Lead for physical health in a community mental health service.

Educationally, Aby teaches on several postgraduate courses for the university and has contributed to the new high-quality nursing curriculum. She has implemented a number of interactive teaching pedagogies – most recently an immersive theatre simulated event and a drama-based hypothetical street. Aby's areas of interest include wound care, clinical skills, advanced level practice and theatre/drama in education and she has published several articles on these subjects.

Ian Naldrett

Lecturer in Intensive Care Nursing, Advanced DipHE Adult Nursing (Middlesex University), Advanced DipHE Acute Adult Nursing (Middlesex University), BSc (Hons) Healthcare Practice (Acute and Critical care) (St Georges University of London), MSc Professional Practice (Nursing) (University of West London).

Ian is employed as the Lead Nurse for critical care education at the Royal Brompton Hospital and is also a lecturer for ICU nursing at the University of West London (UWL). He has a clinical background in respiratory and cardiothoracic ICU nursing gained at the Royal Brompton Hospital in London, UK. Ian has worked extensively as an Extra Corporeal Membrane

Oxygenation (ECMO) specialist nurse at the Royal Brompton Hospital regional Severe Acute Pulmonary Failure centre. Ian is passionate about the development of critical care nursing. He is well published in books and journals. Ian is a recognised Fellow (FHEA). Ian is a board member of the British Association of Critical Care Nurses (BACCN), National board member Extra Corporeal Life Support Organisation (ELSO), and UK Council Representative – European Federation of Critical Care Nurse Association.

Laura Park
BSc (Hons), RN. Graduate Tutor in Adult Nursing, Department of Healthcare, Northumbria University.

Before joining the academic team at Northumbria University, Laura worked as a Staff Nurse for the NHS. Laura's teaching interests are predominately within teaching clinical skills and simulation within the pre-registration adult nursing program. This passion for clinical skills teaching has resulted in Laura co-creating and developing the skills for a practice website. The website is a repository that houses a number of videos, posters and podcasts that demonstrates to students the correct technique of carrying out a specific clinical skill. In 2016, the website was shortlisted for the Student Nursing Times Awards – Teaching Innovation of the Year. Laura is involved in several research projects. Her PhD study examines the working relationships within interprofessional practice via a constructivist grounded theory methodology. In addition, Laura has been a chapter co-author in a 2018 Nurse Associate book and in a number of journal publications 2018–2019.

Ian Peate
EN(G), RGN, DipN (Lond) RNT, BEd (Hons), MA (Lond) LLM, OBE, FRCN, JP. Principal, School of Health Studies, Gibraltar. Editor in Chief *British Journal of Nursing*. Visiting Professor of Nursing St George's University of London and Kingston University London. Visiting Professor Northumbria University. Visiting Senior Clinical Fellow University of Hertfordshire.

Ian began his nursing a career in 1981 at Central Middlesex Hospital, becoming an Enrolled Nurse working in an intensive care unit. He later undertook three years Student Nurse training at Central Middlesex and Northwick Park Hospitals, becoming a Staff Nurse then a Charge Nurse. He has worked in nurse education since 1989. His key areas of interest are nursing practice and theory, men's health, sexual health and HIV. Ian has published widely; he is Principal, School of Health Studies, Gibraltar, Visiting Professor of Nursing, Visiting Senior Clinical Fellow, Editor in Chief of the *British Journal of Nursing,* Founding Consultant Editor of the *Journal of Paramedic Practice,* Editorial Board Member of the *British Journal of Healthcare Assistants*. Ian was awarded an OBE in the Queen's 90th Birthday Honours List 2016 for his services to Nursing and Nurse Education. He was made a Fellow of the Royal College of Nursing in 2017 in recognition of his contribution to the profession.

Anne Phillips
PhD, MSc in Health Professional Education, Registered Nurse Teacher (NMC RNT), BSc Hons Community Nursing, Diploma District Nursing, Registered Nurse (RN). Queens Nurse, National Teaching Fellow (NTF).

Anne undertook her registered nurse training at St Bartholomew's Hospital, London. She worked as a Staff Nurse in various hospitals across London before working in the community in Ealing. She became a District Nurse, then a Community Diabetes Specialist Nurse. Anne then relocated to Yorkshire to work as a Diabetes Specialist Nurse, then a Lecturer Practitioner delivering the diabetes module at the University of Huddersfield, alongside her clinical DSN role. Following her MSc, she joined the University of York and developed the portfolio of clinically focused diabetes education module and degree opportunities with clinical colleagues. This enabled collaborative working with clinical leaders in diabetes care and a focus on age-appropriate education. Anne was awarded the National Quality in Care 'Outstanding Diabetes

Educator' award in 2014. In 2016, she became a Queens Nurse and also was awarded a National Teaching Fellowship for her work in diabetes education.

Anne joined Birmingham City University as an Associate Professor in Diabetes Care in 2018 and leads the online MSc in Advancing Diabetes Care. She works internationally with colleagues across India in research and education, and also works clinically with Birmingham University Hospitals Trust.

Anne edited *Principals of Diabetes Care: Evidence based practice for healthcare professionals* by Quay Books, published in 2017 in its 2nd edition.

Claire Pryor

MSc Advancing Healthcare Practice, PGC Advanced Practice (Clinical), PGC Teaching and Learning in Professional Practice, NMC Teacher (NMC/TCH), V300 Independent Prescriber, Grad Cert Practice Development, Fellow Higher Education Academy (FHEA), Registered Nurse Adult (RN).

Claire Pryor is a Senior Lecturer in Adult Nursing at Northumbria University. Claire's educational interests lie predominantly in nursing care for the older person and she is module lead for non-medical prescribing. Her teaching activity spans both adult pre- and post-registration professional development.

Claire's specialist areas of interest include delirium and delirium superimposed on dementia, which forms the basis of her PhD research, and integrating physical health and mental healthcare education and service provision.

Prior to lecturing, Claire worked in a variety of primary and secondary care settings including acute medical assessment, critical care, intermediate care, and as an older person's nurse practitioner in a mental health setting.

Matthew Robertson

BSc (Hons) Operating Department Practice, Graduate Tutor, Department of Nursing, Midwifery and Health.

Matthew is a registered Operating Department Practitioner with the HCPC. He is also a member of the College of Operating Department Practitioners. Matthew completed his BSc (Hons) at the University of Central Lancashire in Operating Department Practice, where he was able to experience a range of complex surgical specialities. Once qualified, Matthew was employed by Newcastle Hospitals within the Cardiothoracic Surgical Department where I undertook the role of the scrub practitioner, specialising in paediatric and congenital cardiac surgery.

Matthew commenced employment at Northumbria University in November 2017 and since then he has developed a specialist interest in Human Factors within the perioperative environment and is completing a PhD on this topic, focussing on staff well-being and stress management. Recently, Matthew has had several publications regarding 'the care of the surgical patient' and has written two book chapters on the use of analgesics in practice and other related pharmacology. Matthew also sits as a registrant panel member for the Health and Care Professionals Tribunal Service and provide expertise on the disciplinary cases that are presented to me and the rest of the panel.

Leah Rosengarten

MSc Practice Development, BSc (Hons), Nursing Studies (Child). Lecturer Children and Young People's Nursing, Northumbria University.

After qualifying as a Children's Nurse in 2012 from the University of Teesside, Leah began work as a Staff Nurse on the Children and Teenage Cancer Unit at the Great North Children's Hospital, Newcastle. Leah worked on this unit for six years while studying for her MSc in Practice Development, part time. In 2018, Leah commenced a year secondment as a Children and Young People's Nursing Lecturer at Northumbria University, before accepting a permanent position in 2019. Leah's areas of interest include oncology, human factors and continuing professional development and she has recently commenced her PhD.

Emma Senior

Emma is an NMC registered teacher, nurse and health visitor with over 10 years of experience in the NHS and 10 years' teaching experience with Northumbria University. She began her nurse career in theatres specialising in women and children's health before qualifying as a health visitor in 2006. She then went on to work as a Sexual Health Advisor across North Yorkshire where she was able to work collaboratively with a range of services and organisations which included the military, primary care and secondary education.

Emma joined higher education in 2009, taking her first post as a Senior Lecturer/Practitioner taking the lead in implementing a workforce development initiative called Northumbria Integrated Sexual Health Education (NISHE) for post-qualified nurses across County Durham & Darlington – and then project managed the delivery across the South West of England with the University of West England. This involved the development and delivery of e-learning educational materials along with supporting academic staff and students in their practice setting. In 2012, Emma joined the pre-registration nurse team where she has been able to introduce, develop and co-ordinate e-learning packages on the program.

Along with teaching pre-registration healthcare, Emma has maintained her post-registration nurse teaching within sexual health, safeguarding and public health within the Specialist Community Public Health Nurse Program. During her time at Northumbria University, Emma was a part of the workforce development team working in collaboration with external partners to create education packages to develop the workforce. In 2015, Emma became involved and is Program Lead for Northumbria University's innovative program for Professional Non-Surgical Aesthetic Practice, which has been a trail blazer nationally.

Emma's key areas of interest are public health, sexual health, military families and technology enhanced learning. Emma has published widely in journals and is Fellow of the Higher Education Academy.

Laura Stavert

MPharm, PgDip Clinical Pharmacy, PGCert Independent Prescribing, MRPharmS, Advanced Pharmacist Practitioner Cumbria, Northumberland Tyne and Wear NHS Foundation Trust.

Laura began her training in 2005 as a Pharmacy undergraduate at The Robert Gordon University (RGU) in Aberdeen before completing pre-registration training at the Royal Infirmary of Edinburgh in 2009 and developing a range of skills across a number of clinical specialities, including a passion for mental health and medicines of the elderly. After qualification in 2010, she completed a number of basic grade rotations at the Western General Hospital in Edinburgh before taking up a specialist role in mental health services with Cumbria, Northumberland Tyne and Wear NHS FT in 2012. Laura began in a specialist role in the mental health of older adults in 2016 before qualifying as an independent prescriber in 2017.

Laura now has an advanced practice role working in the community with older adults with functional and organic mental health disorders. She currently teaches on the V300 Independent Prescribing course at the University of Sunderland and hopes to pursue a doctorate in the near future.

Hayley Underdown

Nurse Neurological Intensive Care, BSc (Hons) Critical Care, DipHE Adult Nursing.

Hayley embarked on her nursing career in 2002 where she began her Diploma of Higher Education in Adult Nursing at the University of Hertfordshire. Upon qualifying as a nurse in 2005, Hayley started work as a Band 5 Staff Nurse on the acute medical unit.

Hayley then went on to work in cardiothoracic and vascular intensive care at St Mary's Hospital in Paddington, London. She worked there for two and a half years, before moving to Charing Cross

Hospital in London where she worked as a Charge Nurse and the Senior Charge Nurse in the neuro-intensive care unit. After five years at Charing Cross Hospital, Hayley relocated to Perth, Western Australia. While in Perth she worked for five years in a general intensive care unit and coronary care unit at St John Of God Hospital in Murdoch. Hayley currently works at the Royal Perth Hospital in a 50-bedded acute medical unit as a Staff Development Nurse in clinical education.

Hayley has had a strong passion for critical care nursing. Her key interests are clinical and nurse education, service improvement and patient experience.

Elaine Walls

Senior Lecturer, Health and Life Sciences, Northumbria University.

Elaine first qualified as a Children's Nurse in 1996, from the Bolton and Salford School of Nursing. Upon qualification, Elaine worked at Newcastle General Hospital, rotating between paediatric intensive care and the children's bone marrow transplant unit. In 2001, Elaine commenced a Nurse Specialist post for children pre- and post-bone marrow transplant for immunological conditions. This involved national work, alongside presenting developments with international world specialists at European Bone Marrow Transplant Conferences. Elaine then went on to work in paediatric oncology and completed further study to qualify as a Health Visitor in 2007, working across Northumberland and South Tyneside. Following completion of a Masters degree in Public Health, Elaine trained as a Community Practice Teacher for post-registration specialist public health students in Northumberland and was responsible for their practice training and development, working in partnership with Northumbria University. In 2017, Elaine joined Northumbria University as a part time Lecturer on secondment alongside her clinical role. In 2018, Elaine joined the children's nursing team at Northumbria University and currently teaches across pre-registration nursing and post-registration specialist and prescribing programs.

Elaine has been involved in research with Newcastle University, is currently studying for her own PhD and has achieved several publications within academic journals.

David Waters

RN, BSc (Hons), PGDip, MA Ed, PgCert Research. Associate Professor and Head of Department, Department of Post-Qualifying Healthcare Practice, School of Nursing and Midwifery Birmingham City University.

David is an experienced nurse and academic, with a clinical background in cardiac care, critical care and aeromedical repatriation. He currently leads the post-qualifying portfolio, within the School of Nursing and Midwifery at Birmingham City University. He is currently undertaking a PhD, exploring the impact of errors within a critical care setting.

Carol Wills

MSc Multidisciplinary Professional Development and Education, PGDip Advanced Practice, BSc (Hons) Specialist Community Public Health Nursing (SCPHN) (Health Visiting), DipHE Adult Nursing, Registered Nurse (RN), Enrolled Nurse (EN), Registered Health Visitor (HV), Community Practitioner Prescriber (NP), Registered Lecturer/Practice Educator (RLP), Senior Fellow (SFHEA), Subject and Program Leader Non Medical Prescribing at Northumbria University.

Carol began her career undertaking enrolled nurse training in 1983 at Hexham Hospital in Northumberland. She then worked within neurotrauma at Newcastle General Hospital and then spent several years in coronary care and intensive care at Hexham Hospital. This experience and additional training to complete registered nurse qualification then stimulated her to focus on primary care and prevention of ill health. Carol worked as a Practice Nurse and Nurse Practitioner in Newcastle city centre and as a Staff Nurse within Northumberland community nursing teams before going on to complete a Health Visiting degree and working in Newcastle as a Health Visitor for several years. During this time, she undertook several leadership and teaching roles including Immunisation Training Co-Ordinator, Community Practice Teacher and Trust Lead Mentor.

Carol has been a Senior Lecturer at Northumbria University since 2002 and has led several post-graduate professional programs including the MSc Education in Professional Practice (NMC Teacher Program), PGDip SCPHN and the Non-Medical Prescribing Program. She has also undertaken national roles including Policy Advice Committee member and Treasurer for the UK Standing Conference SCPHN Education and Subject Expert for several quality approval panels and external examiner roles. Her key areas of interest and research are around developing learning and teaching and advanced level practice.

Preface

The overarching aim of this text is to provide the reader with an understanding of the fundamentals associated with pharmacology and the adult patient and in so doing enhance patient safety and patient outcomes. This book will help readers develop their competence and confidence within the field of pharmacology as related to the adult care setting, enabling them to recognise and respond compassionately to the needs of those they offer care to. The contributors to the text are all experienced clinicians and academics who have expertise in their sphere of practice.

The Nursing and Midwifery Council (NMC) in the UK is required to establish standards of proficiency that each nurse must achieve prior to being admitted to the professional register demonstrating safe and effective practice. The standards of proficiency for registered nurses and the standards of proficiency for nursing associates have been established (NMC 2018a, b respectively). The NMC (2018a) standards have been designed in such a way as to ensure that pre-registration nurses are 'prescriber ready' when they have successfully completed their undergraduate nursing program (Prydderch 2019).

If undergraduate, pre-registration nurses are to be 'prescriber ready' there is a need for those nurses to be prepared in order to practice as safe and accountable practitioners. *The Fundamentals of Adult Nursing Pharmacology* will help nurses add to their repertoire of skills as they acquire appropriate pharmacological knowledge. While there is an absolute need to ensure that much emphasis is placed on the principles of safe drug administration in the nursing curricula, there is also a need to ensure that students are equipped with the pharmacological foundations related to the bigger issues associated with medicines management. *The Fundamentals of Adult Nursing Pharmacology* provides the reader with an overview of the key issues that will enable them to begin to understand the complexities associated with pharmacology that they will face as well as the exciting challenges that are ahead of them.

Clause 18 of the NMC's (2018c) The Code of Profession Conduct requires all of those whose name appears on their professional register to ensure that if they advise people, prescribe, supply, dispense or administer medicines then they must do this within the limits of their training and competence. They must do this with respect to the law, guidance produced by the NMC and other relevant policies and regulations. In order to comply with the NMC's requirements and other guidance, the nurse must have an understanding of the fundamentals of pharmacology. Professional guidance has been co-produced by the Royal Pharmaceutical Society (RPS) and the Royal College of Nursing (RCN) (2019) and provides principles-based guidance to ensure the safe administration of medicines and has also been endorsed by the Royal College of General Practitioners.

There are 18 chapters in your book: the early chapters provide a broader discussion of pharmacology including a general overview of medicines management, legal aspects, pharmacodynamics and pharmacokinetics. Information and discussion concerning the use of prescribing reference guides, the various medicinal formulations, and the importance of preventing, noticing and responding effectively to adverse drug reactions are provided. Analgesics and antibacterials are given individual chapters and the remaining chapters adopt a systems approach.

When you are looking at the table of contents of this text this it might make you feel a little swamped and you could be forgiven for thinking: how on earth am I going to remember, recall and apply all of this information? There are a number of features in the text that will help you with your learning.

Each chapter is fully referenced and evidence based; the chapters begin with an aim and learning outcomes, providing you with an overall flavour of chapter content. At the beginning and the end of each chapter are a range of learning features that test your knowledge including multiple choice questions. This approach has been adopted to enhance learning and recall.

In most chapters there are a number of boxed features that can assist the reader in applying this complex subject area to their practice. The Clinical Considerations boxes address clinical issues related to chapter content. The Skills in Practice feature offers a 'how to do . . .' component. The Episodes of Care feature uses a case study approach, linked to chapter content that can occur in any care setting. Some chapters feature a glossary of terms and a further reading list is provided at the end of every chapter to encourage you to delve deeper.

As a healthcare student, your learning is not about rote learning and being able to remember. It is more than this: it is about applying that learning to the various situations you will find yourself in, ensuring that the patient, the person you have been given the privilege to offer care and support to, is at the heart of all you do. The goal should be to take your learning further, to develop, to discover and be curious. In this text you will learn and develop your own strategies that will help guide you so as to shape the way you study and learn, changing the way you think as you become a life-long learner with a myriad of transferable skills.

Life-long learning means just that: the continual pursuit of more knowledge as you develop personally and professionally; learning does not stop once you have graduated and had your name entered on to the professional register. Information and the acquisition of information does not stand still, new information is always being generated and applied in the nursing and medical fields. In the area of pharmacology, there are always new drugs being discovered and developed.

References

Nursing and Midwifery Council (2018a). *Future nurse: the standards of proficiency for registered nurses*. www.nmc.org.uk/globalassets/sitedocuments/education-standards/future-nurse-proficiencies.pdf (accessed September 2019).

Nursing and Midwifery Council (2018b). *The standards of proficiency for nursing associates*. www.nmc.org.uk/globalassets/sitedocuments/education-standards/nursing-associates-proficiency-standards.pdf (accessed September 2019).

Nursing and Midwifery Council (2018c). *The Code. Professional standards of practice and behaviour for nurses, midwives and nursing associates*. www.nmc.org.uk/globalassets/sitedocuments/nmc-publications/nmc-code.pdf (accessed September 2019).

Prydderch, S. (2019). *Preparing pre-registration nurses to be 'prescriber ready'*. Aspirational or achievable reality. Nurse Education Today. doi: 10.1016/j.nedt.2019.03.009.

Royal Pharmaceutical Society and the Royal College of Nursing (2019). *Professional guidance on the administration of medicines in healthcare settings*. https://www.rpharms.com/Portals/0/RPS%20document%20library/Open%20access/Professional%20standards/SSHM%20and%20Admin/Admin%20of%20Meds%20prof%20guidance.pdf?ver=2019-01-23-145026-567 (accessed September 2019).

Acknowledgements

Ian would like to thank his partner Jussi Lahtinen for his ongoing support and Mrs. Frances Cohen for her help and encouragement. Thanks also to Magenta Styles at Wiley for her inspiration.

Barry would like to thank Professor Ian Peate for his continued encouragement support and friendship helping me to grow as an academic, an editor, a writer and for always believing in me. I would also like to thank my partner Jose, my mum Tina, Dad Ray and Sisters Melanie and Sonia for being my family. I would like to thank all of the contributory writers who have written book chapters. Working and dedicating your own time to writing for publication is no easy task. I applaud your dedication and thank you on behalf on the readership. Finally, I would like to thank Wiley and the team working behind the scenes for their continuous support on all aspects of the publication process.

Prefixes and suffixes

Prefix: A prefix is positioned at the beginning of a word to modify or change its meaning. Pre means 'before'. Prefixes may also indicate a location, number or time.

   Suffix: The ending part of a word that changes the meaning of the word.

Prefix or suffix	Meaning	Example(s)
a-, an-	not, without	analgesic, apathy
ab-	from; away from	abduction
abdomin(o)-	of or relating to the abdomen	abdomen
acous(io)-	of or relating to hearing	acoumeter, acoustician
acr(o)-	extremity, topmost	acrocrany, acromegaly, acroosteolysis, acroposthia
ad-	at, increase, on, toward	adduction
aden(o)-, aden(i)-	of or relating to a gland	adenocarcinoma, adenology, adenotome, adenotyphus
adip(o)-	of or relating to fat or fatty tissue	adipocyte
adren(o)-	of or relating to adrenal glands	adrenal artery
-aemia	blood condition	anaemia
aer(o)-	air, gas	aerosinusitis
-aesthesi(o)-	sensation	anaesthesia
alb-	denoting a white or pale color	albino
-alge(si)-	pain	analgesic
-algia, -alg(i)o-	pain	myalgia
all(o-)	denoting something as different, or as an addition	alloantigen, allopathy
ambi-	denoting something as positioned on both sides	ambidextrous
amni-	pertaining to the membranous foetal sac (amnion)	amniocentesis
ana-	back, again, up	anaplasia
andr(o)-	pertaining to a man	android, andrology
angi(o)-	blood vessel	angiogram
ankyl(o)-, ancyl(o)-	denoting something as crooked or bent	ankylosis
ante-	describing something as positioned in front of another thing	antepartum

Prefix or suffix	Meaning	Example(s)
anti-	describing something as 'against' or 'opposed to' another	antibody, antipsychotic
arteri(o)-	of or pertaining to an artery	arteriole, arterial
arthr(o)-	of or pertaining to the joints, limbs	arthritis
articul(o)-	joint	articulation
-ase	enzyme	lactase
-asthenia	weakness	myasthenia gravis
ather(o)-	fatty deposit, soft gruel-like deposit	atherosclerosis
atri(o)-	an atrium (especially heart atrium)	atrioventricular
aur(i)-	of or pertaining to the ear	aural
aut(o)-	self	autoimmune
axill-	of or pertaining to the armpit (uncommon as a prefix)	axilla
bi-	twice, double	binary
bio-	life	biology
blephar(o)-	of or pertaining to the eyelid	blepharoplast
brachi(o)-	of or relating to the arm	brachium of inferior colliculus
brady-	slow	bradycardia
bronch(i)-	bronchus	bronchiolitis obliterans
bucc(o)-	of or pertaining to the cheek	buccolabial
burs(o)-	bursa (fluid sac between the bones)	bursitis
carcin(o)-	cancer	carcinoma
cardi(o)-	of or pertaining to the heart	cardiology
carp(o)-	of or pertaining to the wrist	carpopedal
-cele	pouching, hernia	hydrocele, varicocele
-centesis	surgical puncture for aspiration	amniocentesis
cephal(o)-	of or pertaining to the head (as a whole)	cephalalgy
cerebell(o)-	of or pertaining to the cerebellum	cerebellum
cerebr(o)-	of or pertaining to the brain	cerebrology
chem(o)-	chemistry, drug	chemotherapy
chol(e)-	of or pertaining to bile	cholecystitis
cholecyst(o)-	of or pertaining to the gallbladder	cholecystectomy

Prefix or suffix	Meaning	Example(s)
chondr(i)o-	cartilage, gristle, granule, granular	chondrocalcinosis
chrom(ato)-	colour	hemochromatosis
-cidal, -cide	killing, destroying	bactericidal
cili-	of or pertaining to the cilia, the eyelashes	ciliary
circum-	denoting something as 'around' another	circumcision
col(o)-, colono-	colon	colonoscopy
colp(o)-	of or pertaining to the vagina	colposcopy
contra-	against	contraindicate
coron(o)-	crown	coronary
cost(o)-	of or pertaining to the ribs	costochondral
crani(o)-	belonging or relating to the cranium	craniology
-crine, -crin(o)-	to secrete	endocrine
cry(o)-	cold	cryoablation
cutane-	skin	subcutaneous
cyan(o)-	denotes a blue colour	cyanosis
cyst(o)-, cyst(i)-	of or pertaining to the urinary bladder	cystotomy
cyt(o)-	cell	cytokine
-cyte	cell	leukocyte
-dactyl(o)-	of or pertaining to a finger, toe	dactylology, polydactyly
dent-	of or pertaining to teeth	dentist
dermat(o)-, derm(o)-	of or pertaining to the skin	dermatology
-desis	binding	arthrodesis
dextr(o)-	right, on the right side	dextrocardia
di-	two	diplopia
dia-	through, during, across	dialysis
dif-	apart, separation	different
digit-	of or pertaining to the finger (rare as a root)	digit
-dipsia	suffix meaning '(condition of) thirst'	polydipsia, hydroadipsia, oligodipsia
dors(o)-, dors(i)-	of or pertaining to the back	dorsal, dorsocephalad
duodeno-	duodenum	duodenal atresia
dynam(o)-	force, energy, power	hand strength dynamometer

Prefix or suffix	Meaning	Example(s)
-dynia	pain	vulvodynia
dys-	bad, difficult, defective, abnormal	dysphagia, dysphasia
ec-	out, away	ectopia, ectopic pregnancy
-ectasia, -ectasis	expansion, dilation	bronchiectasis, telangiectasia
ect(o)-	outer, outside	ectoblast, ectoderm
-ectomy	denotes a surgical operation or removal of a body part; resection, excision	mastectomy
-emesis	vomiting condition	hematemesis
encephal(o)-	of or pertaining to the brain; also see cerebr(o)-	encephalogram
endo-	denotes something as 'inside' or 'within'	endocrinology, endospore
enter(o)-	of or pertaining to the intestine	gastroenterology
eosin(o)-	red	eosinophil granulocyte
epi-	on, upon	epicardium, epidermis, epidural, episclera, epistaxis
erythr(o)-	denotes a red colour	erythrocyte
ex-	out of, away from	excision, exophthalmos
exo-	denotes something as 'outside' another	exoskeleton
extra-	outside	extradural hematoma
faci(o)-	of or pertaining to the face	facioplegic
fibr(o)	fibre	fibroblast
fore-	before or ahead	forehead
fossa	a hollow or depressed area; trench or channel	fossa ovalis
front-	of or pertaining to the forehead	frontonasal
galact(o)-	milk	galactorrhoea
gastr(o)-	of or pertaining to the stomach	gastric bypass
-genic	formative, pertaining to producing	cardiogenic shock
gingiv-	of or pertaining to the gums	gingivitis
glauc(o)-	denoting a grey or bluish-grey colour	glaucoma
gloss(o)-,glott(o)-	of or pertaining to the tongue	glossology
gluco-	sweet	glucocorticoid
glyc(o)-	sugar	glycolysis
-gnosis	knowledge	diagnosis, prognosis

Prefix or suffix	Meaning	Example(s)
gon(o)-	seed, semen; also, reproductive	gonorrhoea
-gram, -gramme	record or picture	angiogram
-graph	instrument used to record data or picture	electrocardiograph
-graphy	process of recording	angiography
gyn(aec)o-	woman	gynaecomastia
haemangi(o)-	blood vessels	haemangioma
haemat(o)-, hem-	of or pertaining to blood	haematology
halluc-	to wander in mind	hallucinosis
hemi-	one-half	cerebral hemisphere
hepat- (hepatic-)	of or pertaining to the liver	hepatology
heter(o)-	denotes something as 'the other' (of two), as an addition, or different	heterogeneous
hist(o)-, histio-	tissue	histology
home(o)-	similar	homeopathy
hom(o)-	denotes something as 'the same' as another or common	homosexuality
hydr(o)-	water	hydrophobe
hyper-	denotes something as 'extreme' or 'beyond normal'	hypertension
hyp(o)-	denotes something as 'below normal'	hypovolemia
hyster(o)-	of or pertaining to the womb, the uterus	hysterectomy, hysteria
iatr(o)-	of or pertaining to medicine, or a physician	iatrogenic
-iatry	denotes a field in medicine of a certain body component	podiatry, psychiatry
-ics	organized knowledge, treatment	obstetrics
ileo-	ileum	ileocecal valve
infra-	below	infrahyoid muscles
inter-	between, among	interarticular ligament
intra-	within	intramural
ipsi-	same	ipsilateral haemiparesis
ischio-	of or pertaining to the ischium, the hip joint	ischioanal fossa
-ismus	spasm, contraction	hemiballismus
iso-	denoting something as being 'equal'	isotonic
-ist	one who specializes in	pathologist

Prefix or suffix	Meaning	Example(s)
-itis	inflammation	tonsillitis
-ium	structure, tissue	pericardium
juxta- (iuxta-)	near to, alongside or next to	juxtaglomerular apparatus
karyo-	nucleus	eukaryote
kerat(o)-	cornea (eye or skin)	keratoscope
kin(e)-, kin(o)-, kinaesi(o)-	movement	kinaesthesia
kyph(o)-	humped	kyphoscoliosis
labi(o)-	of or pertaining to the lip	labiodental
lacrim(o)-	tear	lacrimal canaliculi
lact(i)-, lact(o)	milk	lactation
lapar(o)-	of or pertaining to the abdomen wall, flank	laparotomy
laryng(o)-	of or pertaining to the larynx, the lower throat cavity where the voice box is	larynx
latero-	lateral	lateral pectoral nerve
-lepsis, -lepsy	attack, seizure	epilepsy, narcolepsy
lept(o)-	light, slender	leptomeningeal
leuc(o)-, leuk(o)-	denoting a white colour	leukocyte
lingu(a)-, lingu(o)-	of or pertaining to the tongue	linguistics
lip(o)-	fat	liposuction
lith(o)-	stone, calculus	lithotripsy
-logist	denotes someone who studies a certain field	oncologist, pathologist
log(o)-	speech	logopaedics
-logy	denotes the academic study or practice of a certain field	haematology, urology
lymph(o)-	lymph	lymphedema
lys(o)-, -lytic	dissolution	lysosome
-lysis	destruction, separation	paralysis
macr(o)-	large, long	macrophage
-malacia	softening	osteomalacia
mammill(o)-	of or pertaining to the nipple	mammillitis
mamm(o)-	of or pertaining to the breast	mammogram
manu-	of or pertaining to the hand	manufacture
mast(o)-	of or pertaining to the breast	mastectomy
meg(a)-, megal(o)-, -megaly	enlargement, million	splenomegaly, megametre
melan(o)-	black colour	melanin

Prefix or suffix	Meaning	Example(s)
mening(o)-	membrane	meningitis
meta-	after, behind	metacarpus
-meter	instrument used to measure or count	sphygmomanometer
metr(o)-	pertaining to conditions of the uterus	metrorrhagia
-metry	process of measuring	optometry
micro-	denoting something as small, or relating to smallness	microscope
milli-	thousandth	millilitre
mon(o)-	single	infectious mononucleosis
morph(o)-	form, shape	morphology
muscul(o)-	muscle	musculoskeletal system
my(o)-	of or relating to muscle	myoblast
myc(o)-	fungus	onychomycosis
myel(o)-	of or relating to bone marrow or spinal cord	myeloblast
myri-	ten thousand	myriad
myring(o)-	eardrum	myringotomy
narc(o)-	numb, sleep	narcolepsy
nas(o)-	of or pertaining to the nose	nasal
necr(o)-	death	necrosis, necrotizing fasciitis
neo-	new	neoplasm
nephr(o)-	of or pertaining to the kidney	nephrology
neur(i)-, neur(o)-	of or pertaining to nerves and the nervous system	neurofibromatosis
normo-	normal	normocapnia
ocul(o)-	of or pertaining to the eye	oculist
odont(o)-	of or pertaining to teeth	orthodontist
odyn(o)-	pain	stomatodynia
-oesophageal, oesophag(o)-	gullet	gastroesophageal reflux
-oid	resemblance to	sarcoidosis
-ole	small or little	arteriole
olig(o)-	denoting something as 'having little, having few'	oliguria
-oma (sing.), -omata (pl.)	tumour, mass, collection	sarcoma, teratoma
onco-	tumour, bulk, volume	oncology
onych(o)-	of or pertaining to the nail (of a finger or toe)	onychophagy

Prefix or suffix	Meaning	Example(s)
oo-	of or pertaining to an egg, a woman's egg, the ovum	oogenesis
oophor(o)-	of or pertaining to the woman's ovary	oophorectomy
ophthalm(o)-	of or pertaining to the eye	ophthalmology
optic(o)-	of or relating to chemical properties of the eye	opticochemical
orchi(o)-, orchid(o)-, orch(o)-	testis	orchiectomy, orchidectomy
-osis	a condition, disease or increase	ichthyosis, psychosis, osteoporosis
osseo-	bony	osseous
ossi-	bone	peripheral ossifying fibroma
ost(e)-, oste(o)-	bone	osteoporosis
ot(o)-	of or pertaining to the ear	otology
ovo-, ovi-, ov-	of or pertaining to the eggs, the ovum	ovogenesis
pachy-	thick	pachyderma
paed-, paedo-	of or pertaining to the child	paediatrics
palpebr-	of or pertaining to the eyelid (uncommon as a root)	palpebra
pan-, pant(o)-	denoting something as 'complete' or containing 'everything'	panophobia, panopticon
papill-	of or pertaining to the nipple (of the chest/breast)	papillitis
papul(o)-	indicates papulosity, a small elevation or swelling in the skin, a pimple, swelling	papulation
para-	alongside of, abnormal	paracyesis
-paresis	slight paralysis	hemiparesis
parvo-	small	parvovirus
path(o)-	disease	pathology
-pathy	denotes (with a negative sense) a disease, or disorder	sociopathy, neuropathy
pector-	breast	pectoralgia, pectoriloquy, pectorophony
ped-, -ped-, -pes	of or pertaining to the foot; -footed	pedoscope
pelv(i)-, pelv(o)-	hip bone	pelvis
-penia	deficiency	osteopenia

Prefix or suffix	Meaning	Example(s)
-pepsia	denotes something relating to digestion, or the digestive tract	dyspepsia
peri-	denoting something with a position 'surrounding' or 'around' another	periodontal
-pexy	fixation	nephropexy
phaco-	lens-shaped	phacolysis, phacometer, phacoscotoma
-phage, -phagia	forms terms denoting conditions relating to eating or ingestion	sarcophagia
-phago-	eating, devouring	phagocyte
-phagy	forms nouns that denote 'feeding on' the first element or part of the word	hematophagy
pharmaco-	drug, medication	pharmacology
pharyng(o)-	of or pertaining to the pharynx, the upper throat cavity	pharyngitis, pharyngoscopy
phleb(o)-	of or pertaining to the (blood) veins, a vein	phlebography, phlebotomy
-phobia	exaggerated fear, sensitivity	arachnophobia
phon(o)-	sound	phonograph, symphony
phot(o)-	of or pertaining to light	photopathy
phren(i)-, phren(o)-, phrenico	the mind	phrenic nerve, schizophrenia
-plasia	formation, development	achondroplasia
-plasty	surgical repair, reconstruction	rhinoplasty
-plegia	paralysis	paraplegia
pleio-	more, excessive, multiple	pleiomorphism
pleur(o)-, pleur(a)	of or pertaining to the ribs	pleurogenous
-plexy	stroke or seizure	cataplexy
pneumat(o)-	air, lung	pneumatocele
pneum(o)-	of or pertaining to the lungs	pneumonocyte, pneumonia
-poiesis	production	haematopoiesis
poly-	denotes a 'plurality' of something	polymyositis
post-	denotes something as 'after' or 'behind' another	post-operation, post-mortem
pre-	denotes something as 'before' another (in [physical] position or time)	premature birth

Prefix or suffix	Meaning	Example(s)
presby(o)-	old age	presbyopia
prim-	denotes something as 'first' or 'most important'	primary
proct(o)-	anus, rectum	proctology
prot(o)-	denotes something as 'first' or 'most important'	protoneuron
pseud(o)-	denotes something false or fake	pseudoephedrine
psor-	itching	psoriasis
psych(e)-, psych(o)	of or pertaining to the mind	psychology, psychiatry
-ptosis	falling, drooping, downward placement, prolapse	apoptosis, nephroptosis
-ptysis	(a spitting), spitting, haemoptysis, the spitting of blood derived from the lungs or bronchial tubes	haemoptysis
pulmon-, pulmo-	of or relating to the lungs	pulmonary
pyel(o)-	pelvis	pyelonephritis
py(o)-	pus	pyometra
pyr(o)-	fever	antipyretic
quadr(i)-	four	quadriceps
radio-	radiation	radiowave
ren(o)-	of or pertaining to the kidney	renal
retro-	backward, behind	retroversion, retroverted
rhin(o)-	of or pertaining to the nose	rhinoplasty
rhod(o)-	denoting a rose-red colour	rhodophyte
-rrhage	burst forth	haemorrhage
-rrhagia	rapid flow of blood	menorrhagia
-rrhaphy	surgical suturing	nephrorrhaphy
-rrhexis	rupture	karyorrhexis
-rrhoea	flowing, discharge	diarrhoea
-rupt	break or burst	erupt, interrupt
salping(o)-	of or pertaining to tubes, e.g. Fallopian tubes	salpingectomy, salpingopharyngeus muscle
sangui-, sanguine-	of or pertaining to blood	exsanguination
sarco-	muscular, flesh-like	sarcoma
scler(o)-	hard	scleroderma
-sclerosis	hardening	atherosclerosis, multiple sclerosis
scoli(o)-	twisted	scoliosis

Prefix or suffix	Meaning	Example(s)
-scope	instrument for viewing	stethoscope
-scopy	use of instrument for viewing	endoscopy
semi-	one-half, partly	semiconscious
sial(o)-	saliva, salivary gland	sialagogue
sigmoid(o)-	sigmoid, S-shaped curvature	sigmoid colon
sinistr(o)-	left, left side	sinistrocardia
sinus-	of or pertaining to the sinus	sinusitis
somat(o)-, somatico-	body, bodily	somatic
-spadias	slit, fissure	hypospadias, epispadias
spasmo-	spasm	spasmodic dysphonia
sperma(to)-, spermo-	semen, spermatozoa	spermatogenesis
splen(o)-	spleen	splenectomy
spondyl(o)-	of or pertaining to the spine, the vertebra	spondylitis
squamos(o)-	denoting something as 'full of scales' or 'scaly'	squamous cell
stat.	statim	at once
-stalsis	contraction	peristalsis
-stasis	stopping, standing	cytostasis, homeostasis
-staxis	dripping, trickling	epistaxis
sten(o)-	denoting something as 'narrow in shape' or pertaining to narrowness	stenography
-stenosis	abnormal narrowing in a blood vessel or other tubular organ or structure	restenosis, stenosis
stomat(o)-	of or pertaining to the mouth	stomatogastric, stomatognathic system
-stomy	creation of an opening	colostomy
sub-	beneath	subcutaneous tissue
super-	in excess, above, superior	superior vena cava
supra-	above, excessive	supraorbital vein
tachy-	denoting something as fast, irregularly fast	tachycardia
-tension, -tensive	pressure	hypertension
tetan-	rigid, tense	tetanus
thec-	case, sheath	intrathecal
therap-	treatment	hydrotherapy, therapeutic
therm(o)-	heat	thermometer

Prefix or suffix	Meaning	Example(s)
thorac(i)-, thorac(o)-, thoracico-	of or pertaining to the upper chest, chest; the area above the breast and under the neck	thorax
thromb(o)-	of or relating to a blood clot, clotting of blood	thrombus, thrombocytopenia
thyr(o)-	thyroid	thyrocele
thym-	emotions	dysthymia
-tome	cutting instrument	osteotome
-tomy	act of cutting; incising, incision	gastrotomy
tono-	tone, tension, pressure	tonometer
-tony	tension	
top(o)-	place, topical	topical anaesthetic
tort(i)-	twisted	torticollis
tox(i)-, tox(o)-, toxic(o)-	toxin, poison	toxoplasmosis
trache(a)-	trachea	tracheotomy
trachel(o)-	of or pertaining to the neck	tracheloplasty
trans-	denoting something as moving or situated 'across' or 'through'	transfusion
tri-	three	triangle
trich(i)-, trichia, trich(o)-	of or pertaining to hair, hair-like structure	trichocyst
-tripsy	crushing	lithotripsy
-trophy	nourishment, development	pseudohypertrophy
tympan(o)-	eardrum	tympanocentesis
-ula, -ule	small	nodule
ultra-	beyond, excessive	ultrasound
un(i)-	one	unilateral hearing loss
ur(o)-	of or pertaining to urine, the urinary system; (specifically) pertaining to the physiological chemistry of urine	urology
uter(o)-	of or pertaining to the uterus or womb	uterus
vagin-	of or pertaining to the vagina	vagina
varic(o)-	swollen or twisted vein	varicose
vasculo-	blood vessel	vasculotoxicity
vas(o)-	duct, blood vessel	vasoconstriction

Prefix or suffix	Meaning	Example(s)
ven-	of or pertaining to the (blood) veins, a vein (used in terms pertaining to the vascular system)	vein, venospasm
ventricul(o)-	of or pertaining to the ventricles; any hollow region inside an organ	cardiac ventriculography
ventr(o)-	of or pertaining to the belly; the stomach cavities	ventrodorsal
-version	turning	anteversion, retroversion
vesic(o)-	of or pertaining to the bladder	vesical arteries
viscer(o)-	of or pertaining to the internal organs, the viscera	viscera
xanth(o)-	denoting a yellow colour, an abnormally yellow colour	xanthopathy
xen(o)-	foreign, different	xenograft
xer(o)-	dry, desert-like	xerostomia
zo(o)-	animal, animal life	zoology
zym(o)-	fermentation	enzyme, lysozyme

Abbreviations

Some abbreviations used in prescriptions

Abbreviation	Latin	English
a.c.	ante cibum	Before food
ad lib.	ad libitum	To the desired amount
b.d. or b.i.d.	bis in die	Twice a day
c.	cum	With
o.m.	omni mane	Every morning
o.n.	omni nocte	Every night
p.c.	post cibum	After food
p.r.n.	pro re nata	Whenever necessary
q.d.	quaque die	Every day
q.d.s.	quaque die sumendum	Four times daily
q.i.d.	quater in die	Four times daily
q.q.h.	quater quaque hora	Every four hours
R.	recipe	Take
s.o.s.	si opus sit	If necessary
stat.	statim	At once
t.d.s.	ter die sumendum	Three times daily
t.i.d.	ter in die	Three times daily

Chapter 1

Introduction to pharmacology

Ian Peate

Aim

The aim of this chapter is to provide the reader with an introduction to therapeutic pharmacology and the key issues surrounding medicines management.

Learning outcomes

After reading this chapter, the reader will be able to:

1. Discuss the importance of patient assessment in association with medicines management
2. Understand the role of the Code and other professional duties
3. Appreciate the importance of the proficiencies of pre-registration nurse education related to medicines management
4. Acknowledge and respect patient preference

Test your knowledge

1. What is the nursing process?
2. Describe the keys skills that are associated with patient assessment.
3. Discuss the role and function of the Nursing and Midwifery Council.
4. What does medicines optimisation mean?
5. Discuss risk management strategies in medicines management.

Fundamentals of Pharmacology: For Nursing and Healthcare Students, First Edition. Edited by Ian Peate and Barry Hill.
© 2021 John Wiley & Sons Ltd. Published 2021 by John Wiley & Sons Ltd.

Introduction

There has been a vast increase in the use of therapeutic agents for medical treatment. The administration of medicines is a common yet important clinical activity. The way in which a medicinal product is administered can determine whether the patient gains any therapeutic benefit or if they will experience any adverse effects from their medicines. The volume and complexity of medication administration contributes to the actual and potential risk of medication errors, which will have a negative impact on a person's health and wellbeing.

The key requirement of a healthcare provider is to 'do no harm', and this is particularly important when the nurse is working with people who have been prescribed medication. The administration of medicines is but one part of the nurse's role; an understanding of pharmacology is essential if the nurse is to provide care that is safe and effective. As well as an understanding of pharmacology, the nurse is also required to work with patients and their families in explaining how to administer the medication, explaining the anticipated effects, the action(s) of the medications and the potential adverse reactions or side effects.

Patient assessment

When a patient is admitted to a healthcare facility (regardless of the setting), an initial assessment must be undertaken which has to include a detailed medication history. Information must be obtained from the patient (and, if appropriate, the patient's family), and information may also be collected from the patient's pharmacy and/or the general practitioner with their permission. In addition, any medications that have been brought in by the patient must be documented and kept in a safe location. At all times, local policy and procedure must be adhered to.

Assessment is the first stage in the planning of care, it is associated with the process of gathering information in order to make decisions about appropriate interventions (Ballantyne, 2015). During the assessment stage, the patient's story is listened to and the nurse–patient relationship is strengthened, ensuring that the patient is truly at the heart of all that is done. The nursing process is a systematic, developing, dynamic approach, that is cyclical in nature, and as such assessment must not be seen as a one-off activity: it is not linear by nature; it is ongoing.

When assessing needs – and this also relates to assessing needs and the use of medications – data is gathered, analysed and organised, and the data is acted upon as critical thinking skills and the mobilisation of resources are used to achieve goals and outcomes that have been set, when possible, in partnership with the patient (Stonehouse, 2017).

Having undertaken patient assessment, a diagnosis is formulated, a plan of care is devised relating to the needs that have emerged following assessment, care is provided using a holistic approach, and finally all that has been done is evaluated to establish efficacy. See Figure 1.1: a systematic approach to care.

The safety and success of medicines administration is based on ongoing nursing assessment. All healthcare providers have a professional duty to ensure that they offer care that is safe and effective (Nursing and Midwifery Council (NMC), 2018a). As well as professional obligations, there are also requirements that must be given due diligence in order to ensure that patient safety is paramount. There is much legislation regarding medicines (see Chapter 3), and the nurse must also adhere to the laws of the country in which they are working.

The skills of assessment require the nurse to undertake a physical and psychological assessment of the person's needs. The nurse obtains a patient history and carries out a physical examination (if required) to identify needs. There are a number of components associated with assessment. Assessment requires the nurse to:

- observe the patient
- undertake a clinical examination
- gather data

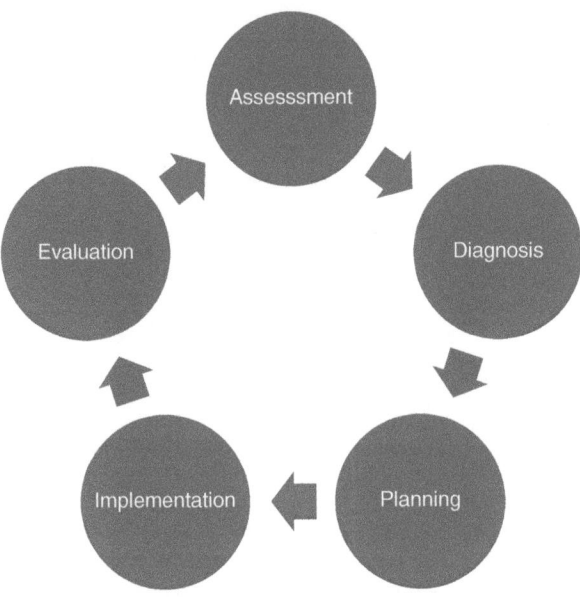

Figure 1.1   A systematic approach to care provision.

- communicate
- undertake various measurements.

Clinical judgment is used to determine the type of assessment required. It is important during the assessment phase to ensure the use of a framework to guide the process as this will help to provide structure and order.

The NMC has suggested that newly qualified nurses will be able to go on a prescribing course soon after their initial pre-registration education; in order to do this, there is a need to include more prescribing theory in undergraduate nursing programmes allowing nurses to prescribe from a limited formulary. It is important to note that nurses will not prescribe at the point of entry to the register (when their pre-registration nurse education is complete), but will complete a post-registration qualification in order to prescribe (NMC, 2018b).

All nursing professionals must practise in line with the requirements of The Code (NMC, 2018a), the professional standards of practice and behaviour that nurses, midwives and nursing associates are required to uphold.

The Code of Conduct

The NMC is the nursing and midwifery regulator for England, Wales, Scotland, Northern Ireland and the Islands. It exists to protect the public and it does this in a number of ways. The NMC sets the standards of education, training and conduct that nurses and midwives are required to adhere to so as to deliver high-quality healthcare. The NMC ensures that nurses and midwives keep their skills and knowledge up to date (through revalidation; NMC, 2017) and uphold the standards of the Code (NMC, 2018a). Where an allegation is made about a nurse's standard of practice or behaviour, the NMC have processes in place to investigate those allegation: they take action if concerns are raised about a nurse's fitness to practice.

The Code sets out in detail the professional standards that nurses must uphold and all nurses, regardless of setting, are required to align their practice and behaviour to the Code. The values and principles that are set out in the Code are not negotiable or discretionary.

All nurses will exercise professional judgment in their work as they offer care to people, including the care that is associated with medicines and medicines management: each nurse

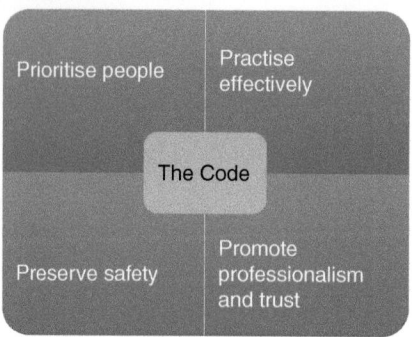

Figure 1.2 The Code. Source: Olympus America, Inc. With permission.

is accountable for their actions and omissions. Nurses are required to uphold the Code within the limits of their competence associated with the contribution they make to overall care provision. Practising within your sphere of competence and your scope of practice is key to the underpinning principle of the Code – to protect the public – and must be upheld at all times.

The Code is made up of a series of statements that taken together imply what good practice looks like. It makes clear that the interests of patients and service users come first, that care is safe and effective and that it promotes trust through professionalism (see Figure 1.2).

Clause 18 of the Code is specifically related to medicines. Nurses are required to advise on, prescribe, supply, dispense or administer medicines that are within the limits of their training and competence, the law, and in relation to NMC guidance and other relevant policies, guidance and regulations. In order to do this, the nurse must:

- Prescribe, advise on, or provide medicines or treatment, including repeat prescriptions (only if the nurse is suitably qualified) if the nurse has enough knowledge of that person's health and is satisfied that the medicines or treatment serve that person's health needs.
- Adhere to appropriate guidelines when providing advice on using controlled drugs and recording the prescribing, supply, dispensing or administration of controlled drugs.
- Ensure that the care or treatment that the nurse advises on, prescribes, supplies, dispenses or administers for each person is compatible with any other care or treatment that the person is receiving, including (where possible) over-the-counter medicines.
- Take all steps to keep medicines stored securely.
- Wherever possible, avoid prescribing for yourself or for anyone with whom you have a close personal relationship.

It should be noted that prescribing is not within the scope of practice of everyone on the NMC register. Nurses who have successfully completed a further qualification in prescribing and recorded it on the NMC's register are the only people on the register that can prescribe.

The Nursing and Midwifery Council's Standards of Proficiency

In 2018, the NMC published future nurse proficiencies for registered nurses (NMC, 2018b) and for nursing associates (NMC, 2018c) along with a range of other revised and updated standards. The standards of proficiency provide the education and training standards that underpin all aspects of nurse education delivery and management.

The standards make significant changes to proficiencies for nurses, introducing a new education framework. The standards of proficiency are designed to enable nurses to meet the changing health needs of the population, to provide them with more clinical autonomy where appropriate, and to prepare them for leadership roles in the sphere of care provision ensuring the nurse is fit for purpose. The standards are based on the following requirements (platforms) to:

- be an accountable professional;
- promote health and prevent ill health;
- assess needs and plan care;
- provide and evaluate care;
- lead and manage nursing care and work in teams;
- improve safety and quality of care;
- coordinate care.

As well as understanding the principles of safe and effective administration and optimisation of medicines and adhering to local and national policies, the nurse must also demonstrate proficiency and accuracy when they are calculating dosages of prescribed medicines. The nurse has to demonstrate knowledge of pharmacology and the ability to recognise the effects of medicines, allergies, drug sensitivities, side effects, contraindications, incompatibilities, adverse reactions, prescribing errors and the impact of polypharmacy – and also over-the-counter medication usage. See Table 1.1 for the procedural competencies for nurses (registered and associate) that are essential for best practice, evidence-based medicines administration and efficacy.

Table 1.1   Registered nurse procedural competencies and the procedural competencies required by the nursing associate

The registered nurse	The nursing associate
• Undertake initial and continued assessments of people receiving care and their ability to self-administer their own medications. • Understand the various procedural routes under which medicines can be prescribed, supplied, dispensed and administered; and the laws, policies, regulations and guidance that underpin them. • Make use of the principles underpinning safe remote prescribing and directions for the administration of medicines. • Undertake accurate drug calculations for a variety of medications. • Undertake accurate checks, including transcription and titration, of any direction to supply or administer a medicinal product. • Apply professional accountability so as to ensure the safe administration of medicines to those who are receiving care. • Administer injections using intramuscular, subcutaneous, intradermal and intravenous routes and manage injection equipment. • Administer medications using a range of routes. • Administer and monitor medications using vascular access devices and enteral equipment. • Recognise and respond to adverse or abnormal reactions to medications. • Undertake safe storage, transportation and disposal of medicinal products.	• Continually assess people who are receiving care and their ongoing ability to self-administer their own medications. • Know when and how to escalate any concerns. • Perform accurate drug calculations for a variety of medications. • Use professional accountability in order to ensure the safe administration of medicines to those receiving care. • Administer medication via oral, topical and inhalation routes. • Administer injections using subcutaneous and intramuscular routes and manage injection equipment. • Administer and monitor medications using enteral equipment. • Administer enemas and suppositories. • Manage and monitor effectiveness of symptom relief of medications. • Recognise and respond to adverse or abnormal reactions to medications and know when and how to escalate any concerns. • Undertake safe storage, transportation and disposal of medicinal products.

Source: Adapted, NMC (2018b and c).

Medicine management and standards

Nurses and health and social care staff often manage medicines on behalf of those people who use their services. It is a requirement of care providers to promote the safe and effective use of medicines. If healthcare organisations fail to do this, the Care Quality Commission (CQC) (2018) suggest that this poses real risks to people who may be vulnerable, including:

- older people;
- people with reduced mental capacity, reduced mobility or a sensory impairment;
- people who rely on help to take their medicines.

Medicine management standards provide nurses with a framework for safe practice. All nurses must read and comply with these standards, and undergraduate students must also be familiar with them. The requirements laid out in the various standards consider issues essential for the safe management of all medications and also include controlled drugs.

Episode of care: Mental health

Mr. Murphy, an 80-year-old man, has vascular dementia and lives in a care home; he relies on the care home staff to manage his medicines safely.

Mr. Murphy was admitted to hospital after he had displayed signs of a venous thromboembolism and he was discharged four days later; he was prescribed and was taking anticoagulant therapy. When he was discharged from hospital, he was discharged with an 18-day supply of medicine. The care home staff failed to order a new prescription for Mr. Murphy after the 18 days lapsed. The systems within the care home had failed to identify that the medication was not given for between 30 and 33 days.

Mr. Murphy was taken back into hospital with a pulmonary thromboembolism and deep vein thrombosis. He was in hospital for over three months where he eventually died.

The care home had failed to adhere to local policy and procedure that helps to minimise medication errors. Regulations and standards are put in place to prevent people from receiving unsafe care and treatment and prevent avoidable harm or risk of harm. Medicines must be supplied in adequate quantities, managed in a safe way and administered appropriately to ensure that people are safe.

In England, the Health and Social Care Act 2008 (Regulated Activities) Regulations 2014: Regulation 12, for example, aims to prevent people from receiving unsafe care and treatment and prevent avoidable harm or risk of harm. Those who provide care must undertake a risk assessment with regards to people's health and safety when receiving care or treatment and make sure that their staff have the appropriate qualifications, competence, skills and experience to maintain people's safety. If an organisation fails to comply with laws and regulations, they may be prosecuted.

Clinical considerations

Managing medicines in care homes

The National Institute for Health and Care Excellence (NICE) (2014) has published guidelines that address good practice for managing medicines in care homes. The guideline aims to promote the safe and effective use of medicines in care homes, and it offers advice on processes for prescribing, handling and administering medicines. The guideline also recommends how care and services relating to medicines should be provided to those people who are living in care homes.

The Nursing and Midwifery Council (2010) previously issued standards and guidance for the administration of medicines; however, they no longer do this. Professional guidance produced

Clinical considerations

Managing medicines for those receiving social care in the community

The National Institute for Health and Care Excellence (NICE) (2017) has published guidelines that cover medicines support for adults who are receiving social care in the community. It aims to ensure that people who receive social care are supported to take and look after their medicines effectively and safely at home. Guidance offers advice on assessing if people will require help with managing their medicines, who should provide medicines support, and how health and social care staff should work together.

by the Royal Pharmaceutical Society (RPS) (2018a) provides a framework for the safe and secure handling of medicines; this replaces the NMC's previous standards. This guidance uses an all professional approach providing information and advice for all healthcare professionals on medicines management and administration. The RCN and RPS (2019) have co-produced Guidance on the Administration of Medicines in Healthcare Settings, offering principles-based guidance to ensure the safe administration of medicines by healthcare professionals.

In 2017, Higher Education England issued advisory guidance for Nursing Associates with regards to the administration of medicines. The guidance plays a key part in ensuring the Nursing Associate is able to work safely and appropriately with regards to medicine and as part of the nursing team.

As well as the various standards, advice and guidance issued, NHS trusts and other organisations will have also prepared their own guidance on how to safely and effectively handle medicines. The healthcare worker should always check and follow this local guidance when providing care that is related to the administration of medicines.

It should also be remembered that there may be a need to consult other sources of guidance concerning specific areas of practice, such as:

- NICE;
- publications by the British National Formulary;
- the Royal College of Nursing;
- the four UK Health and Social Care Departments;
- specialist associations, such as the British Association of Sexual Health and HIV, UK Oncology Forum;
- the World Health Organization.

Clinical considerations

Managing oxygen in care homes

Oxygen is a medical gas and as such should be treated as a medicine.

Home oxygen therapy is commonly used in care homes. It involves breathing oxygen mixed with air from a cylinder or machine. It is often prescribed for those people who have respiratory conditions, such as chronic obstructive pulmonary disease that can result in low oxygen levels in the blood. Home oxygen therapy can be given via:

- nasal cannulae
- face mask
- tracheostomy mask.

The oxygen is delivered via tubing or mask from an oxygen cylinder, an oxygen concentrator or a ventilator.

Oxygen is prescribed on a home oxygen order form. The form contains details of how the oxygen is to be used. The prescriber sends the home oxygen order form to the oxygen supplier who then arranges delivery.

Staff at the care home should tell the person prescribing the oxygen about any changes in a person's clinical condition; this then allows the prescriber to amend and organise for a new home oxygen order form, if required.

The person's care plan should include information about home oxygen therapy. This should include who it is who will be monitoring the person who is using the oxygen.

The care plan (documentation) should also address the administration of oxygen. This has to include flow rate, frequency and duration of use; the prescriber's details should also be included. Each time staff administer oxygen, these details should be checked to ensure that the oxygen is being administered correctly.

If the person is self-administering the oxygen, a risk assessment has to be carried out (individual risk assessments should include information about the potential dangers of having and using oxygen in the care home). A copy of the risk assessment should be kept in the person's care plan.

Local policy and procedure must be adhered to at all times. The tubing and masks must be clean and in good condition and replaced when needed. Tubing and masks must only be used for the person the oxygen was prescribed for.

Staff have to be trained and deemed competent to manage home oxygen therapy.

As with all medications, oxygen cylinders have an expiry date. The expiry date has to be checked to ensure that out-of-date cylinders are not used.

If equipment is no longer in use or it is out of date, it should be returned to the oxygen supplier.

Medicines optimisation

The term medicines optimisation is generally used to encompass a more people-centred approach to the use of medicine as part of a person's care (NICE, 2015). It is essential that patients get the best quality outcomes from medicines: medicines play an important role in maintaining health, preventing illness, managing chronic conditions and curing disease – all against a backdrop of significant economic, demographic and technological change. There is evidence to suggest that there is an urgent need to get the essentials of medicines use right. Medicines use is too often sub-optimal and a step change is needed in the way that all health-care professionals offer support to patients in order to get the best possible outcomes from their medicines (Royal Pharmaceutical Society, 2013).

Medicines optimisation is concerned with ensuring that the right patients get the right choice of medicine, at the right time. When healthcare providers focus on patients and their experiences, there is much potential to help patients improve their outcomes, take their medicines correctly, avoid taking unnecessary medicines, reduce wastage of medicines and improve medicines safety. Medicines optimisation can help to encourage patients to take ownership of their treatment. In order to ensure medicines optimisation reaches its full potential, this requires a multidisciplinary team working approach. Healthcare professionals work together to individualise care, monitor outcomes, review medicines and support patients when needed.

Medicines management is different to medicines optimisation in a number of ways; most importantly it focuses on outcomes and patients as opposed to process and systems. Focusing on improved outcomes can help to ensure that patients and the NHS get better value from their investment in medicines. Medicines optimisation considers how it is that patients use medicines over time. This can involve stopping some medicines as well as starting others and utilising opportunities that may arise for lifestyle changes and nonmedical therapies to reduce the need for medicines.

Patient beliefs and medicines

Patients' beliefs and preferences about medication prescribing may affect medication adherence. Clyne et al. (2017) point out that patients' beliefs about treatment are a critical influence on prescription medication use. Patients may influence prescribing decisions on the basis of their expectations or, in some cases, their unwillingness to take medicines. Patients' strong beliefs in medicines, their expectations and resistance to change are cited as important barriers to prescribing.

Bearing in mind the important role that beliefs can play in medication use, it is important for the nurse to acknowledge this and to explore the beliefs of patients. Non-adherence can result in morbidity and mortality, unnecessary health costs, unnecessary investigations and changes in treatment regimens. Neame and Hammond (2005) conclude that people with strong beliefs in the necessity of taking medication to maintain their health were found to be more adherent to treatment, and those with higher levels of concern about medication, commonly about the dangers of dependence and long-term side effects, were more likely to be non-adherent.

A Scandinavian study (Mårdby et al., 2009) considered beliefs, not of patients but of doctors and nurses in an outpatient setting; their aim was to explore general beliefs about medicines among doctors and nurses. They concluded that nurses saw medicines as more harmful and less beneficial than did doctors. The profession's different beliefs about medicines are important factors for adherence to medicines, just as patients' beliefs are.

There are many reasons for non-adherence and one reason may lie between the expectations of health professionals and the behaviour of patients where there is a failure to recognise that the views and expectations of patients are key factors associated with medicine taking. Patients' beliefs and goals must be at the centre of decision-making about their medicines, so the process of selecting and providing care has to be one of partnership and negotiation between the patient and health professionals.

Patients are invited to make informed decisions about all aspects of their care, and this comes with support from health professionals. In order to make an informed decision, then, these decisions have to be well informed. Health professionals are required to provide information that is appropriate and that fits with the patient's health beliefs, they are also required to offer that information in such a way that it is understandable to each individual. The RPS (2016) provides a framework for reaching a shared decision (see Box 1.1.)

It can be hard to decide how much information to give a patient; for example, which side effects to mention, where to obtain specialised information, as well as where the boundary of

Box 1.1 Reaching a shared decision

- Work with the patient and, if appropriate, carer in partnership to make informed choices, agreeing a plan that respects patient preferences, including their right to refuse or limit their treatment.
- Identify and respect the patient with regards to diversity, values, beliefs and expectations regarding their health and treatment with medicines.
- Routinely assess adherence in a non-judgmental way and understand the different reasons that non-adherence may occur (this may be intentional or non-intentional) and how best to offer support.
- Build a therapeutic relationship with the patient that encourages two-way effective communication.
- With the patient and carer, explore satisfactory outcomes for the patient/carer.

Source: Adapted RPS (2016)

responsibility lies between the health professional and the patient. Chapter 3 of this book addresses some of the ethical and legal issues that are associated with medicines management and pharmacology.

Concordance, adherence and compliance are terms that reflect fundamentally different approaches to care. When applied in its strict scientific definition, compliance is a useful term; however, it can also infer 'nurse or doctor knows best' and may be interpreted as condescending whereby patients do as they are told or advised. Compliance describes a patient's behaviour and concordance implies a process. It is appropriate, therefore, to refer to non-compliant patients, but not to non-concordant patients. The relationship between the patient and the health professional is non-concordant, not the patient. NICE (2009) have determined that adherence presumes an agreement between the prescriber and patient about the prescriber's recommendations. Adherence to medicines is defined as the extent to which the patient's action matches the agreed recommendations. When there is non-adherence, this has the potential to limit the benefits of medicines resulting in a lack of improvement, or a deterioration in health and wellbeing. The economic costs, suggest NICE (2009), are not only limited to wasted medicines but will also include the knock-on costs that arise from increased demands for healthcare if the person's health deteriorates.

Honouring individual choices and beliefs are the hallmarks of professional healthcare providers (NMC, 2018a). Being aware of the individual's values, acceptance of these values and asking or seeking clarification are essential if the person is to be respected. This can also have a positive impact on medicine adherence.

Clinical considerations

Medicines management

In the UK, one in four adults experience mental health problems in their lifetime, with one in six experiencing a diagnosable mental health problem in any one year (Mental Health Foundation, 2016). People with mental health problems may die prematurely; the life expectancy of someone with bipolar disorder or schizophrenia is 15–20 years less than the general population (Hjorthø et al., 2017). Often this is because their physical health suffers due to the fact that they are unable to cope and deal with their long-term condition in a regular and coherent way. The main risks that are specific to those with mental health conditions in terms of premature death include diabetes, obesity, hypertension, lack of exercise and smoking. It is estimated that one in three of the 100 000 people who die avoidably each year in England has a mental illness (Royal Pharmaceutical Society, 2018b).

Many of the medicines that are used to treat mental health problems are also associated with health risks. Pharmacists are experts in medicines and their use and can ensure that people get the best outcomes from their medicines, help to reduce adverse events, minimise any avoidable harm and unplanned admissions to hospital, while also ensuring that resources are used in an efficient way to deliver the standard and level of care that those with mental health conditions deserve. A multidisciplinary approach to medicines optimisation is advocated.

Discussing with patients their experiences of medicines use – for example, their views about what medicines mean to them, how medicines impact on their daily life, whether or not they are able to take their medicines – is a prerequisite that is demonstrated when promoting medicine optimisation.

Conclusion

Medicines are used more than any other intervention by patients as they strive to manage their medical conditions. The number of medicines prescribed, as well as the complexity of the medicines regimens that patients take, are and will continue to increase.

Nurses are involved in the management of medicines in almost every practice setting. Medicines management includes the safe and cost-effective use of medicines in clinical practice, with greatest patient benefits, while at the same time minimising potential harm. It is essential that nurses have knowledge of the regulatory, professional, and legal and ethical frameworks that oversee the prescribing, storage, administration, and safe disposal of drugs and ensure they comply with them. The nurse must have a sound understanding of the wider field of therapeutic pharmacology, a key aspect of clinical practice aiming to provide safe and effective care through a sound understanding of how the use of drugs cause action and effect.

Glossary

Autonomy	Is concerned with self-determination and is a person's ability to make choices on the basis of that person's own preferences, beliefs and values.
Capacity	An ability to understand, deliberate and communicate a choice in relation to a specific healthcare decision at a particular time.
Competence	The achievement and application of knowledge, intellectual capacities, practice skills, integrity, and professional and ethical values needed for safe, accountable, compassionate, and effective practice as a registered practitioner.
Compliance	Medication compliance refers to the degree or extent of conformity to the recommendations about day-to-day treatment by the healthcare provider with regards to timing, dosage and frequency.
Conduct	A person's moral practices, actions, beliefs and standards of behaviour.
Evidence-based practice	The conscious consideration and the application of the best available evidence along with the healthcare provider's expertise and a person's values and preferences in making healthcare decisions.
Guidance	A principle or criterion that guides or directs action. Guideline development emphasises using clear evidence from the existing literature, as opposed to expert opinion alone, as the basis for advisor materials.
Health and wellbeing	A state of complete physical, social and mental wellbeing; not just the absence of disease or infirmity. It is a positive concept that emphasises personal resources as well as physical capabilities.
Regulations	A rule or law designed to control or govern conduct.
Standards	Authoritative statements developed, monitored and enforced by, for example, healthcare regulators to describe the responsibilities and conduct expected of registrants. The standards are based on the principles and that underpin professional practice.
Therapeutic	Relating to therapeutics, the branch of medicine concerned specifically with the treatment of disease. The therapeutic dose of a drug is the amount needed to treat a disease.

References

Ballantyne, H. (2015). Developing nursing care plans. *Nursing Standard* **30** (26): 51–57.

Care Quality Commission (2018). Learning from safety incidents. https://www.cqc.org.uk/guidance-providers/learning-safety-incidents (accessed September 2020).

Clyne, B., Cooper, J.A., Boland, F. et al. (2017). Beliefs about prescribed medication among older patients with polypharmacy: a mixed methods study in primary care. https://bjgp.org/content/67/660/e507 (accessed September 2020).

Higher Education England (2017). Advisory guidance. administration of medicines by nursing associates. https://www.hee.nhs.uk/sites/default/files/documents/Advisory%20guidance%20-%20 administration%20of%20medicines%20by%20nursing%20associates.pdf (accessed September 2020).

Hjorthøj, C., Stürup, A.E., McGrath, J.J. et al. (2017). Years of potential life lost and life expectancy in schizo-phrenia: a systematic review and meta-analysis. *Lancet Psychiatry* **4** (4): 295–301.

Mårdby, A., Åkerlind, I., and Hedenrud, T. (2009). General beliefs about medicines among doctors and nurses in out-patient care: a cross-sectional study. *BMC Family Practice* **18** (10): 35. doi: 10.1186/1471-2296-10-35.

Mental Health Foundation (2016). Fundamental health facts about mental health 2016. https://www.mentalhealth.org.uk/sites/default/files/fundamental-facts-about-mental-health-2016.pdf (accessed September 2020).

National Institute for Health and Care Excellence (2014). Managing medicines in care homes. https://www.nice.org.uk/guidance/sc1/evidence/full-guideline-pdf-2301173677 (accessed September 2020).

National Institute for Health and Care Excellence (2015). Medicines optimisation: the safe and effective use of medicines to enable the best possible outcomes. www.nice.org.uk/guidance/ng5/resources/medicines-optimisation-the-safe-and-effective-use-of-medicines-to-enable-the-best-possible-outcomes-pdf-51041805253 (accessed September 2020).

National Institute for Health and Care Excellence (2017). Managing medicines for adults receiving social care in the community. www.nice.org.uk/guidance/ng67 (accessed September 2020).

Neame, R. and Hammond, A. (2005). Beliefs about medications: a questionnaire survey of people with rheumatoid arthritis. *Rheumatology* **44** (6): 762–767.

Nursing and Midwifery Council (2010). Standards for medicines management. https://www.nmc.org.uk/standards/standards-for-post-registration/standards-for-medicines-management/ (accessed September 2020).

Nursing and Midwifery Council (2017). Revalidation. https://www.nmc.org.uk/globalassets/sitedocuments/revalidation/how-to-revalidate-booklet.pdf (accessed September 2020).

Nursing and Midwifery Council (2018a). The Code: Professional standards of practice and behaviour for nurses, midwives and nursing associates. https://www.nmc.org.uk/standards/code/ (accessed September 2020).

Nursing and Midwifery Council (2018b). Standards of proficiency for registered nurses. https://www.nmc.org.uk/globalassets/sitedocuments/education-standards/future-nurse-proficiencies.pdf (accessed September 2020).

Nursing and Midwifery Council (2018c). Standards of proficiency for nursing associates. https://www.nmc.org.uk/globalassets/sitedocuments/education-standards/nursing-associates-proficiency-standards.pdf (accessed September 2020).

Royal College of Nursing and Royal Pharmaceutical Society (2019). *Guidance on the Administration of Medicines in Healthcare Settings*. London: RCN and RPS.

Royal Pharmaceutical Society (2013). Medicines optimisation: helping patients to make the most of medicines. good practice guidance for healthcare professionals in England. https://www.rpharms.com/Portals/0/RPS%20document%20library/Open%20access/Policy/helping-patients-make-the-most-of-their-medicines.pdf (accessed September 2020).

Royal Pharmaceutical Society (2016). A competency framework for all prescribers. https://www.rpharms.com/Portals/0/RPS%20document%20library/Open%20access/Professional%20standards/Prescribing%20competency%20framework/prescribing-competency-framework.pdf (accessed September 2020).

Royal Pharmaceutical Society (2018a). Professional guidance on the safe and secure handling of medicines. https://www.rpharms.com/recognition/setting-professional-standards/safe-and-secure-handling-of-medicines/professional-guidance-on-the-safe-and-secure-handling-of-medicines (accessed September 2020).

Royal Pharmaceutical Society (2018b). Utilising pharmacists to improve the care for people with mental health problems. https://www.rpharms.com/Portals/0/RPS%20document%20library/Open%20access/Policy/RPS%20England%20mental%20health%20policy%202018.pdf (accessed September 2020).

Stonehouse, D. (2017). Understanding the nursing process. *British Journal of Healthcare Assistants* **11** (8): 388–391.

Further reading

British Pharmacological Society
www.bps.ac.uk
The BPS exists to promote and advance pharmacology in all its forms.

Royal Pharmaceutical Society
www.rpharms.com

The RPS gives pharmacy a clear, strong voice in all healthcare discussions and decisions across Britain.
   They also publish the British National Formulary.

The Nursing and Midwifery Council
www.nmc.org.uk

Better and safer care for people is at the heart of what the NMC does, supporting the healthcare professionals on their register to deliver the highest standards of care.

Multiple choice questions

1. What are the five phases of the nursing process:
    (a) Assess, diagnose, plan, implement, evaluate
    (b) Assess, diagnose, predict, implement, evaluate
    (c) Assess, diagnose, plan, implement, identify
    (d) Assess, detect, plan, implement, evaluate
2. Assessment requires the nurse to:
    (a) Observe the environment, undertake a clinical examination, gather data and
        communicate
    (b) Consult the BNF, observe the patient, perform a clinical examination, gather
        data
    (c) Observe the patient, perform a clinical examination, gather data and
        communicate
    (d) Use the skills of observation, calculate risk, perform a clinical examination,
        gather data and communicate
3. The role of the NMC is to:
    (a) Regulate hospitals or other healthcare settings
    (b) Regulate healthcare assistants
    (c) Regulate nurses and midwives
    (d) Regulate nurses, midwives and pharmacists
4. How many key clauses are there in the NMC's Code:
    (a) 22
    (b) 24
    (c) 25
    (d) 23
5. The registered nurse is required to:
    (a) Act in the patient's best interests
    (b) Undertake accurate drug calculations for a variety of medications
    (c) Uphold the values of the profession
    (d) All of the above
6. What might be the benefits of medications self-administered by the patient:
    (a) Staff have more time for other duties
    (b) The patient gains more control
    (c) There is reduction in the number of medication errors
    (d) There is less risk of infection
7. Medicine management standards provide healthcare workers with:
    (a) Legal protection
    (b) An ability to opt out of medicines administration
    (c) A framework for safe practice in medicines management
    (d) The opportunity to prescribe controlled drugs

8. Oxygen is:
    (a) Safe to use in any circumstance and does not require a prescription
    (b) A medical gas and has no side effects
    (c) A medical gas and as such should be treated as a medicine
    (d) Only used in high-dependency units and never in a patient's home
9. In order to maintain people's safety, staff have to:
    (a) Have passed an in-house course concerning competence
    (b) Have the appropriate qualifications, competence, skills and experience to maintain people's safety
    (c) Be registered with a regulatory body
    (d) Be skilled in CPR
10. Medicines management is different to medicines optimisation as it:
    (a) Focuses on outcomes and patients rather than process and systems
    (b) Focuses on patients and families as opposed to just the patient
    (c) Is governed by the health or social care regulator
    (d) It only applies in community settings
11. In order to enable a shared decision about treatment:
    (a) The healthcare provider's values and beliefs are key
    (b) Patients' beliefs and preferences about medicines must be understood
    (c) The professional regulator's Code has to be paramount
    (d) The patient must sign a consent form
12. The safe use of medicines is the responsibility of:
    (a) The pharmacist
    (b) The patient
    (c) The registered practitioner
    (d) All of the above
13. The terms 'non-compliance' or 'non-adherence' have been criticised for:
    (a) Being sexist
    (b) Suggesting an unequal, paternalistic relationship between health professionals prescribing medication and their patients
    (c) Suggesting an equal, relationship between health professionals prescribing medication and their patients
    (d) Failing to address the age of the patient
14. A therapeutic relationship is:
    (a) A helping relationship based on mutual trust and respect
    (b) A healing relationship
    (c) A curative relationship based on the use of medicines
    (d) None of the above
15. The four core governing principles concerning the safe and secure handling of medicines (Royal Pharmaceutical Society) are:
    (a) Assess, implement, improve, assure
    (b) Establish assurance arrangements, ensure capacity and capability, seek assurance, continually improve
    (c) Establish insurance, ensure capacity and capability, seek assurance, continually improve
    (d) Establish assurance arrangements, ensure asepsis, seek assurance, continually improve
    (e) Establish assurance arrangements, ensure capacity and capability, seek validation, continually improve

Chapter 2

How to use pharmaceutical and prescribing reference guides

Claire Pryor and Annette Hand

Aim

This chapter aims to introduce the reader to commonly used pharmaceutical and prescribing reference guides and their use in practice. Specific focus is placed on the British National Formulary (BNF) and other reference guides used in clinical practice.

Learning outcomes

After reading this chapter, the reader will:

1. Be aware of the different pharmaceutical and reference guides that may be used in practice
2. Understand how to navigate the BNF (both in print and electronic formats)
3. Recognise the different prescribing reference guides available (local and national)
4. Discuss the benefits of using pharmaceutical and prescribing reference guides in practice

Test your knowledge

1. How many times a year is the print version of the BNF updated?
2. What schedule of controlled drug is Midazolam?
3. What is a General Sales List (GSL) medication?
4. Where will you find national prescribing guidelines for managing chronic constipation in adults?
5. Can whiskey be prescribed on an NHS prescription?

Fundamentals of Pharmacology: For Nursing and Healthcare Students, First Edition. Edited by Ian Peate and Barry Hill.

Introduction

The world of medications is vast and learning about them can be daunting for all nursing and healthcare students (as well as registered professionals). The people you care for may have extensive lists of medications you need to be able to review, administer, and consider interactions and monitor the effects of these.

Professional bodies have specific standards of practice in relation to medicines and pharmacological knowledge and this will relate to the practitioner's role. The Nursing and Midwifery (NMC) Code (NMC 2018a) states in Standard 18 that nurses and nursing associates must

> Advise on, prescribe, supply, dispense or administer medicines within the limits of your training and competence, the law, our guidance and other relevant policies, guidance and regulations.
>
> (Nursing and Midwifery Council, 2018a)

Further guidance is issued for nursing associates. The NMC stipulates the requirement for nursing associates: as per Section 3:16 of their standards of proficiency, they must:

> demonstrate the ability to recognise the effects of medicines, allergies, drug sensitivity, side effects, contraindications and adverse reactions.
>
> (Nursing and Midwifery Council, 2018b)

In order to fulfil these requirements, healthcare professionals must have a level of pharmaceutical knowledge and an awareness of how to and where to find appropriate information to support practice. In a sea of new products and complex regimens, where can you turn for up-to-date, clear and concise information to guide your practice? There are numerous guides, websites, texts and resources that are readily available. Ensuring a robust and evidence-based selection of these is paramount, but the choice is also personal. Some are web based, some print, and a new evolution of healthcare apps for professionals means that there is a selection for all user preferences.

This chapter aims to introduce you to using pharmaceutical and prescribing reference guides with a specific focus on the BNF and other pharmaceutical reference guides. These guides are vital and valuable resources to draw upon to ensure safe, accountable and evidence-based care that is matched to the needs and wishes of the people you care for.

Skills in practice

You are a first-year student on your first placement; with your practice supervisor you are assessing a new patient on admission. They give you a list of medication they take and it has lots of names on it that are new to you. You want to impress your supervisor and find out about them for your next shift. How do you do this? Where do you turn?

Your supervisor suggests you look them up and points you to a paper copy of the BNF. Upon opening it, it appears confusing, full of sections and symbols, and you are unsure how to find the information you need.

- Open a paper copy of the BNF and find the last drug you discussed or saw in practice.
- Can you locate it?
- What form does it come in?
- What are the side effects?
- Are there any interactions?
- Can it be bought at the supermarket?

These are some considerations you may have when supporting people with medication. Pharmaceutical reference guides will help you navigate this complex process and support your evidence-based practice.

The British National Formulary

Produced by the Joint Formulary Committee, the BNF is one of the most commonly used and reliable sources of information on medication. It offers comprehensive details on individual medications, groups of medications, uses, side effects and interactions and can assist with decision-making. The BNF is an essential tool for all practitioners; it is a repository of almost all drugs that are used in British healthcare settings (Young and Pitcher, 2016). The nurse should ensure they are familiar with its use, making it the go-to guide for any queries regarding drugs. A joint publication of the Royal Pharmaceutical Society and British Medical Association, it is devised to offer all healthcare professionals contemporary information on medications and their uses. The information provided is sourced from summaries of product characteristics for medications, literature, consensus guidelines and peer review and employs a grading system of A–E and levels of evidence to help readers understand the strength of evidence underpinning the associated recommendations given (Joint Formulary Committee, 2019a).

Paper copy BNF

Two types of BNF are available for practitioners: the BNF and the BNF for children (BNFc). Ensuring that you use the most appropriate type for your practice area is essential as medications, recommendations, licensing, legislation and monitoring differ for adults and children. The BNF is published in paper copy bi-annually in September and March and the BNFc is published in paper copy once a year in September. There are electronic versions (as discussed later) which are frequently updated, so it is always advisable to use the electronic version to ensure the most up-to-date information is accessed.

As a health professional you are accountable for using the most up-to-date evidence base for your practice. This means ensuring that you only use the current version of the BNF and that which relates to your practice area and patient group. You should consider:

- that previous versions may have outdated information or even sections that have been removed;
- the implications of advising your patient on their medication regimen if the information source you have chosen is out of date. What are the potential risks to the patient? What could this mean for your practice and accountability?

How to navigate the BNF

At first glance, the BNF can be overwhelming; however, with a little practice it quickly becomes a fast and reliable way to gather information for yourself, patients and those you work with.

The current BNF print versions are organised into four main sections:

- front matter
- chapters
- appendices
- back matter.

Careful attention should be paid to the font colour (see Table 2.1), images and symbols used in the BNF as these all convey pertinent information.

Front matter

The front matter of the BNF gives quick access to information such as how to use the BNF, the layout of information throughout chapters, and significant changes that have taken place

Table 2.1   Font colour and information purpose.

Text format	Information use
Black	Information on treatment summary and therapeutic uses
Colour block	Information on drug-specific information

since the previous edition. General guidance is given on prescribing and the requirements of legal prescriptions, both handwritten and computer issued. Special attention is paid to controlled drugs, alongside adverse reactions to drugs, and it offers guidance on recognition and reporting.

A general overview of specific patient-centred considerations is given in relation to prescribing in hepatic (liver) and renal (kidney) failure, as well considerations for pregnancy, elderly and palliative care. Each section has a broad overview followed by specific considerations. For example, in prescribing for palliative care, specific information is provided on pain, wider symptom control and continuous subcutaneous infusions.

Chapters

The main body of the BNF is divided into systems chapters (i.e. gastrointestinal system) and follows the same structure.

Some drugs and chapters have a *class monograph*. A class monograph includes information that is common to all drugs within a particular class. It is important to read these in conjunction with the *drug monograph*, which gives information relating to that drug in particular. Class monographs are identified by a flag in a circle ⬤. If the drug you are seeking advice on has an associated *class monograph* it will be indicated by a tab with a flag symbol and the page number where the *class monograph* can be found ▰1234 .

Access a copy of the current BNF and open the gastrointestinal system chapter. It starts with a clear contents section indicating what can be found in the chapter and is followed by information on the associated diseases, conditions and disorders, treatment summaries and individual medication information. Focusing on constipation, find and read the description of the condition and its associated overview and management.

The *classification* of the individual drug is indicated in blue (e.g. Laxatives: Bulk-forming laxatives) with the drug name and *drug monograph* sited below. The *drug monograph* provides comprehensive information on the drug all in one concise section. Pertinent guidance is offered relating to drug action, indications and dose, adjustments and interactions, safety information, contraindications, signposting to the correct section of interactions, side effects and medicinal forms.

Drug class monographs have been created by the publishers of the BNF. Where there is common information relating to a class of drugs, the shared properties are contained in a drug class monograph. Drug class monographs are emphasised by a circled flag symbol next to the title of the drug class monograph. The corresponding individual drug monographs generally follow the drug class monograph; these are highlighted by a non-circled flag symbol (see Figure 2.1).

In the example in Figure 2.1, the monograph depicted displays a flag, this indicates that the drug class monograph for Beta-adrenoceptor blocker (systemic) should be consulted in tandem.

Within the drug monograph the following are also highlighted:

- Drug classification: may be based on pharmaceutical class – for example, opioids – but may also be related to the use of the drug, such as for a cough suppressant.
- Indication and dose: all the information that relates to an individual drug; for example, drug action, indication and dose, contraindications, cautions, interactions, side effects, allergies and so on.
- Specific preparation name: if the dose varies with a specific preparation or formulation, it appears under the heading of the preparation name.
- Evidence grading: this reflects the strength of recommendation applied.
- Legal categories: applied to those preparations that are available only on a prescription issued by an appropriate practitioner and preparations that are subject to the prescription requirements of the Misuse of Drugs Act.

The information found in the *medicinal forms* section of the monograph is vital for healthcare professionals to be able to understand the various routes of administration, supply and

Class monograph ❶

CLASSIFICATION ❷

⚑ 1234

Drug monograph ❶   ❸ 01-Jun-2016

(Synonym) another name by which a drug may be known

- DRUG ACTION how a drug exerts its effect in the body

  - INDICATIONS AND DOSE
  Indications are the clinical reasons a drug is used. The dose of a drug will often depend on the indications
  Indication
  ▸ ROUTE
  ▹ Age groups: [Child/Adult/Elderly]
    Dose and frequency of administration (max. dose)
  SPECIFIC PREPARATION NAME ❹
  Indication
  ▸ ROUTE
  ▹ Age groups: [Child/Adult/Elderly]
    Dose and frequency of administration (max. dose)
  DOSE EQUIVALENCE AND CONVERSION information around the bioequivalence between formulations of the same drug, or equivalent doses of drugs that are members of the same class
  PHARMACOKINETICS how the body affects a drug (absorption, distribution, metabolism, and excretion)
  POTENCY a measure of drug activity expressed in terms of the concentration required to produce an effect of given intensity
  DOSES AT EXTREMES OF BODY-WEIGHT dosing information for patients who are overweight or underweight

- UNLICENSED USE describes the use of medicines outside the terms of their UK licence (off-label use), or use of medicines that have no licence for use in the UK

  IMPORTANT SAFETY INFORMATION
  Information produced and disseminated by drug regulators often highlights serious risks associated with the use of a drug, and may include advice that is mandatory

- CONTRA-INDICATIONS circumstances when a drug should be avoided
- CAUTIONS details of precautions required
- INTERACTIONS when one drug changes the effects of another drug; the mechanisms underlying drug interactions are explained in Appendix 1
- SIDE-EFFECTS listed in order of frequency, where known, and arranged alphabetically
- ALLERGY AND CROSS-SENSITIVITY for drugs that carry an increased risk of hypersensitivity reactions
- CONCEPTION AND CONTRACEPTION potential for a drug to have harmful effects on an unborn child when prescribing for a woman of childbearing age or for a man trying to father a child; information on the effect of drugs on the efficacy of latex condoms or diaphragms
- PREGNANCY advice on the use of a drug during pregnancy
- BREAST FEEDING EvGr advice on the use of a drug during breast feeding ⒶＳ ❺

- HEPATIC IMPAIRMENT advice on the use of a drug in hepatic impairment
- RENAL IMPAIRMENT advice on the use of a drug in renal impairment
- PRE-TREATMENT SCREENING covers one off tests required to assess the suitability of a patient for a particular drug
- MONITORING REQUIREMENTS specifies any special monitoring requirements, including information on monitoring the plasma concentration of drugs with a narrow therapeutic index
- EFFECTS ON LABORATORY TESTS for drugs that can interfere with the accuracy of seemingly unrelated laboratory tests
- TREATMENT CESSATION specifies whether further monitoring or precautions are advised when the drug is withdrawn
- DIRECTIONS FOR ADMINISTRATION practical information on the preparation of intravenous drug infusions; general advice relevant to other routes of administration
- PRESCRIBING AND DISPENSING INFORMATION practical information around how a drug can be prescribed and dispensed including details of when brand prescribing is necessary
- HANDLING AND STORAGE includes information on drugs that can cause adverse effects to those who handle them before they are taken by, or administered to, a patient; advice on storage conditions
- PARENT AND CARER ADVICE for drugs with a special need for counselling
- PROFESSION SPECIFIC INFORMATION provides details of the restrictions certain professions such as dental practitioners or nurse prescribers need to be aware of when prescribing on the NHS
- NATIONAL FUNDING/ACCESS DECISIONS details of NICE Technology Appraisals and SMC advice
- LESS SUITABLE FOR PRESCRIBING preparations that are considered by the Joint Formulary Committee to be less suitable for prescribing
- EXCEPTION TO LEGAL CATEGORY advice and information on drugs which may be sold without a prescription under specific conditions

- MEDICINAL FORMS
  Form
  CAUTIONARY AND ADVISORY LABELS if applicable
  EXCIPIENTS clinically important but not comprehensive [consult manufacturer information for full details]
  ELECTROLYTES if clinically significant quantities occur
  ▹ Preparation name (Manufacturer/Non-proprietary)
    Drug name and strength pack sizes PoM ❻ Prices

  Combinations available this indicates a combination preparation is available and a cross reference page number is provided to locate this preparation

Figure 2.1   Extract drug class monograph.

dose schedule considerations. Alongside this, the medicinal forms section shows the legal category of the drug indicated by a specific category abbreviation or controlled drug schedule abbreviation. Table 2.2 demonstrates the abbreviations and their meanings. In practice, this information may make the difference between generating prescriptions, or giving health advice. The variance between categories may be determined by the drug itself, the dose and amount to be dispensed (see Box 2.1).

Table 2.2   Abbreviations of medication categories.

Category	Description
P – pharmacy-only medicine [P]	A product that may only be sold in a registered pharmacy under the supervision of a registered pharmacist, e.g. bisacodyl suppositories
PoM – prescription-only medicine [PoM]	A product that may only be sold or supplied to the public on a practitioner's prescription, e.g. warfarin tablets
GSL – general sales list [GSL]	A product that may be sold from a retail outlet without the supervision of a registered pharmacist, e.g. NiQuitin 2 mg medicated chewing gum
CD – controlled drug [CD1] [CD2] [CD3] [CD4-1] [CD4-2] [CD5]	A product that is controlled by the Misuse of Drugs Act 1971 and is listed in Schedule 2 or 3 of the Misuse of Drugs Regulations 2001 as amended, which may be subject to specific restrictions relating to supply, prescription, storage, record-keeping, labelling, and destruction; e.g. morphine sulphate (modified release tablets) 60 mg oral tablet
ACBS – Advisory Committee on Borderline Substances	A product that may be prescribed for the treatment of certain conditions. Prescriptions for these products must be endorsed 'ACBS'. e.g. gluten-free bread

Box 2.1 Paracetamol sales

Paracetamol 500 mg tablets in 16 tablet packs are available as GSL and can be purchased without supervision of a pharmacist. Pharmacists may sell packs of a maximum of 32 tablets as pharmacy only (P) drugs: requiring supervision of a pharmacist. Over 32 tablets per pack are prescription only medication (PoM). This example shows that while the drug itself remains the same, other factors (in this instance, quantity) may impact on the classification of a medication. Other licensing considerations may change the legal status of the medication as well, even if the drug remains the same (Joint Formulary Committee, 2019b).

Skills in practice

Using the BNF index, locate docusate sodium.

- What is the drug classification?
- What are the cautions associated with this drug?
- Is this drug harmful in pregnancy?
- Is the drug available as an enema?

Back matter

The back matter of the BNF contains a number of appendices which offer detailed supplementary information on drug interactions, borderline substances, cautionary and advisory labels, and wound management products and elasticated garments. It also includes specific formularies for dental practitioners and the nurse prescribers formulary (for registered and qualified community practitioner prescribers).

Interactions

As a practitioner and professionally accountable for your actions, you must ensure that you know how to review and find out information on potential interactions. A comprehensive list of drugs with known interactions is found in Appendix 1 (as signposted to in the drug monograph). Appendix 1 provides tables and details of specific medications, medication combinations, and their associated pharmacodynamic effects. Each drug or group is listed twice, by name alphabetically and with the specific drug or group that it interacts with.

Borderline substances

In some conditions, such as coeliac disease, food products and toilet preparations may have characteristics of drugs. These products are reviewed and determined by the Advisory Committee on Borderline Substances (ACBS), as such, they may be treated as a prescribed medication. Some examples are enteral feeds, nutritional supplements, gluten free or low protein foods, and nutritional supplements given to treat metabolic diseases (e.g. maple syrup urine disease) alongside toilet preparations for topical use (for example, E45° or Aveeno Cream® for the treatment of dermatitis).

Nutritional supplements are common in care settings. Providing support with supplement drinks and puddings, for example, may form part of your everyday practice, but these should be treated as medication and prescribed based on individual patient need as with any medication.

Clinical considerations

You are looking after a lady for an extended period of time. It is common to offer her a supplement pudding as she only eats small amounts. You support her with her eating and drinking. On discussion with your practice supervisor, you realise this is not prescribed for her and she is being prepared for a transfer of care to a community care setting.
What implications does this practice have? Jot down your initial thoughts.

1. For her (both now and post transfer of care)?
2. For you as a healthcare professional or student?
3. For discharge planning?
4. For the doctors responsible for her medications?

Revisit these considerations and your initial thoughts when you have explored more about the legal and ethical considerations, as well as pharmacokinetics and pharmacodynamics.

Cautionary and advisory labels for dispensed medication

Many medications come with cautionary or advisory information that should be added by pharmacists when dispensing the requested medication. Appendix 3 has a list of approved cautionary and advisory labels, each with a specific code number. The number associated with the label is found in the *drug monograph* in the *medicinal forms* section below the preparation chosen. It is important to advise the patient on the additional advice or directions given for taking their medication. A full list of the labels and wording is found both in Appendix 3 and in the back pages of the print BNF.

Skills in practice

- Using the index, find olanzapine in the BNF.
- Using the drug monograph, find the medicinal form section.
- Identify the cautionary and advisory label number given for oral tablets.
- Use Appendix 3 to identify what the label states.
- What additional information is provided?
- How would you discuss this with the patient?

Wound management products and elasticated garments

Appendix 4 offers details of products that are used for wound management and garments that require a prescription. Best practice and clinical recommendations should be consulted to ensure the most appropriate item is chosen. Often in acute or inpatient settings, the clinical environment has a stock of regularly used dressings or bandages or other medicinal devices, such as surgical adhesive tapes. These remain individual prescribed patient items and should be considered as such on discharge or transfer of care. It is essential that the supply of wound care products, and associated treatment information, should be prepared and documented as per any other medication or medical product or device. This information is paramount for community care providers, practice nurses and general practitioners in order to maintain high-quality care standards.

Emergency care protocols, units, conversions and abbreviations

The BNF print version acts as a reference guide for practitioners in emergency situations. The adult advanced life-support algorithm and an overview of community-based medical emergency management provides a valuable resource in emergency situations.

Conversions and unit tables are presented as a reference followed by the cautionary and advisory label wordings discussed previously. The inside back page lastly provides a guide to the abbreviations and symbols used which are internationally recognised.

Online and mobile application BNF

In an increasingly paper-free healthcare system, you may not have access to paper copies of the BNF. The BNF has an online platform accessed via the National Institute for Health and Care Excellence (NICE), or via Medicines Complete (https://about.medicinescomplete.com) as well as an offline app that can be used on smart phones and tablets. The BNF online https://bnf.nice.org.uk or BNF for children https://bnfc.nice.org.uk is updated monthly and as such is often more up-to-date than the print version and does not require a specific log-in. The app is automatically updated monthly (when connected to wi-fi).

When you visit the home page of the BNF online (via NICE), you are presented with clear options for navigation. All the same information is held online as in print – but navigation is different. Drugs (as drug monographs), interactions and treatment summaries can be searched for by browsing an alphabetised list or the search bar at the top of the webpage. The home page also has a 'type' organisation where quick access to areas such as wound management, borderline substances and nurse prescribers' formularies can be found.

Searching for atenolol (for example) and opening its page displays information under the atenolol drug monograph. A table of contents is provided for rapid navigation of the subsections available. On scrolling down the opening page, indications and dose are clearly presented alongside routes of administration. Next, licensing information, safety information and contraindications are displayed.

Contra-indications

For all BETA-ADRENOCEPTOR BLOCKERS (SYSTEMIC)

Figure 2.2   Contraindication and class monograph.

Cautionary and advisory labels are indicated when a medicinal form is selected both by label number and the associated text. In addition, the schedule of any controlled drug is clearly documented in its medicinal form information.

Associated class monograph information is integrated throughout the chosen drug monograph and indicated by the phrasing 'for all . . ..' An example of this can be seen in the contraindications for atenolol (Figure 2.2).

Searching for interactions is managed within a dedicated interactions section by an initial drug search and then matching to a subsequent alphabetical list. The associated interaction is discussed in terms of potential effects of the interaction, signposting to relevant additional sections of the BNF such as 'Drugs and driving' in 'Guidance for prescribing' and has associated hyperlinks for ease of use. Severity of interactions are defined using terms of severe, moderate, mild and unknown to support decision-making alongside the type of evidence underpinning the interaction information.

Key to safe and accountable practice is the recognition and reporting of suspected adverse reactions or effects of medication. The BNF supports active reporting of adverse reactions by both healthcare professionals and patients themselves or their carers. Using the *Yellow Card Scheme*, the Medicines and Healthcare Products Regulatory Agency (MHRA) collects information on medications, vaccines, herbal treatments, medical devices, defective medications, and – from 2016 – counterfeit or fake healthcare products and e-cigarettes. The print copy of the BNF and BNFc have a small supply of yellow cards in the back matter; alternatively concerns can be raised using the UK MHRA Yellow card webpage https://yellowcard.mhra.gov.uk. Chapter 7, Adverse Drug Reactions in this book provides more details of this.

MIMS (Monthly Index of Medical Specialities)

Within a primary care setting, you may also come across the MIMS prescribing guide. This is an up-to-date prescribing reference for healthcare professionals and it is available both in print and online. MIMS is updated constantly online, to reflect the latest approved prescribing information, along with the addition of new drugs and formulations, and also removes products that are no longer available. The printed version of MIMS is produced quarterly and includes all the updates from the corresponding three months of online updates. MIMS is primarily intended for use by GPs and nurses working within primary care. A subscription is required for nurses who wish to receive the print version. All other prescribing healthcare professionals – such as paramedics, dietitians and physiotherapists – need to subscribe to MIMS to access either the online or print versions. MIMS is a helpful prescribing resource and provides:

- News on changes that affect medicines and prescribing.
- Drug information for branded and generic products, updated daily.
- At-a-glance drug comparison tables including dosing and monitoring regimens, available presentations, prices, potential sensitisers and compatible devices.
- Quick-reference summaries of key clinical guidance from authoritative national bodies, including NICE and the Scottish Intercollegiate Guidelines Network (SIGN).
- Online drugs shortages tracker showing branded and generic medicines that are out of stock.
- Online visual guides to help you identify, compare, and recommend diabetes and respiratory devices.

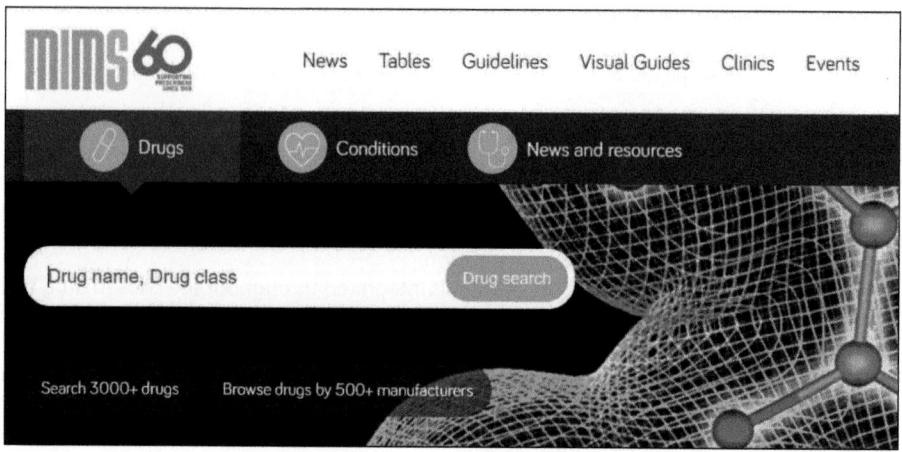

Figure 2.3   Home page of MIMS online. (Source: www.mims.co.uk).

MIMS provides concise summaries of prescribing information for branded and generic products that can be prescribed in the UK, including devices listed in the section on permitted appliances within the Drug Tariff. Drugs that are blacklisted (i.e. not on the Drug Tariff and therefore not prescribable on the NHS) are not listed and no information is given on the unlicensed or off-label use of drugs.

The print edition of MIMS also includes a selection of the most popular drug reference tables. The full range of tables and drug listings are available online, together with at-a-glance summaries of national treatment guidance and helpful visual guides to diabetes and respiratory devices; there is also a prescribing resource centre for specific disease areas. The legal class categories in MIMS are the same as those within the BNF and listed in Table 2.2.

How to use MIMS online

When you visit the home page of MIMS online (see Figure 2.3), you are able to search for drugs (by drug name or drug class), browse news and resources by disease areas (from an A to Z list), or search for news, tables or guidance on any condition or drug. You are also able to search for drugs by manufacturer. Searching for a drug only returns a list if there is more than one hit (i.e. multiple drugs matching the search term and/or drugs matching the search term appearing in multiple sections), otherwise you are taken to the drug entry. Clicking on a drug will display all the different preparations, legal class, indications and dose recommendations for adults and children (where appropriate). The drug listing page will also display helpful links to any related guidelines or related conditions.

Skills in practice

1. Search for paracetamol within the drug search box.

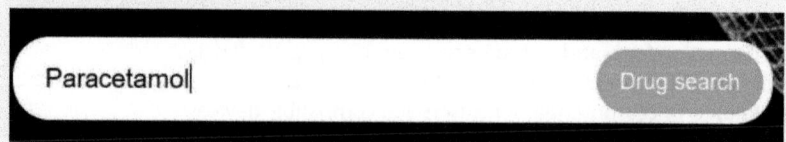

2. You will see that paracetamol-containing products can be used for a number of different clinical conditions (migraine, pain and fever), with different strengths, formulations and combinations.

3. When paracetamol is combined with another product it is still important to understand the strengths of the individual compounds.
   - Clink on co-codamol: you can see there is always 500 mg of paracetamol within one co-codamol capsule, but the dose of codeine phosphate could be 8, 15 or 30 mg.
4. Each form of paracetamol is only licensed for specific indications.
   - Clink on paracetamol infusion: you can see this would only be used as a short-term treatment for moderate pain and fever when other routes are inappropriate.
5. For each paracetamol preparation, there may be different contraindications.
   - Click on paracetamol/ibuprofen (combogesic): you will see the contraindications are alcoholism, aspirin/anti-inflammatory allergy, active or history of gastrointestinal bleeding or peptic ulcer, severe cardiac, hepatic or renal failure, cerebrovascular or other active bleeding, blood formation disturbances and pregnancy (third trimester).

Searching within news and resources, you will find links to relevant tables and summaries of national guidelines, as well as any information about the condition that has been in the news. You can use the filters on the right-hand side to find the results of a particular type (for example, news) or from a particular year.

Many abbreviations are used in healthcare and it is important that you familiarise yourself with these to ensure you understand what they mean. Abbreviations are used within prescribing guides and in practice and it is always best to check what an abbreviation means if you are unsure. A list of the abbreviations used in MIMS can be found at the front of every print issue and online.

Clinical considerations

- You are asked to administer a medication in 'S-C' form.
- Do you get a glass of water for your patient, or an injection/infusion set?
- What would the implications be of not understanding the correct abbreviation?

Be aware that sometimes the same abbreviation is used to mean different things. For some healthcare practitioners, the abbreviation 's-c' or 's/c' could be colloquially used to mean subcutaneous; but within the BNF 's/c' represents sugar coated, and in MIMS 's-c' is used for sugar coated. Note here that the abbreviation is not used to represent the route of administration. It is paramount that you are aware of the formal abbreviations in use and not colloquial, historical interpretations or slang. This is explored further in Chapter 4 of this book, Medicines Management and the Role of the Healthcare Provider.

Electronic Medicines Compendium

The electronic medicines compendium (emc) contains up-to-date, easily accessible information about medicines licensed for use in the UK and can be found at www.medicines.org.uk/emc. The emc has more than 14 000 documents, all of which have been checked and approved by either the UK or European government agencies which license medicines. These agencies are the UK MHRA and the European Medicines Agency (EMA). The emc is updated continually and you are able to browse for medicines, or active ingredients, using the A–Z buttons. The emc contains regulated and approved information on medicines available in the UK including:

1. Summaries of Product Characteristics (known as SPCs or SmPCs).
   A SmPC informs healthcare professionals on how to prescribe and use a medicine correctly. A SmPC is based on clinical trials that a pharmaceutical company has carried out and gives

information about dose, use and possible side effects. A SmPC is always written in a standard format.

2. Patient Information Leaflets (PILs, Package Leaflets or PLs).
   A PIL is the leaflet that is included in the pack with any medicine. The PIL is a summary of the SmPC and is written for patients.

3. Risk Minimisation Materials (RMMs).
   RMMs are resources for healthcare professionals that aim to optimise the safe and effective use of a medicine. RMMs can come in a number of forms, such as educational programs, prescribing or dispensing guides, patient brochures, or alert cards.

4. Safety Alerts.
   Safety alerts are issued by the Regulator and/or marketing authorisation holder and contain important public health messages or safety critical information about a medicine.

5. Product Information.
   This is any additional information about a product. It may include important information such as change of packaging or issues related to stock levels.

Within the emc, there are also audio and video resources that provide additional information in a user-friendly manner, promoting the safe an effective use of a medicine. For example, a video clip may demonstrate how to administer a certain medicine correctly.

What can be prescribed on an NHS prescription?

There are hundreds of medicinal products and devices (or appliances) available to treat and manage illnesses, conditions and diseases. A medicinal product is defined as an item which is not considered to be appliance and could be a drug, food, toiletry or type of cosmetic (Pharmaceutical Services Negotiating Committee (PSNC) https://psnc.org.uk/dispensing-supply/dispensing-a-prescription/medicinal-products). An approved medical device will carry the CE mark (Conformité Européene), which signifies that it conforms to the appropriate regulatory standards. Not all of these medical products, devices or appliances are available from the NHS. On receiving a prescription, pharmacy staff will check whether or not an item is allowed to be prescribed on the NHS prior to dispensing using the Drug Tariff.

The Drug Tariff

The Drug Tariff is produced monthly by the Pharmaceutical Directorate of the NHS Business Services Authority and the NHS Prescription Services for the Secretary of State. It is supplied primarily to pharmacists and doctor's surgeries and is available in print and online; any healthcare professional can view the most up-to-date online version. Only fully licensed and approved medications and devices, found on the Drug Tariff, can be prescribed within the NHS (unless for research purposes). Information on the Drug Tariff can be found on either the PSNC or the NHS Prescription Services websites. Within each of these sites you will find information on how to use the Drug Tariff, the Drug Tariff Preface and the information within the different Parts of the Drug Tariff. The Drug Tariff Preface is an important section as each month as it contains valuable information on additions, deletions and any other alterations to the Drug Tariff.

What The Drug Tariff does

The Drug Tariff outlines information such as:

- what will be paid to pharmacies for the NHS services provided (for example, the cost of drugs and appliances supplied against an NHS prescription);

- rules that need to be followed when dispensing items;
- drug and appliance prices.

How to tell if a medicinal product is allowed on prescription

The 'blacklist' can be found in Schedule 1 to the NHS Regulations 2004 and is found in the Drug Tariff (part XVIIIA); it is a list of medicinal products which cannot be prescribed on the NHS. Any medicinal product not on the 'blacklist' can be prescribed on the NHS. Whiskey, for example, is not on the blacklist, so a prescription for this item would be passed for payment by NHS Prescription Services. The prescriber may, however, be questioned during the auditing process about the appropriateness of prescribing this item at NHS expense. As a general rule, if a branded (proprietary) product is listed on the 'blacklist' it cannot be prescribed on the NHS. Many of the medicinal products on the 'blacklist' are available over the counter for people to buy, while some do not have enough evidence to show their efficacy.

The PSCN flow chart (Figure 2.4) can be used to help identify whether an item is allowed to be dispensed on an NHS prescription form. Different practitioners may use different prescription pads or resources (seen below as FP10, FP10SS, FP10SP*).

If a medicinal product, or device, is prescribed that is not on the Drug Tariff, it cannot be dispensed.

Skills in practice

Go to the Drug Tariff (https://www.nhsbsa.nhs.uk/pharmacies-gp-practices-and-appliance-contractors/drug-tariff) and see which of the following products are blacklisted and should not be prescribed on the NHS.

- ferrous sulfate compound tablets BP
- Gaviscon granules
- Lemsip flu strength
- senokot tablets.

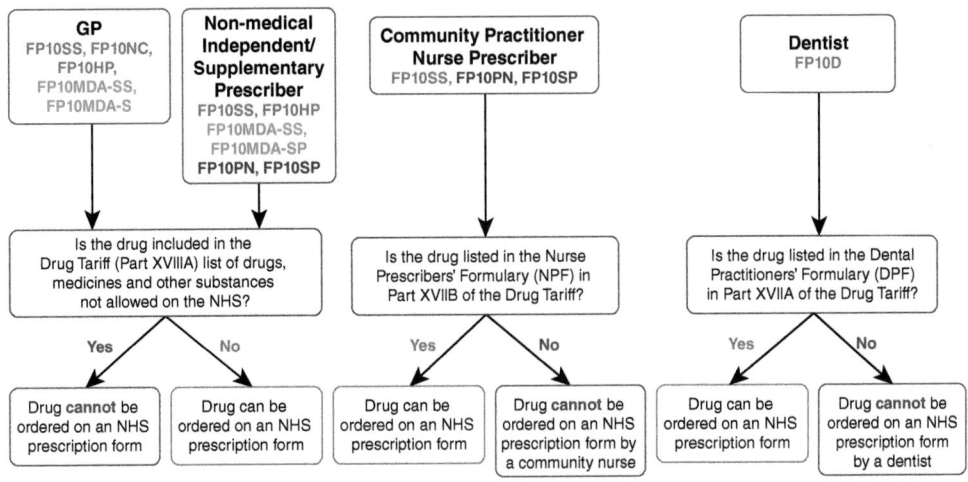

Figure 2.4   How to determine if a drug or devise can be prescribed on the NHS.

Other guides to prescribing

The Joint Royal Colleges Ambulance Liaison Committee (JRCALC) clinical guidelines

The Joint Royal Colleges Ambulance Liaison Committee Clinical (JRCALC) Guidelines is a help-ful resource for paramedics and other healthcare professionals, in emergency care, on the road and in the community. JRCALC combines expert advice with practical guidance to ensure uni-formity in the delivery of high-quality patient care. The book, available as either a comprehen-sive reference edition or pocket guide, covers a wide range of topics, from resuscitation, medical emergencies, trauma, obstetrics and medicines, to major incidents and staff wellbe-ing. It includes an extensive UK drugs formulary and Page for Age drugs tables to assist in making medicines administration simple. A digital version, via an app, of the official JRCALC guidelines is also available for pre-hospital clinicians to download.

Clinical considerations

- There are also numerous prescribing and drug handbooks available, predominantly devel-oped and produced for healthcare staff within the United States (US).
- They can be a useful resource, but be aware the recommended medicines within these guides will not be based on UK NICE/SIGN guidelines and/or the medicinal products may not even have a license to be used within the UK.

Prescribing Drug Therapy

You may also come across other prescribing guides (in electronic and paper format) such as 'Prescribing Drug Therapy'. This guide is written for Advanced Practice Registered Nurse (APRN) students and practitioners in the US who prescribe drugs for acute, episodic and chronic health problems. This guide provides details on treatment details for more than 600 diagnoses for healthcare providers in all primary care settings. Drug information is presented in a con-densed and summary format for ease of use. The print format includes an eBook with digital updates to assure immediate access to essential information.

The guide is simple to use with diagnoses listed alphabetically. For each diagnosis there is a list of:

- medicinal treatment recommendations;
- drug choices listed by generic name;
- Food and Drug Administration (FDA) pregnancy category;
- generic and over-the-counter availability;
- adult and paediatric dosing regimens;
- brand names, forms of dosage and additives;
- other clinically useful information, such as laboratory values to be monitored, patient teaching points and safety information.

Prescribing Drug Therapy also has an alphabetical cross-reference index of drugs by generic and brand name, with FDA pregnancy category and controlled drug schedule.

The evidence base to prescribing: prescribing guidelines

There are many medications that can be used to treat the same condition; it is important to know which drug to use and when. To assist with choosing the most appropriate medica-tion, in terms of efficacy, safety and cost effectiveness, clinical guidelines (where available) must be adhered to. Clinical guidelines are systematically developed statements to assist practitioners and patients make decisions about the most appropriate healthcare for specific clinical circumstances. Guidelines provide recommendations for effective practice in the management of clinical conditions where variations in practice are known to occur and where effective care may not be delivered in a uniform way. There are many guidelines available, but most are based on a consensus of 'expert opinion' or a non-systematic review of the scientific literature. Prescribing clinical guidelines can be local or national (Table 2.3 provides some examples).

NICE prescribing guidance

NICE is a non-departmental public body that provides national guidance and advice to improve health and social care in England.

NICE guidelines make evidence-based recommendations on a wide range of topics including:

- preventing and managing specific conditions;
- improving health;
- managing medicines in different settings;
- providing social care and support to adults and children;
- planning broader services and interventions to improve the health of communities.

Within each NICE guideline, there are recommendations regarding the care (including medications) and services that are suitable for most people with a specific condition or need. NICE guidelines are used by NHS England and NHS clinical commissioners to develop services and are a reference guide for healthcare professionals, with recommendations about medications that should and should not be prescribed. The guidelines also cover areas that patients should be able to manage themselves and obtain, if necessary, appropriate over-the-counter medications.

Table 2.3   Examples of local and national prescribing guidelines.

Local Guidance	National Guidance
<ul><li>to your team, service or condition you are working within</li><li>NHS organisation/employer</li><li>geographical region</li></ul>	<ul><li>NICE or SIGN guidance</li><li>national networks</li><li>clinical groups</li><li>charities</li></ul>

Clinical considerations

- In your area of practice, choose a medical condition that you are familiar with.
- Check to see if there is a local (to your Trust/employer) and/or national guideline for this condition.
- Is the guidance the same as within the BNF?
- Are there are any differences in recommendations? If so, think why this may be.

Scottish Intercollegiate Guidelines Network (SIGN)

The SIGN was formed to improve the quality of healthcare for patients in Scotland by reducing variation in practice and outcome. SIGN collaborate with a network of clinicians, other health and social care professionals, patient organisations and individuals to develop evidence-based guidelines. SIGN guidelines are based on a systematic review of the scientific literature and are aimed at aiding the translation of new knowledge into action. The guidelines are intended to:

- help health and social care professionals and patients understand medical evidence and use it to make decisions about healthcare;
- reduce unwarranted variations in practice and make sure patients get the best care available, no matter where they live;
- improve healthcare across Scotland by focusing on patient-important outcomes.

NICE and SIGN both produce patient booklets that are a lay translation of the clinical guidelines. These booklets explain the recommendations in the clinical guideline and help to make patients aware of the treatment they should expect to receive. They are intended to:

- help patients and carers understand the latest evidence about diagnosis, treatment and self-care;
- empower patients to participate fully in decisions about the management of their condition in discussion with healthcare professionals;
- highlight where there are areas of uncertainty in the management of their condition.

Conclusion

This chapter has provided an overview of the main pharmaceutical and prescribing reference guides used within clinical practice. Guidance has been given to encourage you to start to navigate the BNF in particular, to ensure you know where to find all the information needed about any medicinal product or device in order to ensure safe and effective practice. The differences between paper based and online versions have been highlighted to ensure you are aware where to access the most up-to-date and accurate drug information.

References

Joint Formulary Committee (2019a). How BNF publications are constructed: Assessing the evidence [Online]. https://bnf.nice.org.uk/about/how-bnf-publications-are-constructed.html (accessed 17 September 2019).

Joint Formulary Committee (2019b). British National Formulary: How to use BNF publications online [Online]. London: Joint Formulary Committee. https://bnf.nice.org.uk/about/how-to-use-bnf-publications-online.html (accessed 17 September 2019).

Nursing and Midwifery Council (2018a). The Code: professional standards of practice and behaviour for nurses, midwives and nursing associates [Online]. www.nmc.org.uk/standards/code (accessed 20 September 2019).

Nursing and Midwifery Council (2018b). Standards of proficiency for nursing associates [Online]. https://www.nmc.org.uk/standards/standards-for-nursing-associates/standards-of-proficiency-for-nursing-associates/ (accessed 20 September 2019).

Young, S. and Pitcher, B. (2016). *Medicine Management for Nurses at a Glance*. Oxford: Wiley.

Further reading

Electronic Medicines Compendium www.medicines.org.uk/emc

National Institute for Health and Care Excellence (NICE) Information on Medicines and Prescribing www.nice.org.uk/about/nice-communities/medicines-and-prescribing

Joint Royal Colleges of Ambulance and Liaison Committee (JRCACLC) www.jrcalc.org.uk

Scottish Intercollegiate Guidelines Network (SIGN) www.sign.ac.uk

UK Drug Tariff https://www.nhsbsa.nhs.uk/pharmacies-gp-practices-and-appliance-contractors/drug-tariff

Multiple choice questions

1. Which of the following are all pharmaceutical reference guides?
   - (a) MIMS, NICE and emc
   - (b) SIGN, BNF and MIMS
   - (c) BNF, MIMS and emc
2. What does the BNF stand for?
   - (a) British National Formulary
   - (b) British National Formulations
   - (c) Branded National Formulary
3. How many times a year is the BNF published?
   - (a) Once
   - (b) Twice
   - (c) Three times
4. Does the BNF detail all the information necessary for prescribing and dispensing?
   - (a) Yes, always
   - (b) Not always
   - (c) No
5. What does PoM stand for?
   - (a) Pharmacy-only medicine
   - (b) Prescribed oral medicine
   - (c) Prescription-only medicine
6. MIMS is primarily intended for use in which healthcare setting?
   - (a) All healthcare settings
   - (b) Primary care
   - (c) Secondary care
7. Within MIMS, how are you able to search for a drug?
   - (a) By drug name
   - (b) By condition
   - (c) By manufacturer
   - (d) All of the above
8. What does the abbreviation p.c. mean?
   - (a) Before food
   - (b) With food
   - (c) After food
9. Where will you find the 'blacklist'?
   - (a) Within the BNF
   - (b) Within the Drug Tariff
   - (c) Within NICE
10. On a device, what does the CE mark signify?
    - (a) That the device has been tried and tested and is safe to use
    - (b) That the device can be prescribed
    - (c) That the device has copyright protection
11. How often is the Drug Tariff updated?
    - (a) Continually
    - (b) Weekly
    - (c) Monthly

12. Which document informs healthcare professionals on how to prescribe and use a medicine correctly?
    (a) A clinical trial paper
    (b) Product information
    (c) Summaries of product characteristics

13. A PIL is a medicine leaflet written for whom?
    (a) Healthcare professionals
    (b) Pharmacy staff
    (c) Patients

14. Where will you find the most up-to-date information about the use of medicines?
    (a) BNF/MIMS paper copy
    (b) BNF/MIMS online
    (c) NICE guidance

15. You find an outdated BNF being used within a clinical area, what should you do?
    (a) Nothing, it is still safe to use an outdated BNF
    (b) Nothing, as it is not your place to say anything
    (c) Speak to a senior member of staff to get it replaced with an up-to-date version

Chapter 3

Legal and ethical issues

Claire Leader, Emma Senior and Deborah Flynn

Aim

The aim of this chapter is to examine the legal and ethical considerations that are related to pharmacology and medicines management in contemporary healthcare settings.

Learning outcomes

By the end of this chapter, the reader will be able to:

1. Define commonly used legal and ethical concepts
2. Identify situations where legal and ethical considerations are required to make defensible decisions
3. Explain how legal and ethical considerations influence the decision-making process
4. Apply legal and ethical considerations to a variety of scenarios likely to be encountered in modern healthcare settings

Test your knowledge

1. According to UK law, what must be established in order to prove a case of negligence?
2. Can a wife consent to treatment on behalf of their husband who lacks capacity?
3. What is the meaning of beneficence in relation to ethics?
4. Can healthcare professionals provide treatment for children without the consent of their responsible parent in an emergency situation?
5. What is a professional body's primary function?

Fundamentals of Pharmacology: For Nursing and Healthcare Students, First Edition. Edited by Ian Peate and Barry Hill.
© 2021 John Wiley & Sons Ltd. Published 2021 by John Wiley & Sons Ltd.

Introduction

This section will introduce readers to fundamental ethical principles relating to nursing and healthcare, as well as some of the key legal concepts with which healthcare professionals should become familiar in order to ensure that decisions around pharmacology have a legal and ethical basis.

Any decisions made about pharmacology require consideration of various issues: what you are legally obliged to do, what you are professionally guided to do and what is in the best interests of the person within the situation. In practice, the three usually exist together; but before considering them as a whole, let's start with the fundamentals and look at them separately.

This chapter will consider the three components that underpin high-quality decision-making in pharmacology:

- the law
- ethical principles and theories
- regulatory bodies.

The law

Laws exist to protect patients and the public. Recent years have seen changes in the culture within healthcare in the United Kingdom (UK), with a notable rise in litigation. Unlike some countries, where there is a 'no-blame' process for medico-legal cases, the UK system operates a 'fault criterion' whereby fault has to be established for the complainant to prove a case. Clinical negligence claims quadrupled between 2007 and 2017 (National Health Service Improvement (NHSI), 2019) leading to an exponential growth in the number of cases involving healthcare professionals who are forced to defend their practice in a court setting. Failing to monitor a particular drug therapy, failure to recognise the prescription of a contraindicated drug, failure to warn patients of adverse effects and neglecting to protect a patient from harm are all examples of pharmacology cases whereby blame could be laid. As our professional remit grows, so does the legal expectation. Given the amount of resources and information health professionals have access to, the defence of lack of knowledge is wholly insufficient.

Laws originate from two sources: Common Law, sometimes referred to as 'Case' Law, and Statute Law known as 'Acts of Parliament'.

Common Law or Case Law refers to cases that are tried in courts of law, whereby a judge will give rule to a set of legal precedents. Common Law is constantly changing due to the ways in which judges interpret the law and use their knowledge of legal precedent and common sense as well as applying the facts of the case. Common Law safeguards that the law remains common throughout the land, and can be divided into either Criminal or Civil Law.

Statute Law or Acts of Parliament is law which is written down and codified into law. Acts begin as bills which then become Acts once the bills have been heard and possibly amended in the House of Commons and House of Lords before receiving 'Royal Assent'. The Acts can either be private or public. Private Acts may apply to detailed locations within the UK or they may grant specific powers to public bodies, such as local authorities. Public Acts are the laws that affect the whole of the UK or one or more of its constituent countries: England, Wales, Scotland and Northern Ireland.

Healthcare and the law in the UK are strongly entwined. The laws created to protect the health of an individual can be seen when under the care of the hospital and its medical team, through to public health and the legal requirements of health and safety. Across the UK, the laws and charters that exist have been created to ensure that the rights and health interests of the individual are protected throughout the duration of their medical care. Healthcare professionals therefore have a legal duty to act with reasonable care when providing services. This 'Duty of Care' is defined as a 'legal obligation imposed on individuals or organisations that they take reasonable care in the conduct of acts that could foreseeably result in actionable harm to another' (Samanta and Samanta, 2011, p. 89). This includes prescribing drug therapy and drug administration, as well as consent, negligence and confidentiality – to name but a few. Failure to act with reasonable care could result in healthcare staff being held responsible in both criminal and civil courts.

Clinical considerations: The Bolam test

The majority of litigation in relation to medical malpractice comes under the category of negligence.

When considering cases of clinical negligence, courts will assess whether the health professional or organisation in question acted in line with the practice accepted as proper by a body of health professionals specialising in the specific field under scrutiny. This is known as the 'Bolam' test. The case (Bolam v Friern Hospital Management Committee, 1957), involved a patient who had suffered a fractured hip during electroconvulsive therapy (ECT). No relaxant or other restraint had been given to the patient in preparation for the treatment. The case explored this, along with the information the patient had been offered. The question was asked of a group of similar professionals and it was assessed that the practitioner had not been negligent as he had acted in accordance with accepted practice at that time. This set the standard and the Bolam test is now utilised in cases of negligence as a benchmark for whether the professional concerned acted in a reasonable manner. However, a judge can still make the assessment that the body of opinion is not reasonable.

There are several Acts or Laws that affect the provision of medicines which are illustrated on this timeline (see Figure 3.1).

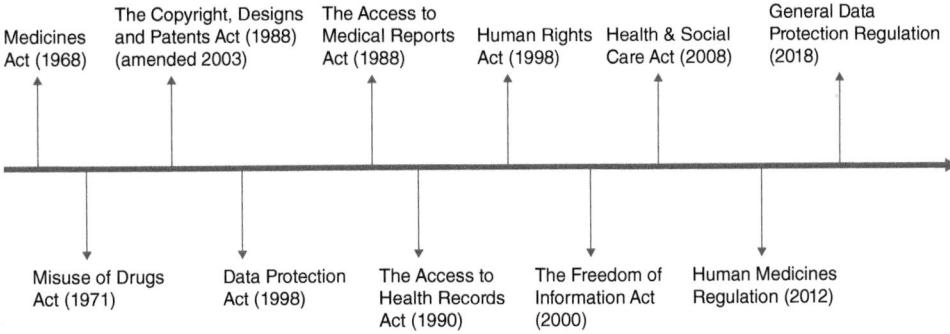

Figure 3.1   Acts or laws affecting the provision of medicines.

Ethical principles and theories

Making ethical decisions is about deciding on the right way to act in a given situation; this is underpinned by the moral values held by an individual or group. In 1979, Beauchamp and Childress (2009) developed a four-point theoretical framework to be used as a method of analysing ethical dilemmas in clinical medicine. The framework included beneficence, non-maleficence, autonomy and justice. These principles remain in healthcare along with the addition of a further two principles. Today the following ethical principles apply:

- beneficence
- non-maleficence

- autonomy
- justice
- veracity
- fidelity.

The principles outlined here are commonly felt to underpin judgments that health profes-sionals believe to be right. First, *beneficence,* whereby we should endeavour to do good. This extends to protecting others and defending their rights, preventing harm and helping oth-ers. It is argued by some, such as Pellegrino (1988), that beneficence is the only fundamental principle within healthcare ethics and that the sole purpose of medicine should be to heal. By this assumption, medicines such as contraception, and treatments for conditions such as infertility, erectile dysfunction or aesthetics, could fall beyond its purpose. However, the notion of 'healing' is complex and dynamic, referring to more than just the rectifying of an immediate physical ailment or condition. Contraception, fertility treatment and plastic sur-gery support health and wellbeing in a myriad of direct and indirect ways, physically as well as psychologically, which is why the endeavour of beneficence is not as straight forward as it would first appear.

In practice, in order to do good, medical interventions and treatments can often carry a risk of harm and therefore require justification. *Non-maleficence* means that by our actions, we should do others no harm. The principle of non-maleficence therefore cannot be absolute and must be balanced against beneficence. For example, when treating patients with cytotoxic chemotherapy drugs for cancer, we balance beneficence (the potential to do good and eradi-cate the cancer) against non-maleficence and the risk of the chemotherapy itself to cause the patient's condition to deteriorate, possibly leading to death.

It is also generally believed that people should have the right to make decisions about what is right for them, provided they have sufficient capacity or understanding to do so. This principle is a respect for the *autonomy* of the individual and relates to enabling patients to make self-determined decisions regarding their care. Consent to treatment is a fundamental component of ethical patient care in addition to a legal requirement. It involves a genuine agreement (verbal or written) to receive treatment under circum-stances where the patient has been assessed as competent, has been fully informed and where there is no undue pressure exerted (Herring, 2018). Beauchamp and Childress (2009) have argued that no decision can be truly autonomous, as patients rarely have the relevant knowledge to hold a full understanding of treatment options and, as such, are vulnerable to the coercion of health professionals who feel that they are best placed to make decisions in the interests of their patients (paternalism). However, increasingly patient groups have sought to increase autonomy for patients through changes in poli-cies and practices which decrease the potential for coercion and increase patients' free-dom to act (Williamson, 2010). An example of this has been seen in recent years, as a greater emphasis has been placed on models of shared decision-making between health professionals and patients. The shared decision-making approach seeks a balance between paternalistic care and the informed consent approach. Paternalistic care is where decisions about care are made by health professionals (predominantly doctors) and patients passively receive the care prescribed. This model does not factor in patients' own values and beliefs and can lead to patients feeling greater distress where there is a negative outcome (Stewart and Brown, 2001). The informed consent approach offers patients greater responsibility and will often involve health professionals offering patients all of the information required and then leaving them to make the decision unsupported. This can lead to patients feeling abandoned and unsure, creating anxiety and distrust (Corrigan, 2003; Deber et al., 2007). The shared decision-making approach involves health professionals and patients working together to devise a plan of care that is in line with the best available evidence as well as the values and beliefs of the individual patient, aligning to the principle of true autonomy.

Clinical considerations

A shared decision-making approach to care has been shown to benefit patients in terms of their active engagement in the treatment plan or taking the prescribed medications (Edwards and Elwyn, 2009). As such, it is an ethical approach to care which has also been shown to reduce the incidences of medico-legal claims where there is a negative outcome (Studdert et al., 2005). As health professionals, we should always aim to fully involve patients in decisions about drug treatments to maximise engagement and increase the potential for success.

Health professionals also abide by the principle of *justice,* which is the belief that people should be treated fairly, equally and reasonably. At its heart, justice is about equality; but how equality is determined can be ambiguous and problematic in healthcare. An example of the difficulties posed within this principle is often seen in relation to the fair and equal distribution of resources: 'distributive justice'. A drug for a specific condition may be available within one healthcare trust but the same drug is not available to patients with the same or similar condition in another trust. Sometimes colloquially labelled the 'postcode lottery', this occurs as a result of differing priorities for resources among those who make difficult commissioning decisions about resources on a local level.

Health professionals should also be honest and tell the truth to enable someone to have the full information relevant to them in order to make full rational choices about their care. This is known as *veracity* and involves conveying accurate and objective information to the patient. Giving patients full information regarding treatment options is the most common application of the veracity principle. Disclosures of medication errors are also an obvious example of veracity, and the recent introduction of the 'Duty of Candour' guidance for health professionals (NMC and GMC, 2015) highlights the importance of the veracity principle. Informing patients when something has gone wrong, apologising, and offering a remedy are measures that are advised by Sir Robert Francis in his report on the failings of the Mid-Staffordshire Health Trust (2013). Francis (2013) stated that candour and transparency are key components of a safe and effective culture for patient care. However, in reality, true veracity is a complex notion. Returning to the example of the drug that is available in one health trust and not another, health professionals engage in such rationing 'inconspicuously' (Williamson, 2010, p. 201) without necessarily informing patients that they are being denied something that could benefit them. Aside from the greater ethical issues concerned with who makes the decisions and how they are implemented, there is the more immediate concern relating to veracity and the decision on whether to inform patients.

Finally, the principle of *fidelity* requires the act of loyalty and trustworthiness; it involves keeping our promises, performing our duties and doing what is expected of us within our relationships with patients. This principle can be conflicted where the health professional's loyalty or obligation may be torn between their patients and colleagues or the organisation for which they work. Conflict may also arise as a result of the patient lacking capacity to make an informed choice and the health professional being compelled to override the wishes of their patient in their best interests.

Clinical considerations: Consent to treatment (adults)

Adults with capacity: The authority to treat comes solely from the patient. According to UK law, consent by proxy is not permitted for the care or treatment of adults who have the capacity to make an informed decision.

Adults lacking capacity: Where a patient does not have the mental capacity to make an informed decision regarding their care due to an impairment or disturbance to the functioning of the mind – e.g. acute confusional state, dementia, brain injury, being unconscious – then under the Mental Capacity Act (MCA, 2005) the health professional can decide upon the treatment that is deemed in the best interests of the patient without the consent of the next of kin.

Section 3(1) of the MCA (2005) sets out the following benchmarks by which to assess an adult's capacity:

a. If they are unable to understand the information given to them relating to the decision.
b. They are unable to retain the information.
c. They are unable to weigh the information as part of the decision-making process.
d. They are unable to communicate their decision.

When ethical dilemmas in practice are met, consideration needs to be given to which principles are in conflict to then consider which is more important. In helping to resolve ethical dilemmas, ethical theories are called upon. Several exist, including:

- utilitarian/consequentialism
- deontological ethics
- virtue ethics
- nursing ethics.

Utilitarian or consequentialism theory considers the rightness of an act as that which, when considering the costs and benefits, creates the greatest good for the greatest number. For example, the issue of immunisation is currently a controversial one with a minority of parents deciding to opt out of immunisation programs for their children. This puts children and other vulnerable members of society at risk of developing some diseases that were previously eradicated in the UK, e.g. measles (Public Health England, 2019), with the associated implications to the individuals, wider society and to the health service. The utilitarian perspective would be that all eligible children should be immunised irrespective of the views/wishes of their parents. Utilitarianism would not be concerned with the autonomy of the individual (the right to not give consent to the vaccine) as this is arguably in conflict with the greater good.

Clinical considerations: Consent to treatment – children

Sixteen to seventeen-year-olds with capacity: According to Section 8(1) of the Family Law Reform Act (1969), consent can be sought from the child for medical and dental treatment. However, those with parental responsibility may still consent on the child's behalf.

Sixteen to seventeen-year-olds lacking capacity: Anyone with parental responsibility can consent on behalf of a child who lacks capacity. In situations where those with parental responsibility do not consent to treatment, but where treatment is felt to be in the best interests of the child, a court order may be obtained. In an emergency situation, treatment may still be provided without parental consent where it is deemed a necessity (Glass v UK, 2004).

Under sixteen years of age: An assessment of the child relating to 'Gillick' competence (Gillick v West Norfolk and Wisbech Area Health Authority, 1985) would determine whether the child has sufficient maturity and understanding of what is involved to enable them to make a decision to consent to treatment or not.

Deontological ethics, or deontology, is an approach to ethics that determines goodness or rightness from examining acts rather than the consequences of the act as in utilitarianism. Deontologists look at rules and duties. For example, the act may be considered the right thing to do even if it produces a bad consequence, if it follows the *rule* that 'one should do unto others as they would have done unto them'. According to deontology, we have a *duty* to act in a way that does those things that are inherently good as acts. In this approach, the duty of care to the individual takes priority over any other considerations. Going back to our example of immunisations, children are, in reality, not forced to have immunisations where parents have opted out. Health professionals have a duty to ensure that any care given is consented to (within the parameters of the MCA 2005 as outlined above). Without this consent we cannot inject a live vaccine into a child no matter what the potential implications might be for wider society. So the act itself is good (abiding by rules of consent), but the consequence may be a negative one (the child contracting measles and passing this on to others). For deontologists, the ends or consequences of our actions are not important, nor are our intentions. Duty is the key consideration. However, it is not always clear what one's duty is. While we may agree that our duty is to 'do no harm', there will be instances where health professionals will have to override this with their duty of care.

Virtue ethics focuses on how we ought to behave, and how we should think about relationships, rather than providing rules or formulas for ethical decision-making. It considers the virtues a 'good' person would have: honesty, compassion, generosity and courage, for example (Velasquez et al., 1988). With the common good in mind, these virtues will be applied to actions and decisions. A group of virtues can be accredited to particular roles or professions, and it could be argued that nurses are attracted to the profession because they already function according to these virtues.

This leads us to nurse ethics. The focus of nursing ethics is on developing a caring relationship and seeking a collaborative relationship with the person. Recently, care, compassion, courage, communication, commitment and competence (the 6 Cs Department of Health, 2012) have been highlighted as the required virtues of nurses. Common themes of nursing ethics emphasise respect for the autonomy of the individual and maintaining the dignity of the client by promoting choice and control over their environment.

What is deemed to be right is not therefore bound by absolute rules or duty, or purely the greatest good, but also considers the virtues that individuals and society value. The ethical views held by society affect healthcare laws and how they are implemented. As society's moral values alter, legislation follows. An example of this was in 1967 when UK society's beliefs changed regarding abortions. It became largely accepted that in some cases they were necessary for saving women's lives as well as reducing the potential for suffering (psychologically as well as physically) of the woman and her pre-existing family, and so the Act was introduced (Abortion Act, 1967).

Regulatory bodies

In order to practice, healthcare professionals are aligned to a regulatory body such as the Nursing and Midwifery Council (NMC) or the Health and Care Professions Council (HCPC). The purpose of a regulatory body is primarily to protect the public, and as such they are established and based upon a legal mandate. Their function is regulatory and to impose requirements, restrictions and conditions – as well as offering a means of support and guidance to professionals. They also set standards in relation to practice activities, securing compliance and enforcement of their practitioners. Regulatory bodies have traditionally provided their practitioners with ethical guidance in the form of a 'code' or an 'oath', such as the NMC Code of Conduct (2018) or the Hippocratic Oath for doctors. A word of caution though; codes such as the NMC Code of Conduct (2018) could be viewed as merely being concerned with specifying rules of responsibility and conduct rather than focusing specifically on ethics.

Within healthcare, regulatory bodies have a duty to protect, promote and maintain the health and safety of the public. They do this by ensuring proper standards are in place in order to practice. Such standards define the overarching goals and the expected role and duties of their practitioners through listing the obligations associated with their individual responsibilities and skill set. The overarching goals are aspirational and represent an optimal position ethically, thus encouraging the individual to strive towards the optimal position. Healthcare professionals, like the public and their patients, possess their own values and beliefs which in turn influence their practice.

Imagine yourself working in a very busy gynaecological outpatients and you are required to administer mifepristone (medically induced abortion) to a young intravenous drug user (IVDU), currently sofa surfing among friends. Your service user is advised to return in between 24 and 48 hours for the second medication – misoprostol, to complete the treatment. She does not return. You notice certain client groups tend not to return to the clinic and you begin to think about why this is the case, using the principles of ethical professional practice, beneficence (do good) and non-maleficence (do no harm).

Within this scenario, there is a possibility the service user's care has been affected by the healthcare professionals implicit bias (IB) towards certain social groups. Several authors have emphasised that a well-meaning, egalitarian (fair) minded individual can have implicit biases which demonstrate the imbalance between their unconscious ways of thinking and how they explicitly perceive themselves treating people (Fitzgerald and Hurst, 2018; Lang et al., 2016). The elements of IB are one's perceived stereotypes (a mental picture of what one thinks, knows and expects) and prejudices (feelings) associated with certain categories of people, learnt through a shared culture, which over time slips into one's unconsciousness, which means it is hidden (Lang et al., 2016). As Stone and Moskowitz (2011) explained, this means the healthcare professionals are unaware of their biases, which impacts on the quality of care delivered, seen in how they may judge and behave towards particular groups (Kelly and Roedderts, 2008). Merino et al. (2018) highlighted over 60% of healthcare professionals harbour variants of IB towards marginalised/vulnerable groups. Examples of vulnerable or marginalised groupings can be based on: gender, age weight, homelessness, ethnicity, immigration status, socio-economic status, educational achievement, mental ill-health, sexual orientation, IVDUs, disabilities and social circumstances – or anyone rendered vulnerable in certain situations (Fitzgerald and Hurst, 2018).

There is a consensus that stereotyping saves cognitive resources in stressful environments, a situation healthcare professionals often find themselves in (Hall, 2017). Drawing on these stereotypes enables the healthcare professional to make timely decisions based on the minimal information available in times of fatigue, tiredness, heavy workload, uncertainty and inadequate support (Stone and Moskowitz, 2011). Nonetheless, it remains that there is a clear link between IB and the quality of care delivered and how it potentially influences the healthcare professionals ability to engage in person-centred care (Merino et al., 2018). Fitzgerald and Hurst (2018) stated that a healthcare professionals IB behaviour towards marginalised groups can impact on the service user's access to healthcare service by producing false diagnoses, non-referral to appropriate services, limiting treatment options or withholding of treatment. Goyal et al. (2015) detailed how IB may have contributed to the creation of health disparities, as African-American children were less likely to receive adequate pain management post-appendectomy than their white counterparts. IB influences within clinical interactions can leave the service user feeling uncomfortable as they pay attention to the healthcare professionals non-verbal mannerisms, such as eye contact, physical closeness and speech errors which can demonstrate the healthcare professionals dislike or unease of dealing with particular clientele (Stone and Moskowitz, 2011). This in turn may not only impede patient–healthcare professional communication, but may also affect patient concordance and willingness to seek future care.

Puddifoot (2017) highlighted that IB can cause an ethical dilemma, demonstrated earlier, as there is potential to do harm within these client groups through the healthcare professionals judgment and behaviour based on their IB. Positive beneficence requires the healthcare professional to consider benefits for others alongside balancing the risks (Baillie and Black, 2015), which is compromised through the harbouring of IB. Such behaviours are in direct contradiction of the professional regulatory bodies' codes of professional performance; therefore, the healthcare professional should reflect upon how they interact with certain client groups to develop awareness of any implicit biases they may have (Lang et al., 2016). Additionally, Stone and Moskowitz (2011) recommend learning courses to expand the healthcare professionals cultural competence by learning about IB.

There are a number of guidelines set out by various professional bodies in relation to pharmacology. The General Medical Council (GMC) have outlined expectations of doctors' ethical prescribing practices which aim to provide more detailed advice on how to apply ethical principles when prescribing and managing medicines (2013). Additionally, largely in response to the withdrawal of the Medicines Management standards by the NMC (2015), the Royal Pharmaceutical Society and the Royal College of Nursing collaborated in developing the 'Professional Guidance on the Administration of Medicines in Healthcare Settings' (2019). These standards seek to promote patient safety in relation to the administration of medicines by acknowledging the importance of guidance for health professionals that is enabling and supportive while being clear and concise. The document recognises the importance of a commitment to ethics, values and principles which put patients first. It is incumbent upon the individual healthcare professional to ensure that they are familiar with the most current guidance related to their own sphere of practice to ensure that ethical and legal considerations are applied.

Clinical considerations

All healthcare professionals have a responsibility to ensure that they are familiar with legislation related to the prescribing, storage and administration of medicines within their sphere of practice. A list of key documents that will support you in the development of knowledge in this area is offered in the Further Reading section.

Research

The legal and ethical standards which govern research into pharmacological treatments are very specific to the context of clinical drug trials. During the Second World War, Jewish prisoners in Nazi concentration camps were used as subjects in medical experiments against their will, leading to permanent disfigurement, disability, trauma and in many cases death. In response to these atrocities, the Nuremberg Code (1947) was developed as international guiding ethical principles for the conduct of research involving human participants. They include principles of informed consent, non-coercion and the right to withdraw, as well as the importance of robust protocols underpinned by beneficence. These principles were later encapsulated within the Declaration of Helsinki (World Medical Association, 2008) and further legislation has evolved to ensure the safety of human participants in clinical trials including: Data Protection Act (2018), Human Tissue Act (2004) and the Medicines for Human Use (Clinical Trials) Regulations (2004) as well as the Human Rights Act (1998).

Research is an important mechanism for healthcare professionals to ensure that the drug treatments we offer patients are thoroughly tested for safety and efficacy. Additionally, there is strong evidence emerging that research-active hospitals have better patient outcomes, highlighting the importance and the responsibility healthcare providers have to offer their service users the opportunity to be involved in clinical trials (Ozdemir et al., 2015). It is essential that legislation enables clinical researchers to conduct clinical trials in the endeavour of medical advancement, while ensuring that participants are fully informed of the potential risks and benefits, are not coerced into consenting to participate, and are aware of their right to withdraw from participating at any time. The guiding principle is that the wellbeing and safety of the participants is paramount and takes priority over any other consideration.

Research Ethics Committees (RECs) have the remit to review any proposed research that involves human participants. Made up of a number of lay-people and professionals experienced in their own field, it is the responsibility of the REC to interrogate the research protocol and to identify any aspects of the research consent and treatment processes which may pose an unacceptable risk to participants or the public. Approval from a REC is essential before a trial can go ahead. As the trial progresses, researchers will also need to seek ethical approval to make any amendments to the protocol, which may be something as minor as a change of wording within a participant information sheet, to something more substantial such as a change in the dose of medication to be administered. These changes will be implemented in line with Good Clinical Practice (GCP) principles (MHRA, 2012).

Despite these safeguards, there are notable incidences that have occurred in recent years related to the conduct of some clinical trials. For example, in 2006, volunteers in an early phase drug trial at the Northwick Park Hospital became seriously ill. The story became headline news after six participants reacted badly to the medication, suffering a severe immune response leading to organ failure and one participant requiring the amputation of his fingers. This led to a full investigation and the resulting report changed a number of practices in the running of drugs trials which sought to prevent this from happening again (Expert Scientific Group on Phase One Clinical Trials, 2006).

Fortunately, however, the ethical and legal frameworks which surround clinical research, limit these incidents and provide principles and guidance for the safe conduct of research and researchers.

Skills in practice: How to use medical ethics

Not all decisions are made easily, and, in some cases, there are multiple factors that influence decision-making, such as personal experience, religion, regulatory codes, legal issues and so on. In practice, a practitioner will use a combination of all such factors to reach a decision; this is sometimes described as a systematic study of moral choices. In the first instance, the code of behaviour or conduct presented by a regulatory body is considered correct. Within healthcare, there are many examples of ethical decision-making process which include varying numbers of steps to follow. Overall, there is the general adoption of principle-based ethics to guide decision-making practice within healthcare, which is evident in this example.

Step 1 – Ability to recognise an ethical issue. Ask yourself: could this scenario or decision cause harm or damage to someone or some group? Are there choices between different alternatives; for example, a good and bad alternative or, maybe, two bads or two goods? Is this situation bigger than what is efficient? Or what is legal? What are your initial gut reactions? By considering the scenario on an emotive level you can recognise your own assumptions, values and biases so that you can set them aside before analysing the situation critically.

Step 2 – Gathering the facts. What facts are already known? What other relevant facts need to be gathered? Who are the relevant stakeholders within this scenario and its outcome? Has everyone involved been consulted? Are some concerns more important than others?

Step 3. Evaluation of alternative options or actions. Includes questions from a range of approaches. From a utilitarian approach ask: which actions/option do the least harm and produce the most good? Considering the deontological approach – which actions/option best respects all stakeholder rights? From a nursing approach, which actions/option treat people proportionately or equally? Which actions/option best serve the whole community and not just some if its members? From a virtue approach, also consider which actions/option lead me based on the type of person I want to be?

Step 4. Make the decision. When all approaches have been considered, which actions/option best addresses the scenario? Which action/option is best based on all the stakeholder core values? Consider what others might say when you have shared your chosen actions/option, can you justify your choice?

Step 5. Carry out the actions/option chosen and reflect on the outcome. Plan how your decision can be implemented with the upmost care, pay attention to any concerns raised by all of the stakeholders. Implement your plan and evaluate. Reflect on the results of your choice of decision and what have you learned from this specific scenario. Consider how the ethical problem could be prevented in the future.

Episode of care

Paul is a 65-year-old man who has attended the walk-in centre with a suspected oral infection. He is allergic to penicillin so is prescribed metronidazole 200 mg twice daily for seven days. However, he smells strongly of alcohol and it states in his previous notes that he has had multiple admissions with alcohol-related injuries and has a chronic alcohol addiction. You as the nurse query this with the doctor who has prescribed the antibiotics, knowing that the British National Formulary (Joint Formulary Committee, 2019) indicates that alcohol and metronidazole are contraindicated and can cause a severe reaction. The doctor states that she has discussed this with Paul and he is aware that he must refrain from drinking alcohol for the course of the treatment. Consider this from an ethical perspective. While the treatment may be doing 'good' (beneficence), it has the potential to do harm (maleficence). It is imperative that health professionals discuss medication plans prior to treatment to ensure that patients are aware of the impact this will have on their daily activities. In Paul's case, it is highly unlikely that he will refrain from alcohol and could either take the metronidazole regardless, risking an adverse reaction, or he may decide to not take the antibiotics and risk further infection and possible sepsis. Key message? Ensure every decision made fully involves the patient and aligns with their own values and lifestyle.

Episode of care

Maya is an 85-year-old woman who lives alone. She is usually independent with all of her activities of living and, although she does not like to leave the house, she is usually in good physical and mental health. Her daughter visits her three times a week and has noticed some increased confusion over the past few days. Today she has visited and felt it necessary to call the GP as Maya is extremely confused and smells strongly of malodorous urine. The GP refers her to the acute admissions unit with a suspected Urinary Tract Infection (UTI). Further tests are undertaken in hospital, but the admissions team decide to prescribe intravenous (IV), broad-spectrum antibiotics to treat the UTI as per the guidance from the National Institute for Health and Care Excellence (NICE NG109, 2018), which they hope will also alleviate the acute confusional state. However, Maya becomes very distressed when the nurse attempts to cannulate and Maya's daughter states that she does not consent to her mother receiving IV antibiotics. Maya has been assessed as an adult lacking capacity by health professionals. In accordance with the Mental Capacity Act (2005), she is cannulated and receives the IV antibiotics. Over the course of the next 24 hours her condition improves and her acute confusional state dissipates. The health professionals have acted in accordance with legal standards. They have also balanced their duty to respect Maya's autonomy with their duty of care in ensuring beneficence (doing good by giving the required treatment in Maya's best interests) and non-maleficence (doing no harm by omitting care that was in her best interests).

Conclusion

This chapter has sought to outline the fundamental legal and ethical principles relating to pharmacology in healthcare. The three key components that underpin high-quality decision-making with and for patients in our care are related to the law, ethical principles and regulatory bodies. A variety of legislation has been discussed to offer an understanding and insight into how healthcare professionals manage and administer medicines within the confines of the law. The interplay of legislation, ethical principles and professional regulation is a fine balance that health professionals seek to strike in order to optimise the safety and efficacy of treatment.

Working in healthcare requires an acknowledgement of the areas of ambiguity and conflict that may be encountered; and while we seek to always 'do good', there are countless situations where this endeavour may be obstructed by other considerations such as patients' capacity or the wider public interest.

Acknowledgement of the issues that have been outlined within this chapter and a deeper understanding of how to apply the knowledge of ethical principles will ultimately improve practice and provide safer and higher quality patient care. It is incumbent upon all health professionals (and students) to act with integrity within these frameworks and to make individualised decisions which are in the patients' best interest and, wherever possible, fully informed.

References

Abortion Act (1967). Abortion Act. www.legislation.gov.uk/ukpga/1967/87/contents (accessed 19 September 2019).

Baillie, L. and Black, S. (2015). *Professional Values in Nursing*. Florida, USA: Taylor & Francis Group.

Beauchamp & Childress (2009). *Principles of Biomedical Ethics*, 6e. Oxford: Oxford University Press.

Bolam v Friern Hospital Management Committee (1957). 1 WLR 583.

Corrigan, O. (2003). Empty ethics: the problem with informed consent. *Sociology of Health and Illness* 25 (3): 768–792.

Data Protection Act (2018). Data Protection Act. www.legislation.gov.uk/ukpga/2018/12/contents/enacted (accessed 19 September 2019).

Deber, R., Kraetschmer, N., Urowitz, S. et al. (2007). Do people want to be autonomous patients? Preferred roles in treatment decision-making in several patient populations. *Health Expectations* 10: 248–258.

Declaration of Helsinki (2008). Ethical principles for medical research involving human subjects. https://www.who.int/bulletin/archives/79%284%29373.pdf (accessed 19 September 2019).

Department of Health (2012). Compassion in practice. https://www.england.nhs.uk/wp-content/uploads/2012/12/compassion-in-practice.pdf (accessed 19 September 2019).

Edwards, A. and Elwyn, G. (eds.) (2009). *Shared Decision-Making in Health Care. Achieving Evidence-Based Patient Choice*. Oxford: Oxford University Press.

Expert Scientific Groups on Phase One Clinical Trials (2006). Final Report. https://webarchive.nationalarchives.gov.uk/20130105143109/www.dh.gov.uk/prod_consum_dh/groups/dh_digitalassets/@dh/@en/documents/digitalasset/dh_073165.pdf (accessed 19 September 2019).

Family Law Reform Act (1969). Family Law Reform Act. www.legislation.gov.uk/ukpga/1969/46 (accessed 12 September 2019).

Fitzgerald, C. and Hurst, S. (2018). Implicit bias in healthcare professionals: a systematic review. *BMC Medical Ethics* 18 (19): 1–18.

Francis, R. (2013). *Report of the Mid Staffordshire NHS Foundation Trust Public Enquiry*. London: Stationary Office.

General Medical Council (2013). Good practice in prescribing and managing medicines and devices. https://www.gmc-uk.org/-/media/documents/prescribing-guidance_pdf-59055247.pdf?la=en (accessed 19 September 2019).

Gillick v West Norfolk and Wisbech area Health Authority and Department of Health and Social Security (1985). Landmark decision for children's rights. *Childright* 22: 11–18.

Glass v United Kingdom (2004). App. No 61827/00, 39 Eur. H.R.Rep. 15.

Goyal, M.K., Kuppermann, M., Cleary, S. et al. (2015). Racial disparities in pain management of children with appendicitis in emergency departments. *JAMA Pediatrics* 169 (11): 996–1002.

Hall, A. (2017). Using legal ethics to improve implicit bias in prosecutorial discretion. *Journal of the Legal Profession* 42 (1): 111–126.

Herring, J. (2018). *Medical Law and Ethics*. Oxford: Oxford University Press.

Human Rights Act (1998). Human Rights Act. www.legislation.gov.uk/ukpga/1998/42/contents (accessed 19 September 2019).

Human Tissue Act (2004). Human Tissue Act. www.legislation.gov.uk/ukpga/2004/30/contents (accessed 19 September 2019).

Joint Formulary Committee (2019). British National Formulary. https://bnf.nice.org.uk (accessed October 2019).

Kelly, D. and Roedderts, E. (2008). Racial cognition and the ethics of implicit bias. *Philosophy Compass* 3 (3): 522–540.

Lang, K.R., Dupree, C., Kon, A. et al. (2016). Calling out implicit bias as a harm in pediatric care. *Cambridge Quarterly of Healthcare Ethics* 25: 540–552.

Medicines & Healthcare products Regulatory Agency (2012). *Good Clinical Practice Guide*. London: TSO.

Medicines for Human Use (Clinical Trials) Regulations (2004). Medicines for Human Use. www.legislation. gov.uk/uksi/2004/1031/contents/made (accessed 19 September 2019).

Mental Capacity Act (2005). Mental Capacity Act. www.legislation.gov.uk/ukpga/2005/9/contents (accessed 19 September 2019).

Merino, Y., Adams, L., and Hall, W.J. (2018). Implicit bias and mental health professionals: priorities and direction for research. *Psychiatric Services* **69** (6): 723–725.

National Health Service Improvement (2019). Clinical negligence and litigation. https://improvement.nhs. uk/resources/clinical-negligence-and-litigation (accessed 4 September 2019).

National Institute of Health and Care Excellence (2018). Guideline 109 Urinary Tract infection (lower): anti-microbial prescribing. www.nice.org.uk/guidance/ng109 (accessed 4 September 2019).

Nuremberg Code (1947). Trials of war criminals before the Nuernberg [sic] military tribunals volume 2 "The medical case". https://www.loc.gov/rr/frd/Military_Law/pdf/NT_war-criminals_Vol-II.pdf (accessed 19 September 2019).

Nursing & Midwifery Council (2015). Standards for medicines management. http://NMC.org.uk.

Nursing & Midwifery Council (2018). The Code: Professional standards of practice and behaviour for nurses, midwives and nursing associates. www.nmc.org.uk/globalassets/sitedocuments/nmc-publications/ nmc-code.pdf (accessed 19 September 2019).

Nursing & Midwifery Council and General Medical Council (2015). Openness and honesty when things go wrong: the professional duty of candour. https://tinyurl.com/zpdk7mk (accessed July 2020).

Ozdemir, B.A., Karthikesalingam, A., Sinha, S. et al. (2015). Research activity and the association with mortality. *PLoS One* **10** (2): e0118253. https://doi.org/10.1371/journal.pone.0118253.

Pellegrino, E.D. (1988). *For the Patient's Good: The Restoration of Beneficence in Health Care*. Oxford University Press.

Public Health England (2019). *Measles: guidance, data and analysis* available at: https://www.gov.uk/government/ collections/measles-guidance-data-and-analysis#epidemiology (accessed 12 September 2019).

Puddifoot, K. (2017). Dissolving the epistemic/ethical dilemma over implicit bias. *Philosophical Explorations* **20** (1): S73–S93.

Royal Pharmaceutical Society and Royal College of Nursing (2019). Professional guidance on the administration of medicines in healthcare settings. https://www.rpharms.com/Portals/0/RPS%20document%20 library/Open%20access/Professional%20standards/SSHM%20and%20Admin/Admin%20of%20 Meds%20prof%20guidance.pdf?ver=2019-01-23-145026-567 (accessed 19 September 2019).

Samanta, J. and Samanta, A. (2011). *Medical Law*. Basingstoke: Palgrave Macmillan.

Stewart, M. and Brown, J. (2001). Patient-centredness in medicine. In: *Evidence-Based Patient Choice* (eds. A. Edwards and G. Elwyn). London: Oxford University Press.

Stone, J. and Moskowitz, G.B. (2011). Non-conscious bias in medical decision-making: what can be done to reduce it. *Medical Education* **45**: 768–776.

Studdert, D., Mello, M., Sage, W. et al. (2005). Defensive medicine among high-risk specialist physicians in a volatile malpractice environment. *JAMA: The Journal of the American Medical Association* **293**: 2609–2617.

Velasquez, M., Andre C., Shanks, S. et al (1988). Ethics and virtue. https://www.scu.edu/ethics/ethics-resources/ethical-decision-making/ethics-and-virtue (accessed 19 September 2019).

World Medical Association (2008). World Medical Association Declaration of Helsinki. Ethical Principles for Medical Research Involving Human Subjects. https://www.wma.net/wp-content/uploads/2016/11/ DoH-Oct2008.pdf (accessed 19 September 2019).

Williamson, C. (2010). *Towards the Emancipation of Patients. Patients' Experiences and the Patient Movement*. Bristol: Policy Press.

Further reading

Useful reads: Medical Protection www.medicalprotection.org/uk/hub/ethics.

Specialist Pharmacy Service (2018). Medicines Matters: A guide to the prescribing, supply and administration of medicines (in England) (2018). https://www.sps.nhs.uk/wp-content/uploads/2018/10/ Medicines-Matters-september-2018-1.pdf

Royal Pharmaceutical Society and Royal College of Nursing (2019). Professional Guidance on the Administration of Medicines in Healthcare settings). https://www.rpharms.com/Portals/0/RPS%20 document%20library/Open%20access/Professional%20standards/SSHM%20and%20Admin/ Admin%20of%20Meds%20prof%20guidance.pdf?ver=2019-01-23-145026-567.

Royal Pharmaceutical Society (2018). Professional Guidance on the safe and secure handling of medicines. https://www.rpharms.com/recognition/setting-professional-standards/safe-and-secure-handling-of-medicines/professional-guidance-on-the-safe-and-secure-handling-of-medicines? welcome=true.

Multiple choice questions

1. Common Law is also known as:
   (a) Criminal Law
   (b) Case Law
   (c) Statute Law
   (d) All of the above

2. Failure to act with reasonable care could result in healthcare staff being held responsible in which courts:
   (a) Criminal Court
   (b) Civil Court
   (c) Civil and Criminal Court
   (d) Family Court

3. What year did the Medicines Act become statute?
   (a) 1966
   (b) 1967
   (c) 1968
   (d) None of the above

4. Utilitarian theory considers:
   (a) The greatest good for the greatest number
   (b) Your duty of care takes priority over any other considerations
   (c) How we ought to behave and seek relationships
   (d) All of the above

5. When adopting principle-based ethics to guide your decision-making, where do you need to gather the facts from?
   (a) From all the stakeholders involved within the scenario
   (b) From what is already known
   (c) From other facts that are relevant from other scenarios
   (d) All of the above

6. Sensitive topics such as abortion can lead to the practitioner having _____ dilemma:
   (a) an Ethical
   (b) a Clinical
   (c) a Legal
   (d) All of the above

7. Implicit means:
   (a) Hidden
   (b) Obvious
   (c) Available
   (d) Explicit

8. Elements of Implicit Bias include:
   (a) Stereotypes
   (b) Prejudices
   (c) Stereotypes and prejudices
   (d) Impartialities

9. Healthcare professionals harbour a _____ level of implicit bias as the general population:
   (a) Lower
   (b) Higher

    (c) Equal

    (d) None of the above

10. The influences of implicit bias on the practitioner's professional behaviour include:

    (a) Making the client feel uncomfortable

    (b) Helping them access services

    (c) Correct diagnoses and treatment

    (d) Patient concordance

11. What is the Bolam test?

    (a) A test to assess patients' capacity

    (b) The opinion of a professional body as to whether the action was accepted practice

    (c) An assessment of competency of a patient under 16

    (d) All of the above

12. Shared decision-making:

    (a) Is an approach to care that increases patient engagement in treatment

    (b) Improves patient engagement with care and treatment

    (c) Reduces medico-legal claims

    (d) All of the above

13. What is distributive justice in relation to healthcare?

    (a) The fair and equal distribution of health resources

    (b) The 'postcode lottery'

    (c) An assessment of patient need

    (d) All of the above

14. Why is research in healthcare so important?

    (a) To test drugs for safety and efficacy

    (b) To develop better treatments for patients

    (c) To improve outcomes for patients

    (d) All of the above

15. What must professionals do in order to abide by the 'Duty of Candour'?

    (a) Tell the patient when a serious incident has occurred

    (b) Inform patients and their families of everything related to the patient's care at all costs

    (c) Apologise to patients

    (d) All of the above

Find out more

The following is a list of considerations, guiding legislation and ethical frameworks for safe and effective practice. Find out more about each of these and make notes in the section provided about what each of these involve and how it impacts upon the care of patients.

The consideration	Your notes
Mental Capacity Act (2005)	
Burden of proof for negligence	

The consideration	Your notes
Human Medicines Regulation (1971)	
Research Ethics Committee	
Northwick Park drug trials controversy	

Chapter 4

Medicines management and the role of the healthcare provider

Annette Hand and Carol Wills

Aim

The aim of this chapter is to provide the reader with an introduction to medicines management and the role of the healthcare provider.

Learning outcomes

After reading this chapter, the reader will:

1. Understand the term 'medicines management' and the role of the healthcare provider
2. Be able to appraise the health professional's role in managing medicines safely and effectively
3. Acknowledge the role of regulatory and advisory bodies in the management and optimisation of medicines
4. Be able to apply the principles of medicine optimisation

Test your knowledge

1. Which Act provides the legal framework governing the use of Controlled Drugs?
2. What do the 9Rs stand for?
3. What activities are included within medicines management?
4. What does the term Patient Group Direction (PGD) stand for?
5. How do you verity the identification of a patient prior to medicines administration?

Fundamentals of Pharmacology: For Nursing and Healthcare Students, First Edition. Edited by Ian Peate and Barry Hill.
© 2021 John Wiley & Sons Ltd. Published 2021 by John Wiley & Sons Ltd.

Introduction

This chapter will support learning in relation to medicines management and the role of the healthcare provider. Medicines are the most common intervention in healthcare and are vital in treating or managing many illnesses and conditions. As more people are taking more medicines it is paramount, for patients, healthcare professionals and organisations, that medicines are used appropriately. Population growth and increases in the numbers of older people push up the volume of medicines prescribed, partly due to older people being more likely to have long-term health conditions, such as cardiovascular problems, arthritis or diabetes (Duerden et al., 2013). Effective and safe medicines management is a key responsibility for many healthcare professionals, and it is important that individuals keep up to date with new guidelines and regulations within this ever-expanding area of care.

A raft of public health and government policies in the 1990s identified the varied quality of health and care services across the UK and set out how this should be addressed so that all patients, no matter where they lived, would be offered prompt and fair access to high-quality services and treatments. Since then, changes within legal frameworks, government and the National Health Service (NHS) have enabled this to happen across the United Kingdom (UK) and various systems and targets introduced to enhance and monitor the quality of services provided.

Currently, all health and social care organisations in the UK are assessed and monitored by an Independent Regulator of Health and Social Care to determine if they provide proper and safe care; this includes the use of medicine. In England the regulator is the Care Quality Commission (CQC), in Wales it is the Health Care Inspectorate Wales (HIW), in Scotland the Healthcare Improvement Scotland and the Regulation and Quality Improvement Authority in Northern Ireland (RQIA). These regulators will inspect and assess the quality of care for people and whether they are safe, effective, caring, responsive and well led. Each service is then rated as outstanding, good, requires improvement or inadequate. Follow the Clinical Consideration to explore the rating of the service you are currently working within. All health professionals have an important role in the provision of quality services.

Clinical considerations

Visit your organisation's website or the regulators website to access its latest inspection report. What was the outcome of the report?

- Were any areas rated as good or requires improvement?
- What is/would your role be within this provision?

Medicines management

Medicines management involves the safe and cost-effective use of medicines in clinical practice, with maximum patient benefits while minimising potential harm. NHS spending on medicines was estimated to cost £17.4 billion in 2016/17 and is said to be increasing at a rate of 5% each year (Ewbank et al., 2018). This has been said to be unsustainable and health professionals need to explore how this can be managed. The human cost, however, when things go wrong with medications include increased use of health services, preventable admissions to hospital, serious harm and ultimately death. It is estimated that 70% of errors are identified before they reach the patient and essentially all healthcare providers must minimise the risk and incidence of harm.

In the UK, laws and regulations, such as The Medicines Act (1968; Department of Health, 2013), Human Medicines Regulations (2012) and The Prescription Only Medicines (Human Use) Order

(1997), are in place which dictate and promote safe and effective medicines management at each stage of the medicines journey. Essential elements include:

- manufacturing and marketing
- procurement and sale
- selection
- supply
- prescribing
- handling and administration
- medicine optimisation
- storage and disposal.

These essential elements will be explored in the following sections.

Manufacturing, marketing, and procurement and sale

NHS medicine policies in the UK require that either the European Medicines Agency (EMA) (the European Union regulatory body) or The Medicines and Healthcare Products Regulatory Agency (MHRA) (the UK regulatory body) approve products and medical devices before they can be supplied to patients. Safety, effectiveness and quality of the manufacturing process are assessed and must meet stringent requirements before they are approved for sale and assigned a marketing authorisation. The marketing authorisation is assigned according to the licensed indication and degree of risk of the product, the pack size, and whether its supply needs to be supervised and monitored by a health professional. The Medicines Act (1968; Department of Health, 2013) and subsequent Human Medicines Regulations (2012) allow the product to then be available to the public by:

1. Prescription as a Prescription only Medicine (PoM), meaning that the product can only be supplied by a prescription from an appropriate health professional and issued by a pharmacist. A Controlled Drug (CD) is also a PoM.
2. As a Pharmacy (P) only product, which can be bought in the presence and supervision of a pharmacist, e.g. chemist or in-store pharmacy within a supermarket.
3. As a General Sales List product (GSL), which means it can be bought in a retail outlet, e.g. supermarket or garage shop.

Pharmacy and GSL items are often referred to as 'Over-the-Counter' (OTC) products, which is a general term meaning they can be purchased in a retail outlet and do not need a prescription. Further details on drug classifications can be found within Chapter 2 of this text.

Following marketing approval, new products may be scrutinised for clinical and cost effectiveness by the National Institute for Health and Care Excellence (NICE) or The Scottish Intercollegiate Guidelines Network (SIGN) to determine whether the NHS will provide them. If NICE or SIGN approve them for NHS use, commissioners (e.g. NHS England or Clinical Commission Groups for England and Health Boards in Scotland and Wales) must make them available for patients. Many new products or changes in the use of the product will be assigned a black triangle like this:

This alerts healthcare practitioners that there is limited experience in the use of this product so all suspected adverse reactions must be reported to the MHRA (this process is discussed further within Chapter 7).

Not all products and devices require assessment by NICE, so these may be considered by NHS commissioners who can decide if they wish to make them available to patients. This may then lead to the procurement or purchasing of products dependent on a variety of factors, which include local priorities, budgets and timeliness of NICE approval. Procurement of medicines and medical devices for the NHS are undertaken by regional pharmacy purchasing groups who aim to obtain the best price possible for the NHS and enter into contracts for supply to NHS Trusts and other organisations. These will be included in the national Drug Tariff (a list of medicines and devices that can be prescribed within the NHS) and then agreed for purchase at a local level, usually via Drugs and Therapeutic Committees.

Independent organisations (e.g. non-NHS pharmacies) may choose specific products that they wish to offer for sale to the general public. These are restricted to pharmacy only and GSL products depending on their status, as discussed previously, but also may have restrictions on the amount or dosage which can be sold. For example, the MHRA discourage multibuy or large quantities of analgesia being sold; for example, Paracetamol, which can result in liver damage if recommended dosages are exceeded. Shopkeepers thus limit purchase of these to 32, or in some cases 16 tablets per pack.

Selection

Where there are many products or devices available to treat a condition, an NHS organisation, or your employer, will decide which of these products are to be prescribed and will be included in the local formulary. This ultimately means that some products will be available for supply in some parts of the UK but not all. Selection will be based upon a range of measures including the evidence available to support the product's effectiveness and the cost of supplying the product in comparison to similar products.

Some products which have been licensed for several years are manufactured by several companies, with the result that an identical drug which is therapeutically equivalent has several proprietary or trade names. An example of this is Ibuprofen; this is its non-proprietary or generic name, but it can also be supplied with a proprietary name of Brufen or Nurofen. Not only can this cause confusion and possible medication errors, but it is generally more cost-effective for the NHS to supply, or for the patient to buy a generic product. Compare the proprietary and non-proprietary forms of ibuprofen in the Clinical Considerations box to understand the differences in cost.

Clinical considerations

Find out how much a pack of 16, 200 mg tablets of each of these products is in your local pharmacy or shop.	Nurofen	Brufen	Ibuprofen
Check the product information on the packet, do they contain the same amount of the same active ingredient?			
Which is the cheapest?			

The NHS Business Services Authority analyse prescribing trends and state that 81% of all drugs in primary care are already prescribed generically, which generates significant savings for the NHS (NHS Business Services Authority, 2018). They also highlight, however, that for medicines optimisation there are further savings that could be realised to help provide even better value care. This also includes the NHS spending on products which can otherwise be bought by patients from a pharmacy or supermarket, such as paracetamol. The NHS currently spends around £136 million a year on prescriptions for such medicines (NHS, 2018). Prescriptions are generally not issued for OTC medicines which are used to treat a range of minor health conditions; however, there are those with chronic ill health who may still have OTC medicines prescribed as part of their care pathway (e.g. paracetamol for pain). All healthcare professionals have a responsibility to help the NHS to deliver an effective and value-for-money service.

Supply

Medicines and medicinal products may be supplied to patients in a variety of ways. These are incorporated within legislation under the Medicines Act (1968) and The Prescription Only Medicines (Human Use) Order (1997), and subsequent changes include patient-specific directions, prescriptions, PGDs and exemptions.

The Clinical Considerations box asks that you think about how patients are supplied with medicines/medical devices in your current practice.

Clinical considerations

Are these provided through patient-specific directions, prescriptions or patient group directions?

1. Tick the boxes below that apply.
2. Give an example product or clinical situation for each process that you identify.

Patient-specific direction

Prescription

Patient group direction

Patient-specific directions

These are written instructions for the supply and/or administration of medicines for a named patient. This may be within a Medications Administration Record Chart (MAR Chart)/ Kardex or within medical notes.

Prescriptions

A prescription is a written instruction or order for the supply of a product by an appropriate healthcare professional to a named patient, and must meet the legal requirements of The Prescription Only Medicines (Human Use) Order (1997). You may be familiar with these if you have been working in a primary care environment or have visited your general practitioner (GP) or dentist and have needed a product prescribed. Prescriptions may be handwritten or electronic.

Patient group directions

PGD is a set of written instructions that allow some registered health professionals to supply and/or administer specified medicines to a pre-defined group of patients, without them having to see a prescriber first (such as a doctor or non-medical prescriber) (MHRA PGD Guidance 2017). Supplying and/or administering medicines under PGDs is reserved for situations in which this offers an advantage for patient care, without compromising patient safety. PGDs are used across a wide variety of healthcare settings. They are particularly useful in primary care for immunisations (for example, primary to pre-school immunisations and seasonal influenza), in sexual health clinics and emergency care environments.

PGDs are developed by multidisciplinary groups including a doctor, a pharmacist and a representative of any professional group expected to supply the medicines under the PGD (NICE, 2017). Legal requirements of a PGD are stated within the Human Medicines Regulations (2012). The legal categories of medicines that can be supplied under a PGD are:

- prescription only (PO)
- pharmacy (P)
- GSL.

Any unlicensed medicines, dressings, appliances, and devices are not allowed to be supplied under a PGD. Each PGD will reference the area that it covers and provide clear parameters in which the PGD may be used.

Before using a PGD, health professionals should ensure that they:

- have undertaken the necessary initial training and continuing professional development;
- have been assessed as competent and authorised to practice by the provider organisation;
- have signed the appropriate documentation;
- are using a copy of the most recent and in-date final signed version of the PGD;
- have read and understand the context and content of the PGD.

When supplying and/or administering a medicine under a PGD, health professionals should follow local organisational policies and act within their code(s) of professional conduct and local governance arrangements.

Exemptions

A range of healthcare professionals are permitted to administer specified licensed medicines under the Human Medicines Regulations (2012 schedule 17 and amendments 2016). These include (within occupational health schemes), midwives, paramedics and optometrists. Orthoptists, chiropodists and podiatrists can undertake further training to undertake a wider range of exemptions. Other exemptions cover a range of situations, such as emergency use of asthma inhalers in schools and access to medicines in a pandemic. It is important that you understand your organisation's policies with respect to administration of specific medicines to save a life in an emergency. Follow the Skills in Practice box to understand your role within an emergency.

Skills in practice

Refer to your organisation's anaphylaxis policy.
What does it say **you** can do and what products can **you** administer in an emergency?

Prescribing

Doctors and dentists are currently the only healthcare professionals who are able to prescribe on registration. The new Nursing and Midwifery Council (NMC) standards for education mean that undergraduate nurses who are studying on NMC validated pre-registration nursing courses will be prescriber ready (NMC, 2018). This means that they will be ready to undertake a prescribing program 12 months post-registration (NMC, 2018). There are a range of health-care professionals within the UK who have the right to prescribe medications. Since 1992, non-medical prescribing has been permitted within the United Kingdom (Cope et al., 2016). Multiple changes in legislation and professional regulation has enabled nurses, midwives, pharmacists, physiotherapists, chiropodists, podiatrists, diagnostic radiographers and advanced paramedics to become independent prescribers on successful completion of an accredited prescribing program and registration of their qualification with their regulatory body. This extension of prescribing responsibilities to other healthcare professional groups is likely to continue where it is safe to do so and there is a clear patient benefit (Royal Pharmaceutical Society [RPS], 2016). There are currently two forms of prescribing: independent prescribing and supplementary prescribing.

An independent prescriber is a practitioner, who is responsible and accountable for the assessment of patients with undiagnosed or diagnosed conditions and can make prescribing decisions to manage the clinical condition of the patient. Nurse independent prescribers can prescribe any medicine or product listed within the British National Formulary (BNF) as well as unlicensed medicines and any CDs (within schedules II–V) if they are competent to do. For other healthcare professionals with prescribing rights, such as physiotherapists and advanced paramedics, there some restrictions, particularly around the CDs they can prescribe.

Dietitians and therapeutic radiographers can undertake an accredited program to qualify and register as supplementary prescribers, enabling them to prescribe against an agreed clinical management plan (CMP). Supplementary prescribing is described by the Department of Health (2005) as: 'a voluntary partnership between an Independent Prescriber and a supplementary prescriber' (e.g. nurse, pharmacist) 'to implement an agreed patient-specific clinical management plan (CMP) with the patient's agreement'.

In 2016, the RPS published a Competency Framework for all Prescribers to support all prescribers to prescribe effectively (Royal Pharmaceutical Society, 2016). This framework consolidated existing profession specific prescribing frameworks and updated the competencies into a single common framework that is relevant to all prescribers, regardless of professional background. Medicines management is an evidence-based approach to prescribing and balances the safety, tolerability, effectiveness, cost and simplicity of treatments. This also includes:

- giving unbiased information about medicines and treatments;
- supporting practitioners and patients to make best use of medicines.

This means ensuring all prescribers draw on the appropriate evidence to identify the most appropriate, effective and cost-efficient treatment which is suitable and agreeable with the individual patient including where they are advised on the purchase and use of OTC products. These issues will be explored further with the Optimising Medicines for Patients section.

Prior to 2019, nurses and midwives had their own specific medicine management standards, produced by the Nursing and Midwifery Council (NMC, 2008). Due to the increasing number of healthcare professionals involved in medicines management, a more consistent approach was required that all healthcare professionals could follow. From January 2019, all healthcare professionals are required to follow the RPS (2018) Professional Guidance on the Safe and Secure Handling of Medicines and the RPS (2019) Professional Guidance on the Administration of Medicines in a Healthcare Setting. These guidance documents ensure consistent, safe and effective medicine administration and handling of medicines. Alongside this guidance, most local NHS Trusts and other employers will also have their own guidance or policies which employees should always check and follow when considering their actions related to medicines management.

Handling and administration

The online professional guidance document Safe and Secure Handling of Medicines (RPS, 2018), accredited by NICE, provides details on the four core governance principles that underpin a framework for the safe and secure handling of medicines. This guidance applies to all healthcare settings and covers all pharmacists and other health professionals whose role involves handling medicines. The document provides comprehensive guidance on obtaining medicines, their transport, receipt, manufacture or manipulation and storage. It also includes information on the issuing of medicines, and their removal or disposal. Additional guidance is provided on the storage of medicines, the handling of CDs and the safe and secure handling of medicines in theatres. This guidance also helps organisations to ensure that they adhere to regulations laid down by the Health and Safety Executive (HSE), to ensure prevention of work-related death, injury and ill health of employees, as some of these elements can expose healthcare practitioners to the risk of harm.

Professional guidance on the Administration of Medicines in Healthcare Settings was co-produced by the RPS and the Royal College of Nursing (RCN) (RPS, 2019). This document provides principles-based guidance to ensure the safe administration, covert administration and transcribing of medicines by registered healthcare professionals. The principles within the guidance can also be applied in any healthcare setting by any person administering medicines.

The guidance recommends that:

> Those administering medicines are appropriately trained, assessed as competent and meet relevant professional and regulatory standards and guidance.
>
> (RPS, 2019, p.3, no. 8)

Each NHS Trust, or other employer, will have their own policies and procedures for the medicines administration process, which may differ slightly, so it is very important that you check these before administering any medication. An example medicines administration procedure is outlined in Box 4.1.

Box 4.1 Example of a medicine administration procedure

This may include (but is not limited to):

1. Checking the identity of the patient.
2. The prescription meets legal requirements, is unambiguous and includes where appropriate the name, form (or route of administration), strength and dose of the medicine to be administered.
3. That issues around consent have been adhered to.
4. Allergies or previous adverse drug reactions (ADRs) have been checked and recorded.
5. The directions for administration (e.g. timing and frequency of administration, route of administration and start and finish dates where appropriate) are clear.
6. Any ambiguities or concerns regarding the direction for administration of the medicine are raised with the prescriber or a pharmacy professional without delay.
7. Any calculations needed are double-checked where practicable by a second person and uncertainties raised with the prescriber or a pharmacy professional.
8. The identity of the medicine (or medical gas) and its expiry date (where available) have been checked.
9. That any specific storage requirements have been maintained.
10. Confirm that the dose has not already been administered by someone else.

Your employing organisation will ensure that any risks associated with handling or administration of medicines have been identified, and procedures should be in place to minimise any risks. Your employing organisation should also ensure that any necessary equipment and devices, required to aid the administration of medicines, are available and well maintained. Follow the Clinical Considerations box to understand the medicine administration procedure within your organisation.

Clinical considerations

Refer to your organisation's policy on medicine administration procedure. How does this compare with the example in Box 4.1?

A prescriber will first document what drug is to be given, and at what time(s). Some NHS Trusts and employers will use a paper-based medication chart to record this while many areas are now moving over to electronic medication records, primarily to improve patient safety. In terms of administration, the guidance states:

> Before administration, the person administering the medicine must have an overall under- standing of the medicine being administered and seeks advice if necessary, from a pre-scriber or a pharmacy professional.
>
> (RPS, 2019, p. 4, no. 14)

This means that prior to administering a medicine, you should have an understanding of what the medication is used for and how it works, the route of administration, potential side effects and circumstances when you should not give the medication. You need to be familiar with resources that will help you to find out this information. Chapter 2 of this book provides you with the details you need to know to be able to look up a medicine, either electronically or via a paper-based system – for example, the BNF – that will provide you with key information.

The correct medicine administration procedure must then be followed to ensure the right patient gets the right medication at the right time. To support this further, a systematic approach has been developed for medicines administration, referred to as the 9Rs, or nine rights of medication administration (Elliott and Liu, 2010).

The 9 Rs

1. *Right patient*: The identity of the patient must be verified by checking their name, address and date of birth – both with the patient and on their chart. Extra care needs to be taken in patients who are unable to identify themselves; for example, the unconscious patient or those with cognitive impairment.
2. *Right drug:* Many drugs look the same, have similar names and even similar packaging. Without careful checking, the wrong medication could be administered by mistake.
3. *Right route*: The same medicine is often available for administration using a variety of routes, but dose and onset of action can be different according to which route has been chosen. The correct route of medicine administration needs to be confirmed prior to giving it to the patient. At times, healthcare professionals are required to use their clinical decision-making skills before administering the medicine via a variety of routes; so, the prescription might say subcutaneous/intramuscular – and the healthcare professional must use critical thinking with regard to the most appropriate route.
4. *Right time*: Medication needs to be given at the prescribed time in order to ensure stable levels of drug within the body and avoid unwanted gaps in therapy. If a medication is ordered to be given at particular time intervals, the nurse should never deviate from this time by more than half an hour (Galbraith et al., 2015). If administration of a medications occurs outside this 30-minute window, bioavailability of the medication may be affected (Elliott and Liu, 2010). It is particularly important that critical medications are administered at the prescribed time as a delay could cause potential harm to the patient.
5. *Right dose:* The dose to be administered will be stated on the prescription. Best practice would suggest that you check the dose of the medication in a pharmaceutical guide (such as the BNF) to ensure it is the correct dose. Some medications will require you to carry out a dose calculation before administration. Variables such as age, weight, condition or specific biochemical markers need to be considered to determine the dose that needs to be given. Once the dose has been confirmed, it may be necessary to calculate how this dose will be given. This may involve calculating how many capsules, or how much liquid, will need to be administered to deliver the correct dose.
6. *Right documentation:* It is very important that records of administration, or a medication being withheld or declined by the patient, are completed at the time or as soon as possible thereafter, and that all records are clear, legible and auditable (NMC Code, 2018). If a medication is not administered, or has been refused, details of the reason why (if known)

should be included in the record and reported to the prescriber, or healthcare team, where appropriate. Look at the Clinical Consideration that follows and consider your actions.

7. *Right action:* Before you administer any medication, you must first ensure that is prescribed for an appropriate reason. This requires knowledge and understanding of the medical condition(s) of your patient and the action of the drug(s) to be administered. Where possible, you should state to the patient the action of the medication and the reason for which it is prescribed, as this may help to avoid a medication error (Elliott and Liu, 2010).

8. *Right form:* Medications are available in different forms, such as tablets, capsules, caplets, syrup, suppositories and ampoules for intravenous administration. It is important that the route of administration is clear (e.g. oral) and that the right form of medication is administered to avoid harm to the patient. It is also important that any specific instructions are given to patients; for example, not to chew enteric-coated tablets as they are designed to dissolve in the alkaline environment of the small intestine, and some drugs are enteric-coated because the active ingredient will irritate the stomach mucosa if they dissolve there (Adams and Koch, 2010).

9. *Right response:* Once a medication has been administered, patients should be monitored for any side effects, adverse effects or adverse reactions and, if they occur, these should be managed and documented appropriately. It is also important to understand that some patients will also need to be monitored to ensure the intended effect or efficacy of the medication is achieved; for example, assessment of blood glucose level for the patient with diabetes or blood pressure monitoring for patients with hypertension (Bruen et al., 2017).

If you are in any doubt about administering a medication, consult the prescriber or pharmacy professional for further information or advice.

Clinical considerations

Doris, a 64-year-old lady admitted with uncontrolled epileptic seizures, has declined her laxatives, as she states she has moved her bowels four times that day already. Doris has also declined her sodium valproate as she says it makes her feel sick.
What action do you need to take for:

- the laxative
- the sodium valproate?

Special consideration: Controlled drugs and critical medications

Some medications, due to their potential to be misused and the harm that this can cause, are classified as CDs. With regards to CDs there will be additional requirements that you must follow regarding their use. The Misuse of Drugs Act 1971, and its associated regulations, detail the legal framework governing the use of CDs. NICE have produced the guideline Controlled Drugs: Safe Use and Management (NG46) (2016) which provides further details on the systems and processes that must be in place in all healthcare environments (except care homes) for managing the use of CDs. Your Trust/employer may also have additional policies/procedures related to CDs that you will need to follow.

Any medication should be administered in a timely manner, but there are some medications that must not be omitted, or their administration delayed, as this has the potential to cause harm to the patient. The Specialist Pharmacy Service (2017) has updated the National Patient Safety Agency (NPSA) Rapid Response Report 'Reducing harm from omitted and delayed

Table 4.1   The potential risks of missed medication.

Risk 1	Risk 2	Risk 3
Nil or negligible patient impact with nil or minor intervention required; no increase in length of stay	Significant short-term patient impact with moderate intervention required; increase in length of hospital stay possible	Significant or catastrophic long-term patient impact with ongoing intervention required; long increase in length of stay possible
• There is no or negligible risk of patient impact • No or minor intervention necessary • There is no possibility of an increase in the length of hospital stay	• There is a risk of significant short-term patient impact • Subsequent moderate intervention is required • A resultant long increase (1–15 days) in the length of hospital stay is possible	• There is a risk of significant long-term patient impact • There is a risk of catastrophic patient impact (i.e. death) • Subsequent ongoing professional intervention is required • A resultant very long (>15 days) increase in the length of hospital stay is possible

medicines in hospital' (February 2010). This document highlights the need for rapid access to medications that are critical for patients with the risks of delay, or omission, for each drug in the BNF are categorised using a traffic light system (see Table 4.1). Medication that fall into the Risk 3 category are classified as 'critical medications' due to the consequences to the patient if they are missed or omitted.

Critical medicines include groups of medicines such as:

- antimicrobials
- anticoagulants
- antiepileptic agents
- anti-Parkinsonian agents
- immunosuppressants
- insulin.

Any omission or delay in the administration of a critical medicine must be discussed with the prescriber (or relevant physician) and reported as a patient safety incident (PSI).

Groups requiring special considerations

There are several groups which require additional considerations when prescribing, administering and monitoring medicines. This section will explore issues related to prescribing, administering and monitoring medicines for pregnant and breast-feeding women and older people, although there are others that you may need to consider; for example, prescribing for people with hepatic impairment.

For women that are pregnant or breast-feeding and for the older population, special considerations need to be given within the medicines management process to ensure the safety of the patient.

Pregnancy and breast-feeding

Many drugs can cross the placenta and may also be transferred in breast milk. It is reported that over 90% of pregnant women take OTC or prescription medications (Adam et al., 2011) and this is of increasing concern as the number of women with pre-diagnosed morbidities enter pregnancy (Murk and Seli, 2011). Most medicines are contraindicated during pregnancy as there is limited data on the safety/benefit–risk aspects (Clemow et al., 2015) and it is known that some can have a harmful effect on a growing embryo or foetus and the breast-feeding baby. It is useful to distinguish whether the presenting 'condition' is related to the pregnancy or not. Many long-term conditions can affect the progress of the pregnancy and pregnancy can also impact upon long-term conditions (RCN, 2018). It is vital, therefore, that specialist advice is sought via the named midwife or obstetrician/specialist team to ensure that appropriate advice and care can be managed.

Managing medicines during pregnancy is complex and can have major consequences if not managed with caution and expertise. It is therefore important to establish whether someone of childbearing age may be pregnant prior to the prescribing or administration of any medicine. Careful consideration must be given to the benefits and risks of taking medicines, both for the mother and the foetus. Within each edition of the BNF (and online resource) there is an advice section on the specific prescribing issues concerning pregnancy and breast-feeding. General advice is that drugs should only be prescribed if the benefit for the mother is greater than the risk to the foetus, but all drugs should avoided where possible during the first trimester (BNF 78). Drugs which appear to be safe and have been used extensively in pregnancy should be preferred to new or untried drugs, using the smallest effective dose possible. Each trimester (a period of three months) carries specific risks if medicines are taken.

The first trimester is when drugs can cause congenital malformations (teratogenesis) with the greatest risks being between week 3 and 11 of the pregnancy (BNF 78). Unfortunately, the woman may not even be aware of the pregnancy at this point and thus a pregnancy test may be performed for drugs of high risk. Drugs can affect the growth or functional development and can cause toxic effects on the foetus during the *second and third trimester* and may also manifest after birth (BNF 78). A well-documented example is a range of anticonvulsants (used for managing epilepsy and neuropathic pain, etc.) which are known to cause congenital malformations in the early stages of pregnancy – for example, baby born with cleft lip and palate – however data demonstrating the risks for the foetus are not always detailed within the Summary of Product Characteristics or Patient Information Leaflet which causes challenges both for the healthcare professional and pregnant woman in considering best treatment options (Rezaallah et al., 2019).

There is also little information available in identifying the safety of medicines for women who are breast-feeding, and thus little guidance. This can cause confusion for health professionals offering information but also for the breast-feeding woman who may cease breast-feeding earlier than planned rather than pose unknown risks to her child (McClatchey et al., 2017). The potential for harm is inferred through the amount of active drug delivered to the infant, the pharmacokinetic efficiency of the infants' body and the way the drug affects the infant. Some drugs are known to inhibit the infant's sucking reflex (e.g. phenobarbital) and others affect lactation (e.g. bromocriptine) (BNF 78). The BNF identifies where it is known that medicines are contraindicated or where caution is indicated during pregnancy and breast-feeding.

Older people

Special care is required when prescribing for older people. Medicines for Older People, a component document within the National Service Framework for Older People (DH, 2001), describes how to avoid excessive, inappropriate or inadequate consumption of medicines by older people. A large proportion of older people within the UK have multimorbidity, and within this population the use of multiple medicines (polypharmacy) is very common. Polypharmacy occurs when an individual is taking four or more regular medicines (Patterson et al., 2012). Taking multiple medications greatly increases the risk of drug interactions, adverse reactions and can also impact upon compliance. It has been estimated that up to 50% of medicines taken for long-term conditions are not taken as prescribed (NICE, 2009). As a result of this, it is recommended that older people's medications are reviewed regularly and any medicine which is not of benefit should be discontinued. As an individual gets older, what the body does to a drug (pharmacokinetics) changes. The most important effect of age is reduced renal clearance, meaning that older people excrete drugs more slowly, increasing the risk of side effects and adverse reactions (Shi and Klotz, 2011) (see Chapter 5 within this text for further details). The BNF (BNF 78) states the most common adverse reactions to monitor for are:

- confusion
- constipation
- postural hypotension and falls.

As a result of this, the BNF (BNF 78) provides some general principles that need to be followed when prescribing for the older person:

1. Lower doses: start at lower doses (usually 50% of an adult doses) and only increase if needed.
2. Review regularly: Regular medication reviews should be undertaken to determine if the medication is still appropriate/required. It may be necessary to reduce medications of some drugs as renal function declines.
3. Simplify regimens: Medications should only be prescribed when there is a clear indication to do so (for example, not prescribing antibiotics for a viral infection). If possible, medicines should only be prescribed once or twice daily and confusing dosage intervals should be avoided.
4. Explain clearly: Each medication should have clear instructions on how to take it with full directions given.

These are some of the issues which need consideration for medicine management, can you think of any more? The Clinical Considerations box that follows will help you to explore this further.

Clinical considerations

Having read this section, are there any other groups in your practice area that require further considerations prior to prescribing, administering and monitoring of medicines?

Monitoring for side effects

All medicines can have side effects, and if any of these is harmful, the patient is classed as having an ADR (Aronson and Ferner, 2005). The EMA (2017) defines an ADR as 'a response to a medicinal product which is noxious and unintended'. Part of your role within medicines management is to understand, and identify, any ADR as some can occur within minutes of administration, whereas others can present years after treatment (Ferner and McGettan, 2018). Further details on ADRs are discussed in Chapter 7.

Medicine optimisation

Medicines optimisation is another term that is often used; this builds on medicines management, but encompasses all aspects of a patient's medicines journey from the initial prescription through to ongoing review and support. Medicines optimisation is about ensuring that the right patients get the right choice of medicine, at the right time. By focusing on patients and their experiences, the goal is to help patients to:

- improve their outcomes;
- take their medicines correctly;
- avoid taking unnecessary medicines;
- reduce wastage of medicines;
- improve medicines safety.

Table 4.2   Four principles of medicines management.

Principle 1 Aim to understand the patient's experience.
Principle 2 Evidence-based choice of medicines.
Principle 3 Ensure medicines use is as safe as possible.
Principle 4 Make medicines optimisation part of routine practice.

Source: Adapted RPS (2013).

A multidisciplinary approach to medicines optimisation can help encourage patients to take ownership of their treatment (RPS, 2013). The RPS (2013) described four guiding principles for medicines management in practice (see Table 4.2).

Medicines optimisation examines how patients use medicines over time. It may involve stopping certain medicines as well as starting others, and considers opportunities for lifestyle changes and non-medical therapies to reduce the need for medicines. By improving medicine safety and adherence to treatment and reducing waste the medicines optimisation approach ensures patients are supported to get the best outcomes from their medicines (NICE, 2015). The key elements of medicines optimisation are that it:

- Is patient-centred and makes a difference to the patient's outcomes.
- Is a partnership between the healthcare professional and patient.
- Is about listening to the patient's views and opinions, supporting adherence and self-care.
- Is the application of clinical and pharmaceutical expertise and understanding.
- Provides a personalised medication regimen for each patient.
- Encourages communication with other healthcare professionals to ensure continuity across care settings.
- Encourages good governance, including safety, quality and better outcomes.

The healthcare professional therefore has a significant role in ensuring that patients/service users, and their carers, are central to the shared decision-making process in managing their medicines with the ultimate aim of improve health outcomes.

Safety in medicines management

A recent study found an estimated 237 million medication errors occur in the NHS in England every year (Elliott et al., 2018). These errors resulted in avoidable ADRs, causing 712 deaths and contributing to 1708 deaths. Non-steroidal anti-inflammatory drugs (NSAIDs), anticoagulants, and antiplatelets caused over a third of hospital admissions due to avoidable ADRs. Gastrointestinal bleeds were implicated in half of the deaths from primary care ADRs. The report also found that older people were more likely to suffer avoidable ADRs. The cost to the NHS for these avoidable ADRs was £98.5 million per year. This is a huge financial drain on the NHS, but the harm and suffering caused to patients and their families is immeasurable.

The transfer of patients between primary and secondary care is also an area for potential error, and it is estimated that up to 70% of patients may have an unintentional change or medication error (RPS, 2012a). Further risks of errors were identified for people residing in care homes, and recommendations for best practice in managing polypharmacy, repeat prescribing and medication reviews as well as training for staff are advised (RPS, 2012b). NHS England (2018) has since outlined guidance to support safe and effective medicine management practices across primary, secondary and tertiary care, outlining the responsibilities of all professionals.

Medication errors are any PSIs where there has been an error in the process of prescribing, preparing, dispensing, administering, monitoring or providing advice on medicines. These PSIs can be divided into two categories:

1. errors of commission (for example, wrong medicine or wrong dose);
2. errors of omission (for example, an omitted dose or a failure to monitor).

The National Reporting and Learning Systems (NRLS) defines a 'patient safety incident' (PSI) as, 'any unintended or unexpected incident, which could have or did lead to harm for one or more patients receiving NHS care'.

The Central Alerting System (CAS) (managed by the MHRA) is a web-based cascading system for issuing patient safety alerts, important public health messages, and other safety critical information and guidance to the NHS and others, including independent providers of health and social care. Alerts within this system include Medical Device Alerts (MDA) and Drug Alerts. These alerts are cascaded to GP practices, community pharmacists, dispensing GPs, emergency departments, hospital pharmacists (as appropriate), and independent healthcare and social care providers registered with CAS.

Storage and disposal

Medicines are used in all healthcare settings and the safe and secure handling of medicines is essential to ensure patient safety. The Human Medicines Regulations (2012) outline the legal requirements to support this process. Each medicine must be stored according to specific instructions, details of which can be found in the electronic Medicines Compendium (www.medicines.org.uk/emc).

The RPS outline professional guidance within the online Safe and Secure Handling of Medicines document (2018). This advises that all individuals who handle medicines must be competent, legally entitled, appropriately trained and authorised to do the job. Medicines must be kept secure and safeguarded from unauthorised access and stored at a level of security appropriate to their proposed use. The legal category for the medicine will also dictate how it must be stored; for example, CDs must be kept in a secure place with restricted access (Human Medicines Regulations, 2012).

Where products need to be stored at cooler temperatures, the cold chain must be maintained to ensure the integrity of the product is maintained; for example, vaccines deteriorate at room temperatures and thus must be stored in a refrigerator and in cool conditions right until the moment they are administered. Where this has been compromised, a risk assessment must be undertaken to determine whether the integrity of the product has been affected.

Safe handling and disposal of toxic substances, such as cytotoxic drugs, is governed by the HSE (2019) as they present significant risks for those who handle them. The HSE offer practical guidance on meeting the Control of Substances Hazardous to Health Regulations (COSHH) (2002) and how these substances should be safely handled and disposed of in all health and social care environments, including the patient's home.

Any old, unwanted or expired medicines need to be returned to a pharmacy or chemist for safe disposal. Inhalers contain gases which can be harmful to the environment so should not be put in waste bins and must also be returned to a pharmacy/chemist where they can be recycled. Pharmacies are obliged to accept back any unwanted medicines from patients. The pharmacy must, if required by NHS England or the waste contractor, sort them into solids (including ampoules and vials), liquids and aerosols, and the local NHS England team will make arrangements for a waste contractor to collect the medicines from pharmacies at regular intervals. Additional segregation is also required under the Hazardous Waste Regulations.

Conclusions

This chapter has explored the many strands to managing medicines to provide safe, efficient and cost-effective care. All health professionals have a role in this process to ensure they understand and follow the regulations, policies and practices which govern safe prescribing, administration and monitoring of medicines. Medicine management should be a partnership between patients and healthcare professionals to ensure patient-centred outcomes regardless of the health or social care setting.

References

Adams, M. and Koch, R. (2010). *Pharmacology Connections to Nursing Practice*. New Jersey: Pearson.

Adam, M.P., Polifka, J.E., and Friedman, J.M. (2011). Evolving knowledge of the teratogenicity of medications in human pregnancy. *American Journal of Medical Genetics* 157: 175–182.

Aronson, J.K. and Ferner, R.E. (2005). Clarification of terminology in drug safety. *Drug Safety* 28: 851–870.

Bruen, D., Delaney, C., Florea, L., and Diamond, D. (2017). Glucose sensing for diabetes monitoring: recent developments. *Sensors* 17 (8): 1866.

Clemow, B., Nolan, J.D., Michaels, D.L. et al. (2015). Medicines in pregnancy forum: proceedings on ethical and legal considerations. Ethic special section meeting report. *Therapeutic Innovaion and Regulatory Science* 49 (3): 326–332.

Cope, L.C., Abuzour, A.S., and Tully, M.P. (2016). Nonmedical prescribing: where are we now? *Therapeutic Advances in Drug Safety* 7: 165–172.

Department of Health (2005). Supplementary prescribing. https://webarchive.nationalarchives.gov.uk/20070306020119/http:/www.dh.gov.uk/assetRoot/04/11/00/33/04110033.pdf (accessed 29 July 2020).

Department of Health (2013). *The Medicines Act 1968 and the Human Medicines Regulations (Amendment) Order*. London: Department of Health.

Duerden, M., Avery, T., and Payne R. (2013). Polypharmacy and medicines optimisation: making it safe and sound. https://www.kingsfund.org.uk/sites/default/files/field/field_publication_file/polypharmacy-and-medicines-optimisation-kingsfund-nov13.pdf (accessed 22 July 2020).

Elliott, M. and Liu, Y. (2010). The nine rights of medication administration: an overview. *British Journal of Nursing* 19 (5): 300–305.

Elliott, R., Camacho, E., Cambell, F., et al. (2018). Prevalence and economic burden of medication errors in the NHS in England. Rapid evidence synthesis and economic analysis of the prevalence and burden of medication error in the UK.

NHS (2018). Conditions for which over the counter medications should not be prescribed. https://www.england.nhs.uk/wp-content/uploads/2018/03/otc-guidance-for-ccgs.pdf (accessed July 2020).

NHS England (2018). Responsibility for prescribing between primary and secondary/tertiary care. Gateway ref 07573.

European Medicines Agency and Heads of Medicines Agencies (2017). Guideline on good pharmacovigilance practices (GVP): Annex I - Definitions (Rev 4).

Ewbank, L., Omojomolo, D., Sullivan, K. et al. (2018). *The Rising Cost of Medicines to the NHS*. London: King's Fund.

Ferner, R.E. and McGettan, P. (2018). Adverse drug reactions. *BMJ: British Medical Journal* 363 https://doi.org/10.1136/bmj.k4777.

Galbraith, A., Bullock, S., Manias, E. et al. (2015). *Fundamentals of Pharmacology: An Applied Approach for Nursing and Health*. Routledge.

Health and Safety Executive (2019). Control of Substances Hazardous to Health. www.hse.gov.uk/coshh/index.htm (accessed July 2020).

HMSO (1997). Prescription Only Medicines (Human Use) Order 1997. Statutory Instrument 1997, No. 1830. London: HMSO.

McClatchey, A.K., Shield, A., Cheong, L.H. et al. (2017). Why does the need for medication become a barrier to breastfeeding? A narrative review. *Women and Birth* 31 (5): 362–366.

Medicines and Healthcare products Regulatory Agency (2017). Patient group directions: who can use them. https://www.gov.uk/government/publications/patient-group-directions-pgds/patient-group-directions-who-can-use-them (accessed July 2020).

Murk, W. and Seli, E. (2011). Fertility preservation as a public health issue: an epidemiological perspective. *Current Opinion in Obstetrics and Gynecology* 23: 143–150.

NHS Business Services Authority (2018). Medicines Optimisation. Generic Prescribing Key Messages Report. https://www.nhsbsa.nhs.uk/sites/default/files/2018-10/Generic%20Prescribing%20Key%20Messages%20%284%29%20PDF.pdf (accessed 22 July 2020).

NICE (2009). Medicines adherence: involving patients in decisions about prescribed medicines and supporting adherence [CG76]. www.nice.org.uk/guidance/cg76 (accessed July 2020).

NICE (2015). Medicines optimisation: the safe and effective use of medicines to enable the best possible outcomes [NG5]. www.nice.org.uk/guidance/ng5 (accessed July 2020).

NICE (2016). Multimorbidity: clinical assessment and management [NG56]. www.nice.org.uk/guidance/ng56 (accessed July 2020).

NICE (2017). Patient group directions. www.nice.org.uk/guidance/mpg2/chapter/Recommendations#training-and-competency (accessed July 2020).

Nursing & Midwifery Council (2008). Standards for medicines management London: NMC.

Nursing & Midwifery Council (2018). *The Code: professional standards of practice and behaviour for nurses, midwives and nursing associates.* https://www.nmc.org.uk/globalassets/sitedocuments/nmc-publications/nmc-code.pdf (accessed September 2020).

Patterson, S.M., Hughes, C., Kerse, N. et al. (2012). Interventions to improve the appropriate use of polypharmacy for older people. *Cochrane Database of Systematic Reviews* (5): CD008165. https://doi.org/10.1002/14651858.CD008165.pub2.

Rezaallah, B., Lewis, D.J., Zeilhofer, H.F., and Ber, B.I. (2019). Risk of cleft lip and/or palate associated with anti-epileptic drugs: postmarketing safety signal detection and evaluation of information presented to prescribers and patients. *Therapeutic and Regulatory Science* 53 (1): 110–119.

Royal College of Nursing (2018). Medicines management; prescribing in pregnancy. www.rcn.org.uk/clinical-topics/medicines-management/prescribing-in-pregnancy (accessed July 2020).

Royal Pharmaceutical Society (2012a). Keeping patients safe when they transfer between care providers – getting the medicines right; final report. https://www.rpharms.com (accessed July 2020).

Royal Pharmaceutical Society (2012b). Improving pharmaceutical care in care homes. https://www.rpharms.com (accessed July 2020).

Royal Pharmaceutical Society (2013). Medicines optimisation. https://www.rpharms.com/Portals/0/RPS%20document%20library/Open%20access/Policy/helping-patients-make-the-most-of-their-medicines.pdf (accessed July 2020).

Royal Pharmaceutical Society (2016). A competency framework for all prescribers. https://www.rpharms.com/Portals/0/RPS%20document%20library/Open%20access/Professional%20standards/Prescribing%20competency%20framework/prescribing-competency-framework.pdf (accessed July 2020).

Royal Pharmaceutical Society (2018). Professional guidance on the safe and secure handling of medicines. https://www.rpharms.com/recognition/setting-professional-standards/safe-and-secure-handling-of-medicines/professional-guidance-on-the-safe-and-secure-handling-of-medicines (accessed July 2020).

Royal Pharmaceutical Society (2019). Professional guidance on the administration of medicines in healthcare settings. https://www.rpharms.com/Portals/0/RPS%20document%20library/Open%20access/Professional%20standards/SSHM%20and%20Admin/Admin%20of%20Meds%20prof%20guidance.pdf?ver=2019-01-23-145026-567 (accessed July 2020).

Shi, S. and Klotz, U. (2011). Age-related changes in pharmacokinetics. *Current Drug Metabolism* 12 (7): 601–610.

The Human Medicines Regulations (2012). Human Medicines Regulations. http://www.legislation.gov.uk/uksi/2012/1916/contents/made (accessed 22 July 2020).

Further reading

RCN (2019). Medicines management: professional resources. www.rcn.org.uk/clinical-topics/medicines-management/professional-resources.

RCN and RPS (2019).Standards professional guidance on the administration of medicines in healthcare settings. https://www.rpharms.com/Portals/0/RPS%20document%20library/Open%20access/Professional%20standards/SSHM%20and%20Admin/Admin%20of%20Meds%20prof%20guidance.pdf?ver=2019-01-23-145026-567.

Northern Ireland Department of Health (2019). Medicines management. https://www.health-ni.gov.uk/articles/medicines-management.

Care Quality Commission (2019). Issue 5: Safe management of medicines. www.cqc.org.uk/guidance-providers/learning-safety-incidents/issue-5-safe-management-medicines.

NHS Specialist Pharmacy Service (2018). Medicines Matters. https://www.sps.nhs.uk/wp-content/uploads/2018/10/Medicines-Matters-september-2018-1.pdf.

NHS (2019). Medicines optimisation. https://www.england.nhs.uk/medicines/medicines-optimisation.

Multiple choice questions

1. Medicine management could be best described as:
   (a) Senior managers controlling medicines
   (b) Safe, efficient and cost-effective use of medicines
   (c) People managing to open their medicines

2. The PoM is:
   (a) The Price of the Medicine
   (b) The Purpose of the Medicine
   (c) A Prescription only Medicine
3. Patient Group Directions are:
   (a) Maps of the hospital to direct patents
   (b) A list of medicines that can be given to a patient without a prescription
   (c) Written instructions directing registered health professionals to supply/administer specified medicines to a pre-defined group of patients
4. Medicines are regulated by the:
   (a) The Medicines Regulatory Body
   (b) The Medicines and Healthcare Products Regulatory Agency
   (c) Regulatory Agency for Medicines
5. A black triangle is applied to
   (a) Cheaper medicines
   (b) Products where there is limited experience of its use
   (c) Medicines which should not be used
6. A generic medicine is:
   (a) A non-proprietary medicine
   (b) A medicine which can be used for any condition
   (c) A proprietary medicine
7. The legal framework for medicines includes:
   (a) The Human Medicines Regulations 2012
   (b) The Medicines Law 2000
   (c) The Regulations for Medical Use 2012
8. Which of the following is non-propriety drug?
   (a) Brufen
   (b) Ibuprofen
   (c) Nurofen
9. Critical medicines:
   (a) Are important medicines
   (b) Need special care
   (c) Must not be omitted or delayed
10. Before administering a medicine, the healthcare professional must:
    (a) Consult with the prescriber for every patient
    (b) Understand the medicine being administered and seek advice from the prescriber or pharmacy professional if required
    (c) Contact the pharmacist to check the prescription
11. Which of the following Royal Pharmaceutical Society guidance should healthcare professionals adhere to, to direct the administration of medicines?
    (a) The RPS A Competency Framework for All Prescribers
    (b) The RPS Professional Guidance for the Administration of Medicines in Healthcare settings
    (c) The RPS Professional Guidance on the safe and secure handling of medicines.
12. Common adverse reactions in older people include:
    (a) Confusion, constipation, postural hypotension and falls
    (b) Chest pain, headaches and constipation
    (c) Earache, stomach pains and dizziness

13. The Central Alerting System:
    (a) Issues alerts to organisations about healthcare staff
    (b) Alerts healthcare professionals about patients
    (c) Issues patient safety alerts
14. Which of the following bodies analyse the use of NHS medicines?
    (a) The NHS Business Authority
    (b) The NHS Medicines Authority
    (c) The NHS Supply of Medicines Authority
15. Optimising medicines:
    (a) Focuses on the medicine cost
    (b) Focuses on the patient
    (c) Focuses on healthcare professional

Chapter 5

Pharmacodynamics and pharmacokinetics

Barry Hill and Jaden Allan

Aim

The aim of this chapter is to provide the reader with an introduction to pharmacokinetics and pharmacodynamics and the important issues surrounding medicines management.

Learning outcomes

After reading this chapter, the reader will be able to:

1. Acknowledge the professional responsibilities of Registered Nurses (RN) who administer drugs to patients
2. Define and understand the differences between pharmacodynamics and pharmacokinetics
3. Appreciate the complexities of how drugs work differently in every individual

Test your knowledge

1. Describe the professional responsibilities of Registered Nurses who administer medications.
2. Define pharmacodynamics.
3. How many phases of pharmacokinetics are there?
4. What are the phases of pharmacokinetics?
5. Discuss drug interactions and some of the key considerations for 'at risk' groups of patients.

Introduction

This chapter explores the pharmacokinetics and pharmacodynamics of drugs.

Fundamentals of Pharmacology: For Nursing and Healthcare Students, First Edition. Edited by Ian Peate and Barry Hill.
© 2021 John Wiley & Sons Ltd. Published 2021 by John Wiley & Sons Ltd.

Royal Pharmaceutical Society

As new diseases emerge, and older medicines – such as antibiotics – no longer work as well as they once did, the contribution of pharmacology to finding better and safer medicines becomes even more significant in order to improve the quality of life for patients. The Royal Pharmaceutical Society (RPS) is the body responsible for the leadership and support of the pharmacy profession within England, Scotland and Wales. The RPS is the leading society within the United Kingdom (UK), and believes that; 'Pharmacological knowledge improves the lives of millions of people across the world'. They also recommend all healthcare professionals have pharmacological knowledge, as it 'maximises their benefit and minimises risk and harm' (RPS and RCN, 2019). In 2019, the RPS and RCN published the Professional Guidance on the Administration of Medicines in Healthcare Settings (RPS and RCN, 2019). This guidance has replaced all previously published NMC medicines management guidance and should be the key document for all healthcare professionals.

The Nursing and Midwifery Council

The Nursing and Midwifery Council (NMC), who are the regulating body for nurses, nursing associates and midwives, require utilisation of 'critical thinking' and 'clinical judgement' when working with medicines in order to provide patient safety. Registered Nurses should be able to practice as autonomous professionals, exercising their own professional judgment, and should also be able to modify and adapt practice to meet the clinical needs of patients within the healthcare environment.

Consequently, for nurses to think critically, work within their scope of practice, and most importantly improve patient safety when working with medicines, it is imperative that they understand the patient's health condition/s. This is usually in the structure of a medical model including: Presenting Complaint (PC), History of Presenting Complaint (HPC), Past Medical History (PMH), Drug History (DH), Social History (SH), and acknowledge the patient's Ideas Concerns and Expectations (ICE) when providing pharmacological interventions and treatments (Bickly, 2017).

When Registered Nurses directly prepare, administer or have any input into pharmacology and medicines management, it is vital that they understand how medicines work and how they will affect the patient receiving medicinal treatment. The two most popular and well-published terms that are used to explore the effects of medications are pharmacokinetics and pharmacodynamics.

Pharmacokinetics

In its most basic form, pharmacokinetics is 'what the body does to drugs'. Pharmacokinetics can be considered as four processes: the absorption, distribution, metabolism and excretion (ADME) of drugs (Young and Pitcher, 2016), and their corresponding pharmacological, therapeutic or toxic responses.

Pharmacokinetic principles (the ADME process)

Pharmacokinetics describes the influence that the human body has on drugs or foreign chemicals over time (Young and Pitcher, 2016). The key concerns of pharmacokinetics are what the body does to the drug, how drugs are absorbed by the body, how they are distributed to the tissues, how drugs are metabolised by the body (with the liver being the primary organ for metabolisation of drugs) and elimination (primarily by the kidneys and lungs) (see Box 5.1).

Pharmacokinetics is important to our understanding of why drugs are administered via different routes. For example, why is a drug administered orally (PO) via tablet or liquid suspension form, or into the tissues by subcutaneous injection (SC), intramuscularly (IM) or directly

Box 5.1 Four stages of pharmacokinetics: ADME

1. Absorption of drugs into the body   How does it get into the body?
2. Distribution of drugs to the tissues of the body   Where will it go?
3. Metabolism of drugs into the body   How is it broken down?
4. Elimination of drugs from the body   How does it leave?

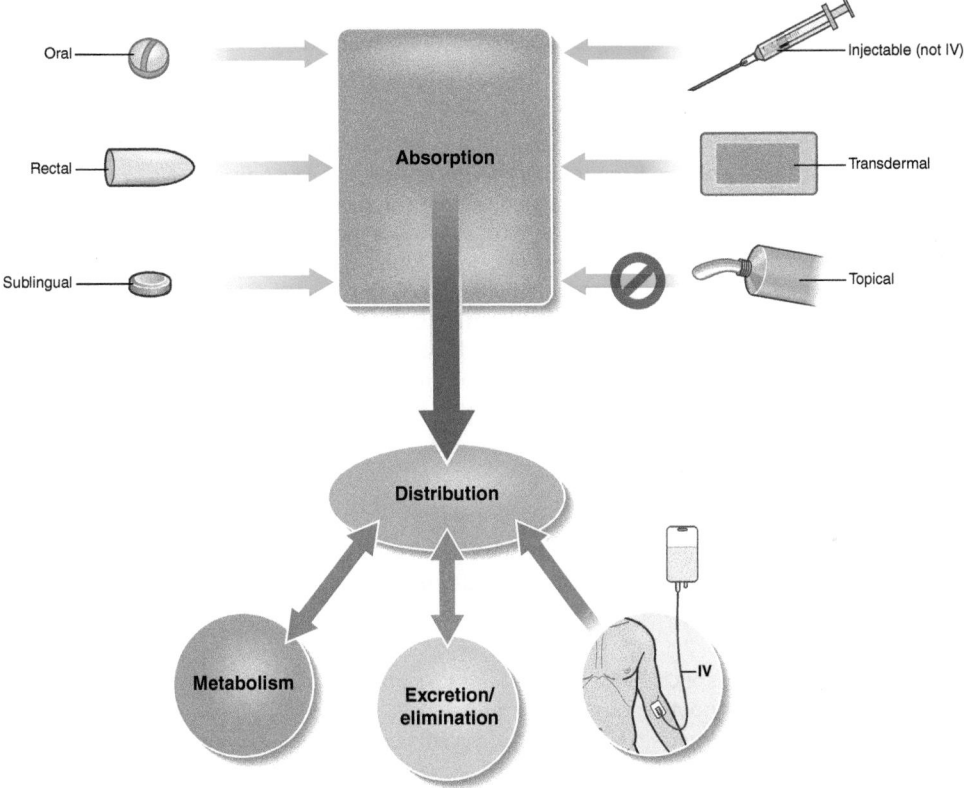

Figure 5.1 An integration of ADME and the routes of administration. Source: Adapted Young and Pitcher (2016).

into the bloodstream by intravenous (IV) injection? Chapter 6 of this text discusses drug formulations.

Pharmacokinetics also helps us appreciate the frequency of drug administration, for example: why are some drugs are administered once a day and others administered twice a day, three times a day, or four times a day, or even continuously via SC, IM or IV infusion via a mechanical pump? When thinking about the organs that work with drugs during the process of ADME, it becomes clear why absent, diseased or aged organs would affect the metabolisation of drugs.

Figure 5.1 integrates the four main features of pharmacokinetics (ADME) and the main routes or administration of medication. Note that the IV route bypasses absorption and the topical route is used to achieve a local effect and minimise absorption.

Phase 1: Absorption

Absorption is defined as the process by which a drug proceeds from the site of administration to the site of measurement (usually blood, plasma or serum). Absorption is the process of a drug/s entering the blood circulation. Le (2019) suggests that drug absorption is determined by the drug's physicochemical properties, formulation and route of administration, i.e. enteral or parenteral. Dosage forms (e.g. tablets, capsules, solutions), consisting of the drug plus other ingredients, are formulated to be given by various routes (e.g. oral, buccal, sublingual, rectal, parenteral, topical, inhalational). Regardless of the route of administration, drugs must be in solution to be absorbed. Thus, solid forms (e.g. tablets) must be able to disintegrate and disaggregate.

Unless given IV, a drug must cross several semi-permeable cell membranes before it reaches the systemic circulation. Cell membranes are biological barriers that selectively inhibit the passage of drug molecules. The membranes are composed primarily of a bimolecular lipid matrix, which determines membrane permeability characteristics.

How drugs cross the cell membrane

Many drugs need to pass through one or more cell membranes to reach their site of action. A common feature of all cell membranes is a phospholipid bilayer, about 10 Nanometer (nm) thick. Spanning this bilayer or attached to the outer or inner leaflets are glycoproteins, which may act as ion channels, receptors, intermediate messengers (G-proteins) or enzymes. Cells obtain molecules and ions from the extracellular fluid, creating a constant in and out flow. The interesting thing about cell membranes is that relative concentrations and phospholipid bilayers prevent essential ions from entering the cell. Therefore, for drugs to move across the membrane these problems must be addressed. In general, this is completed by facilitated diffusion or active transport. In facilitated diffusion, relative concentrations are used to transport in and out. Active transport uses energy (ATP) to transfer molecules and ions in and out of the cells.

Concept of drugs crossing the cell membrane

Cellular signals cross the membrane through a process called signal transduction. This three-step process proceeds when a specific message encounters the outside surface of the cell and makes direct contact with a receptor.

1. A receptor is a specialised molecule that takes information from the environment and passes it throughout various parts of the cell.
2. Next, a connecting switch molecule, a transducer, passes the message inward, closer to the cell.
3. Finally, the signal gets amplified, therefore causing the cell to perform a specific function. These functions can include moving, producing more proteins, or sending out more signals.

Methods of drugs crossing the cell membrane

Passive transport

The most common method for drugs to cross the cell membrane is by passive diffusion. Drug molecules will diffuse down their concentration gradient without expenditure of energy by the cell. However, the membranes are selectively permeable, so the membrane has different effects on the rate of diffusion on different drug molecules. The rate of diffusion can also be enhanced by transport proteins in the membrane by facilitated diffusion. There are two types of transport proteins that carry out the facilitated diffusion: channel proteins and carrier proteins.

Active transport

Active transport is an energy-requiring process. There are also two types of active transport: (1) primary active transport and (2) secondary active transport.

1. *Primary active transport* directly uses energy to transport molecules across a membrane. Occasionally the carrier protein can be an electrogenic pump.
2. *Secondary active transport* (or co-transport), also uses energy to transport molecules across a membrane.

Absorption depends on the administration route and can either be: (i) **enteral,** entering the GastroIntestinal (GI) tract, either by oral administration, feeding tubes, or rectal suppositories. Or **parenteral,** not into the GI tract, such as via injection or topical medicine (such as creams or patches).

To be absorbed, a drug given orally must survive encounters with low pH and numerous GI secretions, including potentially degrading enzymes. Peptide drugs (e.g. insulin) are particularly susceptible to degradation and are not given orally. Absorption of oral drugs involves transport across membranes of the epithelial cells in the GI tract. Absorption is affected by:

- differences in luminal pH along the GI tract;
- surface area per luminal volume;
- blood perfusion;
- presence of bile and mucus;
- the nature of epithelial membranes.

The oral mucosa has a thin epithelium and rich vascularity, which favour absorption; however, contact is usually too brief for substantial absorption. A drug placed between the gums and cheek (buccal administration) or under the tongue (sublingual administration) is retained longer, enhancing absorption.

The stomach has a relatively large epithelial surface, but its thick mucus layer and short transit time limit absorption. Because most absorption occurs in the small intestine, gastric emptying is often rate-limiting. Food, especially fatty food, slows gastric emptying (and rate of drug absorption), explaining why taking some drugs on an empty stomach speeds absorption. Drugs that affect gastric emptying (e.g. parasympatholytic drugs) affect the absorption rate of other drugs. Food may enhance the extent of absorption for poorly soluble drugs (e.g. Griseofulvin), reduce it for drugs degraded in the stomach (e.g. penicillin G), or have little or no effect.

The small intestine has the largest surface area for drug absorption in the GI tract and its membranes are more permeable than those in the stomach. For these reasons, most drugs are absorbed primarily in the small intestine. The intraluminal pH is 4 to 5 in the duodenum but becomes progressively more alkaline, approaching 8 in the lower ileum. GI microflora may reduce absorption. Decreased blood flow (e.g. in shock) may lower the concentration gradient across the intestinal mucosa and reduce absorption by passive diffusion.

Intestinal transit time can influence drug absorption, particularly for drugs that are absorbed by active transport (e.g. B vitamins), that dissolve slowly (e.g. griseofulvin), or that are polar (i.e. with low lipid solubility; e.g. many antibiotics).

To maximise adherence, clinicians should prescribe oral suspensions and chewable tablets for children less than eight years old. In adolescents and adults, most drugs are given orally as tablets or capsules primarily for convenience, economy, stability and patient acceptance. Because solid drug forms must dissolve before absorption can occur, the dissolution rate determines the availability of the drug for absorption. Dissolution, if slower than absorption, becomes the rate-limiting step. Manipulating the formulation (i.e. the drug's form as salt, crystal or hydrate) can change the dissolution rate and thus control overall absorption.

Enteral

Enteral medicines are medicines that enter the GI tract. Oral medicines, such as a tablet or liquid suspension, would normally be administered into the mouth of the patient and would pass into their GI tract. If the oral route is not an option, enteral medications may also be administered via nasogastric tube (NGT) or orogastric tube (OGT). From here, medicine would be absorbed via the GI tract wall and would enter plasma. Any substances that are absorbed via the GI wall will be transported by plasma to the liver via the hepatic portal vein (HPV); this is completed prior to being delivered to the body's tissues and organs. In pharmacology, this process is known as first-pass metabolism.

Parenteral

Drugs given IV enter the systemic circulation directly (Le, 2019). However, drugs injected IM or SC must cross one or more biological membranes to reach the systemic circulation. If protein drugs with a molecular mass > 20 000 g/mol are injected IM or SC, movement across capillary membranes is so slow that most absorption occurs via the lymphatic system. In such cases, drug delivery to systemic circulation is slow and often incomplete because of first-pass metabolism (metabolism of a drug before it reaches systemic circulation) by proteolytic enzymes in the lymphatic system.

Perfusion (blood flow/gram of tissue) greatly affects capillary absorption of small molecules injected IM or SC. Thus, the injection site can affect the absorption rate. Absorption after IM or SC injection may be delayed or erratic for salts of poorly soluble bases and acids (e.g. parenteral form of Phenytoin) and in patients with poor peripheral perfusion (e.g. during hypotension or shock).

Topical

Applying medication to the skin or mucus membranes allows it to enter the body from there. Medication applied in this way is known as topical medication. It can also be used to treat pain or other problems in specific parts of the body.

Topical medication can also be used to nourish the skin and protect it from harm. Some topical medications are used for local treatment and some are meant to affect the whole body after being absorbed through the skin.

Additional factors that can affect how the drug is absorbed are from the drug's formation, extended release versus immediate release, blood flow to the area of absorption, and GI motility for enteral medications. A common example of enteral medication would be Ibuprofen. Common parenteral medications include insulin and heparin. Some medications, such as Penicillin, have both enteral and parenteral formulations. See Table 5.1 and Figure 5.5.

Phase 2: Distribution

Distribution is the drug's dispersion through the body's fluids and tissues as it travels to its site of action (usually blood or plasma). This is dependent on blood flow, both to the area where the drug is to be administered and how perfusion occurs to other areas of the body, as well as protein binding. If a drug binds to protein, they become attached and therefore the drug cannot exert its effect on the body. The more a drug binds to protein, the less of the drug there is available for distribution.

Protein binding

Most drugs are bound to proteins in the blood and transported around the body by venous circulation. When drugs have bound to protein, they become enlarged and cannot enter capillaries and then into tissues to react. Some drugs are tightly bound and are released slowly, meaning that they have a longer duration of action as they are not broken down or excreted by the kidneys. Some drugs are in competition with other drugs at the same protein-binding site, which will change the effectiveness of the drug, or cause toxicity when two or more drugs of the same group are administered together (Karch, 2017).

Table 5.1   Factors that affect absorption of drugs.

Route	Factors Affecting Absorption
Intravenous (IV)	None: direct entry into the venous system
Intramuscular (IM)	Perfusion of blood flow to the muscle Fat content of the muscle Temperature of the muscle: cold causes vasoconstriction and decreases absorption; heat causes vasodilation and increases absorption
Subcutaneous (SC)	Perfusion of blood flow to the tissues Fat content of the tissue Temperature of the tissue: cold causes vasoconstriction and decreases absorption; heat causes vasodilation and increases absorption
Oral (PO)	Acidity of the stomach Length of time in the stomach Blow flow to the gastrointestinal tract Presence of interacting foods or drugs
Rectal (PR)	Perfusion of blood flow to the rectum Lesions in the rectum Length of time retained for absorption
Mucous membranes (sublingual, buccal)	Perfusion or blood flow to the area Integrity of mucus membranes Presence of food or smoking Length of time retained in area
Topical (skin)	Perfusion or blood flow to the area Integrity of skin
Inhalation	Perfusion or blood flow to the area Integrity of lung lining Ability to administer drug properly

Source: Karch (2017).

Blood–Brain Barrier

The Blood–Brain Barrier (BBB) prevents entry into the brain of most drugs from the blood. The BBB is a protective system of cellular activity that keeps many things out, such as foreign invaders and poisons. Drugs that are highly lipid soluble are more likely to pass through the BBB and reach the Central Nervous System (CNS). Drugs that are not lipid soluble are not able to pass the BBB. This is clinically significant in treating brain infections. For example, antibodies are too large to cross the BBB and only certain antibiotics can pass. The BBB becomes more permeable during inflammation, allowing antibiotics and phagocytes to move across it. However, this also allows bacteria and viruses to infiltrate BBB. Most antibiotics are not lipid soluble and therefore cannot treat brain infections as they are unable to cross the BBB. IV medications such as Rifampicin would be used in such cases. The presence of the BBB makes the development of new treatments of brain diseases, or new radiopharmaceuticals for neuroimaging of brain extremely complex. All of the products of biotechnology are large molecule drugs that do not cross the BBB.

Placenta and breast milk

The placenta is the lifeline of the developing foetus (Figure 5.2). It is a semi-permeable barrier through which all nutrients and waste products must pass. Several factors affect a medication's ability to cross the placenta; although many drugs are transported by passive diffusion based on the concentration gradient, conversely, if a medication is hydrophilic, ionised in maternal serum, and highly protein bound, little to no medication will cross. If there is little to

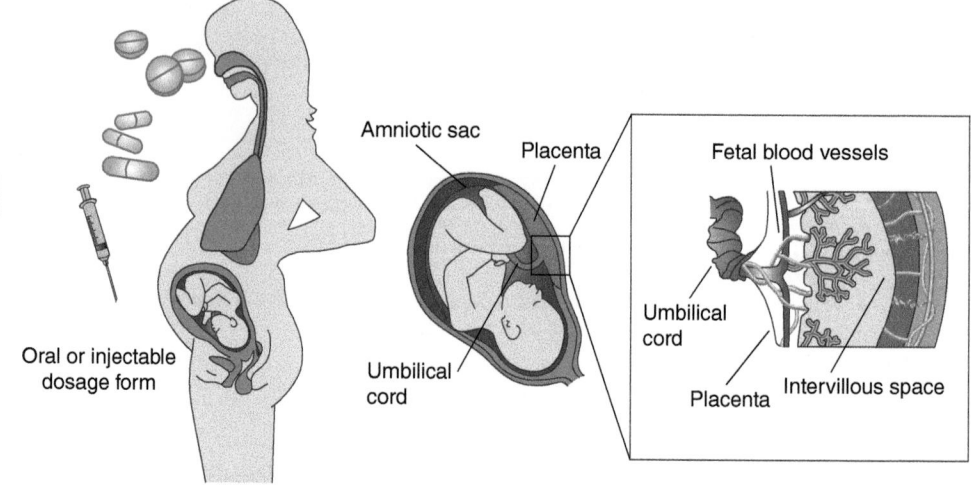

Figure 5.2   Medication delivery to baby during gestation.

no published safety data for a medication, the pharmacist can evaluate these details of a medication to predict the possibility of fetal exposure.

The transfer of medication into human milk shares some of the same principles as crossing the placenta, by passive diffusion. A medication may cross through the placenta into fetal circulation and back on the concentration gradient, just as a drug may pass into milk and diffuse back into the bloodstream as serum concentrations decrease. Certain properties of some medications may cause them to be sequestered into or actively excreted into breast milk (Hale, 2012). Drugs should only be given to pregnant women when the benefit clearly outweighs any risk. Drugs are likely to be secreted into breast milk and therefore have the potential to affect the neonate. All drugs must be checked prior to administration, this includes utilising the British National Formulary (BNF), organisation approved guidelines, and published contemporary medication guides. It is important to recognise that different guides support patients with specific needs, for example there is a renal BNF for patients with renal abnormalities (BNF and NICE, 2019c).

By better understanding the pharmacokinetics and pharmacodynamics of medications during lactation, nurses can assist mothers in making well-informed decisions about medication use during lactation. The most important factor in infant exposure through breast milk is the amount of medication in the mother's serum.

Phase 3: Metabolism (Biotransformation)

Metabolism, sometimes referred to as biotransformation, is recognition by the body that the drug is present and the transformation of the drug into usable parts. Most drugs are metabolised in the liver via the cytochrome P450 family of enzymes. Other organs involved may include the kidneys and intestines.

Drugs can be metabolised by oxidation, reduction, hydrolysis, hydration, conjugation, condensation or isomerisation; whatever the process, the goal is to make the drug easier to excrete. The enzymes involved in metabolism are present in many tissues but generally are more concentrated in the liver. Drug metabolism rates vary among different people. Some people metabolise a drug so rapidly that therapeutically effective blood and tissue concentrations are not reached; in others, metabolism may be so slow that usual doses have toxic effects. Individual drug metabolism rates are influenced by genetic factors, co-existing disorders (particularly chronic liver disorders and advanced heart failure) and drug interactions (especially those involving induction or inhibition of metabolism).

For many drugs, metabolism occurs in two phases.

- Phase I reactions involve formation of a new or modified functional group or cleavage (oxidation, reduction, hydrolysis); these reactions are non-synthetic.
- Phase II reactions involve conjugation with an endogenous substance (e.g. glucuronic acid, sulfate, glycine); these reactions are synthetic. Metabolites formed in synthetic reactions are more polar and thus more readily excreted by the kidneys (in urine) and the liver (in bile) than those formed in non-synthetic reactions. Some drugs undergo only phase I or phase II reactions; thus, phase numbers reflect functional rather than sequential classification.

According to Young and Pitcher (2016), certain drugs only undergo phase 1 metabolism, others only phase II metabolism, and some drugs have no metabolism at all. Some drugs underdo phase II metabolism and then phase I. Certain drugs – such as levodopa, used to treat Parkinson's disease – are inactive in the body until biotransformation takes place. These drugs are known as pro-drugs. Certain drugs, such as the antidepressant fluoxetine, are transformed into metabolites that are also active and these metabolites are partially responsible for the therapeutic activity of the drug agent.

Rate

For almost all drugs, the metabolism rate in any given pathway has an upper limit (capacity limitation). However, at therapeutic concentrations of most drugs, usually only a small fraction of the metabolising enzyme's sites are occupied and the metabolism rate increases with drug concentration (Le, 2019). In such cases, called first-order elimination (or kinetics), the metabolism rate of the drug is a constant fraction of the drug remaining in the body (i.e. the drug has a specific half-life).

First-pass metabolism

The first-pass effect (also known as first-pass metabolism or pre-systemic metabolism) (Figure 5.3) was coined by Rowland (1972) for the phenomenon of drug metabolism whereby the concentration of a drug is greatly reduced before it reaches the systemic circulation.

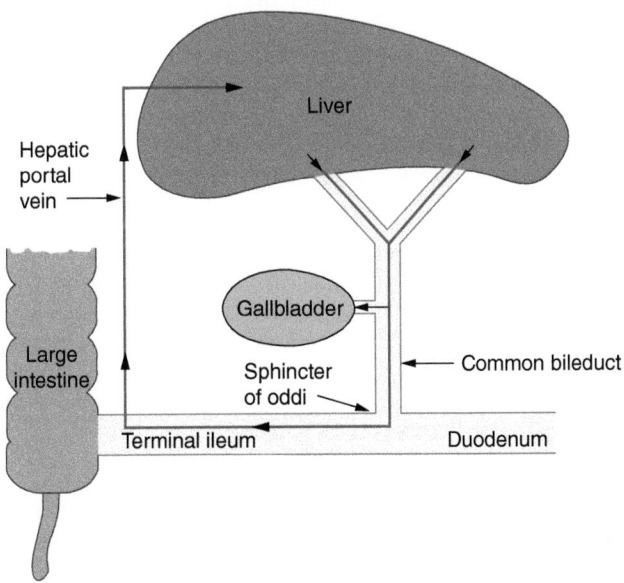

Figure 5.3   Hepatic first-pass metabolism (first-pass effect).

The process of drug metabolism is part of the body's normal response to removal of drugs and chemicals from the circulating system. Hepatic metabolism, or biotransformation, is the main site and method of the process of elimination. This is followed by excretion of the drug and its metabolites from the body. The liver plays an extremely important role in drug removal. When drug molecules are distributed in the blood stream, the plasma flow through the functional units of the liver presents these molecules for biotransformation. This occurs after administration by any route.

The oral route of drug administration is by far the most commonly used route. It is normally accessible and the least invasive route available in most cases. This route is well tolerated and convenient. Many common drugs are available in oral formulations as well as in preparations suitable for administration by other routes. There are very few drugs in the BNF that have no oral formulation.

Hepatic first-pass effect

Drugs given by the oral route are absorbed from the stomach and the small intestine into the HPV. This blood vessel goes directly to the liver. The process of biotransformation begins and the drug will start to be metabolised in preparation for excretion from the body. The drug molecules in the plasma move through circuiting volume. The drug molecules are now metabolised by liver enzymes. The 'first-pass effect' reduces the fraction of the dose administered, which then goes on to reach the systemic circulation and become available for therapeutic effect. This process occurs in the hepatic microsomal enzymes and includes the cytochrome P450 enzymes. For drugs given orally, the amount of first-pass metabolism known to occur has been factored into oral dosing by pharmaceutical companies. This means that the bioavailability, which is a known factor, has been considered when dose and dose ranges are advised in the BNF. It is important, therefore, that prescriber's and people who administer medication must establish any hepatic dysfunction for those receiving oral medications. If there is compromised liver function or a disease such as cirrhosis, then first-pass metabolism will be compromised. This could lead to more active drug entering the systemic circulation due to the reduced liver enzyme functionality and may cause side effects, adverse effects, or toxicity. Drug dosing may need to be reduced in patients in this situation. Some drugs are destroyed by liver enzymes at this first-pass stage and will not enter the general systemic circulation. An example of such a drug is glyceryl trinitrate, which is metabolised completely by the liver and inactivated. Consequently, you will find GTN being given via non oral routes; sublingual being a very good alternative. Not all oral drugs are destroyed by the liver at first pass, but many clinically significant drugs do undergo an extensive first-pass effect. Therefore, the doses of some drugs are considerably higher when given by the oral route compared to their dosing if given intravenously.

Two drugs given together may change the absorption of either one or both of the drugs. For example, a drug that may change the acidity of stomach acid is likely to affect a drug that is dissolved in the stomach. Other drugs can interact and form an insoluble compound that can't be absorbed. Sometimes an absorption interaction can be avoided by separating the administration of each drug by at least two hours (Gersh et al., 2016).

1. The drug is absorbed by the GI tract.
2. Drug absorbed from the GI tract travels immediately to the liver through the HPV.
3. The first-pass effect occurs at this stage. Hepatic first pass occurs when drug absorbed from the GI tract is metabolised by enzymes within the liver to such an extent that most of the active agent does not exit the liver and, therefore, does not reach the systemic circulation.
4. The remaining drug is distributed around the body within blood cells and plasma.

Phase 4: Elimination

Elimination is the irreversible loss of drug from the site of measurement (blood, serum, plasma). Elimination of drugs occur by one or both of:

- metabolism
- excretion.

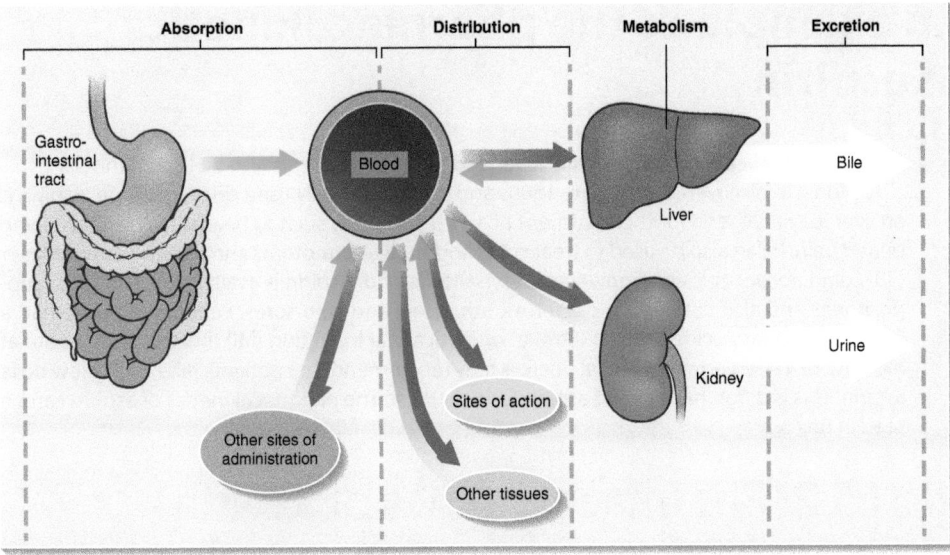

Figure 5.4 Pharmacokinetics (ADME) and the main anatomical structures/physiological systems that are responsible for executing those processes. Source: Adapted Young and Pitcher (2016).

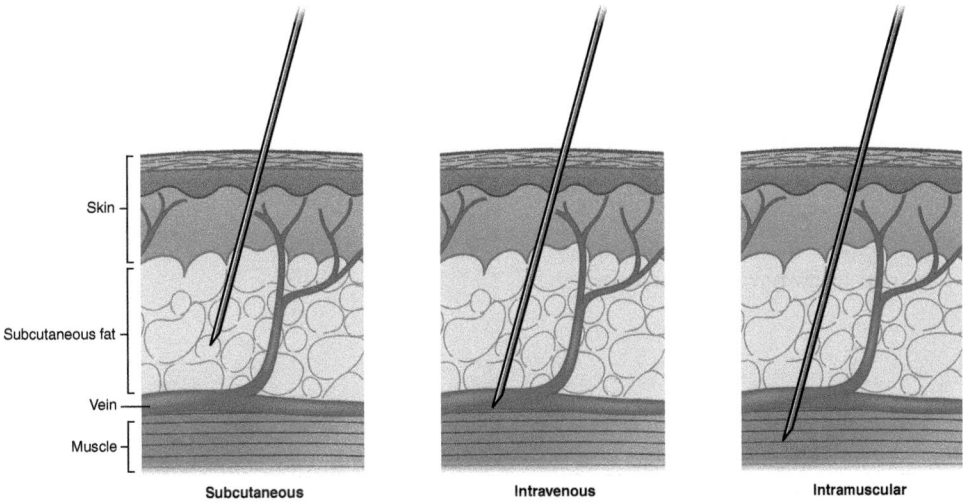

Figure 5.5 Injectable routes of administration. Source: Adapted Young and Pitcher (2016).

Excretion

Excretion is the irreversible loss of a drug in a chemically unchanged or unaltered form. The two principal organs responsible for drug elimination are the kidney and the liver. The kidney is the primary site for removal of a drug in a chemically unaltered or unchanged form (i.e. excretion) as well as for metabolites. The liver is the primary organ where drug metabolism occurs. The lungs, occasionally, may be an important route of elimination for substances of high vapour pressure (i.e. gaseous anesthetics, alcohol). Another potential route of drug removal is via breast milk. Although not a significant route for elimination of a drug for the mother, the drug may be consumed in enough quantity to affect her baby or infant (Figure 5.4).

An example of the pharmacokinetics of aspirin
Aspirin

Aspirin is a medication used for pain, fever and inflammation. It is also a blood thinner.

Aspirin was discovered in the late 1800s and has been widely used since that time. Aspirin is an everyday analgesia for the treatment of aches and pains such as headache, toothache and period pain. It can also be used to treat colds and 'flu-like' symptoms and to bring down a fever (38 °C and above). It is also known as acetylsalicylic acid. Aspirin is available as tablets or suppositories and also comes as a gel for mouth ulcers and cold sores. People who have had a Cerebro Vascular Accident (CVA) (Stroke) or Myocardial Infarction (MI) (heart attack) or are at high risk of a heart attack. Medical doctors may recommend that patients take a daily low dose aspirin. This is different to taking aspirin for pain relief. The pharmacokinetics of aspirin can be seen in Box 5.2.

Box 5.2 Pharmacokinetics of aspirin

A   Aspirin is available in oral forms. When taken, it is absorbed in the gastrointestinal tract.

D   It is distributed to all tissues of the body. In pregnant women, it does cross the placenta to the foetus. It is also passed through breast milk to a nursing infant.

M   In the body, it quickly breaks down into salicylic acid and the liver changes it into metabolites. The half-life of aspirin is only 15–20 minutes. Half-life is the amount of time it takes to decrease the concentration of the drug in the body by half. Once aspirin is broken down into salicylic acid, it has a half-life of six hours. In higher doses, half-life increases and in toxic doses (over dose) it may exceed 20 hours.

E   It is then excreted by the kidneys.

Some of the clinical considerations when thinking about pharmacokinetics can be seen in in the following clinical considerations.

Clinical considerations

Half-life
The half-life of medication is how long it takes for the medication to be reduced by half of its blood concentration level. This is done through metabolisation. It can be affected by the individual's ability to metabolise, such as if the patient has renal failure and liver damage.

Clinical considerations

Steady state
A steady state (SS) is when the amount of drug administered is equal to the amount of drug eliminated within a one dose interval, resulting in a plateau or constant serum drug level. Drugs with a short half-life reach steady state rapidly, while drugs with a long half-life can take days to weeks to reach a steady state.

Clinical considerations

Termination of action

A termination of action is when the medication has stopped its action at the site where it is required. This may be seen in analgesic control; when pain returns, the medication has stopped acting.

Clinical considerations

Therapeutic range

The therapeutic range is similar to the therapeutic index. It is the range area where medication is effective. Linking back to analgesic control, it is the period from when pain is blocked to when it returns.

This can be seen with medication such as paracetamol, where you can repeat the dose of 1 g every four to six hours. Greater dosages can be toxic having exceeded the therapeutic index.

The example of paracetamol and ibuprofen (subject to any contraindications) can be seen in Figure 5.6, where to maintain the therapeutic level (black line) the two medications are used to complement each other, while not exceeding the recommended dose and thus the therapeutic index.

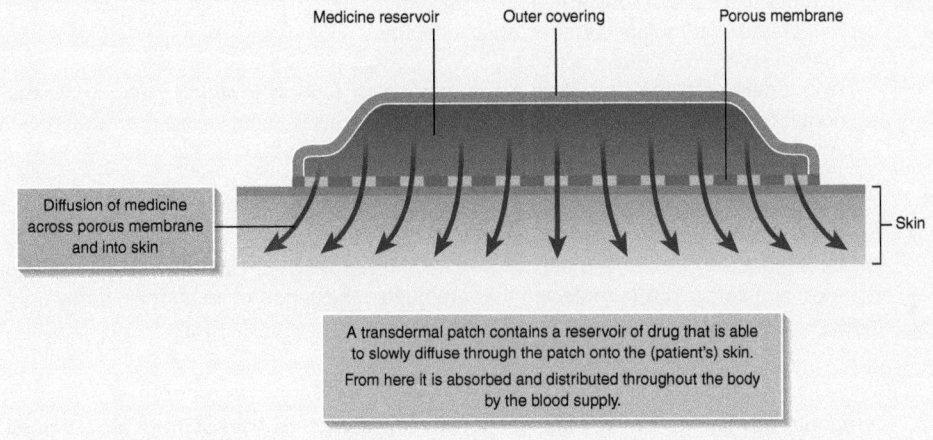

Medicine reservoir   Outer covering   Porous membrane

Diffusion of medicine across porous membrane and into skin

Skin

A transdermal patch contains a reservoir of drug that is able to slowly diffuse through the patch onto the (patient's) skin. From here it is absorbed and distributed throughout the body by the blood supply.

Figure 5.6   Diagram illustrating how a transdermal patch works. Source: Adapted Young and Pitcher (2016).

Routes of drug administration

The sites of drug administration include:

- oral
- sublingual
- rectal
- vaginal
- parenrteal: intravenous, intramuscular and subcutaneous – an illustration can be seen in Figure 5.5
- topical – an illustration can be seen in Figure 5.6 (see Chapter 6 in this book for further information).

Pharmacodynamics

Pharmacodynamics explores what the drug does to the body; specifically, how the drug molecules interact within the body, what they interact with, and how they cause their effects (Young and Pitcher, 2016, p. 21). To expand on this, a drug exerts its biological effects by interacting with the receptors located on tissues and organs throughout the body. The effects of the drug are dependent upon the drug's ability to bind to a variety of the body's receptors (Gersh et al., 2016). For example, if a drug's concentration is increased where many receptors are located, the intensity of the drug's effect will be improved. Therefore, the pharmacological response depends on the drug's ability to bind to its target. The concentration of the drug at the receptor site influences the drug's effect.

One of the key challenges for nurses when studying pharmacodynamics is that drugs are affected by a patient's physiological changes, such as disease, genetic mutations, ageing, and/or by other drugs. These changes are likely to alter the level of binding proteins, or decrease receptor sensitivity (Campbell and Cohall, 2017). It is important that nurses recognise that some drugs acting on the same receptor (or tissue) differ in the magnitude of the biological responses that they can achieve (i.e. their 'efficacy') and the amount of the drug required to achieve a response (i.e. their 'potency'). Drug receptors can be classified based on their selective response to different drugs. Constant exposure of receptors or body systems to drugs sometimes leads to a reduced response; for example, desensitisation.

All medications act in one of four ways (Karch, 2017):

1. To replace or act as a substitute for missing chemicals.
2. To increase or stimulate certain cellular activities.
3. To depress or slow cellular activities.
4. To interfere with the functioning of foreign cells, such as invading microorganisms or neoplasms leading to cell death (drugs that act in this way are called chemotherapeutic agents).

Agonists and antagonists

The terms agonist (a molecule that binds to a receptor causing activation and resultant cellular changes) and antagonist (a molecule that attenuates the action of an agonist) apply only to receptors. See Figure 5.7.

Agonist

An agonist is an example of a drug that interacts with receptors. Agonist drugs are attracted to receptors and stimulate them. Once stimulation has occurred, the agonist binds to the receptor and the drug effect occurs: the outcome of this activity is known as intrinsic activity. Agonists can be full, partial or inverse. Some drugs act on a variety of receptors. These are known as non-selective and can cause multiple and widespread effects (Gersh et al., 2016).

Pleuvry (2004) notes that a full agonist can produce the largest response that the tissue can give. The term 'efficacy' has been used to describe the way that agonists can vary in the response they produce even when occupying the same number of receptors. A high-efficacy agonist produces a maximum response even when occupying a small proportion of the available receptors. The magnitude of response to an agonist is usually proportional to the fraction of receptors that are occupied. As the concentration of an agonist at its site of action increases, so the fraction of occupied receptors rises and, in turn, the magnitude of response rises. A partial agonist cannot fully activate the receptors, irrespective of the concentration available. In contrast to a full agonist, a partial agonist cannot exert a maximal response. Finally, an inverse agonist: the simplest definition is that the compound binds to a receptor but produces the opposite effect from an accepted agonist.

An example of a widely used agonist is Salbutamol. Salbutamol is a β_2 agonist. One easy way to remember the location of β_1 and β_2 cells simply and quickly is that humans have one heart

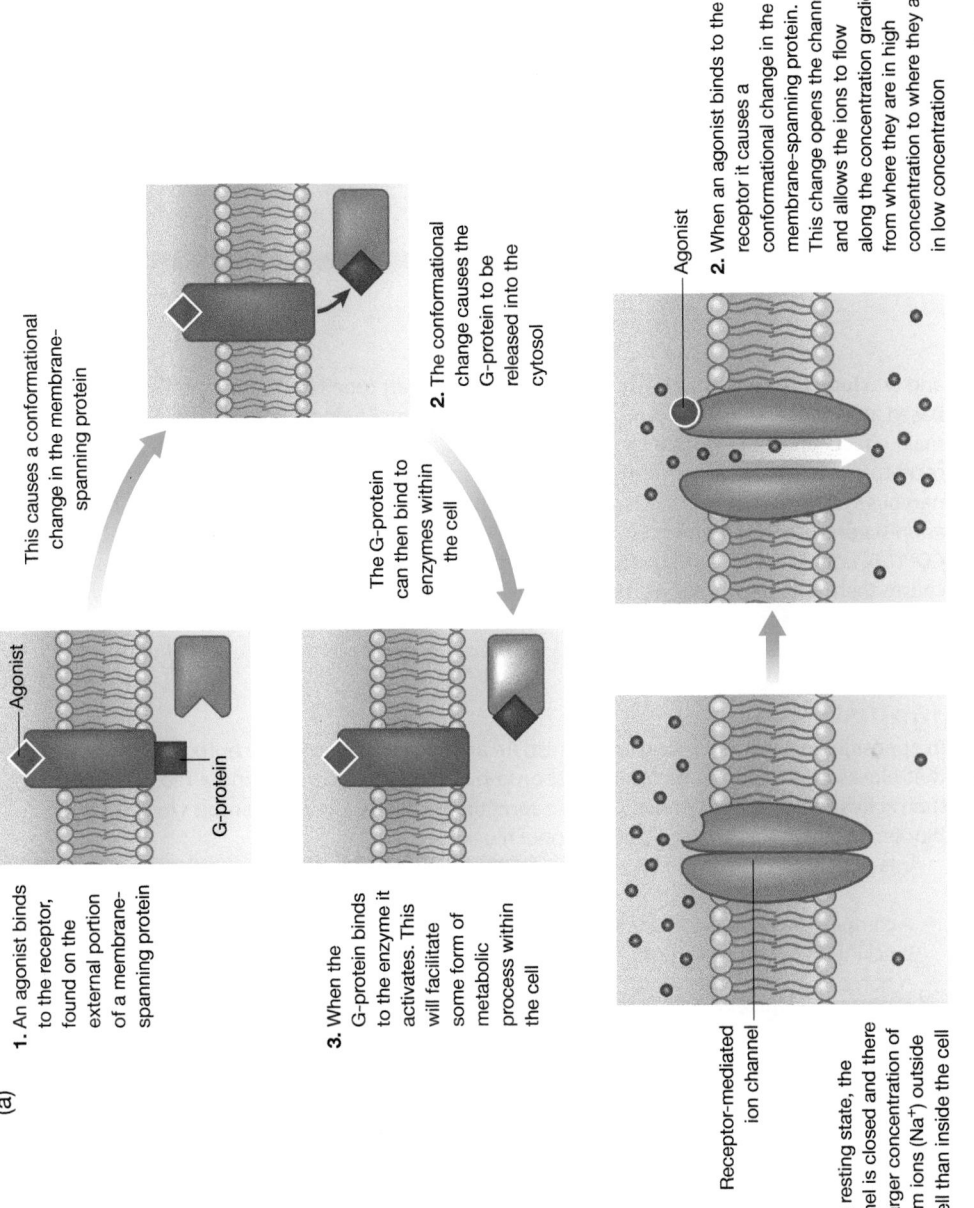

(a)

1. An agonist binds to the receptor, found on the external portion of a membrane-spanning protein

Agonist

G-protein

This causes a conformational change in the membrane-spanning protein

2. The conformational change causes the G-protein to be released into the cytosol

The G-protein can then bind to enzymes within the cell

3. When the G-protein binds to the enzyme it activates. This will facilitate some form of metabolic process within the cell

(b)

Receptor-mediated ion channel

1. In the resting state, the channel is closed and there is a larger concentration of sodium ions (Na⁺) outside the cell than inside the cell

Agonist

2. When an agonist binds to the receptor it causes a conformational change in the membrane-spanning protein. This change opens the channel and allows the ions to flow along the concentration gradient, from where they are in high concentration to where they are in low concentration

Figure 5.7 (a) The step-by-step process of a second messenger system. (b) Step-by-step receptor-mediated ion channel. Source: Adapted Young and Pitcher (2016).

Table 5.2   Examples of opioid by receptor binding.

Full Agonist	Partial Agonist	Mixed Agonist	Antagonist (also known as blockers or reversals)
Codeine	Buprenorphine	Buprenorphine	Naloxone
Fentanyl	Butorphanol	Butorphanol	Naltrexone
Heroin	Pentazocine	Nalbuphine	
Hydrocodone	Tramadol	Pentazocine	
Hydromorphone			
Levorphanol			
Meperidine			
Methadone			
Morphine			
Oxycodone			
Oxymorphone			

and two lungs. β_1 cells are mainly based around the heart (one heart) and β_2 cells are mainly based around the lungs (two lungs). Therefore, Salbutamol being a β_2 agonist would have its main effects on the receptors based within the lungs. β_1 receptors, along with β_2, α_1 and α_2 receptors, are adrenergic receptors primarily responsible for signalling in the sympathetic nervous system. β-agonists bind to the β-receptors on various tissues throughout the body. β_2 agonists are used for both asthma and COPD, although some types are only available for COPD. β_2 agonists work by stimulating β_2 receptors in the muscles that line the airways, which causes them to relax and allows the airways to widen (dilate). Hence why Salbutamol is known as a bronchodilator.

Using opioids as an example, Table 5.2 gives examples of opioid by receptor binding.

Antagonists

In opposition of an agonist is an antagonist. An antagonist is a type of receptor ligand or drug that blocks or dampens a biological response by binding to and blocking a receptor rather than activating it like an agonist. They are sometimes called blockers; examples include alpha blockers, beta blockers and calcium channel blockers.

Antagonists can be competitive or non-competitive:

- A competitive antagonist binds to the same site as the agonist but does not activate it, thus blocking the agonist's action.
- A non-competitive antagonist binds to an allosteric (non-agonist) site on the receptor to prevent activation of the receptor.

Clinical considerations

Confidence in the drug

In clinical practice, all drugs have been tested through rigorous drug research trials prior to being made available for safe prescription and administration (unless patients have provided informed consent and are actively enrolled on early human clinical trials) (see Chapter 4 of this text). These drugs are licensed for use within a recommended dose range. This ensures that patients achieve a good response to their medication, without the need for constant review and titration of their prescription. This is known as the therapeutic index.

Episode of care: Mental health

Mr. Jones is a 32-year-old Welshman with a previous medical history of depression. Mr. Jones has had continuous depression for a year and a half. He has been diagnosed with dysthymia (persistent depressive disorder or chronic depression). Mr. Jones has been feeling tired and can easily become tearful. At times he has a sense of isolation and displays an inability to interact or relate to people around him. Mr. Jones has been prescribed a monoamine oxidase inhibitor (MAOIs) called phenelzine. Mr. Jones had previously been prescribed amitriptyline, which is in the tricyclic antidepressant (TCA) drug classification and acts by blocking the reuptake of both serotonin and norepinephrine neurotransmitters. Mr. Jones could only tolerate amitriptyline for a short time as he felt 'spaced out' and said that he felt worse and had dark thoughts and feelings. Mr. Jones is concerned as he does not recall what was said to him regarding his new medication.

Medications are often utilised after self-help and other therapies or activities, depending on the patient's circumstances (see NICE 2009, 2018).

Clinical considerations

The side effects of medication can be wide ranging, especially when people start a new medication; as a registrant you must understand medicines management including side effects and monitoring the effects of medication. You should report/take action where there is a possible or actual side effect.

Some medications may exacerbate a patient's underlying health condition, and in such cases the nurse must pay diligence to the patient's vital signs to observe any deteriorating signs and symptoms. In this instance, the identified side effects of amitriptyline can be seen in the early stages of treatment and reflect known issues such as blurred vision, dry mouth, low blood pressure on standing, sleepiness and constipation around TCAs such as amitriptyline (MIND, 2016; NHS, 2018a; BNF and NICE, 2019a).

The change to phenelzine and lack of awareness by Mr. Jones should cause concern to the nurse. Patient education on medication is a fundamental underpinning priority to ensure compliance, concordance and management, ensuring up-to-date information on medicines is utilised.

Drug potency and efficacy

The concepts of potency and efficacy are often confused and used interchangeably within the scientific and pharmaceutical industry. It is important that the distinction between the two is understood and that the terms are defined within their correct context. Potency is an expression of the activity of a drug in terms of the concentration or amount of the drug required to produce a defined effect, whereas clinical efficacy judges the therapeutic effectiveness of the drug in humans. Drug potency is also used to compare two drugs. For example, if Drug A and Drug B both produce the same response, but Drug A does this at a lower dose, that means Drug A is more potent than Drug B.

Therapeutic index

The therapeutic index is the range at which a medication is therapeutic to the individual. A drug with a low or narrow therapeutic index (NTI) has a narrow range of safety between an effective dose and a lethal one. Alternatively, a drug with a high therapeutic index will have a wide range of safety and fewer risks of toxic effects. It should be noted that doubling a dose of a drug does not mean that the therapeutic effect will be doubled, but will most likely double the toxic effect. Furthermore, administration above the dose at which the maximum effect is observed will produce no added benefit.

Therapeutic range will rise and fall depending on the medication formulation, its strength and the time it has until it is broken down and metabolised within the body. This process can be affected by the patient's health and organ condition/s, particularly the patient's liver and kidney function. For example, the liver is the principal site of drug metabolism. Although metabolism typically inactivates drugs, some drug metabolites are pharmacologically active. An inactive or weakly active substance that has an active metabolite is called a prodrug, especially if designed to deliver the active moiety (The molecule or ion which is responsible for the physiological or pharmacological action of the drug) more effectively.

Some medication has what is called a NTI, meaning the gap between effective and toxic effect is small. Some examples of drugs that are known to have an NTI can be seen in Box 5.3. Slight changes in medication dose or blood concentration level need to be carefully monitored and recorded (see Boxes 5.4 and 5.5 for examples).

Box 5.3 Narrow therapeutic index examples

Drug Name	Indication	Drug Group
PHENYTOIN	Tonic–clonic seizures, Focal seizures	Anticonvulsants
CARBAMAZEPINE	Focal and secondary generalised tonic–clonic seizures, Primary generalised tonic–clonic seizures	Anticonvulsants
GENTAMICIN	Infection	Aminoglycoside antibiotics
VANCOMYCIN	Infection	Glycopeptide antibiotics
TEICOPLANIN	Serious infections caused by gram-positive bacteria	Glycopeptide antibiotics
LITHIUM	Treatment and prophylaxis of mania, Treatment and prophylaxis of bipolar disorder, Treatment and prophylaxis of recurrent depression, Treatment and prophylaxis of aggressive or self-harming behaviour	Antimanic agents
DIGOXIN	Rapid digitalisation, for atrial fibrillation or flutter	Cardiac glycosides
AMINOPHYLLINE and THEOPHYLLINE	Severe acute asthma or severe acute exacerbation of COPD in patients not previously treated with Theophylline.	Xanthines

Source: Joint Formulary Committee (2019).

Box 5.4 An example of the monitoring requirements of aminophylline (NICE, 2020)

Aminophylline is a stable mixture or combination of theophylline and ethylenediamine; the ethylenediamine confers greater solubility in water. Theophylline is metabolised in the liver. The plasma–theophylline concentration is increased in heart failure, hepatic impairment and in viral infections. The plasma–theophylline concentration is decreased in smokers and by alcohol consumption. Differences in the half-life of aminophylline are important because the toxic dose is close to the therapeutic dose.

Monitoring requirements (Therapeutic Drug Monitoring)

Aminophylline is monitored therapeutically in terms of plasma–theophylline concentrations. Measurement of plasma–theophylline concentration may be helpful and is essential if a loading dose of intravenous aminophylline is to be given to patients who are already taking theophylline, because serious side effects such as convulsions and arrhythmias can occasionally precede other symptoms of toxicity.

In most individuals, a plasma–theophylline concentration of 10–20 mg/L (55–110 μmol/L) is required for satisfactory bronchodilation, although a lower plasma–theophylline concentration of 5–15 mg/L may be effective. Adverse effects can occur within the range 10–20 mg/L and both the frequency and severity increase at concentrations above 20 mg/L.

If aminophylline is given intravenously, a blood sample should be taken four to six hours after starting treatment to measure plasma–theophylline concentration.

With oral use

Plasma–theophylline concentration is measured five days after starting oral treatment and at least three days after any dose adjustment. A blood sample should usually be taken four to six hours after an oral dose of a modified-release preparation (sampling times may vary – consult local guidelines).

Box 5.5 Phenytoin: An example of therapeutic drug monitoring (BNF, 2019b)

Ethnicity

HLA-B (major histocompatibility complex, class I, B) is a human gene that provides instructions for making a protein that plays a critical role in the immune system. HLA-B is part of a family of genes called the human leukocyte antigen (HLA) complex. The HLA complex helps the immune system distinguish the body's own proteins from proteins made by foreign invaders such as viruses and bacteria. The HLA-B*1502 allele is highly associated with the outcome of drug induced Stevens–Johnson syndrome and toxic epidermal necrolysis. HLAB* 1502 allele in individuals of Han Chinese or Thai origin should be avoided unless crucial (as this increases the risk of Stevens–Johnson syndrome). The syndrome is uncommon; however, it is a serious disorder that affects the skin, mucus membrane, genitals, and eyes (NHS, 2018b). The mucus membrane is the soft layer of tissue that lines the digestive system from the mouth to the anus, as well as the genital tract (reproductive organs) and eyeballs. Stevens–Johnson syndrome is usually caused by an adverse random reaction to particular medications. It may also be the result of infection. Often the syndrome starts with flu-like symptoms, and this is followed by a red or purple rash that extends with blister formation. The area of skin that has been affected will eventually die and peel off. Stevens–Johnson syndrome is a medical emergency requiring in-patient treatment, often in intensive care or a burns unit.

In Adults

The usual total plasm–phenytoin concentration for optimum response is 10–20 mg/L (or 40–80 μmol/L). In pregnancy, the elderly, and certain disease states where protein binding may be reduced, careful interpretation of total plasma–phenytoin concentration is necessary; measuring free plasma–phenytoin concentration may be more appropriate.

Source: BNF (2019b) https://bnf.nice.org.uk/drug/phenytoin.html#indicationsAndDoses

Adverse effects

The International Union of Basic and Clinical Pharmacology (IUPHAR) (2019) suggests that the adverse effects of drugs are often dose-related in a similar way to the beneficial effects. Drugs have multiple potential adverse effects, but the concept of the therapeutic index is usually reserved for those requiring dose reduction or discontinuation. Drugs with low therapeutic indices are more difficult to prescribe and hazardous for patients, but they are still preferred if there are no alternative drugs with similar efficacy (e.g. anticancer drugs). The doses of such drugs must be titrated carefully for individual patients to maximise benefits but avoid adverse effects. This is done by monitoring drug effects, either clinically or using regular blood tests (often known as 'therapeutic drug monitoring').

Conclusion

This chapter has introduced the reader to pharmacodynamics and pharmacokinetics of medicines. The reader should now be able to acknowledge the professional responsibilities of registered healthcare professionals who administer drugs to patients; define and understand the differences between pharmacodynamics and pharmacokinetics; and appreciate the complexities of how drugs work differently in every individual.

References

Bickly, L. (2017). *Bates' Guide to History Taking and Physical Examination*, 12e. Walters Kluwer.

BNF and NICE (2019a). Amitriptyline. https://bnf.nice.org.uk/drug/amitriptyline-hydrochloride.html (accessed 8 October 2019).

BNF and NICE (2019b). Phenelzine. https://bnf.nice.org.uk/drug/phenelzine.html (accessed 8 October 2019).

BNF and NICE (2019c). Guidance: prescribing in renal impairment. https://bnf.nice.org.uk/guidance/prescribing-in-renal-impairment.html (accessed 2 October 2019).

Campbell, J.E. and Cohall, D. (2017). Pharmacodynamics – a Pharmacognosy perspective. In: *Pharmacognosy: Fundamentals, Applications, and Strategies* (eds. S. Badal and R. Delgoda), 513–525. New York: Elsevier-Inc.

Gersh, C., Heimgartner, N., Rebar, C., and Willis, L. (2016). *Pharmacology Made Incredibly Easy!* 4the. Philadelphia: Wolters Kluwer.

Hale, T.W. (2012). *Medication and Mother's Milk*, 15e. Amarillo, TX: Hale Publishing.

Health Education England (HEE) (2017). Advisory guidance administration of medicines by nursing associates. https://www.hee.nhs.uk/sites/default/files/documents/Advisory%20guidance%20-%20administration%20of%20medicines%20by%20nursing%20associates.pdf (accessed 2 October 2019).

Karch, A. (2017). *Focus on Nursing Pharmacology*, 7e, 18–19. Philadelphia: Wolters Kluwer.

Le, J. (2019). Drug metabolism. https://www.msdmanuals.com/en-gb/professional/clinical-pharmacology/pharmacokinetics/drug-metabolism (accessed 2 October 2019).

MIND (2016). Information and support. www.mind.org.uk/information-support/drugs-and-treatments/medication/explaining-the-half-life/#.XYZFn-NKiUk (accessed 2 October 2019).

NHS (2018a). Antidepressants. https://www.nhs.uk/conditions/antidepressants (accessed 8 October 2019).

NHS (2018b). Stevens-Johnson syndrome. https://www.nhs.uk/conditions/stevens-johnson-syndrome (accessed 8 October 2019).

NICE (2009). Guideline CG90: Depression in adults with a chronic physical health problem: recognition and management. www.nice.org.uk/guidance/CG91 (accessed 8 October 2019).

NICE (2020). Aminophylline. https://bnfc.nice.org.uk/drug/aminophylline.html (accessed 3 July 2020).

NMC (2018). The NMC Code. https://www.nmc.org.uk/globalassets/sitedocuments/nmc-publications/nmc-code.pdf (accessed 6 February 2019).

Pleuvry, B. (2004). Pharmacology: receptors, agonists and antagonists. *Anaesthesia and Intensive Care Medicine* 5 (10): 350–352.

RPS and RCN (2019). Professional guidance on the administration of medicines in healthcare settings. https://www.rpharms.com/Portals/0/RPS%20document%20library/Open%20access/Professional%20standards/SSHM%20and%20Admin/Admin%20of%20Meds%20prof%20guidance.pdf?ver=2019-01-23-145026-567 (accessed 8 October 2019).

Rowland, M. (1972). Influence of route of administration on drug availability. *Journal of Pharmaceutical Sciences* 61 (1): 70–74. https://doi.org/10.1002/jps.2600610111.

The International Union of Basic and Clinical Pharmacology (IUPHAR) (2019). Pharmacodynamics. https://www.pharmacologyeducation.org/pharmacology/pharmacodynamics (accessed 6 February 2019).

Young, S. and Pitcher, B. (2016). *Medicine Management for Nurses at a Glance*. Chicester, UK: Wiley Blackwell.

Multiple choice questions

1. An accurate definition of pharmacodynamics is
   (a) The study of how a certain concentration of a drug produces a biological effect by interacting with specific targets at its site of action
   (b) The study of how the body affects the given drug
   (c) The study of how a drug affects the body
2. Pharmacodynamics is that they can be affected by physiologic changes due to disease, genetic mutations, aging, and/or other drugs.
   (a) True
   (b) False
3. Drugs usually work in which way:
   (a) To replace or act as a substitute for missing chemicals
   (b) To increase or stimulate certain cellular activities
   (c) To depress or slow cellular activities
   (d) To interfere with the functioning of foreign cells, such as invading microorganisms or neoplasms leading to cell death (drugs that act in this way are called chemotherapeutic agents.
   (e) All of the above
4. What is meant by Medications that have a Narrow Therapeutic Index?
   (a) the gap between effective and toxic effect is large
   (b) the gap between effective and toxic effect is small
   (c) the gap between effective and toxic effect is insignificant
5. Pharmacokinetics is the study of drugs and their corresponding pharmacological, therapeutic, or toxic responses in man and animals. Is this:
   (a) True
   (b) False
6. What does ADME mean?
   (a) absorption, distribution, metabolism and elimination
   (b) absorption, digestion, metabolism and excretion
   (c) administration, distribution, metabolism and excretion
   (d) absorption, distribution, metabolism and excretion
7. What is ADME the process of:
   (a) Pharmacodynamics
   (b) Pharmacokinetics
   (c) Pharmacovigilance
   (d) Pharmacotherapeutics
8. The two principal organs responsible for drug elimination are:
   (a) the spleen and the respiratory system
   (b) the kidneys and the bowel
   (c) the spleen and the bowel
   (d) the kidney and the liver

9. A drug that may change the acidity for the stomach acid is likely to affect a drug that is dissolved in the stomach
    (a) True
    (b) False

10. Active transports uses energy (ATP) to transfer molecules and ions in and out of the cell.

    (a) True
    (b) False

11. Drug potency is an expression of
    (a) how much alcohol is used within the drug
    (b) the activity that judges the therapeutic effectiveness of the drug in humans.
    (c) the activity of a drug in terms of the concentration or amount of the drug required to produce a defined effect

12. Clinical efficacy
    (a) judges the therapeutic effectiveness of the drug in humans.
    (b) is the activity of a drug in terms of the concentration or amount of the drug required to produce a defined effect
    (c) is how ethical it is to administer the drug

13. People of Han Chinese or Thai origin have an increased risk of developing Stevens- Johnson syndrome when taking Phenytoin
    (a) True
    (b) False

14. Another name for biotransformation is:
    (a) Administration
    (b) Distribution
    (c) Metabolism
    (d) Elimination

15. Drugs that are not lipid soluble are
    (a) not able to pass the BBB
    (b) can pass the BBB

Chapter 6

Drug formulations

Hayley Underdown and Nicola Clipperton

Aim

The aim of this chapter is to review the many different drug formulations and the points of consideration involved with the prescribing, dispensing and administering to patients.

Learning objectives

After reading this chapter, the reader will be able to:

1. Identify the many different formulations that medicines are available in
2. Understand the reasons why a certain drug formulation may be selected by the prescriber
3. Acknowledge and appreciate the complexities surrounding the administration of medications via different routes
4. Acknowledge and appreciate the risks and considerations regarding altering medication dose form by crushing/dissolving
5. Understand and accept the professional responsibilities of registered healthcare professionals who administer medications to patients.

Test your knowledge

1. How many different formulations of medications are there?
2. Why is the specific formulation of a medication important and what implications may this have in the care setting?
3. What are the key issues a heath practitioner should take into account when considering the route of a drug administration?
4. What are ACE inhibitors used for and how are they administered? If a patient was to ask you for the rationale for the route of administration, how would you explain it?
5. Discuss the benefits and rationale for sublingual drug administration and when this route may be used in practice.
6. Can you list the '7 rights' to consider when administering medications to patients?

Fundamentals of Pharmacology: For Nursing and Healthcare Students, First Edition. Edited by Ian Peate and Barry Hill.
© 2021 John Wiley & Sons Ltd. Published 2021 by John Wiley & Sons Ltd.

Introduction

This chapter explores the different formulations in which medications are available. In contemporary healthcare, medications are now available in a variety of formulations and preparations. The reason for these many formulations relates to the way in which certain medications work and are broken down and the individual needs of the patient (e.g. age, sex, health condition and so forth). The many different formulations include solid, semi-solid and liquid preparations, all of which can be administered via a variety of routes. Pharmaceutical formulations incorporate the process in which different chemical substances, including the active drug, are combined in order to produce a final medicinal product.

This chapter discusses these many different formulations, gives examples of their use and outlines examples of their administration in the practice setting, alongside the many clinical considerations and implications to be mindful of. It also addresses the issues surrounding the need to alter certain medication formulations in order to make the administration easier for certain patient populations. It is important to remember that when administering any medication to a patient – whether it is a steroid cream to treat their eczema, or an intravenous antibiotic – the 'seven rights of medication administration' (right patient, right drug, right dose, right time, right route, right reason and right documentation) must be adhered to in order to ensure patient safety and eliminate the occurrence of medication errors (Smeulers et al., 2015). Some authors refer to the 'nine rights of medication administration'.

Preparations such as creams, inhalers and drops are referred to as topical medications, meaning that they are directly applied to the site in which they are needed, i.e. eye drops for the treatment of conjunctivitis. The drops are applied directly into the eye, where they are absorbed and work on that specific area of need. Other types of medications that are administered internally in order to take effect are referred to as systemic medications.

A systemic medication is a medication that enters the blood stream. Various medications have different modes of action; for example, if an analgesic (pain killer) is taken for back pain, it is not necessarily carried directly to the site of pain, but works by binding to certain receptors within cell membranes, which then block the pain signals either in the brain or at a more direct level. Chapter 8 of this book provides more detail regarding analgesics.

Intravenous (IV) medications are the fastest way to deliver medicines. The medication enters the bloodstream directly, so does not rely on the patient being able to absorb it via their gut, which is not always achievable. IV medications are usually instantaneous and bring with them many benefits, risks and side effects that need to be considered. IV preparations are often more potent than their oral equivalents.

Oral medications come in the form of tablets and liquids. When in the stomach, they must be absorbed and broken down in order for them to be effective. They are not always directly absorbed in the stomach; some tablets, such as enteric coated medication, may be absorbed further down the intestinal tract and therefore take much longer to enter the bloodstream. Liquid preparations take effect much faster because they do not require the stomach to first break them down (Gautami, 2016).

Each formulation will now be considered in more detail.

Tablets

There are many different varieties of tablet preparations, which work in very different ways. Each has its benefits and its drawbacks. They are made from a pharmaceutical dose of a medication, which is then compressed to form a tablet. They are often coated with a substance such as starch to help them to dissolve once in the digestive tract. A binding agent, lubricating material and flavours are all added to make the medication more palatable and appear more attractive to the consumer (Singh et al., 2012).

Tablets are often, but not always, round and disc like in appearance – they come in various shapes and sizes, which are not always easy to swallow, especially for the older adult. The size and shape of a tablet can have both positive and negative effects on how acceptable it appears to the patient who is about to take it. In addition to this, other factors such as swallowing difficulties (dysphagia), the involvement of caregivers, reticence and polypharmacy are common in the older adult and can provide barriers to the successful administration of a tablet (Liu et al., 2014). Tablets may be required to be cut in half in order to reduce their size and make it easier for them to be swallowed; this is, however, classed as altering or modifying the medication and its dosage form, which can potentially change the bioavailability, toxicity or stability of the medication, so should be avoided without expert advice (Australian Pharmaceutical Advisory Council (APAC), 2006). Many tablets are scored to make cutting easier, either by snapping or using a pill cutter, but it should be noted that it is not considered good practice to halve tablets as it is difficult to get an exact dose. Capsules, controlled release (CR) tablets and enteric coated tablets should never be halved. If there is no other clear solution, occasionally a tablet may be halved if it has been verified by a pharmacist first to ensure there is no other way to administer the medication and this is an acceptable solution. Smaller tablets and those that are not scored are harder to divide, therefore this should not be attempted as the dosage cannot be controlled, (Van der Steen et al., 2010).

There are any number of reasons for prescribing tablets to patients, either for simple one-off pain relief, such as paracetamol for a headache, or the use of certain drug categories, such as angiotensin-converting enzyme (ACE) inhibitors to manage cardiovascular disease. As with any prescription, it is essential to ensure that the tablet is prescribed appropriately, with the correct dose, route, correct medication, for the correct patient, and is not contraindicated for that patient. The relevant checks prior to administration must always be carried out.

Tablets are largely easy to ingest and digest and many patients are capable of self-administering in the community. Disadvantages to tablets include the need for adequate absorption from the gut and the patient needs to be able to tolerate them without adverse side effects. For those patients who are taking a large number of different tablets – polypharmacy – it may be necessary to rationalise their prescriptions and prescribe dual action tablets where possible; such as co-plavix which contains both aspirin and clopidogrel – a dual antiplatelet therapy tablet – rather than prescribing aspirin and clopidogrel separately, meaning there is one single tablet instead of two. This is not always possible, but worth considering, as this will help with patient concordance, especially in the community. Advantages to tablets are that they are a relatively quick and simple way of administering and taking medication. They can be taken outside of a designated healthcare facility, meaning that patients are able to manage a multitude of health conditions in their own homes while maintaining their normal lives. This autonomy is hugely valuable to an individual, as it assists them to take ownership of their own healthcare condition.

Tablets are available in the following preparations:
Dispersible (soluble/effervescent)

These are solid dosage forms which disintegrate in water or another liquid forming a solution or suspension (Liu et al., 2014). They can either be pre-dissolved in water prior to administration or they disintegrate orally. An example is dispersible paracetamol tablets, which are dissolved in water before taking. An advantage of this is that it is easy to take, but it is important to be mindful that once dispersed and administered it is necessary to add some more water to the container, swill it around, and ingest to ensure any residual drug particles are administered, otherwise the dose would be incomplete. Soluble medications make large doses easier to administer as they are easier to swallow than a large tablet or multiple tablets. Effervescent preparations have the added benefit of helping to promote safe swallowing in patients with dysphagia due to the production of carbon dioxide in water – carbonated water has been found to aid swallowing by exciting chemical stimulation in the oral cavity (Michou et al., 2012). Disadvantages include the taste, which is not always deemed palatable by the patient. Additionally, they can require up to 200 mL of water to dissolve adequately, which may be unrealistic. A benefit is that they can be added to a flavoured liquid such as the patient's preferred squash, making them more tolerable and appealing.

Enteric coated/gastro resistant tablets

Enteric coated tablets are coated with a material which does not disintegrate directly in the acidic environment of the stomach, but in the more alkaline medium of the intestines. This ensures that the lining of the stomach is protected from any potentially irritating substances, which over a period of prolonged use could cause gastritis. Another benefit to such a coating is that it takes longer to dissolve – up to two hours, making it ideal for those medications which require a delayed relief action (Singh et al., 2012). Disadvantages to these tablets are that they cannot be chewed or crushed/dissolved, making them unsuitable for any patient who is unable to swallow a whole tablet.

An example of an enteric coated tablet is ibuprofen 200 mg tablets, a non-steroidal anti-inflammatory drug (NSAID), used for the treatment of inflammatory pain, such as pain caused by osteoarthritis and other inflammatory conditions (MIMS, 2019). Ibuprofen, while highly effective, is not suitable for all patient groups, so its appropriateness must always be assessed prior to prescribing and administering.

Modified release tablets (slow release)

Modified release (MR), sustained release (SR) or controlled release (CR) are all terms applied to tablets that deliver their dosage over a prolonged period of time. These tablets are specifically designed to have an altered pattern of drug release compared to regular immediate release (IR) tablets, enabling a specific therapeutic outcome. This medication group have the following abbreviations after their name CR – controlled release, ER – extended release, LA – long acting, SR – sustained release, XL – extra long or XR – extra release. The aim of this formula is to achieve a constant plasma drug concentration. Often this allows a significant reduction in administration frequency of the drug due to its prolonged period of action. This is beneficial to patients with chronic illnesses and disease processes, who require a constant therapeutic plasma concentration of the drug in order to prevent a breakthrough of symptoms; for example, the overnight management of pain in the terminally ill (Aulton, 2008). An example is Oxycontin MR, which comes in a variety of dosages and is designed to be taken every 12 hours. Disadvantages of this tablet preparation include the fact that any adverse side effects are not easily resolved due to the prolonged release nature of the medication (Ummadi et al., 2013). These tablets cannot be crushed or halved – doing so would potentially allow immediate absorption of the full dosage, making them unsuitable for those who are not capable of swallowing effectively (MIMS, 2019). Due to the sustained release characteristics, dose increases need to be made cautiously, in 25–50% increments. The need for breakthrough pain support more than twice a day indicates the need for increasing the dose (eMC, 2019). An advantage of this medication group is the sustained effect, meaning the patient's pain should be well managed for an extended length of time, with minimal need for additional analgesics.

Immediate release tablets (IR)

These are tablets which act immediately upon ingestion for a specific time frame, depending on that particular drug's half-life. Drawbacks to this preparation is that repeated doses throughout a day may be required to maintain its effects, which some patients may find tiresome if required for a long time. Advantages include the drug being relatively short acting, meaning that any adverse side-effects should resolve quicker than if the medication was active for a prolonged amount of time. An example of an IR medication is propranolol 10 mg tablets, used for the management of hypertension, long-term prophylaxis of re-infarction following recovery from myocardial infarction (MI), management of migraine and many other conditions. This is a β-adrenergic blocking drug resulting in a reduced heart rate and blood pressure. The drug reaches peak plasma concentration one or two hours after administration and is rapidly distributed throughout the body (eMC, 2019). This medication is generally taken twice daily.

Capsules

Capsules contain a solid dosage form of a drug, which is enclosed in a hard or soft soluble container. The capsules themselves come in various forms including gelatin, starch and liquid filled. Capsules can appear more attractive to some individuals and some liquid filled capsules are quicker to dissolve once ingested. Some plastic capsules are also suitable to be split open and the powdered contents diluted allowing them to be administered via an enteral feeding tube, but it is essential to clarify the efficacy of this with a pharmacist first. Some capsules are more bulky and harder to swallow, whereas the smooth shape of others makes them easier to swallow; there is a wide selection available. An example of a capsule form medication is Pregabalin 150 mg, a hard gelatin capsule containing granulated powder. Pregabalin is used for the treatment of peripheral and central neuropathic pain in adults (eMC, 2019).

Clinical considerations

Medications administered via enteral feeding systems

It is important to consider that for patients who are unable to swallow tablets or those with enteral feeding systems such as naso-gastric (NG) or percutaneous endoscopic gastrostomy (PEG) tubes, the way in which medications can be administered is altered. It is necessary for the nurse to possess the specialised skills required to administer medications via this route. Not all medications are licensed or formulated to be administered via this route, which would require dissolving or crushing it if it is in tablet or capsule form. Some medications have a liquid formulation, but for those that do not it is essential to discuss with the pharmacist if a medication is suitable for alteration, or what other options are available (Williams, 2008).

The potential consequences involved when manipulating a medication should be recognised, as an action such as crushing will change the way in which the dosage form of the drug is delivered to the patient, as the absorption process will be altered. The result of this could render the drug unstable or could produce increased adverse side effects, fail to reach the site of action and could most importantly make the medication unsafe to administer.

The Royal Pharmaceutical Society (2011) lists the following as potential consequences when splitting, crushing or opening tablets or capsules:

Risks to healthcare workers/carers – potential exposure to the person crushing the medication, which could contain cytotoxic agents, hormones or corticosteroids.

Drug instability – crushing a solid tablet could impact the stability of the drug, either in dosage delivery, absorption alterations or exposure to light.

Changes in pharmacokinetics and bioavailability – crushing changes the bioavailability and pharmacokinetic products of a drug, resulting in adverse side effects or under dosage.

Drug irritation – drugs often have an outer coating applied to minimise irritation, such as oesophageal ulceration.

Bitter taste – a sugar coating is often applied to avoid this.

Dosage form effects – crushing a controlled release preparation will alter the drug release characteristics of the drug, potentially allowing a large dose to be delivered in a short space of time, rather than over an extended period – which makes it potentially toxic with a high risk of adverse effects. The crushing of an enteric coated tablet will also allow the drug to be released too early, or the drug may be destroyed in the stomach or irritate the stomach lining.

It is also imperative to note that the changing of the original preparation of a drug will make it an unlicensed use of the medication, unless there is a clear use for the medication stated in the product's marketing authorisation information (RPS, 2011). Consideration should also be given to the inappropriate or inadequate tablet crushing or dispersing, which can lead to tube blockage when administered via an enteral feeding system. With this in mind, it is imperative to always liaise with a pharmacist and senior members of the multidisciplinary team when faced with this obstacle, in order to review the need for the medication and ensure the most appropriate preparation is supplied in order to be able to administer it to this patient group safely and effectively without complication while adhering to the seven rights of administration.

Chewable

Chewable tablets are intended to be chewed and swallowed by the patient rather than being swallowed whole. They are designed to be palatable and easily chewed. They are especially useful for a patient group such as those who are cognitively impaired, who do not understand the process of swallowing a tablet in its whole form, or for those who are incapable of doing so due to poor swallowing strength. These types of tablets would also be suitable for crushing and diluting to administer via an enteral feeding tube. Chewable tablets are available for many over-the-counter (OTC) medications as well as prescription medications. It is necessary, though, to consider the fact that many chewable tablets require the patient to possess a strong chewing action due to the hardness of the tablet, so those who struggle to chew effectively, or do not have all of their teeth – such as the older adult – may not cope well with this preparation (Peltola and Vehkalahti, 2005).

Chewable tablets come in two categories – those that can be chewed for ease of administration and those which are chewed in order to release the active ingredient (Center for Drug Evaluation and Research (CDER), 2018). An example of a chewable tablet is adcal 1500 mg (calcium carbonate) tablets, which is a supplementary source of calcium often used for those patients with osteoporosis (eMC, 2019). These tablets are large, so being chewable is an advantage.

Buccal/sublingual

Buccal and sublingual medications come in the form of tablets, wafers, films or sprays. To be absorbed buccally, the medication is to be placed in the buccal cavity, high up along the top gum under the upper lip, where it is to remain until fully dissolved. Sublingual medications are placed under the patient's tongue where they should remain until fully dissolved. See Figure 6.1 depicting the sublingual and buccal routes. When used via this route, the medication is absorbed directly into the bloodstream via the oral mucosa. This is a highly efficient way of absorbing medication – peak blood drug levels are usually achieved 3–10 times faster than that of the oral route, (Nerang and Sharma, 2011). An example of a buccal medication is prochloperazine 3 mg tablets, which are effective for treating nausea and vomiting, as well as migraine and dizziness (eMC 2019). Advantages of this medication – given that it is used for

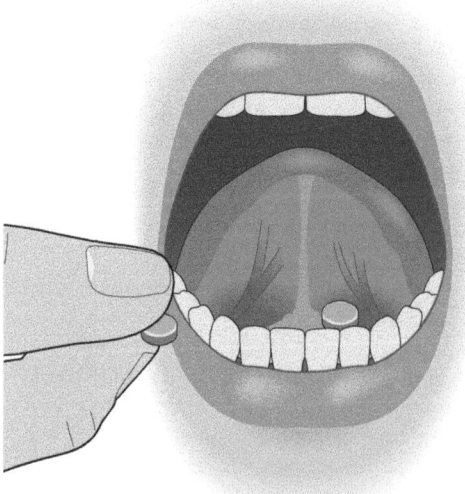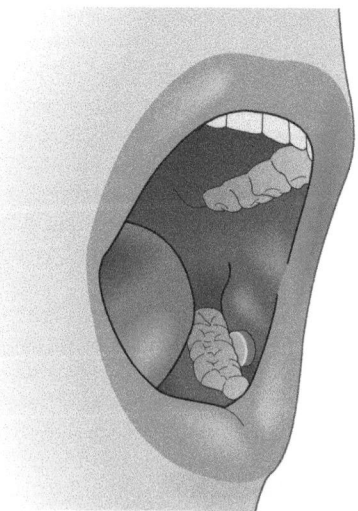

Figure 6.1   Sublingual and buccal routes. Source: Peate and Wild (2014).

96

nausea and vomiting – is that it is far easier to tolerate than having to swallow a tablet with water when a patient is vomiting. Disadvantages include the fact that it can take up to two hours to fully dissolve, which may not feel pleasant to some patients (Cox et al., 2006). These types of medications can also cause local irritation to the gums and mouth.

An example of a sublingual medication is glyceryl-trinitrate (GTN), which comes in both tablet and spray form and is used to treat chest pain, commonly brought on by angina, or experienced by patients experiencing acute coronary syndrome (ACS) or acute myocardial infarction (AMI). GTN is a potent coronary vasodilator, which reduces venous return due to its vasodilating properties, therefore reducing left ventricular load and resulting in pain relief for the patient if the chest pain is coronary in origin. To administer, either a tablet or spray is placed under the patient's tongue where it is left to dissolve. Sprays are becoming increasingly common; it is essential to remember that they are single patient use only, so once opened should remain with that patient with their addressograph attached to avoid cross-contamination. Advantages of sublingual GTN are that it is very fast to work and gives almost immediate relief of symptoms. Disadvantages are the side effects, which can be severe in some patients. It can cause hypotension and a high number of patients report severe headaches after taking it (eMC, 2019). Due to the nature of the medication, the risk to benefit ratio should be closely considered on an individual basis; for those patients experiencing AMI who are also hypotensive, alternative analgesics, such as opioids, may be more appropriate.

The older adult or those who are cognitively impaired may not be cooperative with this medication route as it requires understanding and tolerance to administer effectively. Also, those patients with a dry mouth may need to rinse their mouth with water prior to using this route to assist disintegration and absorption of the tablet.

As well as tablets, medications are available in many other formulations.

Oral
Liquid

Liquid medications include liquids, solutions, suspensions, syrups and mixtures. Liquid medications are commonly used in those patients with dysphagia, particularly in the older adult, as they are easier to swallow (Morris, 2005). Some liquid medications are flavoured so that they are more palatable. Liquid medications vary from thin and watery to thick and gloopy and therefore the consistency of medications needs to be considered by the practitioner prior to administration, particularly in patients with dysphagia who may require thickening agents in order to avoid pulmonary aspiration and choking. Along with the active drug, liquid medications also contain other ingredients to ensure the drug remains active and equally distributed throughout the bottle. Many liquid bottles will state: 'shake well before use', which ensures equal distribution of the medication and avoids the settling of any medication at the bottom of the bottle. Measuring liquid medications can be a source of confusion, with many receptacles available including medicine cups, medicine spoons and syringes. It is important that the practitioner ensures that the dose is correctly measured using a receptacle provided and recommended by their hospital/trust.

Topical
Suspension
Eye drops and ointments

Eye drops and ointments are prescribed and administered to treat acute or long-term eye conditions, including the eye itself and its surrounding structures. An example of an eye drop is latanoprost for the treatment of open-angle glaucoma (Joint Formulary Committee, 2019a). This form of medication remains at the forefront of treatment for eye disease as it is administered directly to the site of injury/disease, therefore making it more effective than other medications, such as oral tablets. As with any medication, it is important that the eye medication be given routinely, as prescribed, for full effect, with the same priority and standards given to that of oral or intrave-nous medication, for example (Shaw, 2014). Eye drops work through a process known as systemic absorption. It is suggested that one drop be administered to the affected eye(s) at five-minute intervals to ensure maximum therapeutic effect (Andrews, 2006). It is important for practitioners to understand that eye drops and ointments, like any other medication, come with contraindica-tions and side effects. It is vital the practitioner is aware of these prior to administration, as stipu-lated by the Royal College of Nursing and the Royal Pharmaceutical Society (RPS, 2019).

Ear drops and ointments

Ear drops and ointments are prescribed and administered to treat acute ear infections or to help with the breakdown of cerumen (ear wax). Due to the anatomy of the inner ear, it is difficult to administer medication to the affected area. Ear drops are an effective form of medication, but should only be used in the presence of obvious infection, confirmed by a doctor, general prac-titioner, clinical nurse specialist, or advanced care practitioner with otoscope – and medications should not be utilised for more than two weeks. It is also important to recognise that patients with a perforated tympanic membrane (eardrum) should refrain from the use of ear drop/oint-ment medication due to the increased risk of ototoxicity (Joint Formulary Committee, 2019b). For the removal of cerumen, the use of ear drops can be effective. For example, olive oil or sodium bicarbonate 5% ear drops are licensed for use to soften ear wax to ease removal.

Nasal drops and sprays

Nasal sprays are commonly used in the treatment of rhinitis. Nasal sprays, such as corticosteroid nasal sprays, are considered first line treatment for allergic rhinitis. For example, the corticoster-oid works to manage nasal congestion and treat symptoms of seasonal rhinitis (hay fever) (Bartle, 2017). Nasal sprays are available as an over-the-counter medication and do not require prescription. They are suitable for young children and adults. Patients with asthma or long-term rhinitis caused by perennial allergens should seek medical attention prior to using nasal sprays. Nasal sprays reduce inflammation and symptoms associated with increased mucus production and nasal congestion. Although some immediate relief can be found, nasal sprays can take a number of weeks to become effective and the relief of symptoms be noted (Scadding et al., 2017). Like eye drops and ointments, nasal sprays also subject to systemic absorption and the bioavailability of the nasal drug. Different nasal sprays have different bioavailability rates and this should be considered before the long-term use of a product (Salib and Howarth, 2003).

Creams and lotions

The skin is the largest organ of the body and its fundamental function is to protect. The skin protects from bacteria and the elements, helps to regulate body temperature and allows the sensations of touch, heat and cold. There are a wide range of skin conditions, such as eczema, psoriasis, and dermatitis, and topical creams and lotions can treat such conditions, when administered properly. The same care should also be taken when administering topical creams as with any other medication (Nicol, 2010).

Examples of topical creams and lotions are:

- Sunblock – to prevent sun damage.
- Antifungal – to treat fungal infections, such as: tinea pedis (athlete's foot).
- Antiviral – to treat viral infections, such as: shingles.
- Antibacterial – to treat bacterial infections, such as: cellulitis.
- Anti-inflammatory – to treat inflammatory conditions, such as: psoriasis,
- Analgesia – to provide local anaesthetic.
- Moisturising – to combat dryness.

It is important that whichever topical cream is chosen, it is appropriate for the presenting condition and administered correctly. Clinical considerations – such as using gloves when applying steroid or antibacterial cream to avoid absorption, or using tubed or pump dispenser antibacterial medication rather than pots to avoid cross-contamination (Dunning, 2005) – all need to be considered when administering topical medications.

Clinical considerations

Topical medications
Healthcare professionals may be called upon to administer topical medications and creams to patients. As described in this chapter, topical medications come in varying forms depending on patient needs. Topical medications are designed to act locally on the affected area through absorption of the skin. It is therefore required that all healthcare professionals wear gloves when administering topical treatments to prevent the absorption of the medication through their hands. Following hand hygiene techniques also will prevent the absorption of the medication. Using clean gloves is sufficient but the use of sterile gloves maybe used when in contact with broken skin to prevent the transmission of microorganisms.

When giving any medication, it is always important to remember the seven Rs of medication administration:

- The right patient
- The right medication (drug)
- The right dose
- The right route
- The right time
- The right reason
- The right documentation.

Patches

This form of medication is applied to the skin, usually through an adhesive disc that allows medication to be absorbed at a slow, consistent rate into the body for systemic effect (Chernecky et al., 2002). A transdermal patch, for example, contains a certain dose of drug that when applied to the skin releases a quantity sufficient enough for a therapeutic dose. Examples of transdermal patches include: fentanyl, nicotine and hyoscine (Hillery et al., 2001). The advantages of patches are that they avoid pre-systemic metabolism, allowing the therapeutic window to be maintained for longer, the reduction of side effects and maintenance of constant dosing. Disadvantages of patches include skin irritation, non-adhesion to the skin and there are a limited number of drugs available in this formulation (Dougherty et al., 2015).

Rectal
Suppositories

A suppository is a solid form of medication prepared for use within the rectum. Once inserted, the suppository is designed to dissolve from its solid form into a liquid through the use of body temperature (Higgins, 2007; Gunning, 2015). Suppositories are useful for local effect, for example: in the treatment of haemorrhoids or faecal impaction, or for systemic effect, for example: analgesia. Suppositories can also be used prior to surgery if a patient is nil-by-mouth or to clean bowel mucosa prior to investigation such as flexible sigmoidoscopy. Care should be taken prior to administering a suppository and contraindications noted, such as low rectal surgery, obstruction, recent radiotherapy or in patients with an increased risk of colonic perforation (Higgins, 2007). Prior to the administration of a suppository, a digital examination of the rectum should be performed to examine the anal canal and rectum for residual solid stool or any abnormalities (Peate, 2015). Conflict has arisen over the technique of inserting a suppository (apex versus blunt end); however, no evidence of statistical significance has been found to support either method (Bradshaw and Price, 2007; Higgins, 2007; Peate, 2015). Practitioners need to understand the differences in type of suppository and their actions in order to gain their full effect (Peate, 2015). For example, if a suppository is to be used as a form of analgesia for systemic effect, it would help if the bowel were emptied prior to its administration in order to ensure its full effect.

Enemata

Enemata are another medication designed for administration via the rectum. Enemas have varying quantities of drugs in a liquid preparation. The enema comes in a plastic container with a tube applicator. The applicator is inserted into the rectum and the container compressed to release the medication. Similar to suppositories, enemas can be used for patients who are pre-surgery or nil-by-mouth and can be used to cleanse the bowel mucosa prior to colonic investigations, such as flexible sigmoidoscopy. However, enema administration has been reported to be more difficult than that of suppositories and therefore it is not widely used (Aulton, 1988).

Vaginal

Pessaries

Similar to suppositories, pessaries are solid forms of medication. Once inserted, the suppository is designed to dissolve from its solid form into a liquid through the use of body temperature. The pessary is usually made up of vegetable oil containing the medication. The medication is gradually absorbed into the vagina as it dissolves. Pessaries can be inserted using the fingers, or with an applicator; they are used for local effect for conditions such as candida or dryness.

Inhalation

Nebulisers

Nebulisation works by a flow of gas; typically, room air or oxygen, passing through a small hole. Rapid expansion of air causes a negative pressure which is sucked up the receptacle, usually a facemask or mouthpiece (Jevon and Humphrey, 2007). Nebulisation creates a mist of the drug particles that are then inhaled. The proportion of drug inhaled and reaching the lungs via nebulisation is approximately 12% (Rees and Kanabar, 2006), which is why nebulised medication doses are usually higher than those administered via an inhaler. In comparison, the proportion of drug inhaled and reaching the lungs when using dry powdered inhalers is up to 40% (Labiris and Dolovich, 2003). The most common nebulised medications are bronchodilators, such as Salbutamol. However, other nebulised medications such as corticosteroids – i.e. beclomethasone – and anticholinergics – for example, Ipratropium Bromide – can also be administered via nebulisation.

Clinical skills in practice

How to administer a nebuliser.
Equipment
Prescription chart containing the relevant prescription.
Nebuliser kit (containing face mask or mouthpiece, nebuliser chamber, tubing).
Gas supply (air or oxygen, depending on the patient condition and the medication being administered – this must be prescribed accordingly).
Medication to be inhaled.

Pre-procedure actions

As with any medications, prior to administering, check the following on the patient's prescription chart:

- Correct patient.
- Correct drug/dose/time/date.
- Correct route/method of administration.
- Validity of prescription – signature of prescriber.
- Legibility of prescription.

If any of the above are absent, unclear or illegible the nurse must not proceed. They should instead rectify this with the prescriber before continuing.

Procedure

- Fully explain the procedure to the patient and ensure they are happy to proceed.
- Wash hands with antibacterial soap or bactericidal alcohol hand gel and apply appropriate personal protective equipment (PPE).
- If not contraindicated, sit patient fully upright, preferably in a chair.
- Perform peak flow rate (PEFR) if not contraindicated and required for the patient's monitoring.
- Assemble the nebulisation kit as per the manufacturer's guidelines and adhere to local policy and procedure.
- Measure any liquid as needed and add the prescribed medication and diluent (if needed) to the nebuliser chamber.
  a. Attach the mouthpiece or mask via the tubing to the medical piped air or oxygen as prescribed.
  b. If the patient has a clinical need for oxygen therapy, this should not be discontinued while the nebuliser is in progress. In this situation, the drug should be nebulised using oxygen. The patient should be monitored with continuous pulse oximetry.
  c. If the patient is hypercapnic or acidotic (e.g. a person with COPD who retains CO_2), the nebuliser should be administered using medical air instead of oxygen.
- Ask the patient to hold the mouthpiece between their lips or apply the facemask and take a slow deep breath.
- After inspiration there should be a brief pause before exhalation.
- Turn on the piped oxygen or air and ensure a mist is formed. A minimum flow of 6–8 L/minute is needed.
- The patient should continue to breathe as above until the nebuliser has finished – optimal nebulisation of approximately 4 mL takes about 10 minutes.
- If appropriate and prescribed, recommence oxygen therapy afterwards at the appropriate rate.
- Make the patient comfortable
- Clean any equipment used and discard any single use containers/pieces of equipment.
- Wash hands.
- Record administration on appropriate charts.

Source: Adapted from Dougherty et al. (2015).

Inhalers

Control or preventer inhalers are used to treat conditions such as asthma and chronic obstructive pulmonary disease (COPD). Inhalers work by inhaling medications designed to work directly on the airways and lungs. Control inhalers usually contain a corticosteroid to reduce inflammation and swelling and the repetitive use of inhalers protects from triggers, reducing the risk of symptoms of asthma. Control inhalers work slowly for long-lasting symptom relief when used daily. Unlike nebulisers, the inhalers work by directly inhaling the medication into the lungs. As the medication is having a direct effect on the target area, the doses of medications are typically smaller than that of nebulised medications. It is therefore important that patients use an effective technique in order to gain the full benefit of their medications. An example of a control inhaler is beclomethasone.

Rescue inhalers work in a similar way to that of control inhalers but are used to treat acute symptoms of asthma or COPD. Unlike control inhalers that have a long-term impact, rescue inhalers work within minutes and last up to a few hours. An example of a rescue inhaler is ventolin.

Injection routes

IV – Intravenous – this is the administration of a medication directly into the bloodstream, usually via a peripheral vein. This is the fastest route of absorption.

IM – Intramuscular – this is the administration of a medication directly into the muscle. Medications administered through this route have a slower rate of absorption than via the IV route, but usually have a slow and even absorption; it may be used for administration of antibiotics.

SC – Subcutaneous – this is the administration of medications into the fat layer of tissue below the skin's surface. This is a slower method of absorption compared with IM injections and is used for insulin, for example.

ID – Intradermal – this is the administration of medications into the dermis, just below the epidermis. This route has the longest method of absorption of all injections and is used mainly for sensitivity tests, for example: tuberculosis (TB). This route is used for these tests as reactions are easy to see and the degree of reaction can also be determined.

Clinical skills in practice

How to give an intramuscular (IM) injection.

Equipment	
Gloves	Pre-filled syringe
Apron	Gauze
Alcohol swab	Procedure tray
Needle	Sharps bin

Undertake the procedure with adherence to local policy and procedure.

Pre-Procedure Actions

1. Inform the patient of the procedure and fully explain the process in order to gain informed consent.
2. Check the drug against the drug chart/prescription and ensure the following:
   a. Right patient
   b. Right drug
   c. Valid prescription
   d. Right dose
   e. Right route

     f. Right date and time of administration
     g. Correct diluent (as necessary)
     h. Valid prescriber's signature
     i. Legible prescription.

If any of the above are absent, unclear or illegible the nurse must not proceed. They should instead rectify this with the prescriber before continuing.

Procedure

3. Don the apron, close the door or draw the curtains and wash hands thoroughly, remembering the six steps of hand hygiene.
4. Expose only the area where the injection is to be administered.
5. Don gloves and undertake an assessment of the skin in the injection area. Be aware of any inflammation, oedema, infection or broken skin. Do not use this area if any of the above are present.
6. Clean the injection site thoroughly with the alcohol swab/stick for 30 seconds and allow to dry for 30 seconds.
7. With your non-dominant hand, stretch back the skin of the injection area.
8. Inform the patient of the injection and insert the needle into the area quickly, with one swift movement, at a 90° angle, until approximately 1 cm of the needle remains visible.
9. Pull back on the syringe plunger and observe for signs of blood. If no blood is aspirated, slowly inject the drug into the area, approximately 1 mL of drug every 10 seconds, to ensure slow and constant infusion of the medication. If blood is noted at any time during the administration, the injection must be stopped, the needle withdrawn, and the procedure completed again from the beginning. The patient must also be informed of the reason for this.
10. Upon completion of injection, wait 10 seconds before withdrawing the needle.
11. Withdraw the needle swiftly, applying pressure with the gauze to the injection site.
12. Cover injection area with a plaster, checking for allergies prior.
13. Make the patient comfortable.

Post-Procedure

14. Where applicable, engage automatic needle re-sheath to prevent needle-stick injury or place directly into sharps bin. Place all other disposable equipment into an orange clinical waste bin.
15. Wash hands post procedure following the six steps of hand hygiene.
16. Document procedure in nursing notes and sign for medication on prescription chart.

Source: Adapted from Dougherty et al. (2015).

Clinical considerations

IV medications

As an advocate for the patient, it is a constant requirement to rationalise the need and the appropriateness of each medication prescribed. Special considerations should be made in order to review the need for IV medications. Things to consider when an IV medication is prescribed include whether this is a necessary route of administration, as it requires the patient to have a peripheral intravenous cannula (PIVC), which brings about its own risks – infection and phlebitis being the main ones. Furthermore, the patient may be receiving IV antibiotics, which after a certain number of doses or a certain length of time could be converted to the oral preparation, signifying the PIVC is no longer required and can be removed. This also changes the situation for the patient, meaning if they are well enough to no longer be in hospital, they can manage their medication in their own home with support of family and/or carers. There are also cost and work-load implications associated with this. Many IV preparations are more expensive than their oral equivalents and IV drug administration requires specific education and preparation in order to be deemed competent in this skill and should be carried out according to local policy and proce-dure. Administration of IV medication requires more time and work than administering an oral tablet. Being mindful of this, each patient's medication chart should be reviewed daily and rationalised appropriately.

Additionally, some IV medications require a central venous catheter (CVC) or peripherally inserted central catheter (PICC) line in order to be administered: this is an invasive procedure. Drugs such as norepinephrine, amiodarone, or highly concentrated drugs require CVC adminis-tration to avoid adverse side effects, such as tissue damage and necrosis, to the administration site. Some such medications also require continuous cardiac monitoring while they are being administered.

Many patients can now be cared for and supported in the community with a PICC line, which is ideal for those patients requiring long-term IV antibiotics, for example, which has a positive impact on hospital bed availability as well as overall patient experience. Previously, patients would be required to remain in hospital for the duration of their treatment, which can be a num-ber of weeks.

Clinical considerations

Dosage differences across formulations

Paracetamol is an analgesic medication commonly utilised as a first-line pain killer. Paracetamol is available in different formulations including oral tablets, liquid, intravenous solutions and rec-tal suppositories.

It is therefore vital that all healthcare professionals understand the differences in drug dos-ages across formulations suitable and seek guidance where unsure.

For example: a standard and maximum dose of paracetamol administered orally in tablet form to adults is 1 g every four to six hours, up to four times daily. Considerations must be considered when giving in different formulations, taking into account the patient's weight.

For example: for adults who weigh less than 50 kg, the maximum intravenous dose is 15 mg/kg every four to six hours. For adults who weigh over 50 kg, the dose remains the same as the oral recommendations.

Recommendations are also in place for patients with known renal or hepatology disorders or those at risk of hepatotoxicity. A maximum daily dose of 3 g can be administered to this patient group. Patients with an estimated glomerular filtration rate (e-GFR) of less than 30 mL/min/1.73 m^2 should have their interval intravenous infusion doses increased to every six hours. Clinical judgment should be used to adjust the dosage accordingly if deemed at risk of toxicity.

It is important that all healthcare professionals familiarise themselves with the differences in dosages across formulations, while remembering that some doses are calculated based on weight and others on co-morbidity/toxicity risk. It is important to check, prior to admin-istration, the cumulative paracetamol dose over the previous 24 hours and seek guidance on dosages from your local ward pharmacist, nurse consultant, matron, doctor or BNF where unsure.

Episode of care: Surgical high dependency unit (HDU)

Valerie is a 68-year-old female who was admitted to the surgical HDU following a laparotomy, radical hysterectomy, bilateral salpingo oophorectomy, appendicectomy, omentectomy and staging for cancer. She was seen by the acute pain service (APS) (a specialised pain management service available in most tertiary hospitals) on day 2 post surgery for a review of her pain management.

Upon review, Valerie was receiving a fentanyl patient-controlled analgesia (PCA) pump and had a transdermal norspan (buprenorphine 5 mcg/h) patch in situ, which was applied at 16.00 hours the previous day. As a result of being on the PCA, 2 L O_2 was prescribed and was being administered via nasal prongs to ensure adequate oxygenation should she become drowsy from the opioid. Valerie also had two vari-vac surgical drains in situ to her abdomen on low suction, which were draining moderate haemo-serous fluid.

Valerie's pain was well controlled up to this point, she had a pain score of 2/10 at rest and she described it as being mild. The APS made recommendations to discontinue Valerie's PCA and prescribed some regular oral analgesics for her to take instead and some as required analgesics and anti-emetics should her pain levels increase, or if she started to experience nausea as a result of the medications. APS also advised to leave the transdermal patch in place for the full seven days as recommended by the manufacturers and outlined in the policy and care-plan for the management of transdermal analgesic patches.

In order to successfully transition Valerie away from her PCA and on to regular oral analgesia, it was recommended that her first oral analgesic be administered two hours prior to taking the PCA away, to ensure it had taken effect before removing the PCA.

The following regimen was prescribed:

Morphine SR 15 mg twice daily, orally (08.00 hours and 20.00 hours)
Paracetamol 1 g four times daily, IV/oral (06.00 hours, 12.00 hours, 18.00 hours and 24.00 hours)
    As required:

Buprenorphine 200–400 micrograms two hourly sublingual tablets
Tramadol 50–100 mg six hourly IV
Ondansetron 4–8 mg eight hourly IV/sublingual
Metoclopramide 10 mg eight hourly IV

Valerie's PCA was discontinued and her pain managed on the above regimen. It was necessary to assess her pain every hour to ensure she was receiving adequate pain relief. She was also assisted to get out of bed and take a short walk with the nursing associate and physiotherapist. This additional activity meant that she required extra analgesia to make her comfortable, on the 'as required' section of the medication chart, which had good effect. She was also provided with a rolled-up towel to press onto her laparotomy incision when coughing to provide support and help her brace her abdominal muscles.

Inadequate pain management post major surgery can have multiple consequences. The patient will not only be reluctant to mobilise – putting them at risk of developing deep vein thrombosis – but they will also be adverse to efficient coughing and deep breathing, which can result in lung consolidation and ultimately lower respiratory tract infection (LRTI) or pneumonia, complicating their recovery and requiring a longer hospital stay. These are all contributors to increased morbidity and mortality within the hospitalised population.

The APS is a valuable resource within the hospital. They offer a prior plan, tailored to the patient's individual needs, which provides the patient with a clear pathway, with backup analgesia already prescribed, resulting in fewer delays and better patient outcomes. A variety of drug preparations and administration routes are utilised to ensure that adequate cover can be achieved in patients who have limited gut absorption, as well as those who can easily tolerate oral ingestion.

Conclusion

This chapter provides the reader with details concerning the different formulations of medication available and their uses. The reader should understand why different formulations are available and now have a wider understanding when entering into practice. This chapter provides the reader with knowledge and guidance concerning the various formulations of drugs, how to administer these safely and correctly and when to raise a concern should a formulation not be appropriate or necessary. At all times, the nurse must ensure that the patient is at the centre of all that is done.

Glossary

Autonomy	A person's ability to make their own choices based on their personal preferences, values and beliefs.
Bioavailability	The degree and rate of which a medication is absorbed into the circulatory system.
BNF	British National Formulary. A pharmaceutical reference book, used by healthcare professionals, containing a wide source of information when prescribing and administering medication.
Compliance	In the context of medications compliance, it refers to the patient's ability to conform to the recommended treatment course prescribed for them, including the relevant times, dosages and frequency of medications.
Digest	The breakdown of material in the alimentary canal into a substance that can be absorbed by the body.
Dispensing	Includes the activities that occur between the time the medication prescription is presented to pharmacy and the time they are presented either to the patient/healthcare professional/carer collecting them from the pharmacy.
Formulations	A mixture of ingredients prepared in a certain way and used for a specific purpose.
Half-life	Relating to drugs, a pharmacokinetic parameter – the time it takes for the total amount of the drug in the body to be reduced by half.
Health-care facility	Any location where healthcare to some degree is provided – ranging in size and speciality.
Health Practitioner	A registered health professional who is licensed to perform within the scope of their registration guidelines and professional abilities.
Ingest	Take a substance into the body by swallowing or absorbing it.
Plasma-concentration	A reflection of the minimum concentration of a drug at the receptor site to achieve the desired pharmacological response/effect.
Prescription medication	A pharmaceutical drug that legally requires a medical prescription to be dispensed.
Professional responsibility	Legal or moral duty of a registered professional to apply their knowledge in ways that benefit society, while preventing harm, within the scope of their practice, and in accordance with the Code of Conduct.
Polypharmacy	The concurrent use of multiple medications by a patient (five or more medications).
Systemic absorption	The process of medication being directly absorbed through the body for therapeutic effect.

References

Andrews, S. (2006). Pharmacology. In: *Ophthalmic Care* (ed. J. Marsden), 45–70. Chichester: Whurr Publishers.

Aulton, M. (ed.) (1988). *Pharmaceutics. The Science of Dosage from Design*. Edinburgh: Churchill-Livingstone.

Aulton, M.E. (2008). *Aulton's Pharmaceutics; The Design and Manufacture of Medicines*, 3e, 99–102. Philadelphia, USA: Churchill Livingstone Elsevier.

Australian Pharmaceutical Advisory Council (APAC) (2006). *Guidelines for Medication Management in Residential Aged Care Facilities.* https://www2.health.vic.gov.au/about/publications/policiesan-dguidelines/apac-medication-management-residential-aged-care-facilities-resource-kit (accessed September 2020).

Bartle, J. (2017). How to use a corticosteroid nasal spray. *Nursing Standard* 31 (52): 41–43.

Bradshaw, A. and Price, L. (2007). Rectal suppository insertion: the reliability of the evidence as a basis for nursing practice. *Journal of Clinical Nursing* 16 (1): 98–103.

Center for Drug Evaluation and Research (CDER) (2018). Quality attribute considerations for chewable tablets guidance for industry. www.fda.gov (accessed August 2019).

Chernecky, C., Butler, S., Graham, P., and Infortuna, H. (2002). *Drug Calculations and Drug Administration*. Philadelphia: WB Saunders.

Cox, L.S., Linnemann, L.D., Nolte, H., Weldon, D., Finegold, I. and Nelson, H.S. (2006) Sublingual immuno-therapy: a comprehensive review https://www.ncbi.nlm.nih.gov/pubmed/16675328 (accessed September 2019).

Dougherty, L., Lister, S., and West-Oram, A. (eds.) (2015). *The Royal Marsden Manual of Clinical Nursing Procedures*, 9e. Oxford: Wiley Blackwell.

Dunning, G. (2005). The choice, application and review of topical treatments for skin conditions. *Nursing Times* 101 (4): 55.

Electronic Medicines Compendium (eMC) (2019). www.medicines.org.uk (accessed August 2019).

Gautami, J. (2016). Liquid Dosage Forms. https://www.scribd.com/document/380330178/Liquid-Dosage-Forms (accessed September 2020).

Gunning, A. (2015). Elimination. In: *The Royal Marsden Manual of Clinical Nursing Procedures*, 9e (eds. S. Lister and L. Dougherty), 133–202. Oxford: Wiley Blackwell.

Higgins, D. (2007). Bowel care part 6 – administration of a suppository. *Nursing Times* 103 (47): 26–27.

Hillery, A., Lloyd, A., and Swarbrick, J. (eds.) (2001). *Drug Delivery and Targeting for Pharmacists and Pharmaceutical Scientists*. Florida: CRC Press.

Jevon, P. and Humphrey, N. (2007). Respiratory procedures. Part 3 – use of a nebuliser. *Nursing Times* 103 (34): 24–25.

Joint Formulary Committee (2019a). *British National Formulary*. London: BMJ Group and Pharmaceutical Press. https://bnf.nice.org.uk/drug/latanoprost.html#cautions (accessed September 2020).

Joint Formulary Committee (2019b). *British National Formulary*. London: BMJ Group and Pharmaceutical Press. https://bnf.nice.org.uk/treatment-summary/ear.html (accessed September 2020).

Labiris, N.R. and Dolovich, M.B. (2003). Pulmonary drug delivery. Part II: the role of inhalant delivery devices and drug formulations in therapeutic effectiveness of aerosolized medications. *British Journal of Clinical Pharmacology* 56 (6): 600–612.

Liu, F., Ranmal, S., Batchelor, H.K., Orlu-gul, M., et al. (2014). Patient-centred pharmaceutical design to improve acceptability of medicines: similarities and difference in paediatric and geriatric populations. https://www.ncbi.nlm.mih.gov/pmc/articles/PMC4210646 (accessed September 2019)

Michou, E., Mastan, A., Ahmed, S., et al. (2012) Examining the role of carbonation and temperature on water swallowing performance: a swallowing reaction-time study. *Chemical Senses*, 37 (9): 799–807. https://doi.org/10.1093/chemse/bjs061.

MIMS (2019). www.mims.com.au (accessed September 2019).

Morris, H. (2005). Administering drugs to patients with swallowing difficulties. *Nursing Times* 101 (39): 28.

Nerang, N. and Sharma, J. (2011). Sublingual mucosa as a route for systemic drug delivery. *International Journal of Pharmacy and Pharmaceutical Sciences*, 3 (2): 18–22. https://innovareacademics.in/journal/ijpps/Vol3Suppl2/1092.pdf (accessed September 2019).

Nicol, N. (2010). Considerations in topical treatments for atopic dermatitis. *Dermatology Nursing* 22 (3): 2–11.

Peate, I. and Wild, K. (2014). *Nursing Practice: Knowledge and Care*, 2nde. John Wiley & Sons.

107

Peate, I. (2015). How to administer suppositories. *Nursing Standard* 30 (1): 34–36.

Peltola, P. and Vehkalahti, M.M. (2005). Chewing ability of the long-term hospitalised elderly. *Special Care in Dentistry*, 25(5): 260–264. https://www.deepdyve.com/lp/wiley/chewing-ability-of-the-long-term-hospitalized-elderly-RrRsfQISDo (accessed September 2020).

Rees, J. and Kanabar, D. (2006). *ABC of Asthma*. Oxford: Blackwell.

Royal Pharmaceutical Society (2019). *Professional Guidance on the Administration of Medicines in Healthcare Settings*. London: RPS.

Royal Pharmaceutical Society (RPS) (2011). Pharmaceutical issues when crushing, opening or splitting oral dosage forms. https://www.rpharms.com/Portals/0/RPS%20document%20library/Open%20access/Support/toolkit/pharmaceuticalissuesdosageforms-%282%29.pdf (accessed July 2019).

Salib, R.J. and Howarth, P.H. (2003). Safety and tolerability profiles of intranasal antihistamine and intranasal corticosteroids in the treatment of allergic rhinitis. *Drug Safety* 26 (12): 863–893.

Scadding, G.K., Kariyawasam, H.H. et al. (2017). BSACI guideline for the diagnosis and management of allergic and non-allergic rhinitis (revised edition 2017; first edition 2007). *Clinical and Experimental Allergy* 47 (7): 856–889.

Shaw, M. (2014). How to administer eye drops and ointments. *Nursing Times* 110 (40): 16–18.

Singh, D.H., Roychowdhury, S., Verma, P., and Bhandari, P. (2012). A review on recent advances of enteric coating. IOSR *Journal of Pharmacy* e-ISSN: 2250–3013, p-ISSN: 2319–4219, 2 (6): 5–11. http://www.iosrphr.org/papers/v2i6/Part_1/B0260511.pdf (accessed September 2020).

Smeulers, M., Verweij, L., Maaskant, J.M., et al. (2015) Quality indicators for safe medication preparation and administration: a systematic review. *PLoS ONE*, 10(4): e0122695. doi:10.1371/ journal.pone.0122695.

Ummadi, S., Raghavendra Rao, N.G., Reddy, M.S., and Nayak, B.S. (2013). Overview on controlled release dosage form. https://pdfs.semanticscholar.org/bc6e/eaec51abc07f4f1b891d2ecc31d063ed05b8.pdf (accessed September 2019).

Van der Steen, K.C., Frijlink, H.W., Schipper, C.M.A., and Barends, D.M., (2010). Prediction of the ease of subdivision of scored tablets from their physical parameters. https://res.mdpi.com/d_attachment/applsci/applsci-09-03066/article_deploy/applsci-09-03066.pdf#page26 (accessed September 2019).

Williams, N.T. (2008). Medication administration through enteral feeding tubes. *American Journal of Health-System Pharmacy*, 65 (24): 2347–2357.

Further reading

National Institute for Health and Care Excellence (NICE) – Medications Management https://www.nice.org.uk/guidance/health-and-social-care-delivery/medicines-management

Nursing and Midwifery Council – www.nmc.org.uk

Royal Pharmaceutical Society – www.rpharms.com

British Pharmaceutical Society – www.bps.ac.uk

Multiple choice questions

1. Enteric coated tablets:
   (a) Disintegrate in the stomach
   (b) Take longer to dissolve and take effect than regular tablets
   (c) Can be crushed
   (d) Are suitable for patients who have difficulty in swallowing
2. Modified release medications:
   (a) Are fast acting
   (b) Are suitable for crushing/dissolving/cutting
   (c) Require less frequent dosages
   (d) Are not suitable for the treatment of chronic pain
3. Sublingual GTN spray:
   (a) Is an ineffective treatment for cardiac chest pain
   (b) Is a potent vasodilator and should be used with caution
   (c) Is suitable for hypovolemic patients
   (d) Can be multipatient use

4. When administering a nebuliser to a COPD patient:
   - (a) High-flow oxygen should be used
   - (b) Oxygen is appropriate if only used at 2 L/min
   - (c) Medical air should be used
   - (d) If they are short of breath, high flow oxygen should be used regardless of their CO_2 levels

5. Patients unable to absorb oral medications due to gut ileus:
   - (a) Should be given their tablets anyway on the offchance that they may absorb them
   - (b) Should receive the equivalent IV preparation for all essential medications
   - (c) Should have all medications ceased until their gut starts to work again
   - (d) Do not require any further investigation and/or monitoring

6. When noticing an error in a medication order, the nurse should:
   - (a) Rectify the error with the prescriber immediately then proceed to administer the medication
   - (b) Continue to administer the medication if they know what the order was intended to say
   - (c) Cross out the mistake and write the correct order next to it themselves
   - (d) Omit the medication and wait until they next see the person who prescribed it before raising it with them

7. When removing a PCA from a patient you should:
   - (a) Just remove it and re-assess their pain in two to four hours before administering any analgesics
   - (b) Tell them they can have some pain relief in a few hours if they like
   - (c) Ensure they have received adequate alternative pain relief prior to removing the PCA and that there is further PRN (pro re nata – taken as required) analgesia prescribed for break-through pain
   - (d) Tell the patient that they no longer need pain relief

8. You are dispensing tablets on a medication round and notice that a patient has been prescribed tablet medication but has dysphagia, you should:
   - (a) Go ahead and give the tablet as prescribed
   - (b) Consider an alternative formulation when administering medication
   - (c) Discuss with the medical team, nurse-in-charge, speech, and language team and pharmacist prior to giving medications
   - (d) Crush the tablet and give it to the patient

9. Which condition below will antiviral lotions/creams treat?
   - (a) Cellulitis
   - (b) Shingles
   - (c) Psoriasis
   - (d) Athletes foot

10. Suppositories can be used for what effect:
    - (a) Analgesia
    - (b) Bowel preparation
    - (c) Local treatment; such as haemorrhoids
    - (d) All of the above

11. What proportion of inhaled drugs via nebulisation reach the lungs?
    - (a) 6%
    - (b) 10%
    - (c) 12%
    - (d) 18%

12. How many 'Rights' of medication administration are there?
    (a) 5
    (b) 6
    (c) 7
    (d) 8

13. When giving an IM injection, what should you do if you pull back on the syringe plunger and notice blood?
    (a) Continue giving the injection
    (b) Continue pulling back on the plunger until no more blood is aspirated
    (c) Stop the procedure for 10 seconds and check again
    (d) Stop the procedure and withdraw the needle

14. When administering eye drops, what is the recommended time interval between drops to ensure maximum effect?
    (a) 30 seconds
    (b) 3 minutes
    (c) 5 seconds
    (d) 60 minutes

15. Oral liquid suspensions should be considered for:
    (a) Patients with dysphagia
    (b) Children
    (c) The elderly
    (d) All of the above

Find out more

The following is a list of some common conditions requiring a variety of medications to be administered via a variety of routes using different drug preparations. Take some time to test your knowledge and write some notes about each condition. Think specifically about the different medications, treatments or therapies the patient will require and how these might be administered/what formulation they are available in, and which route of administration is most appropriate for each patient group. Remember to include aspects of patient care and relate to real practice experiences if applicable – maintaining patient confidentiality at all times.

Condition	Your notes
Eczema	
Pneumonia	
Nausea and Vomiting	
Atrial Fibrillation	
Diabetes Mellitus	

Chapter 7

Adverse drug reaction

Laura Park and Michelle Mitchell

Aim

The aim of this chapter is to provide the reader with an understanding of what is meant by the term adverse drug reaction (ADR) in pharmacology.

Learning outcomes

After reading this chapter, the reader will:

1. Understand what is meant by the term an ADR and why it is important to be aware of it
2. Gain knowledge in the different classifications of ADRs
3. Be able to recognise the signs and symptoms of ADR
4. Understand professional duties when caring for patients and reporting ADRs

Test your knowledge

1. What is your interpretation of an ADR?
2. List how you might recognise symptoms of an ADR.
3. Do you consider ADR to be a common occurrence?
4. Which groups of patients are more vulnerable to experiencing an ADR?

Definition – what is an adverse drug reaction

An adverse drug reaction (ADR) can be defined as 'an appreciably harmful or unpleasant reaction resulting from an intervention related to the use of a medicinal product; adverse effects usually predict hazard from future administration and warrant prevention, or specific treatment, or alteration of the dosage regimen, or withdrawal of the product'

(Coleman and Pontefract, 2016, p. 481).

Fundamentals of Pharmacology: For Nursing and Healthcare Students, First Edition. Edited by Ian Peate and Barry Hill.
© 2021 John Wiley & Sons Ltd. Published 2021 by John Wiley & Sons Ltd.

An ADR as defined by the National Institute of Health and Care Excellence (NICE) (2017) is an unwanted or harmful reaction that transpires after the administration of a drug and is suspected or known to be due to the drug. However, NICE (2017) states that there are other terms that ought to be distinguished; the interchangeable terms 'adverse reaction' and 'adverse effect' are often referred to, yet reflect different opinions; a person experiences an adverse reaction, whereas a drug has an adverse effect. These terms are favoured over other terms, such as 'side effect,' for the reason that they encompass all unwanted effects. They make no assumptions about mechanism, suggest no doubt and avoid the risk of misclassification.

The prevalence of adverse reactions

Neal (2016) states that 5% of acute hospital admissions are a result of adverse drug reactions (ADR) to drugs given in general practice. The percentage of hospital admissions due to ADRs in the UK was estimated by NICE just a year later in 2017 to be 6–7%, with ADRs thought to occur in 10–20% of hospital inpatients; and although rare, ADRs are thought to account for 0.5–1% of hospital inpatient deaths (NICE, 2017). Contributing to 1700 – and directly responsible for approximately 700 – deaths per year, avoidable ADRs collectively cost £98.5 million per year. In addition to treating preventable adverse events, significant costs are paid in covering any litigation expenses (NICE, 2017).

These substantial costs concomitant with preventable medicines-related acute hospital admissions could represent significant savings to the NHS. The treatment and management of possible preventable ADRs that transpire during an inpatient stay, for example, may increase the length of a patients hospital stay by up to three days, consequently resulting in additional costs. The daily cost of a non-elective inpatient bed, for example, is £265, so there may be a saving up to £795 per ADR avoided. A decrease in a patient's length of stay also releases capacity for NHS providers to make better use of hospital beds. NHS litigation has reported that since 2008, there have been 551 successful claims made against NHS trusts where a medication error has been listed as one of the causes. Since 2008, a total cost of £16 572 028 has been awarded in damages, a further £1 643 142 has been paid to cover defence costs and £9 637 309 paid to cover claimant costs (NICE, 2015).

With the aim to decrease the global encumbrance of severe and avoidable medication-related harm by 50% over a five year period, The World Health Organization (WHO) (2017) propelled its third Global Patient Safety Challenge: 'Medication without Harm'.

Type A reactions (categorised below) can be anticipated and may be avoided through increased awareness and vigilance. To achieve this, in adherence to the Nursing and Midwifery Council Code (Nursing and Midwifery Council, 2018), nurses must work cooperatively with other health and care professionals and staff by respecting the skills, expertise, and contributions of colleagues, maintaining effective communication by sharing information, keeping colleagues informed to identify and reduce risk and preserve the safety of those receiving care.

Partnership working is crucial in healthcare and the core of collaborative partnership is of course the patient. There are many terms referred to in the field of partnership working (interprofessional working, collaborative working, multidisciplinary and multiprofessional) (Lewin and Reeves, 2016). In relation to medicine management, using the term working collaboratively means healthcare workers who are professionally regulated working together to achieve the shared goal of ensuring that the patient's treatment, including pharmacological interventions, are safe and effective (Tully and Franklin, 2016). Patients' roles in collaborative healthcare partnerships in relation to medicine management will be endorsed according to the level of exchange in those partnerships. Based on study findings, patients may well become active partners even when conditions for a partnership are not met. Many patients understand that they cannot only participate in self-managing their health and healthcare, but can also actively establish partnerships with the healthcare professionals providing their care (Pomey et al., 2015).

There are also numerous non-registrants, such as healthcare assistants, hospital porters and community care workers, whose work as part of the healthcare multidisciplinary team is vital both within hospitals and in the community. Without them, patient care and safety would be severely affected; although in the majority of cases these individuals do not have direct responsibility for administering patient medication, it is important that they have an awareness of the dangers of drugs and be aware of the symptoms of an ADR. Their responsibility would be to notify the healthcare professional on the ward or GP practice (Lawson and Hennefer, 2010).

The ABCDE classification of adverse reactions

Understanding and differentiating between the different types of ADRs can be complex. To make ADRs easier to understand and to manage, they are classified into subtypes (Young and Pitcher, 2016). An overview of the different classifications (A, B, C, D, E) and their profiles are outlined below.

A – augmented (common)

These reactions are related to the pharmacological actions of the drug. Therefore, they **can be predicted** and are normally dose dependent, meaning they can be alleviated by altering (normally reducing) the drug's dose. The majority of reported ADRs are type A reactions.

An example of an augmented ADR is bleeding from anticoagulants (i.e. warfarin).

B – bizarre (uncommon)

Subtype B reactions are **difficult to predict** due to them being idiosyncratic (i.e. relating to the individual). Type B ADRs are not related to the pharmacological action of the drug or the dose. Type B accounts for about 20% of all ADR and, although more uncommon than type A, are often more serious as they have the potential to be fatal if not recognised and managed quickly.

An example includes anaphylaxis from penicillin.

C – chronic (uncommon)

These are classified as reactions from the biological characteristic and can be predicted from the drug's chemical structure. Reactions persist for a relatively long period of time.

An example includes osteonecrosis of the jaw from the use of bisphosphonates.

Bisphosphonates are used to treat conditions that affect an individual's bones. Bisphosphonates slow both the rate of growth and dissolution, reducing the rate of bone turnover.

D – delayed effects (uncommon and difficult to detect)

These are reactions that occur over time and are usually dose related.

An example includes lomustine (treatment for certain cancers), as it can cause leucopenia up to six weeks after treatment has started.

E – end of treatment effect (uncommon)

These are classified as reactions that occur on withdrawal, i.e. when a drug is stopped abruptly.

An example includes insomnia and anxiety following the withdrawal of benzodiazepines. Benzodiapines are the most commonly used anxiolytics (sedatives).

(Beard and Lee, 2006; Greener, 2014; MHRA, 2015; Schatz and Weber, 2015; Kaufman, 2016; Young and Pitcher, 2016; BNF NICE, 2019a, b).

The signs and symptoms of adverse effects

The fundamental principles for identifying ADRs relate to recognising the relationship between medications and their side effects from various sources of information, such as social media, biomedical literature, medical records and clinical trials (Wang et al., 2019).

Young and Pitcher (2016) recognise that research and audit have clearly demonstrated the importance of ADRs and their prevalence in the causes of morbidity and mortality. Crouch and

Chapelhow (2008) highlight that the causes of an ADR are multifactorial, with common factors including the following:

- Poor prescribing practices; for example, prescribing medications that are known to interact with each other.
- Prescribers' perceptions of the risks associated with prescribing particular medicines.
- Lack of healthcare professionals' education in medicine management.
- Patients' susceptibility to a particular medicine.
- Patients' perceptions of the risks of using medicines.

Lee (2006) highlights that recognising an ADR is an important, but not always an easy, task, emphasising that the vigilance of a nurse or healthcare professional is vital. As nurses are the healthcare professionals that spend the most time with patients, they are very often in the best position to recognise if something is wrong and assess the effects of an ADR so that the drug(s) can be stopped prior to harm occurring (Crouch and Chapelhow, 2008).

It is important to recognise when a patient is experiencing an ADR, or the omission may lead to subsequent prescribing of additional drugs to correct the drug-induced disease. However, these challenges test the diagnostic expertise of the most experienced clinician as it can be difficult to distinguish an ADR from an exacerbation of a patient's existing disease or a possible new health condition, as a result of the clinical picture being complex. However, to identify an ADR, a healthcare professional must first entertain the possibility of an adverse event. If you do not look, you will not find them.

Drugs that most commonly cause ADRs are:
- warfarin
- diuretics
- digoxin
- tranquilisers
- antibacterials
- steroids
- potassium
- antihypertensives
- drugs for treatment of Parkinson's disease
- antineoplastic drugs.

Clinical considerations

Predisposing factors
Certain groups of patients are more vulnerable to ADRs than others and certain factors can influence the likelihood of a patient suffering a reaction.

Polypharmacy	A key factor to consider is multiple drug therapy, which is referred to as polypharmacy. Patients who take multiple medications are more likely to experience side effects linked with one drug that in turn may influence another (a drug reaction).
Age	Those who are at the extremes of age are particularly susceptible to ADRs (Beard and Lee, 2006). Children and neonates, in particular, are at a higher risk of experiencing an ADR, because how their body manages and responds to drugs is different (Kaufman, 2016). Older adults are more vulnerable to an adverse drug reaction than younger adults for numerous reasons. This is often due to those factors that influence pharmacokinetics (absorption, distribution, metabolism and excretion (ADME) and pharmacodynamics in the older patient differs from those in younger adults. In older patients, the liver loses the ability to metabolise drugs. As people age, the amount of water in their body decreases and the volume of fat tissue relative to water increases. Therefore, older people who take medicines that dissolve in water will reach a higher concentration of the medication as there will be far less water to dilute them. Medicines that dissolve in fat accrue more as there is

	moderately more fat tissue to store them. It is also important to note that as people age, an individual's kidneys may be less able to excrete drugs and the liver may be less able to metabolise many drugs. In addition to this, some older people may have concurrent health problems; therefore, they may take several medicines and over-the-counter drugs (as explained in the section above).
Gender	Biological differences between a male and female affect the action of numerous drugs. The anatomical and physiological variations are body composition, body weight, liver metabolism, gastrointestinal tract factors and renal function. Females in contrast to men generally have a lesser bodyweight and smaller size organs, a larger proportion of body fat, a different gastric motility and a lower glomerular filtration rate. The differences may affect the way a body metabolises drugs, therefore altering the pharmacokinetics and pharmacodynamics of the drug, including the absorption, distribution, metabolism and elimination of a drug. Women are at greater risk of an adverse drug reaction. The reason for this is not completely clear; nevertheless, gender-related factors, such as immunological and hormonal factors, the differences in pharmacokinetics, and the general use in the medicines that are taken and used are all factors that may contribute to ADRs (Alder et al., 2016).
Ethnicity	The distinct differences of an individual are controlled by genetic factors. The ethnic background of an individual has a tendency to present certain reactions and is related to the genetic make-up of an individual; therefore, a drug action differs significantly between individuals. Genetic factors can determine an individual's susceptibility and may make the drug act in an entirely abnormal way. Ethnic differences can increase the risk of an adverse drug reaction. For example, an enzyme deficiency of glucose-6-phosphate dehydrogenase is widespread in parts of Southern Europe Africa, Asia and Oceania (Alder et al., 2016). Glucose-6-phosphate dehydrogenase protects an individual's red blood cells from harm caused by medicines such as nitrofurantoin and quinolone antibiotics that may cause haemolytic anaemia (Alder et al., 2016).
Environmental factors	With scant research in the form of studies, it is difficult to ascertain how many individuals are more likely to be affected; however, it is possible in certain individuals that tobacco, alcohol, and diet consumption and other, as yet unknown, factors may influence the response to a drug. For example: smoking is one risk factor of various diseases such as cancer, cardiovascular disease and peptic ulcers. By affecting the metabolic process, it affects liver enzymes, acting as a compelling inducer of the hepatic cytochrome. Many drugs are substrates and their metabolism can be induced in individuals that smoke, resulting in a clinically significant decrease in pharmacologic effects. The drug interaction is not instigated by nicotine; the cause of it is the tobacco, as it stimulates the body's sympathetic nervous system (Alomar, 2014).
Pregnancy	During pregnancy, women are at increased risk of an ADR (Kaufman, 2016). This is due to the pharmacokinetics of many drugs becoming altered, i.e. how the body receives and responds to drugs during pregnancy (da Silva et al., 2019). It is estimated that while pregnant 80% of women will take additional medication (McElhatton, 2006). ADRs during pregnancy have been found to affect the foetus and the breastfed baby, with thalidomide being a well-known example (Kaufman, 2016). While studies into ADR during pregnancy are limited for ethical reasons, there have been studies that estimate the incidence of ADR during pregnancy to be around 10% (da Silva et al., 2019).
An individual's current health status	The status of an individual's current health can also predispose individuals to experience ADRs (Kaufman, 2016). A reduced renal function and liver impairment are two examples of health issues in those who are more at risk of ADRs (Alder et al., 2016). A reduced renal excretion of drugs can lead to toxicity. Changes in the liver metabolism can also affect the risk of adverse drug reactions. Some reactions occur more in the type B category, frequently in patients with liver disease (Schatz and Weber, 2015; Alder et al., 2016). Other conditions that may predispose an individual to an adverse drug reaction include infectious mononucleosis (glandular fever) and immunodeficiency virus (Kaufman, 2016).
Host factors	Host disease may predispose to a certain adverse reaction. For example, patients with infectious mononucleosis are liable to experience a rash if given ampicillin.

Physical signs of an adverse drug reaction may include the following

Acute anaphylaxis

With rapid onset, this may be caused by certain foods (for example, nuts, eggs and fish), by drugs (notably penicillin), by wasp and bee stings, by injection or foreign serum, and by contact with latex rubber:

- feeling light-headed or faint;
- confusion and anxiety;
- breathing difficulties – such as fast, shallow breathing;
- a fast heartbeat;
- wheezing;
- clammy skin;
- collapsing or losing consciousness.

There may also be other allergy symptoms, including an itchy, raised rash (hives), feeling or being sick, swelling (angioedema) or stomach pain. (See Figures 7.1–7.3.)

Rashes

May occur as a result of a drug allergy, but not all rashes which occur when drugs are given are due to an allergy. An example of a non-allergic drug rash is the typical erythematosus rash, which often occurs when ampicillin is taken. See Figure 7.4.

Serum Sickness

Develops after the serum or drug has been administered. The symptoms of serum sickness typically start within one to three weeks of exposure to a new medication. There is usually an urticarial rash with stiffness and swelling of joints, occasionally a mild nephritis, and lymph node enlargement. See Figure 7.5.

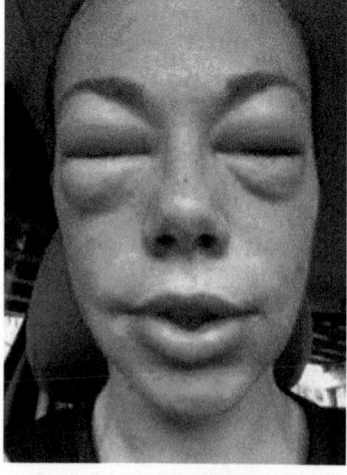

Figure 7.1   Anaphylaxis eyes. Source: ABC News.

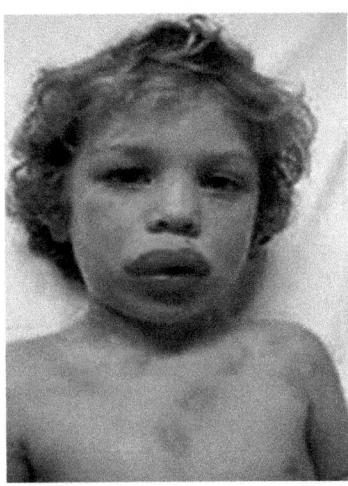

Figure 7.2   Anaphylaxis lips. Source: BBC News.

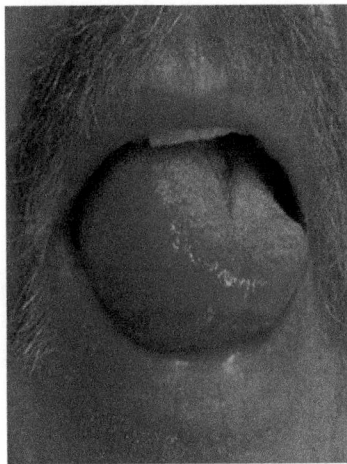

Figure 7.3   Anaphylaxis tongue. Source: BBC News.

Renal Disorders

Damage to the glomerulus by several drugs, including penicillamine and gold, can cause gross proteinuria. Non-steroidal anti-inflammatory drugs (NSAIDs) and angiotensin-converting enzyme (ACE) inhibitors can cause renal failure and there are a number of other types of drug-induced renal disease.

When a reaction to a drug is suspected, the healthcare professional must investigate whether that particular drug is recognised to cause such a reaction, rule out any other explanation, and establish a progressive link between the onset of the reaction and drug administration. When empirical methods fail or produce an uncertain result, the more formal process of using a probability assessment tool will often produce clearer results.

The fundamental principle of recognising an ADR is: when a patient experiences what seems like an exacerbation of an current medical condition, or develops what appears like a new medical problem while being treated for something else, the possibility of an ADR must be added to the investigation of diagnosis.

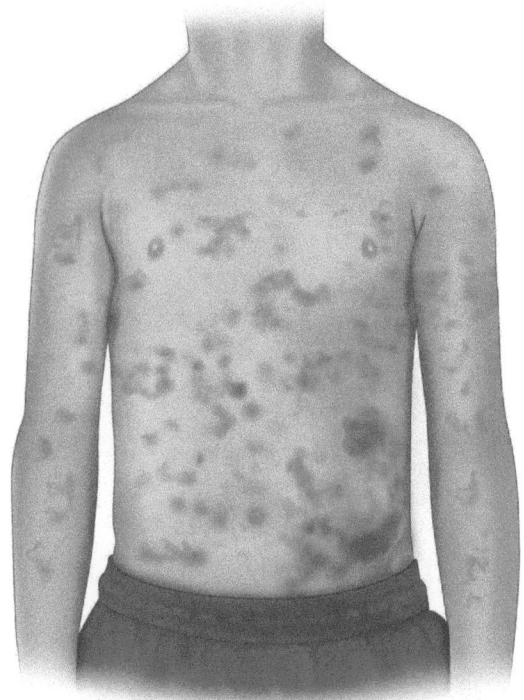

Figure 7.4   Rash. Source: ABC News.

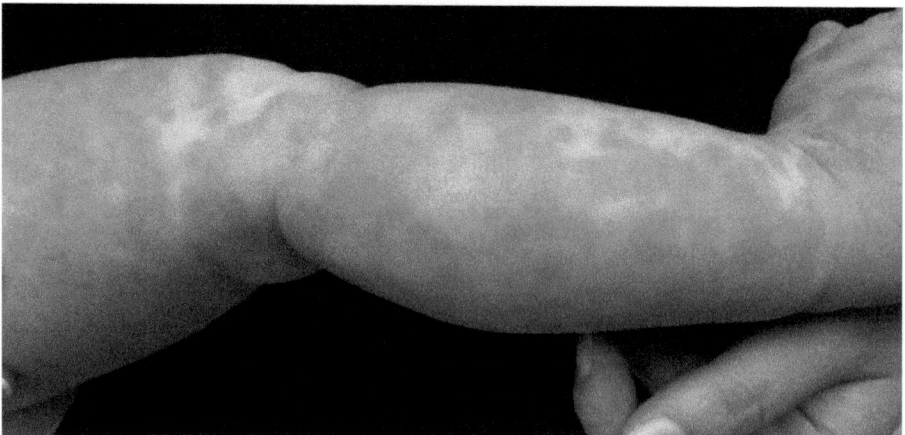

Figure 7.5   Serum sickness. Source: ABC News.

Adverse reaction diagnosis and management

Despite the precautions made to avoid ADRs, they are still a regular occurrence on both a UK and global scale. It is therefore important that all healthcare professionals have an awareness of the signs and symptoms of ADRs that have already been outlined in this chapter. While many ADR reactions have minor symptoms and consequences, there are times where emergency treatment is required for ADRs (Ferner and McGettigan, 2018).

If an ADR is observed, it is important that you remain with the patient and call/arrange for help (Lawson and Hennefer, 2010). If a serious ADR is suspected (an initial assessment can be done using the ABCDE assessment tool), i.e. the reaction is life threatening, then call for emergency help. If in a hospital setting, this can be done by pressing the emergency buzzer or, in the community, by ringing the emergency services (NICE, 2017). If applicable, stop the drug from being administered; i.e., if given via an IV infusion, stop the infusion. Minor ADRs or ADRs with non-life-threatening reactions can, however, be difficult to diagnose as patients often do not link their symptoms with the drug and/or drugs that they are taking. Educating patients about the drugs that they are taking (i.e. making patients aware of a drug's known side effects), what an ADR is, along with taking a detailed drug history can improve patient safety as it can aid the quick identification and management of ADRs (Ferner and McGettigan, 2018).

Examples of drug history questions for suspected ADRs include:

- Have you taken the medication before without experiencing an adverse reaction?
- Did the reaction occur only after the drug was started?
- Did anything else change around the time of the suspected drug (i.e. other treatments/ drugs, disease progression)?

(Coleman and Pontefract, 2016)

For ADRs that are not life-threatening, the following needs to be considered for management:

- Can the ADR be managed in primary care setting (i.e. GP) or does the patient need to be admitted to hospital for treatment?

If the ADR can be managed in a primary care setting, consider the following for management:

- Review and discuss treatment options. This may include stopping the suspected drug if the reaction has caused serious harm or stopping the drug on the request of the patient.
- If the patients still requires treatment, then an alternative treatment needs to be considered.
- If the drug is still required for treatment, then a review of the dose of the drug is required.
- Consider stopping the drug temporarily.
- Manage symptoms of the ADR as appropriate: i.e. the prescribing of other medication is required. If other drugs are prescribed, ensure that the patient is aware of the benefits and harms, if applicable, when prescribing another drug to treat their ADR.
- Record the ADR in the patient's health records and record the ADR through the yellow card scheme.

(NICE, 2017)

Reporting incidents of adverse drug reactions

Patient safety in relation to medicines management is not a new topic. Healthcare professionals can make significant improvements to medicine safety: being knowledgeable and proactive in reporting drug-related incidents in accordance with the reporting systems is vital (NICE, 2015). There is still much to learn about ADRs; this is despite medicines, drugs and treatments being widely tested before their commercial availability, as often pre-licensing trials are too small to uncover the uncommon but important harms and reactions that drugs can have on patients (Dougherty and Lister, 2015; Ferner and McGettigan, 2018). Reporting schemes for ADRs have been found to be significant in continuing to build on drug knowledge, to maximise the benefits from a drug, and to reduce harm (Kaufman, 2016). Pharmacovigilance is the scientific process of, monitoring, assessing, detecting and preventing incidents of ADR (Dougherty and Lister, 2015; Alder et al., 2016); further information on pharmacovigilance can be found in the Skills Practice box.

Skills in practice: What is pharmacovigilance?

Pharmacovigilance is the term applied to the scientific study of drug safety i.e. understanding, monitoring and responding to ADR's (WHO, 2020). The aim of pharmacovigilance is therefore to maintain patient safety by minimising the risks of adverse reactions and to detect/prevent medical errors (WHO, 2014).

Pharmacovigilance is a vital component of every healthcare professional's role and, as discussed, it is often the nurse who will recognise emerging side effects as part of caring for the patients (Tully and Franklin, 2016; Young and Pitcher, 2016).

In 2012, EU legislation provided healthcare professionals and stakeholders with clear guidance on their role and responsibilities with regards to drug safety and surveillance (Coleman and Pontefract, 2016). As both healthcare professionals and patients have a responsibility to report ADRs, it is important that nurses and other healthcare professionals ensure that patients are aware of ADRs and the reporting process.

ADRs in the UK are reported to the Medicines and Healthcare Products Regulatory Agency (MHRA) via the yellow card scheme (Figure 7.6) (Dougherty and Lister, 2015; NICE, 2017; Gregory and Middleton, 2019). The MHRA is an executive agency of the Department of Health and is recognised globally for protecting and improving public health and supporting innovation through research (MHRA, 2019a). The yellow card scheme was introduced in 1964 following the thalidomide incident in the late 1950s (Coleman and Pontefract, 2016). Through reporting, the scheme collects data on all suspected ADRs (this includes both prescribed and self-medicated drugs) in adults and children (NICE, 2017).

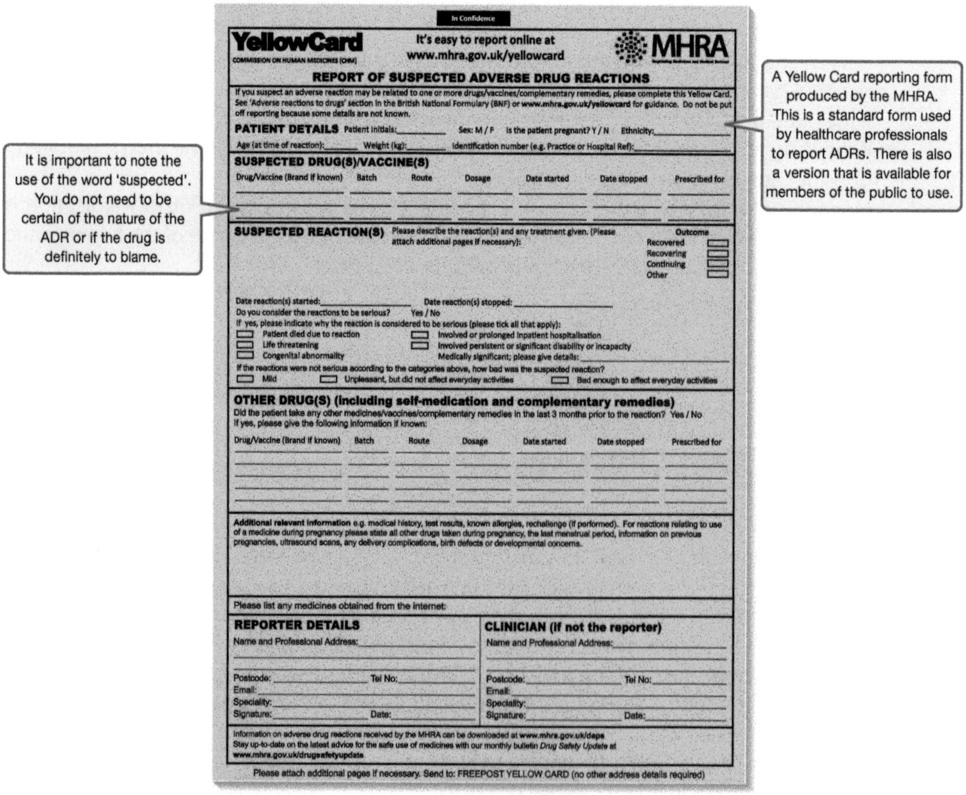

It is important to note the use of the word 'suspected'. You do not need to be certain of the nature of the ADR or if the drug is definitely to blame.

A Yellow Card reporting form produced by the MHRA. This is a standard form used by healthcare professionals to report ADRs. There is also a version that is available for members of the public to use.

Figure 7.6 'Yellow Card' notification for suspected adverse drug reactions. Source: Yellow Card reporting form. © Crown copyright. Reproduced under OGL 3.0.

Skills in practice: Completing a yellow card

How to report an ADR

Reporting suspected ADRs in the UK should be done as soon as possible through the yellow card scheme. The yellow card scheme can be accessed by healthcare professionals or patients in a multitude of ways:

- Electronically through the MHRA www.mhra.gov.uk/yellowcard.
- Via a free mobile yellow card app.
- By writing to FREEPOST YELLOW CARD.
- By emailing yellowcard@mhra.gsi.gov.uk.
- By calling the National Yellow Card Information Service.
  (NICE, 2017)

Yellow cards can be filled out by healthcare professionals or patients for any of the following:

- all medicines
- vaccines
- blood factors
- immunoglobulins
- complementary medicines (homoeopathic/herbal remedies) (NICE, 2017).

Any ADR incidents will additionally need to be documented in the patient's notes (a copy of the yellow card report could be included as part of the documentation). Furthermore, depending on the hospitals medicine management policy, healthcare professionals may be required to complete additional reports/forms and comply with other policy requirements (O'Brien et al., 2011); for example, informing/alerting other healthcare professionals such as ward mangers, clinical matrons and the pharmacy team.

Once information has been reported via the yellow card scheme, the MHRA analyse and collate the data. Reports are then created and distributed via publication, enabling advice, recommendations and warnings associated with ADRs to be made widely available so that actions can be taken to minimise harm (Kaufman, 2016; MHRA, 2015, 2019b).

Following the collation of yellow card data, the MHRA can make the following recommendations:

- Restrict the use of a drug.
- Change a drugs legal status (i.e. from over the counter to prescription only).
- Make amendments to the warning information.
- If risks out weight the benefits, they can remove medicines from the market.

What information is needed to report an ADR using the yellow card scheme?

When completing a yellow card, the following pieces of information are required (it is important to note that within the yellow card document the word **suspected** is used; therefore, healthcare professionals and/or patients do not need to be certain of an ADR incident (Young and Pitcher, 2016):

- The name and full address of the reporter. This is so the MHRA can acknowledge receipt of the report and follow up for further information if required.
- If known, information about the suspected drug that has caused the ADR. This includes route of administration, dose, frequency, dates of administration, and, if applicable, the brand and batch number of the drug.

- If known, information about the suspected reaction or reactions, i.e. when the reaction occurred, seriousness, if any treatment was given, and the outcome of reaction.
- At least one of the following pieces of patient information: sex, age at the time of the reaction, weight, the person's initials, and a local identification number (i.e. hospital number). This information is needed so that the patient can be identifiable to you (but not to the MHRA). Please note that providing this information does not violate patient confidentiality.

If relevant or applicable, the following information should also be included in the yellow card report:

- Test results (include print-outs if necessary).
- Medical history, including allergies.
- Relevant drug information: this should include any information on the drug/drugs taken in the last three months prior to the reaction (this includes over-the-counter and herbal medicines).
- If the patient who experienced the suspected ADR was **not** taking any other drugs/medications.
- Alternatively, if there is no other information to declare, this should be indicated on the form too.

(NICE, 2017)

Despite the accessibility of the yellow card scheme and its ability to reduce harm from ADRs, the system is challenged by underreporting with fewer than 5% of all ADRs estimated as being reported in practice (Coleman and Pontefract, 2016). Steps, however, have been made to encourage the reporting of ADRs via the yellow card scheme. This is in the form of continuous professional development e-learning from the MHRA and the distribution of a monthly drug safety bulletin outlining information about suspected ADRs (General Pharmaceutical Council, 2019).

Episode of care

Mr. Butterfield and Mr. Gent

Mr. Butterfield and Mr. Gent are two gentleman who came separately via ambulance on the same morning to an acute stroke unit with suspected cerebrovascular accidents (CVA). Mr. Butterflied is a 65-year-old retired primary school headmaster. He is married and has recently welcomed his first grandchild. Mr. Gent is 60, widowed and remains in employment as a civil engineer.

From the symptoms they present with and the onset, Mr. Butterfield and Mr. Gent are both potential candidates for thrombolysis. Mr. Butterfield and Mr. Gent both describe their current health status as being fit and well, neither take regular medications (including both prescribed and over-the-counter medications), and they have no reported allergies. Mr. Butterfield does disclose that his father died 20 years ago following a stroke. Both Mr. Butterfield and Mr. Gent from assessment are eligible for thrombolysis.

The majority of strokes are caused when blood clots move to a blood vessel in the brain blocking the flow of blood (Stroke Association, 2019). For such strokes (ischaemic strokes/infarcts), a clot-busting drug can be given, i.e. thrombolysis medication, which aims to dissolve the clot thus allowing blood flow to return (Stroke Association, 2019).

Both Mr. Butterfield and Mr. Gent were given the same batch of thrombolysis medication on the same day with 15 minutes between their start times.

Both Mr. Butterfield and Mr. Gent during the administration of the thrombolysis medication experienced swollen lips, breathlessness and nausea. Mr. Gent additionally presented with a rash to his hands and face. Upon noticing these signs and symptoms of anaphylaxis, the nurse caring for Mr. Gent and Mr. Butterfield pulled the emergency alarm. Both thrombolysis infusions were stopped and urgent care was given, i.e. epinephrine (adrenaline).

The nurse caring for Mr. Gent and Mr. Butterfield completed two separate yellow cards (this was done online) in order to report the incident as an ADR. The nurse additionally documented these incidents in the patients' notes, informed her ward manager and the pharmacy team. The pharmacy team asked for the batch of thrombolysis medication given to Mr. Butterfield and Mr. Gent to be returned to pharmacy and an alternative batch was given to the stroke ward for the next thrombolysis case.

Conclusion

ADRs and their impact on clinical practice have been discussed in this chapter. Having an awareness of ADRs is essential for any healthcare provider in order to improve patient safety and reduce the 5% of patient admissions that ADRs have been reported to cause (Neal, 2016).

While understanding the complexities of the different ADR symptoms, category types and management precautions are important. A significant impact on safe clinical practice outlined in this chapter is simply healthcare professionals being proactive and vigilant in reporting incidences of ADRs via the yellow card scheme. As demonstrated, reporting incidences of ADRs is not exclusive to healthcare professionals, nor does it require an extensive set of skills; it does, however, require awareness. It is, therefore, essential that healthcare students start to develop a sound knowledge of ADRs so that they have the skills to provide information and advice to patients on ADRs and ADR reporting.

References

Alder, J., Astles, A., Bentley, A. et al. (2016). Essential pharmacology: therapeutics and medicines management for non-medical prescribers. In: *The Textbook of Non-Medical Prescribing*, 2ee (eds. D. Nuttall and J. Rutt-Howard), 148–182. Chichester: Wiley-Blackwell.

Alomar, A.J. (2014). Factors affecting the development of adverse drug reactions. *Saudi Pharmaceutical Journal* 22 (2): 83–94.

Beard, K. and Lee, A. (2006). Introduction. In: *Adverse Drug Reactions*, 2e (ed. A. Lee), 1–22. London: Pharmaceutical Press.

BNF NICE (2019a). Bisphosphonates. https://bnf.nice.org.uk/drug-class/bisphosphonates.html (accessed 21 October 2019).

BNF NICE (2019b). Hypnotics and anxiolytics. https://bnf.nice.org.uk/treatment-summary/hypnotics-and-anxiolytics.html (accessed 21 October 2019).

Coleman, J.J. and Pontefract, S.K. (2016). Adverse drug reactions. *Clinical Medicine* 16 (5): 481–485.

Crouch, S. and Chapelhow, C. (2008). *Medicines Management a Nursing Perspective*. Essex: Pearson Edcuation Ltd.

Dougherty, L. and Lister, S. (2015). *The Royal Marsden Manual of Clinical Nursing Procedures, 9th (edn)*. Chichester, West Sussex: John Wiley & Sons, Ltd.

Ferner, R.E. and McGettigan, P. (2018). Adverse drug reactions. *The BMJ* 363: 1–9.

General Pharmaceutical Council (2019). Focus on reporting to the MHRA's yellow card scheme. https://www.pharmacyregulation.org/regulate/article/focus-reporting-mhras-yellow-card-scheme (accessed 29 September 2019).

Greener, M. (2014). Understanding adverse drug reactions: an overview. *Nurse Prescribing* 12 (4): 189–195.

Gregory, J. and Middleton, C. (2019). Medicine Management. In: *Foundations of Adult Nursing*, 2e (ed. D. Burns). London: SAGE.

Kaufman, G. (2016). Adverse drug reactions: classification, susceptibility and reporting. *Nursing Standard* 30 (50): 53–56.

Lawson, E. and Hennefer, D.L. (2010). *Medicines Management in Adult Nursing*. Exeter: Learning Matters Ltd.

Lee, A. (2006). *Adverse Drug Reactions*, 2e. London: Pharmaceutical Press.

Lewin, S. and Reeves, S. (2016). Enacting 'team' and 'teamwork': using Goffman's theory of impression management to illuminate interprofessional practice on hospital wards. *Social Science & Medicine* 72 (10): 1595–1602.

McElhatton, P. (2006). Adverse drug reactions in pregnancy. In: *Adverse Drug Reactions*, 2e (ed. A. Lee), 75–124. London: Pharmaceutical Press.

Medicines and Healthcare Products Regulatory Agency (MHRA) (2015). Guidance on adverse drug reactions: classification of adverse drug reactions. http://www.gov.uk/government/uploads/system/uploads/attachment_data/file/403098/Guidance_on_adverse_drug_reactions.pdf (accessed 20 September 2019).

Medicines and Healthcare Products Regulatory Agency (MHRA) (2019a). About us. https://www.gov.uk/government/organisations/medicines-and-healthcare-products-regulatory-agency/about (accessed 29 September 2019).

Medicines and Healthcare Products Regulatory Agency (MHRA) (2019b). Yellow card. https://yellowcard.mhra.gov.uk/faqs (accessed 20 September 2019).

Neal, M.J. (2016). *Medical Pharmacology at a Glance*, 8the. West Sussex: Wiley Blackwell.

NICE (2015). Medicines optimisation: the safe and effective use of medicines to enable the best possible outcomes. www.nice.org.uk/guidance/ng5 (accessed 29 September 2019).

NICE (2017). Adverse drug reactions. https://cks.nice.org.uk/adverse-drug-reactions#!scenarioRecommendation:3 (accessed 20 September 2019).

Nursing and Midwifery Council (2018). The Code; Professional standards of practice and behaviour for nurses, midwives and nursing associates. https://www.nmc.org.uk/standards/code/read-the-code-online/#fifth (accessed 19 September 2019).

O'Brien, M., Spires, A., and Andrews, K. (2011). *Introduction to Medicines Management in Nursing*. Exeter: Learning Matters Ltd.

Pomey, M.P., Ghadiri, D.P., Karazivan, P. et al. (2015). Patients as partners: a qualitative study of Patients' engagement in their health care. *PLoS ONE* 10 (4): e0122499. doi: 10.1371/journal.pone.0122499.

Schatz S.N. and Weber, R.J. (2015) Adverse drug reactions. https://www.accp.com/docs/bookstore/psap/2015B2.SampleChapter.pdf (accessed 29 September 2019).

da Silva, K.D.L., Fernanades, F.E.M., Pessoa, T.D.L. et al. (2019). Prevalence and profile of adverse drug reactions in high-risk pregnancy: a cohort study. *BMC Pregnancy and Childbirth* 19: 2–6.

Stroke Association (2019). Ischaemic stroke guide. https://www.stroke.org.uk/resources/ischaemic-stroke-guide (accessed 29 September 2020).

Tully, M.P. and Franklin, B.D. (2016). *Safety in Medication Use*. Cornwell: TJ International Ltd.

Wang, C.S., Lin, P.J., Cheng, C.L. et al. (2019). Detecting potential adverse drug reactions using a deep neural network model. *Journal of Medical Internet Research* 21 (2): E11016.

WHO (2014). Reporting and learning systems for medication errors: the role of pharmacovigilance centres. https://www.who.int/medicines/areas/quality_safety/safety_efficacy/emp_mes/en/ (accessed 29 September 2020).

WHO (2020). Pharmacovigilance. https://www.who.int/medicines/areas/quality_safety/safety_efficacy/pharmvigi/en/ (accessed 29 September 2020).

Young, S. and Pitcher, B. (2016). *Medicines Management for Nurses at a Glance*. West Sussex: Wiley.

Further reading

Department of Health and Social Care (2018). Medication errors: short life working group report. A review on the extent of medication errors and recommendations to reduce medication-related harm in England. https://www.gov.uk/government/publications/medication-errors-short-life-working-group-report (accessed 28 September 2019).

Kaufman, G. (2016). Adverse drug reactions: classification, susceptibility and reporting. *Nursing Standard* 30 (50): 53–56.

Medicines and Healthcare Products Regulatory Agency (2019). Yellow card. https://yellowcard.mhra.gov.uk/faqs (accessed 20 September 2019).

NICE (2017). Adverse drug reactions. https://cks.nice.org.uk/adverse-drug-reactions#!scenarioRecommendation:3 (accessed 20 September 2019).

World Health Organisation (2019). Pharmacovigilance. https://www.who.int/medicines/areas/quality_safety/safety_efficacy/pharmvigi/en (accessed 29 September 2019).

Multiple choice questions

1. What ADR category type is most commonly reported?
   (a) B
   (b) E
   (c) A

2. Who can report ADR via the yellow card scheme?
   (a) Patients
   (b) Healthcare professionals
   (c) Both
3. What percentage of ADRs are estimated as being reported in practice?
   (a) 8%
   (b) 12%
   (c) 5%
4. True or false: yellow cards can be completed for homoeopathic remedies?
   (a) True
   (b) False
5. What does category C stand for when describing the types of ADRs?
   (a) Crisis
   (b) Chronic
   (c) Common
6. True or false pregnant: women are more susceptible to experiencing an ADR?
   (a) True
   (b) False
7. What term refers to the scientific study of monitoring drug safety?
   (a) Polypharmacy
   (b) Pharmacodynamics
   (c) Pharmacovigilance
8. What does MHRA stand for?
   (a) Medicine Products and Healthcare Regulatory Agency
   (b) Medicines and Healthcare Products Regulatory Agency
   (c) Management of Healthcare Regulatory Agency
9. Approximately how many avoidable deaths are ADRs directly responsible for per year?
   (a) 700
   (b) 1700
   (c) 7000
10. What drug below does not commonly cause an ADR?
   (a) Warfarin
   (b) Digoxin
   (c) Paracetamol
11. Since 2008, how much money has been awarded in damages following an ADR?
   (a) £1657 000
   (b) £16 572 028
   (c) £166 328 028
12. What percentage of acute hospital admissions are the result of an ADR to drugs given in general practice?
   (a) 5%
   (b) 15%
   (c) 25%
13. The causes of an ADR are multifactorial; which of the following factors are common?
   (a) Lack of healthcare professionals' education in medicine management.
   (b) Patients' susceptibility to a particular medicine.
   (c) Both of the above

14. Which healthcare professional is in the best position to recognise if a patient is suffering from an ADR?
    (a) Pharmacist
    (b) Doctor
    (c) Nurse
15. Which of the following can cause an ADR?
    (a) Contact with latex
    (b) Food
    (c) Both of the above

Chapter 8

Analgesics

Claire Ford and Matthew Robertson

Aim

The aim of this chapter is to provide the reader with an introduction to some of the most common drugs used to manage pain in adults. This chapter will also explore the concept of multimodal analgesic approaches, and discuss the need for comprehensive individualised pain assessments and the importance of incorporating pharmacological and non-pharmacological strategies.

Learning outcomes

After reading this chapter, the reader will:

1. Appreciate the importance of understanding the pharmacology associated with analgesic medications
2. Understand treatment optimisation in order to maintain therapeutic analgesic effects
3. Have a greater awareness of the importance of respecting individual choice and utilising multimodal medication regimens for optimal delivery and person-centred care
4. Recognise the importance of administering the right drug, in the right dose, via the right route, at the right time to manage individuals' pain

Test your knowledge

1. What do you already know about the pathophysiology of pain?
2. How can pain be manifested in adults?
3. In what ways can pain impact on individuals' wellbeing?
4. Name as many definitions of pain as you can and indicate how these differ from one another.
5. Discuss some of the assessment strategies that can be used by healthcare professionals to assess individuals experiencing pain.

Fundamentals of Pharmacology: For Nursing and Healthcare Students, First Edition. Edited by Ian Peate and Barry Hill.
© 2021 John Wiley & Sons Ltd. Published 2021 by John Wiley & Sons Ltd.

Introduction

Pain, which is universally experienced, is one of the most common patient problems and one of the most frequent reasons why individuals seek medical advice (Pasero, 2015). Within the UK, it is estimated that pain affects one out of every four individuals (British Pain Society, 2019). While healthcare professionals are frequently faced with this clinical issue, pain can often be difficult to assess and manage as it is subjective, unique to each individual, and activated by a variety of stimuli, including biological, physical and psychological (Boore et al., 2016). When patients state they are in pain, it is, therefore, every healthcare professionals' duty to listen to what they say (Nursing and Midwifery Council [NMC], 2018; General Medical Council [GMC], 2019; Health and Care Professions Council

[HCPC], 2019), believe that the pain is what they say it is, observe for supporting information using appropriate and varied assessment approaches, and act as soon as possible by utilising suitable management strategies. Pain left untreated (regardless of how it is manifested) can cause significant issues and negatively impact on individuals' physical health (i.e. mobility, sleep pattern, nutritional and hydration status) and emotional wellbeing (i.e. depression or becoming socially withdrawn) (Flasar and Perry, 2014; Mears, 2018).

Pain pathways

The way in which pain is transmitted and modulated by the body, and received and interpreted by the brain, is extremely complex. This process is also associated with a variety of chemicals, neurons and electrical impulses and influenced by psychological and social elements (Ashelford et al., 2016). In order to understand the pharmacokinetics of analgesic drugs, it is important to examine these pain pathways in greater detail. Pain pathways are associated with ascending, descending and modulating processes, and while some medications are effective in interfering with the signals that are being sent to the brain, others could play a role in how the body responds to these signals after they are received and interpreted by the brain. See the illustration of a pain pathway in Figure 8.1.

The first part of the pathway is usually associated with the stimulation of sensory nerve endings, 'nociceptors', by chemicals such as histamines and prostaglandins that are released when tissue injury or irritation occurs (Boyd, 2013). Once activated, these primary sensory neurons then carry impulses via afferent A-delta fibres (wide, myelinated, fast and associated with localised sharp pain) and C fibres (narrow, non-myelinated and slower) towards the central nervous system (CNS) (Todd, 2016). These terminate in the dorsal horn of the spinal cord and form synapses, where the actions of neurotransmitters (i.e. glutamate and substance-P) continue to transfer the signals along relay neurons to the somatosensory cortex (Ashelford et al., 2016). The perception of the pain signals in the brain can be influenced by a wide array of factors, including psychological, physical, social and pharmacological, and the response to the perceived pain signals could be in the form of emotional reactions and physiological responses, which activate the descending inhibitory efferent pathways (Smith and Muralidharan, 2014). Signals are transmitted from the brain, back to the dorsal horn, where nerve endings are activated to release neurotransmitters (noradrenaline, serotonin and endorphins) which bind to the afferent pain fibres, inhibiting the synaptic transmission to the relay neurons. It is in the descending pain pathway that opioids have been recognised as being the most effective medication, by inhibiting the synaptic transmission between the pain fibres. However, the way in which this occurs is different from the body's natural inhibitory mechanism. Opioid peptides, once bound to the appropriate receptors (mu – μ, kappa – κ and delta – δ), modulate pain input in two ways: by releasing a large number of calcium ions which block the pre-synaptic terminal; and by opening potassium channels which flood the synapse and hyperpolarise the neurons, preventing signals from passing across the synapse (Bannister, 2019).

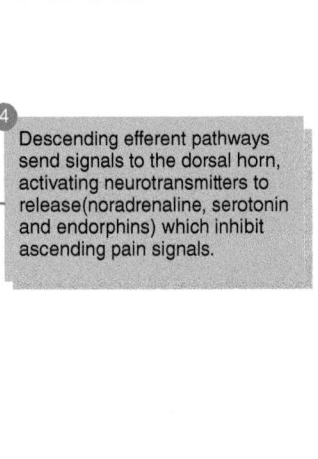

③ The perception of the pain signals in the somatosensory cortex can be influenced by psychological, physical and social factors.

④ Descending efferent pathways send signals to the dorsal horn, activating neurotransmitters to release(noradrenaline, serotonin and endorphins) which inhibit ascending pain signals.

② Primary sensory neurons carry impulses via afferent A-delta and C fibres, which terminate in the dorsal horn of the spinal cord. Neurotransmitters continue signals to the brain.

① Stimulation of nociceptors by chemicals(histamine and prostaglandins) released when tissue injury or irritation occurs (i.e. heat, cold, chemicals).

Figure 8.1 Pain pathway.

Definitions and categories of pain

Before pain can be treated, it is necessary to understand and determine which type of pain the patient is experiencing, as the choice of analgesic should be tailored to the type of pain and personal preferences of the individual. See Figure 8.2 for the different types of pain. The first worldwide accepted definition of pain is from The International Association for the Study of Pain (IASP), which declares that pain is 'an unpleasant sensory and emotional experience associated with actual or potential tissue damage' (Merskey and Bogduk, 1994, p. 209). However, pain is not always directly linked to the amount of trauma as it can also be associated with psychological and emotional issues (Rodriguez, 2015). It is therefore multilayered and the most commonly used classifications are separated by duration (acute or chronic), type (nociceptive, neuropathic and psychogenic) and site (somatic and visceral) (see Figure 8.2). Some overlap, and patients may present with one or more.

- **Acute:** serves a protective purpose, is of short duration (less than three months), and is reversible. It is predominantly nociceptive in nature, involves sensory processes and is treated very effectively with analgesics (Turk and Melzack, 2011; Kettyle, 2015).
- **Chronic:** serves no protective purpose and persists past the initial healing stage, usually more than three months. It is largely neuropathic, associated with an array of changes to

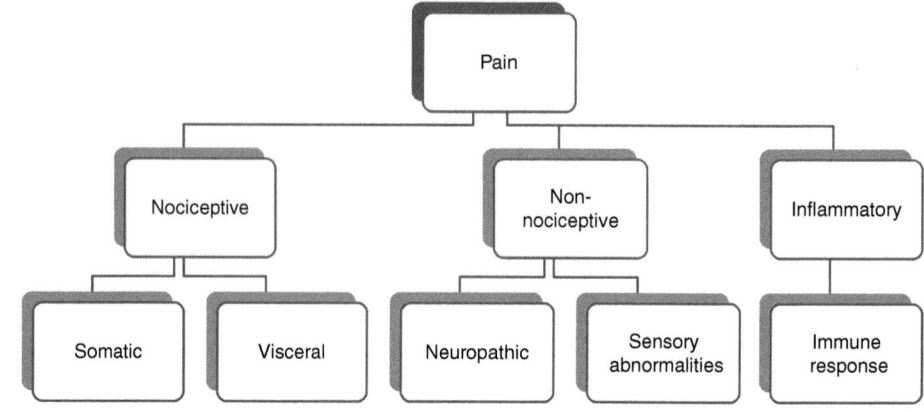

Figure 8.2   Types of pain. Source: Adapted Cunningham (2017).

the peripheral and central sensory pathways, typically connected with chronic disease, and usually treated alongside psychological measures due to its extremely subjective nature (Tornsey and Fleetwood-Walker, 2012; Koneti & Perfitt, 2019).

- **Nociceptive:** is the most frequently experienced type of pain. It is a primitive sensation, protective in nature and involves the passing of information through primary afferent fibres to the cerebral cortex via pain receptors, referred to as 'nociceptors', which are stimulated and activated by tissue damage resulting from heat, cold, stretch, vibration or chemicals (Solaro and Uccelli, 2016; Mears, 2018).
- **Neuropathic:** is more degenerative in nature and usually occurs as a result of pain related to sensory abnormalities that can result from damage to the nerves (a nerve infection) or neurological dysfunction (a disease in the somatosensory nervous system). This type of pain may not be diagnosed immediately as it can manifest itself in various ways and can often be confused with acute persistent pain. Neuropathic pain is often managed via multimodal analgesic approaches (Colvin and Carty, 2012; Old et al., 2016).
- **Inflammation:** stimulation of nociceptive processes by chemicals released as part of the inflammatory process (Cunningham, 2017).
- **Somatic:** is a large part of the body's natural defence mechanism and is associated with nociceptive processes activated in skin, bones, joints, connective tissues and muscles (VanMeter and Hubert, 2014).
- **Visceral:** is a sensation and nociceptive process activated in the organs (i.e. stomach, kidneys, gallbladder) transmitted via the sympathetic fibres, and linked to conditions such as irritable bowel syndrome and dysmenorrhoea (Boore et al., 2016).
- **Referred:** is pain that is felt in the skin that lies over an affected organ, or in an area some distance from the site of disease or injury (Patton and Thibodeau, 2016).

Importance of individualised pain assessments

Individuals react to pain in varying ways; for some, pain is seen as something that should be endured, while for others it can be a debilitating problem that impedes their ability to function. Therefore, in order to ensure an effective and individually tailored holistic management plan is developed, it is important to understand how the pain is uniquely affecting the individual from a biopsychosocial perspective (Flasar and Perry, 2014). In order to do this, healthcare profession- als use a range of tools, such as the skills of observation (the art of noticing), questioning

130

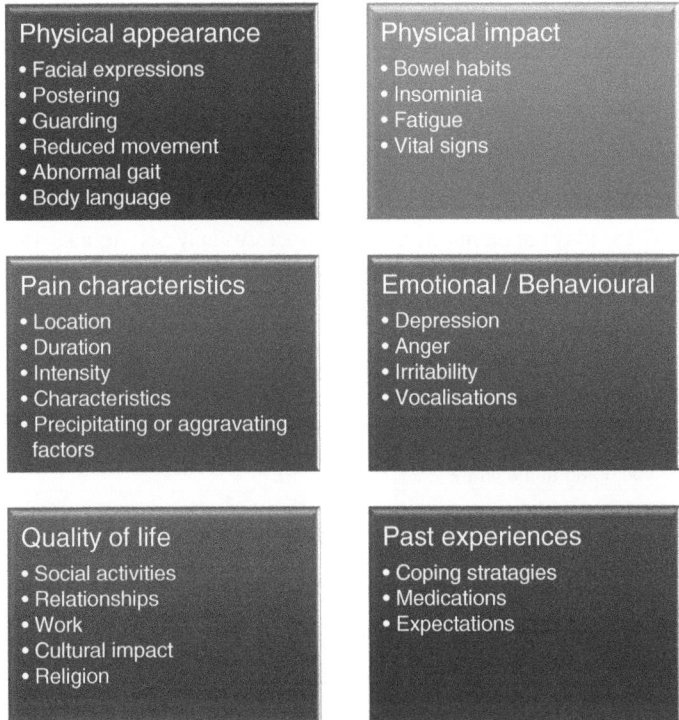

Physical appearance
- Facial expressions
- Postering
- Guarding
- Reduced movement
- Abnormal gait
- Body language

Physical impact
- Bowel habits
- Insominia
- Fatigue
- Vital signs

Pain characteristics
- Location
- Duration
- Intensity
- Characteristics
- Precipitating or aggravating factors

Emotional / Behavioural
- Depression
- Anger
- Irritability
- Vocalisations

Quality of life
- Social activities
- Relationships
- Work
- Cultural impact
- Religion

Past experiences
- Coping stratagies
- Medications
- Expectations

Figure 8.3 Example of assessment domains. Source: Adapted Kettyle 2015 and Cunningham 2017.

techniques, active listening and interpretation. Another strategy often employed by health-care professionals is the assessment and measurement of vital signs. Bendall et al. (2011) were able to demonstrate a correlation between patients' pain scores and changes in vital signs and concluded that a respiratory rate of over 25 breaths per minute was of crucial importance when predicting pain severity. Tachycardia (over 100 beats/minute) and systolic hypertension (over 140 mmHg) have also been identified as clinically important when assessing patients of all ages. This becomes even more relevant when attempting to take observations from a patient who is sedated or is unconscious; key indicators (such as the respiratory rate and heart rate) will help in identifying patients' pain when they are unable to verbalise (Erden et al., 2018). It is important to remember that no one skill is superior, rather it is the accumulation of information gathered via the various methods that enables a healthcare professional to determine if a patient is in pain and understand how this pain is affecting them physically, psychologically, socially and culturally (Cunningham, 2017) (see Figure 8.3).

Assessment tools

While vital observations and behavioural manifestations may indicate that a patient is in pain, questioning, measurement and interpretation skills will assist with determining the intensity, severity and effect of the pain on the patient's wellbeing and quality of life. This process can be aided by the use of specifically designed tools, which act as prompts for healthcare professionals and facilitate the assessment of one or more dimensions.

Unidimensional tools

The Visual Analogue Scale (VAS), Numerical Rating Scale (NRS) and Verbal Rating Scale (VRS) can be quick, easy to use, regularly repeated and do not require complex language.

Multidimensional tools

Ask for greater information and measure the quality of pain via affective, evaluative and sensory means. The McGill Pain Questionnaire (MPQ) is one example and this is often used to assess individuals who are experiencing chronic pain.

Mnemonics

OPQRST and SOCRATES are just two examples of mnemonic aids that can be useful and require no equipment as they use mental assessment processes only. See Figure 8.4 for further details on the above mnemonic examples and the following Clinical Considerations box for additional information that needs to be taken into consideration when in clinical practice regarding the use of assessment tools.

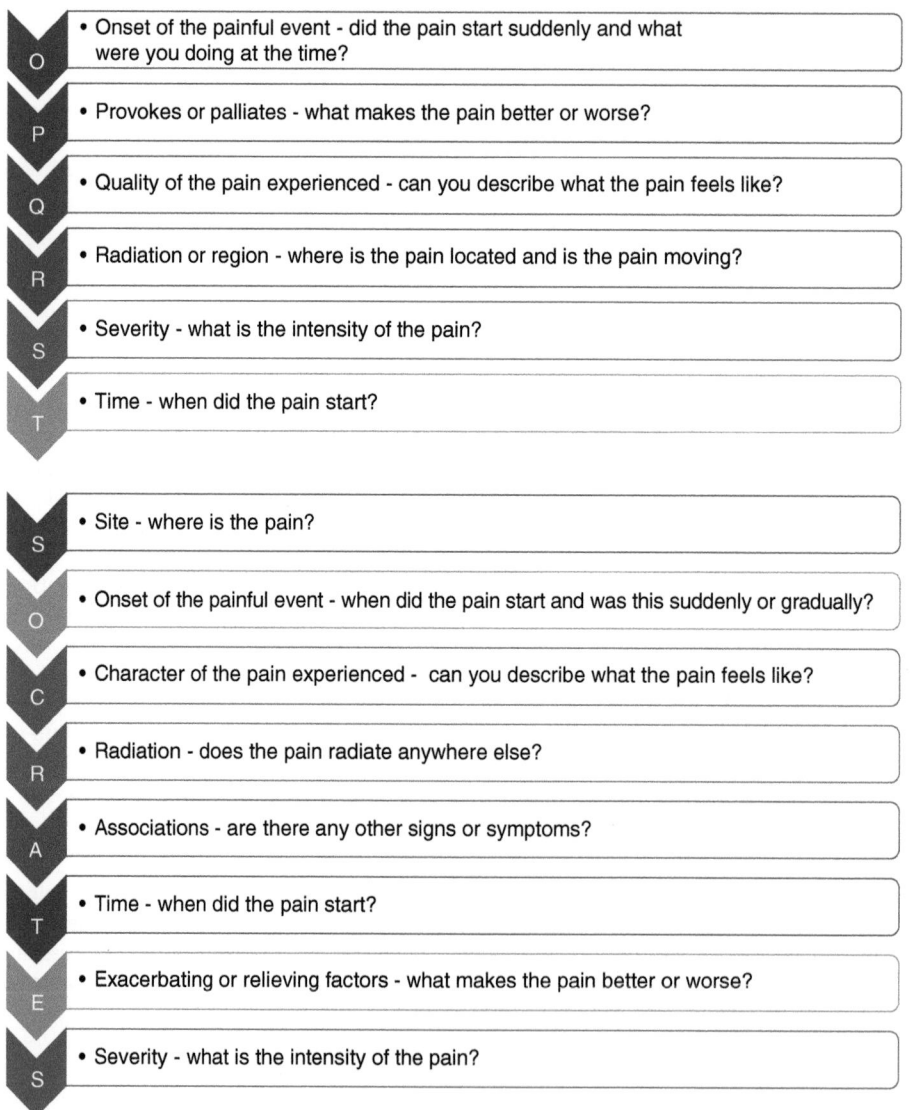

O
• Onset of the painful event - did the pain start suddenly and what were you doing at the time?

P
• Provokes or palliates - what makes the pain better or worse?

Q
• Quality of the pain experienced - can you describe what the pain feels like?

R
• Radiation or region - where is the pain located and is the pain moving?

S
• Severity - what is the intensity of the pain?

T
• Time - when did the pain start?

S
• Site - where is the pain?

O
• Onset of the painful event - when did the pain start and was this suddenly or gradually?

C
• Character of the pain experienced - can you describe what the pain feels like?

R
• Radiation - does the pain radiate anywhere else?

A
• Associations - are there any other signs or symptoms?

T
• Time - when did the pain start?

E
• Exacerbating or relieving factors - what makes the pain better or worse?

S
• Severity - what is the intensity of the pain?

Figure 8.4   Example of mnemonics used for assessment of pain.

Clinical considerations

Person-centred and tailored approach

Regardless of which tool or mnemonic is used, as pain presentations are often unique, pain assessment will be unsuccessful if the healthcare professional fails to ascertain and interpret the signs and symptoms, uses the assessment tools inappropriately, and does not apply a person-centred approach to the overall assessment process, i.e. using the wrong tool for the wrong patient.

Multimodal management strategies

One of the primary goals is to pre-empt and prevent pain from occurring in the first instance; however, if pain cannot be avoided (as in the case of surgery), optimal analgesic management is vital. The word analgesia – 'to be without the feeling of pain' – is derived from the Greek language, and in terms of pain management relates to medication and alternative interventions (Law and Rudall, 2013). Hence, pain management plans should incorporate a multimodal approach using a range of pharmacological and non-pharmacological strategies (see the following Clinical Considerations box) in order to successfully and holistically treat patients' pain (Flasar and Perry, 2014). A combination approach is also recommended for pharmacological management, as several drugs have morphine sparing properties, which increases the effect of opioids; therefore, the use of adjuvants is recommended (Boyd, 2013). Boore et al. (2016) state that this is an effective way to manage pain, but stress that the decisions about which management strategies to use also need to take into consideration the context of the clinical situation, the patient's level of acuity, the environment and physical space and the availability of resources. The clinical decisions associated with analgesic administration must also be made in line with Royal Pharmaceutical Society (RPS) (2019) recommendations, which state that any HCP administering medicines must possess a comprehensive understanding of the drug itself and an awareness of the potential risks and side effects.

Clinical considerations

Non-pharmacological strategies

Pharmacological treatments are not the only strategy at healthcare professionals' disposal, and true holistic management cannot be achieved without the incorporation of other non-pharmacological therapies. Some of these interventions are longstanding, are engrained in some traditional medical practices and, when used correctly, can enhance patients' feelings of empowerment and involvement (Flasar and Perry, 2014). However, due to limited resources, funding, space, time, knowledge of use and personal beliefs, some therapies are not fully utilised or embraced (Cullen and MacPherson, 2012). These can be placed into three main groups, (see Figure 8.5 below), and the choice of which to use will depend upon patients' preferences and existing coping mechanisms. The following strategies have been highlighted as they align with the fundamental core values of care and compassion and require very little in terms of resources or time.

- **Distraction:** This can take various forms, i.e. talking to the patient about their specific hobbies. This basic skill often requires no equipment, can be done anywhere, and is a useful way of taking the patient's mind off their pain.
- **Imagery/meditation:** This management technique takes distraction therapy one step further by utilising a more structured approach.
- **Therapeutic touch and massage:** For centuries, the therapeutic placing of hands has proven to be a useful skill, and has beneficial physiological (stimulation of A-beta fibres which restrict pain pathways) and psychological properties (Kettyle, 2015).
- **Environment:** Sound, lighting and the temperature of the patient's immediate environment have been shown to heighten or reduce perceptions of pain.

Psychological / Emotional	Physical	Alternative

• Spiritual
• Relaxation
• Information
• Breathing
• Music
• Distraction
• Imagery
• Cognitive Behavioural
  Therapy
• Yoga
• Tai chi
	• Heat and cold
	• Exercise
	• Massage
	• Body position / comfort
	• Art therapy
	• Rest
		• Acupuncture
		• Acupressure
		• Electrostimulation
		• Herbs
		• Reflexology
		• Biofield therapies
		  (i.e. raki)

Figure 8.5   Example of non-pharmacological management strategies. Source: Modified from Cunningham (2017).

Pharmacological management

One very effective strategy that healthcare professionals have within their management arsenal is the use of pharmacological treatments; and the choice depends on whether the pain is nociceptive, neuropathic, inflammatory or of mixed origin. There are three main categories: opioids, non-opioids/non-steroidal anti-inflammatories and adjuvants/co-analgesics (see Figure 8.6). The most efficient pharmacological regimen for moderate to severe pain (i.e. cancer-related pain) often incorporates a combined approach, by administrating a specific drug in conjunction with adjuvants or co-analgesics (see Figure 8.7).

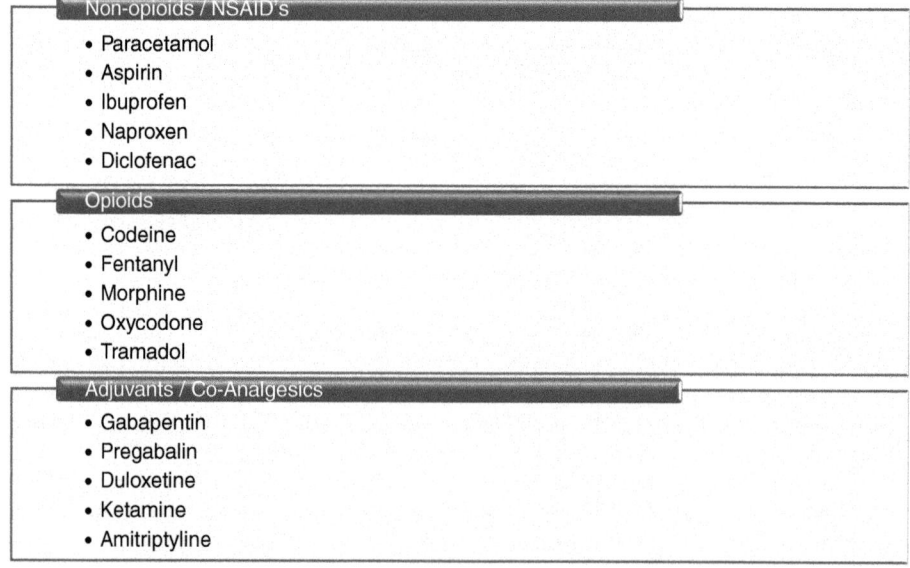

Non-opioids / NSAID's
- Paracetamol
- Aspirin
- Ibuprofen
- Naproxen
- Diclofenac

Opioids
- Codeine
- Fentanyl
- Morphine
- Oxycodone
- Tramadol

Adjuvants / Co-Analgesics
- Gabapentin
- Pregabalin
- Duloxetine
- Ketamine
- Amitriptyline

Figure 8.6   Classifications of pharmacological analgesics (examples). Source: Modified from Smith and Muralidharan (2014).

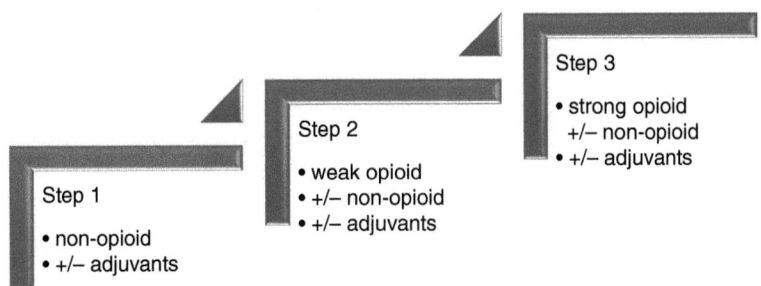

Figure 8.7   Analgesic ladder. Source: Modified from World Health Organisation (2018).   135

N.B. It is very important that the most appropriate drug is used to treat individuals' pain and the decision of which analgesic to choose should (whenever possible) be made in partnership with the patient (NMC, 2018; GMC, 2019; HCPC, 2019; RPS, 2019).

Non-opioids

The most widely used and safest analgesic (when taken correctly) is paracetamol, which can also be used as an antipyretic (Boyd, 2013). See Table 8.1 for further details of the pharmacokinetics, pharmacodynamics and common side effects of oral paracetamol. The recommended oral dose is 500 mg to 1 g, every four to six hours with a maximum of 4 g in 24 hours. While these are normally administered orally, an effective way to bypass the absorption process, especially for drugs with a high degree of first-pass metabolism, is to deliver the drug directly into the circulatory system via intravenous (IV) infusion (Neal, 2016). IV paracetamol is therefore often used due to its ease of administration and rate of effectiveness. It can also be administered rectally.

Pharmacodynamics and pharmacokinetics

During the activation of nociceptors, prostaglandins, which are converted from arachidonic acid by cyclooxygenases (COX) enzymes, bind to receptors and stimulate pain fibres to transmit signals more frequently, causing an increase in pain messages being sent to the brain. The exact mechanism of action is not fully understood (Young and Pitcher, 2016); however, it is believed that paracetamol can hinder the production of prostaglandin centrally rather than peripherally. Following oral administration, paracetamol is rapidly absorbed from the gastrointestinal tract, with its systemic bioavailability being dose-dependent and ranging from 70% to 90%. Its rate of oral absorption is predominantly dependent on the rate of gastric emptying, being delayed by food. It distributes rapidly and evenly throughout most tissues and fluids and has a volume of distribution of approximately 0.9 L/kg. 10%–20% of the drug is bound to red blood cells. Paracetamol is metabolised in the liver by conjugation with glucuronic and sulfuric acid and 85%–95% is excreted in the urine within 24 hours.

Notable contraindications, cautions and side effects

There are very few side effects associated with paracetamol; however, if taken in excess it can lead to serious hepatotoxicity (see the following Clinical Considerations box). When an overdose is suspected, the antidote 'N-acetylcysteine' should be administered. Caution is advised for anyone with renal or hepatic impairment and heavy alcohol consumption can increase the risk of hepatotoxicity.

Table 8.1 Examples of non-opioids and non-steroidal anti-inflammatory drugs (NSAIDs) and the pharmacodynamics, pharmacokinetics and common side effects

Medication type	Acetaminophen	Salicylic Acid Derivatives	Propionic Acid Derivatives	Selective COX-2 Inhibitors	Others
Medication name	Paracetamol	Aspirin	Ibuprofen	Celecoxib	Diclofenac
Route of administration	Oral, rectal or intravenous infusion	Oral or rectal	Oral or topical	Oral	Oral, intramuscular injection, rectal, topical, intravenous infusion
Dose (oral)	500–1 g up to 4 g daily	300–900 mg	600 mg up to 1.8 g daily	200–400 mg daily	75–150 mg daily
Frequency and timings (oral)	4–6 hours	4–6 hours	4–6 times a day	1–2 times a day	1–3 times a day
Onset/duration	15–60 minutes/6 hours	30–60 minutes or 1–8 hours for coated tablets/12 hours	1–2 hours/5–10 hours	1 hour/8 hours	1 hour/12 hours
Common side effects	No common side effects	Indigestion	Heartburn and indigestion	Indigestion, diarrhoea, flatulence, dizziness and swollen ankles	Gastrointestinal disorders
Absorption (A)	Rapidly absorbed from the gastrointestinal tract	Rapidly by passive diffusion in the gastrointestinal tract	Rapidly absorbed from the upper gastrointestinal tract	Rapidly absorbed from the gastrointestinal tract	Absorbed from the gastrointestinal tract but due to the first-pass metabolism, only 50% of the drug reaches systemic circulation unchanged
Distribution (D)	Distributes evenly throughout tissues and fluids – the volume of distribution is approximately 0.9 L/kg	Binds to albumin in the plasma and distributes rapidly into body fluid compartments. The volume of distribution is 10.5 L/kg	Binds to albumin in the plasma – the volume of distribution is 0.1 L/kg	Binds to albumin in the plasma – the volume of distribution is 400 L	Binds to albumin in the plasma – the volume of distribution is 1.4 L/kg
Metabolism (M)	Predominately in the liver by conjugation with glucuronic and sulfuric acid	Mainly in the liver by conjugation with glucuronic acid	Ibuprofen is rapidly metabolised in the liver	Mainly in the liver by conjugation with carboxylic and glucuronic acid	Predominately in the liver by conjugation with glucuronic and sulfuric acid
Excretion (E)	Excreted in the urine	Excreted in the urine	Excreted in the urine	Predominantly excreted in the foeces and urine	60–70% is eliminated in the urine and 30% is eliminated in the foeces

Source: Adapted BNF 2019.

Clinical considerations

The right combination

Some medications, such as paracetamol, are often found in combination medication (i.e. co-codamol) that can be purchased over the counter. Care must be taken, as they may contain drugs that the patient may be unaware of and this could lead to inadvertent overdose.

Non-steroidal anti-inflammatories (NSAIDs)

NSAID drugs are used not only for their anti-inflammatory actions but also for their analgesic and antipyretic properties. They are not effective for individuals experiencing visceral pain associated with the abdomen and chest, but can be given as an adjuvant for individuals experiencing severe pain, due to their opioid-sparing effects. These are usually administered orally, but can also be administered via the rectal route or topically. There are a wide variety of NSAIDs, each with their own chemical composition; however, they are very similar in terms of the analgesic effect. One example of each type of NSAID and the pharmacokinetics, pharmacodynamics, common side effects and recommended corresponding dosages can be found in Table 8.1.

Pharmacodynamics and pharmacokinetics

NSAIDs act on two enzymes: COX-1 which is expressed in the platelets, the gastrointestinal tract, the kidneys and is always present in the body, and COX-2 which is found in the kidneys, the CNS and is mainly induced in response to trauma (Smith and Muralidharan, 2014; Young and Pitcher, 2016). They restrict the synthesis of prostaglandin (which increases pain signals) both centrally and peripherally, but more effectively peripherally, at the site of the inflammation (Neal, 2016).

Notable contraindications, cautions and side effects

Prostaglandin has beneficial effects in maintaining renal blood flow and keeping the lungs open; therefore, care must be taken with individuals with asthma, the elderly, and those with poor renal function. Prostaglandin suppression can also result in gastrointestinal damage, nausea, gastritis, dyspepsia, and in severe cases gastric bleeding and ulcerations (Boyd, 2013). Oral NSAIDs should, therefore, be taken with or after food and drugs may be enteric-coated. For NSAIDs which are COX-2 selective, gastrointestinal side effects can be reduced; however, inhibiting COX-2 can also increase cardiovascular risk and therefore they are not used routinely.

Opioid agonists

Opioids are a class of drug naturally found within the opium poppy plant; however, some opioids can also be created synthetically and semi-synthetically. See Table 8.2 for further details of the pharmacokinetics, pharmacodynamics and common side effects of opioids. Stronger opioids (i.e. morphine) are indicated for the treatment of severe pain and weaker opioids (i.e. codeine) are often prescribed to manage mild to moderate pain. These will be discussed in greater detail later in this chapter.

Pharmacodynamics and pharmacokinetics

Opioids bind to opioid receptors located within the CNS, the brain, the spinal cord and peripherally in the gastrointestinal tract. Once the opioids attach to the receptors, they block pain signals and release large amounts of dopamine throughout the body (Schumacher et al., 2015).

Table 8.2 Examples of opioids and the associated pharmacokinetics, pharmacodynamics and common side effects.

Medication type	Opioids				
Medication name	Codeine	Dihydrocodeine	Tramadol	Morphine	Fentanyl
Route of administration	Oral, intramuscular injection	Oral, deep subcutaneous or intramuscular injection	Oral, intramuscular injection, intravenous injection or infusion	Oral, intramuscular, subcutaneous, or intravenous injection or infusion, rectal	Intravenous injection or infusion, transdermal patches
Dose	Oral – 30–60 mg Maximum 240 mg/daily	Oral – 30–60 mg Maximum 240 mg/daily	Oral – 50–100 mg Maximum 400 mg	IV – 5 mg initially, adjusted according to response	IV – 50–200 mcg/kg higher dose for anaesthesia
Frequency and timings	4–6 hours orally	4–6 hours orally	4 hours orally	4 hours IV, slower with titration	4–6 hours IV
Onset/duration	30–60 minutes/6 hours	30–60 minutes/6 hours	Up to 60 minutes/6 hours	6–30 minutes (depending on route)/4 hours	2–10 minutes/6 hours
Common side effects	Nausea and vomiting, constipation, cardiac arrhythmias (prolonged use)	Nausea and vomiting, constipation, paralytic ileus, abdominal pain	Seizures, serotonin syndrome	Nausea and vomiting, constipation, delirium, dependence	Respiratory depression
Absorption (A)	Absorbed by the gastrointestinal tract, with a bioavailability of around 60%	Low bioavailability in the gastrointestinal tract, approximately 20% due to first-pass metabolism	Rapidly absorbed in the gastrointestinal tract, bioavailability of 75%	Almost complete absorption in the upper intestine, approximately 95% bioavailability	Short distribution phase, high concentration of fentanyl found in well-perfused areas (lungs, brain, liver)
Distribution (D)	Extensively distributed into the tissues and plasma – the volume of distribution is 3–6 L/kg	Distributed evenly into the tissues and plasma – the volume of distribution is 3–6 L/kg	High affinity for tissue, distributed evenly – the volume of distribution is 2.6–2.9 L/kg	Low transfer for plasma, distributed most effectively in high alkaline areas, e.g. upper intestine – the volume of distribution is 5.3 L/kg	80% distributed in plasma – IV volume of distribution is 4 L/kg
Metabolism (M)	70–80% of the oral dose is metabolised in the liver	Hepatic pre-systemic metabolism into active metabolite dihydromorphine	Extensive first-pass metabolism, from which there are 23 metabolites	Significant first-pass metabolism in the liver	Metabolised in the liver into a number of inactive metabolites
Excretion (E)	Renal elimination and urinary excretion – 90% after 6 hours	Renal elimination and urinary excretion	Hepatic elimination, metabolites excreted through urine (90%) and foeces (10%)	Renal elimination of morphine and metabolites, excreted through urine	Renal elimination of metabolites and urinary excretion

Source: Adapted BNF (2019).

There are four different types of opioid receptor which have designated Greek letters (mu – μ, kappa – κ and delta – δ) and different analgesics bind to these receptors in a variety of ways, which explains why there is a wide range of benefits and side effects associated with opioid use (Barber and Robertson, 2012). See the Clinical Considerations box for additional information that needs to be taken into consideration when in clinical practice and caring for individuals with a head injury.

Opioids are metabolised primarily by the liver, but also in the brain and the kidneys, and approximately 87% is excreted after 72 hours (MacKenzie et al., 2016). All opioids are able to cross the blood–brain barrier (BBB); however, those that can cross the BBB more easily (due to poor lipid solubility and protein binding) tend to be more potent (Schumacher et al., 2015).

Notable contraindications, cautions and side effects

Caution should be taken when administering opioid analgesics, as there are several cautions and contraindications to be aware of. First, it is of note that repeated opioid administration could result in opiate dependence. The National Institute for Health and Care Excellence (NICE) produced a document specifically focusing on opioid dependence, stating that signs of physical and psychological dependence can appear in as little as 2–10 days (NICE, 2019). It is also worth recognising that individuals may experience increased tolerance to the potency of an opiate with repeated usage, which may then develop into a dependence where pain cannot be managed with the medication prescribed (British National Formulary [BNF], 2019). However, the BNF (2019) state that dependence is no deterrent for the control of severe pain.

Pain management is always complex with patients with hepatic impairment due to the adverse reactions caused by the opioids. These reactions can result in sedation, constipation and sudden onset of hepatic encephalopathy (defined as a spectrum of neuropsychiatric abnormalities in patients with liver dysfunction). It is suggested that opioids are avoided or the dose is reduced in patients with hepatic impairment (BNF, 2019). The effect of an opioid analgesic is also prolonged and increased where renal impairment is present, and there may be an increase in cerebral activity. It is suggested that in these instances, opioid use should be avoided, or the dose reduced (BNF, 2019).

One of the most serious side effects is an increase in respiratory depression, which, if not treated, could result in a significant brain injury, cardiac arrest or death (Lee et al., 2015). To treat respiratory depression, an opioid antagonist 'naloxone' – also known as an opiate reversal agent – should be administered (see the following Clinical Considerations box). When injected intravenously, the effects of this agent occur within two minutes of administration. The mode of action for naloxone is not fully understood, but it is thought to be a competitive opioid receptor antagonist, so it has a higher affinity to the receptor sites in the CNS, especially the mu receptor (Wang et al., 2016). Naloxone is primarily metabolised by the liver and its metabolites are excreted in the urine (Lynn and Galinkin, 2017).

Clinical considerations

Opioids and serious head injury

If a serious head injury has occurred, there may be a concern about intracranial pressure. In order to obtain accurate neurological observations, the healthcare professional will need to check the pupils of the individual are equal and reactive to light. In this instance, opioids should be avoided as they can have an impact on the individual's pupillary response (causing pin-point pupils – see below) and therefore the healthcare professional would not be able to gain a true reading of the patient's neurological condition (Kosten et al., 2018).

N.B. Pin-point pupils are caused by opioid drugs as they stimulate the oculomotor nerves which shrink the diameter of the pupil. This phenomenon is still utilised as a vital diagnostic tool when testing for opioid overdose, as other causes of non-consciousness tend to cause the pupils to dilate.

Clinical Considerations

Naloxone is very short-acting, with a half-life of approximately 30–80 minutes, which is shorter than the average half-life of some opiates. As a consequence, repeated administration may be necessary.

Other side effects such as nausea and vomiting, constipation, itching and drowsiness are generally proportionate to the type and strength of the opioid (Young and Pitcher, 2016). Specific types of opioids will now be explored in greater detail.

Codeine phosphate

Codeine phosphate is often referred to as a weak opioid as it is a less potent analgesic than some of its counterparts, such as morphine and fentanyl. It is a naturally occurring opioid agonist with analgesic, antidiarrhoeal and antitussive properties (BNF, 2019). If codeine is taken orally, 30–60 mg every four hours is indicated with a maximum dosage of 240 mg/day. Codeine can also be given by intramuscular injection; the same dosage applies.

Pharmacodynamics and pharmacokinetics

Codeine will bind to many opioid receptor sites within the CNS and gastrointestinal system, causing a reduction in the release of neurotransmitters (Dubin and Patapoutian, 2010). Codeine has an advantage over morphine as it is well absorbed when administered orally, due to its bioavailability. However, the analgesic effect of this drug does not increase above a certain range, so higher quantities do not provide increased analgesia (Barber et al., 2012).

Notable contraindications, cautions and side effects

The dosage of codeine should be reduced in elderly individuals with renal or hepatic impairment (BNF, 2019). When administered over an extended period, codeine can also increase the risk of developing cardiac arrhythmias. In individuals at greater risk of these conditions, such as the elderly, regular electrocardiograms (ECG) are recommended (Li and Ramos, 2017).

Dihydrocodeine

Dihydrocodeine is a semi-synthetic opioid agonist which also possesses antitussive properties. This opioid is used to treat moderate to severe pain as well as severe dyspnoea. The recommended oral dose is 30 mg every four to six hours and for administration via intramuscular injection 50 mg is suggested every four to six hours (BNF, 2019). Like many of the other opioids, dihydrocodeine can be used in combination with other medications (i.e. co-drydamol contains dihydrocodeine and paracetamol) (Wiffen et al., 2016).

Pharmacodynamics and pharmacokinetics

Once administered, dihydrocodeine is metabolised to dihydromorphine, a highly active metabolite with a high affinity for the mu-opioid receptor. The bioavailability of dihydrocodeine is relatively low (approximately 20%) if administered orally, this may be due to poor gastrointestinal absorption; this highlights the substantial role pre-systemic metabolism plays in reducing the bioavailability of this opioid (BNF, 2019).

Notable contraindications, cautions and common side effects

Caution must be used when administering dihydrocodeine to a patient with a history of pancreatitis as codeine-based medications have been linked with acute pancreatitis (Hastier et al., 2000). Additionally, when this drug is broken down into dihydromorphine, an individual can be placed at greater risk of the cardiovascular side effects of opioids such as arrythmias and hypotension if they are elderly and have severe right sided heart failure (cor pulmonale) (BNF, 2019).

Tramadol

Tramadol is a synthetic opiate analgesic indicated to treat moderate to moderately severe pain and has central analgesic properties similar to that of morphine (see below), although not as potent. In June 2014, tramadol was classified as a schedule three controlled drug (Stannard, 2019). The initial oral dosage is 100 mg followed by 50–100 mg every four to six hours; the maximum daily dose is 400 mg. If administered intravenously, an initial loading dose of 100 mg is recommended, followed by 50 mg every 10–20 minutes, up to a total maximum of 250 mg (including initial dose) in the first hour, after which 50–100 mg every 4–6 hours is recommended (BNF, 2019).

Pharmacodynamics and pharmacokinetics

Tramadol has a unique dual mode of action, acting both as a central opiate agonist and as a CNS reuptake inhibitor of norepinephrine and serotonin. It is therefore not surprising that due to tramadol's broad range of pain and inflammation targets, it has been shown to be effective for a number of pain types, such as neuropathic pain, post-operative pain, lower back pain, as well as pain associated with labour, osteoarthritis, fibromyalgia and cancer (Beyaz et al., 2016). Tramadol is primarily metabolised by the liver and the metabolites are excreted by the kidneys in urine.

Notable contraindications, cautions and side effects

As tramadol may cause seizures, particularly if high doses of the drug are being used, it is contraindicated in individuals with poorly controlled or uncontrolled epilepsy (Beyaz et al., 2016). A secondary side effect of tramadol is serotonin syndrome, which is more commonly seen when taking antidepressants (SSRIs). However, a link has now been found between tramadol and serotonin syndrome, due to tramadol's mode of action. Tramadol binds with the mu-opioid receptor in the CNS and inhibits the serotonin reuptake pathways, resulting in a build-up of serotonin in the CNS (Beakley et al., 2015). This has the potential to result in symptoms such as high body temperature, agitation, increased reflexes, tremor, sweating and dilated pupils (Hassamal et al., 2018).

Morphine

Morphine is a naturally occurring strong opioid that offers analgesia for severe pain as well as having the effect of euphoria and mental detachment. Due to morphine's potency, it has a duration of analgesia of approximately four to six hours – compared to some of the weaker opiates that have a duration of two to four hours or less (BNF, 2019). Morphine is often described as the 'prototypical opioid', creating a standard that other opioids are compared against (Barber and Robertson, 2012). Initially, 5 mg every four hours is indicated for morphine via a slow intravenous injection (see the Skills in Practice box for details on how to insert a peripheral cannula for the administration of intravenous analgesic medications). The dosage can be adjusted according to individual response and more frequently during titration (BNF, 2019). For oral morphine, 10 mg every four hours is the recommended dose, and this should be adjusted depending on the response of the individual.

Pharmacodynamics and pharmacokinetics

Morphine predominantly binds to the mu and delta-opioid receptors found within the CNS, which in turn inhibit the voltage-gated channels needed for the pain signals to reach the brain.

Contraindications, cautions and side effects

Nausea and vomiting are common side effects; therefore, oral morphine should be administered after a meal or with food and it may be necessary to prescribe anti-emetic (anti-sickness) medication (Smith and Laufer, 2014). Morphine has also been shown to have a noted effect on the gastrointestinal system as it slows the motility rate of the gastrointestinal tract, which often leads to constipation (BNF, 2019). The reason for this is that there are also opioid receptors within the GI tract and when the agonists bind with them, it decreases gastric emptying and stimulates pyloric tone (Nelson and Camilleri, 2016). It is of note that any oral medication taken may take longer to absorb if it is being taken alongside morphine. To relieve the symptoms of opioid-induced constipation, high fibre foods, hydration and gentle exercise are recommended.

Fentanyl

Fentanyl is a strong synthetic opioid analgesic, which is approximately 100 times as potent as morphine. Consequently, fentanyl is only indicated for severe chronic pain and is mainly utilised within operating departments and critical care, as part of the general anaesthetic. Fentanyl can be administered via transdermal patches for chronic pain; the two most common patches release fentanyl at 12 or 25 mcg per hour and these should be replaced every 72 hours in a new location (BNF, 2019). If fentanyl is being administered through an intravenous infusion, 3–4.8 mcg/kg/h is recommended and this will need to be increased for individuals receiving assisted ventilation (10 mcg/kg over 10 minutes, then 6 mcg/kg/h, adjusted according to the response of the individual) (BNF, 2019).

Pharmacodynamics and pharmacokinetics

As a mu-opioid receptor agonist, fentanyl binds to these receptors 50–100 times more strongly than morphine; it also binds with the delta and kappa receptors, but not as strongly (Brzakala & Leppert, 2019). Once fentanyl has successfully bound with the opioid receptors, it causes an influx of calcium ions (charged particles) into the cell, causing hyperpolarisation and the inhibition of nerve activity.

Contraindications, cautions, and side effects

Due to the potency of fentanyl, respiratory depression is a real concern; therefore, it is suggested that all opioids, especially fentanyl, should only be administered where an opioid antagonist is present and the individual's respiratory rate should also be closely monitored (Hill et al., 2019).

Adjuvants and co-analgesics – gabapentinoids

Gabapentinoids, such as pregabalin and gabapentin, are indicated for neuropathic pain and the treatment of focal seizures. For neuropathic pain, the recommended oral dose is to be administered in increasing levels of: day one, 300 mg once; day two, 300 mg twice; day three, 300 mg three times throughout the day (BNF, 2019).

Pharmacodynamics and pharmacokinetics

Gabapentin was developed to mimic the neurotransmitter GABA; however, it does not bind to the GABA receptors in the CNS. Instead, it has been found to bind to an auxiliary subunit $(\alpha_2\delta - 1)$ of voltage-gated calcium channels, which can be found at the synaptic terminals of 'excitable cells' such as muscle, neurons and glial cells (Kukkar et al., 2013). The gabapentin then inhibits calcium channels by reducing the number of available channels and preventing the neuropathic pain response from continuing to the brain (Fornasari, 2017).

Notable Contraindications, Cautions and Side Effects

Caution needs to be applied to individuals who have a history of psychotic illness, as the listed potential side effects of gabapentin may aggravate their condition (BNF, 2019).

Inhalation analgesics

Nitrous oxide (N_2O), commonly referred to as entonox, is a well-established anaesthetic and analgesic gas mixture. The combination of 50% nitrous oxide and 50% oxygen is found obstetric and maternity departments, trauma scenarios, and is frequently used for the maintenance of anaesthesia (BNF, 2019). When inhaled, it provides pain relief as well as anaesthetic properties such as sedation.

Pharmacodynamics and pharmacokinetics

The precise mechanism of action for the anaesthetic properties of nitrous oxide remains unknown; however, the most prevalent explanation is that the N_2O inhibits the pain receptors on the ascending pain pathway, blocking the neurons that carry the pain response via the afferent A-delta and C fibres. The analgesic mechanism of N_2O is better understood. The nitrous oxide forces the release of opioid peptides that bind to the opioid receptors in the brain and CNS. This results in the release of opioids in the brainstem, blocking the pain signals on the descending pain pathway (Huang & Johnson, 2016). Nitrous oxide is absorbed via diffusion in the lungs and is eliminated and excreted by respiration with a duration of approximately five minutes (BNF, 2019).

143

Notable contraindications, cautions and common side effects

Nitrous oxide may have a detrimental impact on patients, especially if those patients are experiencing entrapped air (i.e., pneumothorax, an underwater dive, intracranial air following a head trauma or a recent intraocular gas injection) (BNF, 2019). The reason this should be avoided is due to the fact that administered nitrous oxide has the potential to diffuse into these spaces, causing an increase in pressure which has the potential to be harmful and even fatal for the patient (i.e. in the case of a pneumothorax, an increase in pressure would result in compromised respiration).

Local and regional anaesthesia

Local anaesthetics (LA) are used alone for specific regional anaesthesia as well as in combination with a general anaesthetic. They can be used to manage both acute and chronic pain, which make it of vital importance when considering individuals with complex pain management needs (Lirk et al., 2014).

Pharmacodynamics and pharmacokinetics

Every local anaesthetic has different physicochemical properties, but they all share the same mode of action. They block the voltage-gated sodium channels in the axon of nerve cells, halting the transfer of electrons between the nerve cells and interrupting pain signals.

Toxicity

When injecting a local anaesthetic into the subcutaneous tissue, it is vital to aspirate and check position, as injecting the local anaesthetic into a blood vessel can result in complications from the toxic potential of this drug (see the following Clinical Considerations box). Early symptoms of a mild LA toxicity include restlessness, tinnitus, slurred speech and a metallic taste in the mouth (Christie et al., 2015). In the most serious of cases, the local anaesthetic toxicity can enter the systemic circulation and cause a cardiac arrest through the inhibition of the calcium, potassium and sodium channels, stopping the contraction of the heart. Initial signs include tachycardia and hypertension, followed by myocardial depression, vasodilation, hypotension and a multitude of cardiac arrhythmias such as sinus bradycardia, conduction blocks, ventricular tachyarrhythmia and eventually asystole. Systemic local anaesthetic toxicity tends to have a delayed onset, and so any unusual cardiovascular signs after LA administration should be recognised as local anaesthetic systemic toxicity (Christie et al., 2015).

Clinical considerations

To treat LA toxicity, the healthcare professional should assess airway, breathing and circulation in turn. If the individual still has a strong cardiac output, 100% oxygen should be administered and the airway secured, followed by a 20% lipid emulsion intravenous infused, which absorbs toxins in the circulatory system, reducing the amount of toxin that is able to bind to the myocardium (Ciechanowicz and Patil, 2012).

Skills in practice

How to insert a peripheral cannula for the administration of intra-venous analgesic medications

Intravenous cannulation is a technique that involves the insertion of a fine flexible hollow tube, with an inner retractable needle, into a peripheral vein by a competent practitioner and, worldwide, is the most commonly performed invasive procedure (Boyd, 2013). In order to carry out the procedure, additional equipment is required (see Figure 8.8), all of which should be checked prior to carrying out the procedure.

1. Communicate with the patient and provide them with relevant information in order for them to provide informed consent. This will also provide you with the opportunity to talk about previous experiences with cannulation, ascertain if the patient has any allergies to dressings, assess for potential complications, and physically prepare the patient and the environment prior to collecting the equipment.
2. Decontaminate hands, and with the patient's arm in a comfortable and appropriate position, apply the tourniquet 7–10 cm above the chosen site. To encourage venous filling and vein distention, ask the patient to open and close their fist, use gravity by asking the patient to hang their arm down, apply a warm compress or lightly stroke the vein in a downward motion (Phillips and Gorski, 2014).
3. With two fingers, palpate the vein in order to confirm suitability and release the tourniquet.
4. Decontaminate hands, clean the tray/receptacle, and gather the equipment, ensuring that you check for damage and contamination. Place equipment into the clean receptacle using the aseptic non-touch technique (ANTT) (do not touch the key parts – the tip of the cannula and the end of the syringe for flushing).

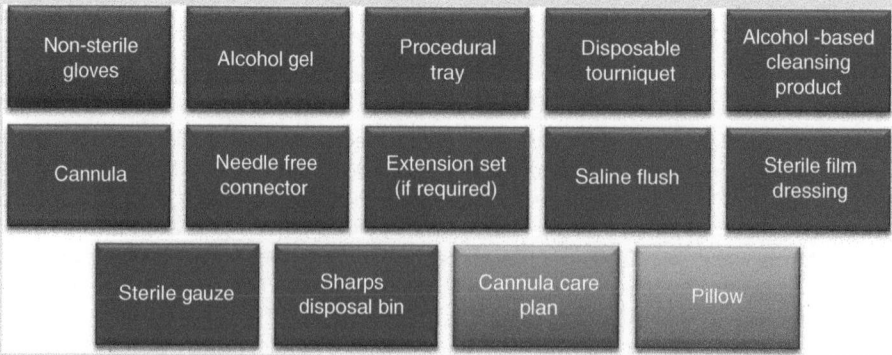

Figure 8.8 Additional equipment that may be required. Source: Modified from Dougherty and Lister (2015).

5. Reapply the tourniquet; do not over tighten as this may obstruct arterial flow.
6. Clean the chosen site with the alcohol-based (2% chlorhexidine in 70% isopropyl alcohol) preparation equipment. Ensure that you abide by the manufacturer's application instructions and allow to dry for 30 seconds. Do not touch the skin or re-palpate the vein after application of the skin preparation (Dougherty and Lister, 2015).
7. While waiting for the skin preparation solution to dry, decontaminate hands and don gloves.
8. Prepare the cannula device by removing the needle guard and assessing the tip for damage.
9. Then with your non-dominant hand, apply traction to the skin and stabilise the vein below the chosen site. Advise the patient that they will feel a sharp scratch.
10. Insert the cannula at an angle of 20–30° (depending on manufacturer's instructions) ensuring that the bevel is up and observe for the first flashback of blood into the cannula.
11. Lower the angle of insertion by dropping the cannula closer to the skin and advance the device slightly.
12. Then continue to advance the cannula 2 mm and draw the stylet back 2–3 mm noting the second flashback in the lumen of the cannula.
13. Slide the cannula over the needle, advancing further into the vein. Keeping traction on the skin will make this process easier.
14. Release the tourniquet, apply pressure beyond the cannula tip, loosen the cap at the end of the stylet, and withdraw the needle, placing it immediately into the sharps waste container. In line with the Health and Safety Executive (2013) regulations, the cannula will have a safety device (active or passive) in place to prevent a sharps injury. Depending on the specific design, it may also have a passive safety feature that prevents the reinsertion of the needle back into the lumen of the cannula, reducing the risk of cannula tip damage. Reapply the cap before releasing pressure and fix the cannula in place with a semi-permeable film dressing.
15. Flush with 0.9% sodium chloride (procedure for how this is undertaken will differ if using an extension set, or an integrated cannula), and ensure patient comfort.
16. Dispose of waste, remove PPE, and decontaminate hands using the appropriate technique (Ford and Park, 2018, 2019).
17. Document your care (via paper-based or electronic platforms) according to Trust guidelines and protocols. This should include, as a minimum standard, your signature, date, and designation, the time, cannula size, site of insertion, the number of insertion attempts, and any noted insertion complications. Further documentation, such as the VIP score, may also need to be completed, depending upon Trust requirements.

(Ford, 2019)

145

Episode of care 1: Regional block

Mrs. Jane Symonds is a 72-year-old woman who was admitted to the emergency department by paramedics who had received a 111 referral after she fell while shopping and sustained a fracture of her lower leg. A pain assessment was undertaken at the scene of the fall and in agreement with Mrs. Symonds, nitrous oxide was administered. On arrival at her local hospital, Mrs. Symonds care was transferred to the Emergency Department nurse practitioner, who arranged diagnostic tests and an assessment by an orthopaedic registrar. They confirmed that she has fractured her tibia and discussed the need for surgery, to stabilise the fracture.

As part of the pre-operative preparations, Jane was visited by an anaesthetic member of staff, who discussed peri-operative analgesic requirements. A shared decision was made to utilise a left lower limb regional block as well as pharmacological strategies. These options were chosen as a regional blockade of the distal nerves of the lower limbs is usually well-tolerated and has a low risk of systemic toxicity and neurological damage. This was administered prior to the general anaesthetic and involved an injection of a local anaesthetic around the nerves in the lower limb in order to achieve complete analgesia in the lower leg and foot. During this procedure, the operating department practitioner used distraction therapy, therapeutic touch and advanced communication skills in order to ensure that her levels of anxiety and procedural pain were limited.

Jane was transferred to the post-anaesthetic care unit where the healthcare professionals closely monitored and assessed her for signs of pain and regional block functioning. As the effects of the blockade began to reduce, Jane was then encouraged to take pharmacological analgesics, which were necessary in order to pre-empt the onset of nociceptive pain. The choice of whether to administer non-opioids, NSAIDs and opioids were dependent on the assessment of the pain and Jane's preferences.

Episode of care 2: Chronic pain

Diane Green is a 30-year-old woman who suffers from endometriosis and chronic pain. Diane has only recently been diagnosed with this condition, after experiencing unexplained visceral pain for many years. She was initially started on a pain management pathway by her GP, which consisted of a combination treatment of paracetamol and ibuprofen to manage the inflammatory response and the pain.

After 10 weeks Diane returned to see her GP as she felt her management plan was not effective. She was then prescribed an additional opioid analgesic, tramadol, which was to be taken alongside the paracetamol and ibuprofen. The GP prescribed a gradually increasing dose, so Diane could make a decision about how much was required in order to manage the pain, up to a maximum daily dose of 400 mg. The potential side effects were explained (nausea and vomiting, dry mouth, drowsiness, addiction and tolerance) and non-pharmacological strategies were discussed including heat packs, massage and warm baths. They also discussed the potential need for a referral to the gynaecologist (surgical options) or involvement of a specialist pain team, if the pain persisted.

Conclusion

Pain management strategies are most successful when they incorporate multimodal approaches, which are chosen in partnership with the patient (see the above Episodes of Care). This is not only to take advantage of the pharmacological benefits of a range of drugs but also to reduce potential side effects and adopt a holistic and partnership approach to pain management. In order to achieve this safely and effectively, healthcare professionals must ensure that their knowledge and understanding of pharmacological management options is varied and up-to-date and, if additional advice is required, that they consult a prescriber or pharmacy professional (RPS, 2019).

References

Ashelford, S., Raynsford, J., and Taylor, V. (2016). *Pathophysiology and Pharmacology for Nursing Students.* London: SAGE.

Bannister, K. (2019). Descending pain modulation: influence and impact. *Current Opinion in Physiology* 11 (1): 62–66.

Barber, P. and Robertson, D. (2012). *Essentials of Pharmacology for Nurses*, 2e. New York: McGraw-Hill Education.

Barber, P., Parkes, J., and Blundell, D. (2012). *Further Essentials of Pharmacology for Nurses*, 1e. New York: McGraw-Hill Education.

Beakley, B., Kaye, A., and Kaye, A. (2015). Tramadol, pharmacology, side effects and serotonin syndrome: a review. *Pain Physician* 18 (1): 195–400.

Bendall, J.C., Simpson, P.M., and Middleton, P.M. (2011). Prehospital vital signs can predict pain severity: analysis using ordinal logistic regression. *European Journal of Emergency Medicine* 18 (6): 334–339.

Beyaz, S., Sonbahar, T., Bayar, F., and Erdem, A. (2016). Seizures associated with low-dose tramadol for chronic pain treatment. *Anaesthesia Essays and Researchers* 10 (2): 376–378.

Boore, J., Cook, N., and Shepherd, A. (2016). *Essentials of Anatomy and Physiology for Nursing Practice*. Los Angeles: Sage.

Boyd, C. (2013). *Clinical Skills for Nurses*. West Sussex: Wiley.

British National Formulary (BNF) (2019). *BNF – 78*. London: BMJ Group and Pharmaceutical Press.

British Pain Society (2019). Pain: Less Campaign. https://www.britishpainsociety.org/painless-campaign (accessed 29 September 2019).

Brzakala, J. and Leppert, W. (2019). The role of rapid onset fentanyl products in the management of breakthrough pain in cancer patients. *Pharmacological Reports* 71 (3): 438–442.

Christie, L., Picard, J., and Weinberg, G. (2015). Local Anaesthetic systemic toxicity. *British Journal of Anaesthesia* 15 (3): 136–142.

Ciechanowicz, S. and Patil, V. (2012). Intravenous lipid emulsion – rescued at LAST. *Association of Anaesthetists of Great Britain and Ireland* 212 (5): 237–241.

Colvin, L.A. and Carty, S. (2012). Neuropathic pain. In: *ABC of Pain* (eds. L.A. Colvin and M. Fallon), 25–30. West Sussex: Wiley.

Cullen, M. and MacPherson, F. (2012). Complementary and alternative strategies. In: *ABC of Pain* (eds. L.A. Colvin and M. Fallon), 99–102. West Sussex: Wiley.

Cunningham, S. (2017). Pain assessment and management. In: *Clinical Skills for Nursing Practice* (eds. T. Moore and S. Cunningham), 104–131. Oxon: Routledge.

Dougherty, L. and Lister, S. (2015). *The Royal Marsden Hospital Manual of Clinical Nursing Procedures*, 9e. West Sussex: Wiley.

Dubin, A. and Patapoutian, A. (2010). Nociceptors: the sensors of the pain pathway. *The Journal of Clinical Investigation* 120 (11): 3760–3772.

Erden, S., Demir, N., Ugras, G. et al. (2018). Vital signs: valid indicators to assess pain in intensive care unit patients? An observational, descriptive study. *Nursing and Health Sciences Journal* 20 (4): 502–508.

Flasar, C.E. and Perry, A.G. (2014). Pain assessment and basic comfort measures. In: *Clinical Nursing Skills and Techniques* (eds. A.G. Perry, P.A. Potter and W.R. Ostendorf), 345–374. London: Elsevier.

Ford, C. (2019). Cannulation in adults. *British Journal of Nursing* 28 (13): 838–841.

Ford, C. and Park, L.G. (2018). Hand hygiene and handwashing: key to preventing the transfer of pathogens. *British Journal of Nursing* 27 (20): 1164–1166.

Ford, C. and Park, L.G. (2019). How to apply and remove medical gloves. *British Journal of Nursing* 28 (1): 65–72.

Fornasari, D. (2017). Pharmacotherapy for neuropathic pain: a review. *Pain and therapy* 6 (1): 25–33.

General Medical Council (2019). Good medical practice. https://www.gmc-uk.org/ethical-guidance/ethical-guidance-for-doctors/good-medical-practice (accessed 14 October 2019).

Hassamal, S., Miotto, K., Dale, W., and Danovitch, I. (2018). Tramadol: understanding the risk of serotonin syndrome and seizures. *American Journal of Medicine* 131 (11): 1382–1383.

Hastier, P., Buckley, M.J., Peten, E.P. et al. (2000). A new source of drug-induced acute pancreatitis: codeine. *The American Journal of Gastroenterology* 95 (11): 3295–3298.

Health and Care Professional Council (2019). Standards of conduct, performance and ethics. https://www.hcpc-uk.org/standards/standards-of-conduct-performance-and-ethics (accessed 14 October 2019).

Health and Safety Executive (2013). Sharp Instrument in Healthcare Regulations 2013: guidance for employers and employees. Health and Safety Executive Publications.

Hill, R., Santhakumar, R., Dewey, W. et al. (2019). Fentanyl depression of respiration: comparison with heroin and morphine. *British Journal of Pharmacology* 14860: 1–12.

Huang, C. and Johnson, N. (2016). Nitrous oxide, from the operating room to the emergency department. *Current Emergency and Hospital Medicine Reports* 4 (1): 11–18.

Kettyle, A. (2015). Pain management. In: *Essentials of Nursing Practice* (ed. C. Delves-Yates), 379–401. London: Sage.

Koneti, K. and Perfitt, J. (2019). Chronic pain management after surgery. *Surgery (Oxford)* 37 (8): 467–471.

Kosten, T., Graham, D., and Nielsen, D. (2018). Neurobiology of opioid use disorder and comorbid traumatic brain injury. *JAMA Psychiatry* 75 (6): 642–648.

147

Kukkar, A., Bali, A., Singh, N., and Jaggi, A. (2013). Implications and mechanism of action of gabapentin in neuropathic pain. *Archives of Pharmacal Research* 36 (3): 237–251.

Laws, P. and Rudall, N. (2013). Assessment and monitoring of analgesia, sedation, delirium and neuromuscular blockade levels and care. In: *Critical Care Manual for Clinical Procedures and Competencies* (eds. J. Mallet, J.W. Albarran and A. Richardson), 340–354. West Sussex: Wiley.

Lee, L., Caplan, R.A., Stephens, L.S. et al. (2015). Postoperative opioid-induced respiratory depression – a closed claims analysis. *Journal of Pain Medicine* 122 (1): 649–665.

Li, M. and Ramos, L. (2017). Drug-induced QT prolongation and Torsades de pointes. *Pharmacy and Therapeutics* 42 (7): 437–477.

Lirk, P., Picardi, S., and Hollmann, M. (2014). Local Anaesthetics: 10 essentials. *European Journal of Anaesthesiology* 31 (11): 575–585.

Lynn, R. and Galinkin, J. (2017). Naloxone dosage for opioid reversal: current evidence and clinical implications. *Therapeutic Advances in Drug Safety* 9 (1): 63–88.

MacKenzie, M., Zed, P., and Ensom, M. (2016). Opioid pharmacokinetics-pharmacodynamics: clinical implications in acute pain Management in Trauma. *Annals of Pharmacotherapy* 50 (3): 209–218.

Mears, J. (2018). Pain management. In: *Acute and Critical Care Nursing at a Glance* (eds. H. Dutton and J. Finch), 10–11. West Sussex: Wiley.

Merskey, H. and Bogduk, M. (1994). *Classifications of Chronic Pain.*, 2nde, 209–214. Washington: International Association for the Study of Pain Task Force on Taxonomy, IASP Press.

Neal, M.J. (2016). *Medical Pharmacology at a Glance*, 8e. West Sussex: Wiley.

Nelson, A. and Camilleri, M. (2016). Opioid-induced constipation: advances and clinical guidance. *Therapeutic Advances in Chronic Disease* 7 (2): 121–134.

NICE (2019). Opioid dependence. https://cks.nice.org.uk/opioid-dependence (accessed 29 September 2019).

Nursing and Midwifery Council (2018). The Code: Professional standards of practice and behaviour for nurses, midwives and nursing associates. https://www.nmc.org.uk/standards/code (accessed 16 August 2019).

Old, E.A., Nicol, L.S.C., and Malcangio, M. (2016). Recent advances in neuroimmune interactions in neuropathic pain: The role of microglia. In: *An Introduction to Pain and its Relation to Nervous System Disorders* (ed. A.A. Battaglia), 123–147. West Sussex: Wiley-Blackwell.

Pasero, C. (2015). Focus issue: innovations in pain management. *Journal of Perianesthesia Nursing* 30 (3): 178–180.

Patton, K.T. and Thibodeau, G.A. (2016). *Structure and Function of the Body.*, 15the. Missouri: Elsevier.

Phillips, L.D. and Gorski, L.A. (2014). *Manual of I.V. Therapeutics: Evidence-Based Practice for Infusion Therapy*, 6e. Philadelphia: F.A. Davis Company.

Rodriguez, L. (2015). Pathophysiology of pain: Implications for perioperative nursing. *AORN Journal* 101 (3): 338–344.

Royal Pharmaceutical Society and Royal College of Nursing (2019). *Professional Guidance on the Administration of Medicines in Healthcare Settings*. London: Royal Pharmaceutical Society.

Schumacher, M., Basbaum, A., and Naidu, R. (2015). Opioid agonists and antagonists. In: *Basic and Clinical Pharmacology* (ed. B. Katzung), 553–574. New York: McGraw-Hill Education.

Smith, H. and Laufer, A. (2014). Opioid-induced nausea and vomiting. *European Journal of Pharmacology* 722 (1): 67–78.

Smith, M.T. and Muralidharan, A. (2014). Pain pharmacology and the pharmacological management of pain. In: *Pain: A Textbook for Health Professionals*, 2e (eds. H. Van Griensven, J. Strong and A.M. Unruh), 159–180. London: Elsevier.

Solaro, C. and Uccelli, M.M. (2016). Pain in multiple sclerosis: From classification to treatment. In: *An Introduction to Pain and its Relation to Nervous System Disorders* (ed. A.A. Battaglia), 345–360. West Sussex: Wiley-Blackwell.

Stannard, C. (2019). Tramadol is not "opioid-lite". *BMJ* 365 (1): 12095.

Todd, A.J. (2016). Anatomy of pain pathways. In: *An Introduction to Pain and its Relation to Nervous System Disorders* (ed. A.A. Battaglia), 13–34. West Sussex: Wiley.

Tornsey, C. and Fleetwood-Walker, S. (2012). Pain mechanisms. In: *ABC of Pain* (eds. L.A. Colvin and M. Fallon), 5–10. West Sussex: Wiley-Blackwell.

Turk, D.C. and Melzack, R. (2011). Prologue. In: *Handbook of Pain Assessment* (eds. D.C. Turk and R. Melzack), 1–2. New York: Guilford Press.

VanMeter, K.C. and Hubert, R.J. (2014). *Gould's Pathophysiology for the Health Professions*, 5the. Missouri: Elsevier.

Wang, X., Zhang, Y., Peng, Y. et al. (2016). Pharmacological characterization of the opioid inactive isomers (+)-naltrexone and (+)-naloxone as antagonists of toll-like receptor 4. *British Journal of Pharmacology* 173 (5): 856–869.

Wiffen, P., Knaggs, R., Derry, S. et al. (2016). Paracetamol (acetaminophen) with or without codeine or dihy-drocodeine for neuropathic pain in adults. *Cochrane Database of Systematic Reviews* 12: 1465–1858.

World Health Organisation (2018). WHO's cancer pain ladder for adults. http://www.who.int/cancer/palliative/painladder/en (accessed 24 July 2019).

Young, S. and Pitcher, B. (2016). *Medicines Management for Nurses at a Glance*. West Sussex: Wiley.

Multiple choice questions

1. Which type of pain originates in the organs?
   (a) Referred
   (b) Somatic
   (c) Visceral
   (d) Nociceptive

2. Which pain assessment strategy is associated with the use of scales?
   (a) Unidimensional tool
   (b) Multidimensional tool
   (c) Mnemonics
   (d) The art of noticing
3. What classification of pharmacological analgesic is aspirin?
   (a) Opioid
   (b) Non-opioid
   (c) Non-steroidal anti-inflammatory
   (d) Co-analgesic
4. NSAIDs are contraindicated in individuals who have a history of . . .?
   (a) Haemorrhoids
   (b) Gastric ulcer
   (c) Hyperthyroidism
   (d) Hypotension
5. Pain within the UK affects approximately how many individuals?
   (a) 1:2
   (b) 1:3
   (c) 1:4
   (d) 1:5
6. Which chemical is associated with the stimulation of nociceptors and is inhibited by NSAIDs?
   (a) Prostaglandin
   (b) Substance-P
   (c) Histamine
   (d) Bradykinin
7. What are A-delta fibres?
   (a) Relay neurons
   (b) Efferent pain fibres
   (c) Afferent pain fibres
   (d) Synapses
8. What is the name of the antagonist drug to reverse the effects of opioid-induced respiratory depression?
   (a) Naproxen
   (b) Naloxone
   (c) Nefopam
   (d) Nefazodone

9. What is the maximum daily dose recommended for oral paracetamol?
   - (a) 4 g
   - (b) 3 g
   - (c) 5 g
   - (d) 2 g

10. Which type of NSAIDs is celecoxib?
    - (a) Paracetamol
    - (b) Salicylic acid derivatives
    - (c) Propionic acid derivatives
    - (d) Selective COX-2 inhibitors

11. How often should fentanyl transdermal patches be changed?
    - (a) 36 hours
    - (b) 24 hours
    - (c) 72 hours
    - (d) 48 hours

12. Which drug causes pinpoint pupils?
    - (a) Paracetamol
    - (b) Naproxen
    - (c) Gabapentin
    - (d) Morphine

13. Which route is not used for the administration of paracetamol?
    - (a) Oral
    - (b) Rectal
    - (c) Intravenous infusion
    - (d) Intramuscular

14. How many different types of opioid receptors are there?
    - (a) 3
    - (b) 4
    - (c) 5
    - (d) 6

15. What is the antidote for paracetamol overdose?
    - (a) N-acetylcysteine
    - (b) N-acetyl-para-aminophenol
    - (c) Naloxone
    - (d) Narcan

Find out more

The following are a list of some of the conditions that are related to acute pain episodes or associated with people who suffer from chronic pain. Take some time and write notes about each of the conditions. Think about the medications that may be used in order to treat these conditions and be specific about the pharmacokinetics and pharmacodynamics. Remember to include aspects of patient care. If you are making notes about people you have offered care and support to, you must ensure that you have adhered to the rules of confidentiality.

The Condition	Your Notes
Fibromyalgia	
Respiratory Depression	
Migraine	
Endometriosis	
Osteoarthritis	

Chapter 9

Antibacterials

Deborah Flynn

Aim

The aim of this chapter is to encourage the reader to develop an understanding and appreciation of the differences in antibacterial use.

Learning outcomes

After reading this chapter, the reader will be able to:

1. Understand how pathogens cause infections and the use of terminology associated with this category of medication
2. Understand the different antibacterial classifications and be able to explain their actions and associated side effects
3. Explain the nursing considerations of each antibacterial classification
4. Understand the nurse's health-promoting role within the use of antibacterial therapy and antimicrobial stewardship

Test your knowledge

1. What is the difference between bacteriostatic and bactericidal treatments?
2. Describe the professional responsibilities of registered healthcare professionals in relation to antimicrobial stewardship.
3. What are the pharmacokinetics of aminoglycosides?
4. What considerations should be taken into account when administering gentamycin?
5. What does the term 'teratogenic' mean?

Fundamentals of Pharmacology: For Nursing and Healthcare Students, First Edition. Edited by Ian Peate and Barry Hill.
© 2021 John Wiley & Sons Ltd. Published 2021 by John Wiley & Sons Ltd.

Introduction

This chapter explores antibacterials. Antibiotics are the miracle drugs of the last two centuries as their actions have reduced mortality rates in previous life-threatening conditions; for example, pneumonia and tuberculosis (World Health Organisation [WHO], 2018a). This trend is jeopardised due to a lack of development and research in antimicrobial treatments (WHO, 2018b), which include antibiotics, antivirals and antifungals. The Parliamentary Office of Science and Technology [POST] (2017) identified infectious disease as creating a significant burden to the Untied Kingdom's health and economic systems, causing 7% of all deaths and being responsible for a large proportion of sick days, respectively.

Microorganisms are omnipresent in the world, but are only seen microscopically. These include bacteria, virus, fungi or protozoa (Barber and Robertson, 2020). Microorganisms live on and inside us; often they are more beneficial than harmful to us; for example, normal body flora is made up of colonised, mostly bacterial, microorganisms acquired through contact with the outside world (Burchum and Rosenthal, 2019). The purpose of normal flora is to prevent the colonisation and spreading of infection by pathogens (Ashelford, Raynsford and Taylor, 2016). A pathogen is a disease producing microorganism (Ashelford, Raynsford and Taylor, 2016). The extent to which they are disease-causing depends on the type of microorganism and its severity or harmfulness (Burchum and Rosenthal, 2019). It is known that pathogenic bacteria such as *Escherichia coli* live harmlessly in the alimentary tract; however, if spread to other bodily regions, they can cause infection; for example, a urinary tract infection (Ashelford, Raynsford and Taylor, 2016). Likewise, in times of vulnerability, normally harmless microorganisms can cause infections, similar to invading microorganisms (Ashelford, Raynsford and Taylor, 2016). Survival of microorganisms depends on the presence of oxygen; aerobic pathogens require oxygen for survival whereas anaerobic pathogens do not (Barber and Robertson, 2020).

Language and terminology

Several authors (Karch, 2017; Burchum and Rosenthal, 2019) highlight the interchangeable use of the terms antimicrobial, antibacterial and antibiotic. They explain that the difference lies in the origin (manufacture) of the drug, as an antimicrobial is a substance, naturally or synthetically produced, which suppresses growth or kills bacteria and other microorganisms, including viruses, fungi, protozoa and rickettsiae (Burchum and Rosenthal, 2019). An antibacterial agent is one that kills bacteria or inhibits their growth, regardless of whether natural or chemically produced, as the therapeutic aim is the same (Ashelford, Raynsford and Taylor, 2016; Burchum and Rosental, 2019). An antibiotic is a natural chemical produced by one type of microorganism that either inhibits growth or kills another microorganism (bacteria); therefore, the terms will be used interchangeably here (Burchum and Rosenthal, 2019). Selective toxicity is the antimicrobial's ability to target certain parts of the microorganism to cause destruction via a number of mechanisms (see Table 9.1), without injuring human cells (Barber and Robertson, 2020). However, sometimes the antimicrobials cannot distinguish between the actions in a pathogen or human cell, due to similarity in function: this leads to the human cells suffering greater injury (Barber and Robertson, 2020).

The goal of antibacterial therapy is to reduce bacteria (infection causing) to a point at where the body's immune system can effectively deal with the microorganisms (Xiu and Datta, 2019). These drugs have certain properties: bactericidal, that is, they directly kill the bacteria; for example, penicillin and aminoglycosides; or, bacteriostatic, that is, they inhibit bacterial growth and rely on the body's immune system to kill the bacteria; for example, tetracycline; or a combination of both properties; for example, aminoglycosides (Barber and Robertson, 2020; Ashelford, Raynsford and Taylor, 2016). The combination of bacteriostatic and bactericidal properties in certain drugs is due to the dosage and serum level concentration of the drug as well as outside influences and the health of the person. Narrow therapeutic index drugs, such as aminoglycosides, rely on the monitoring of the serum concentration as this determines whether they lie within therapeutic range; the aim is to prevent underdosing or drug toxicity (Burchum and Rosenthal, 2019).

As this chapter focuses on antibacterial agents, an understanding of bacteria cell structure and the various mechanisms of antibacterial action need to be considered.

Table 9.1   Classifications of antimicrobials with examples.

Classification	Action	Group	Example
Antibacterial	Disrupt cell wall synthesis (Beta-lactams)	Penicillin	Benzylpenicillin
		Cephalosporins (5 generations)	Cephalexin
		Carbapenems	Imipenem
	Folate interference	Sulphonamides	Trimethoprim
			Co-trimoxazole
	Bacterial DNA inhibition	Quinolones	Ciprofloxacin
	Protein synthesis interference	Tetracyclines	Tetracycline
		Chloramphenicol	
		Aminoglycosides	Gentamycin
		Macrolides	Erythromycin
		Lincosamides	Clindamycin
Antifugal (AF)	Cell membrane damage	Polyene AF	Nystatin
		Imidazole AF	Clotrimazole
		Triazole AF	Fluconazole
Antiviral	Potential inhibition of DNA replication	Anti-HIV	
Antiprotozoal	Either inhibit bacterial reproduction or damage DNA of protozoa	Antimalarials	Quinines
		Miscellaneous	Metronidazole (also used as antibacterial)

Source: Adapted Burchaum and Rosenthal (2019); Karch (2017).

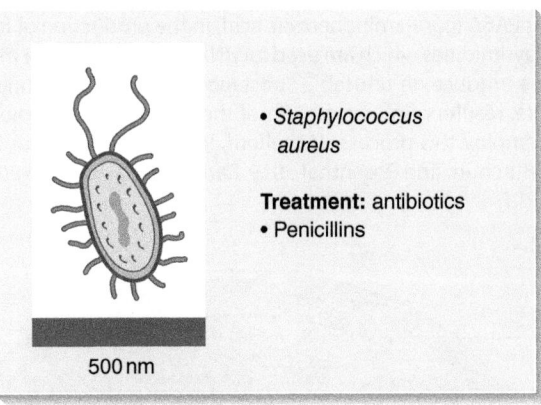

• *Staphylococcus aureus*

Treatment: antibiotics
• Penicillins

500 nm

Figure 9.1   Bacteria. Source: Adapted Young and Pitcher (2016).

Bacteria

Bacteria are invisible to the naked eye, existing inside or outside organisms and they can live independent from a host (Barber and Robertson, 2020) (see Figure 9.1). Bacteria are single-cell microorganisms (prokaryotic) that have no nucleus but contain DNA (Ashelford, Raynsford and Taylor, 2016). They use their enzymes and ribosomes to manufacture proteins that allow their growth and reproduction to occur. Each bacterial type has a different shape: bacilli are rod-shaped, cocci are round-shaped and spirochetes are spiral/corkscrew-shaped (Barber and Robertson, 2020).

Bacteria can be harmless, pathogenic or beneficial to humans (Barber and Robertson, 2020). Beneficial bacteria are, for example, those settled within our intestines; however, bacteria become pathogenic if through pre-existing disease our resistance is lowered or our natural defence system is affected by disease or trauma and it is through the destruction of our normal intestinal flora that these pathogens have the opportunity to invade (Xiu and Datta, 2019).

Superinfections can occur; these are defined by Burchum and Rosenthal (2019, p. 1019) as 'as a new infection that appears during the course of treatment for a primary infection'. This is often seen in cases of drug-resistant microorganisms. There is an increased likelihood of a superinfection occurring in the use of broad-spectrum antibiotics as they destroy greater quantities of normal flora than narrow-spectrum ones (Burchum and Rosenthal 2019). This gives a chance for the rise of pathogens, normally kept in balance by the normal flora, to invade bodily tissues, thus causing an infection; common sites of these infections are the gastrointestinal tract and vulvar area (British Medical Association [BMA], 2018).

Antibacterial mechanisms of action

The following section of the chapter considers the four main mechanisms of actions that were listed in Table 9.1, these are illustrated in Figure 9.2.

Disruption of the cell wall synthesis

Penicillins act on bacterial cell wall synthesis in two ways: firstly, they inhibit the formation of peptidoglycan, which makes up 50% of the cell wall, alongside giving the cellular wall its strength; and secondly, they bind with penicillin-binding proteins (responsible for allowing bacterial growth and division). Due to the greater intracellular osmotic pressure, the bacterial cells swell and burst. Structurally, penicillins contain a β-lactam ring and certain bacteria create enzymes which inactivate penicillin: these are called β-lactamases (penicillinase). Cephalosporins act in a similar manner (Ashelford et al., 2016; Karch, 2017; Burchum and Rosenthal, 2019; Xiu and Datta, 2019; Barber and Robertson, 2020).

Folate interference

Bacterial cells, unlike human cells, must produce their own folic acid for growth and reproduction. The cell uses PABA (para-aminobenzoic acid) in the production of folic acid, necessary for the purines and pyrimidines which are used for RNA, DNA and protein manufacture. For example, sulfonamides produce an unusable substance similar to PABA and this blocks the cell's synthesis of folate, resulting in non-growth of the bacteria. An antibiotic group such as the sulphonamides employ this process (Ashelford, Raynsford and Taylor 2016; Karch 2017; Xiu and Datta 2019; Burchum and Rosenthal 2019; Barber and Robertson 2020).

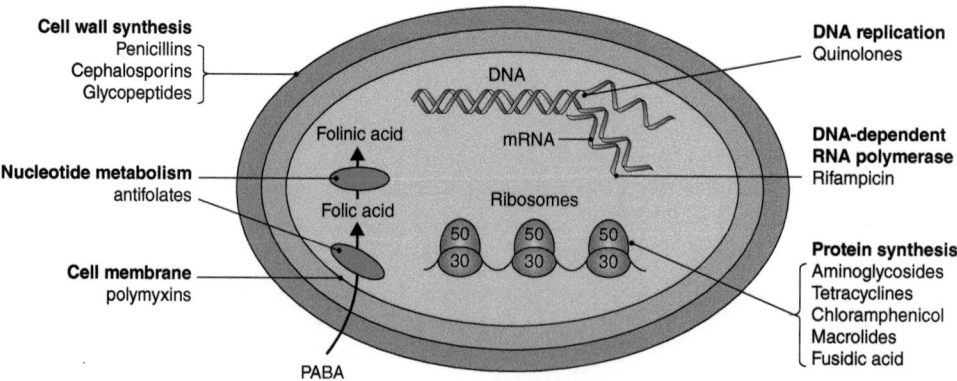

Figure 9.2 Sites of action of different types of antibiotic agent. DNA, PABA, RNA. Source: Xiu and Datta (2019).

Bacterial DNA inhibition

Bacterial cells' DNA (deoxyribonucleic acid) is supercoiled and requires enzymes for certain parts to be uncoiled for replication that are necessary for survival. Antibiotic groups, such as fluroquinolones, interfere with this process (Ashelford, Raynsford and Taylor, 2016; Karch, 2017; Burchum and Rosenthal, 2019; Xiu and Datta, 2019; Barber and Robertson, 2020).

Protein synthesis interference

The initiation of bacterial protein synthesis occurs via their ribosomes, which are different to humans Protein synthesis inhibitors, such as aminoglycosides, bind irreversibly to ribosome 30S causing disruptions either in the initiation of the process, or by creating misreading of the genetic code, or by ending the protein synthesis process before completion (Ashelford, Raynsford and Taylor, 2016; Karch, 2017; Burchum and Rosenthal, 2019; Xiu and Datta, 2019; Barber and Robertson, 2020).

157

Choosing the right treatment

The right drug for the right bug.

(Burchum and Rosenthal, 2019, p. 1042).

The Joint Formulary Committee British National Formulary (Joint Formulary) (2019) suggests one key factor of choosing the right treatment is to establish the causative microorganism; a specimen will need to be sent to a laboratory for culture and sensitivity testing. For means of identification, microorganisms are subjected to gram staining as part of culture testing (Cattini and Kiernan, 2020). During this process, gram-negative bacteria cell walls lose the strain or become decolourised (Ashelford et al., 2016). On the other hand, gram-positive bacteria cell walls retain the strain or resist decolourisation (Ashelford et al., 2016). The next part, sensitivity testing, is to determine the appropriate therapy.

There are two main categories of antibiotics, based on the spectrum of their activity: broad spectrum and narrow spectrum. Table 9.2 below details the main differences with examples.

Another key factor that must be given much consideration, is the patient. The clinician must take note of the patient's allergy history, liver (hepatic) and kidney (renal) function, susceptibility to disease, route tolerance (for example, ability to swallow), severity of illness, race and ethnicity (influence on pharmacokinetics due to differing genetics [Zurlinden and Reisfeld, 2017]), age, concomitant medication intake and pregnancy status, if breast-feeding, or taking oral contraceptives (Joint Formulary Committee, 2020a). POST (2017) states that inappropriate prescribing of antibiotics increases antimicrobial resistance (AMR).

Antimicrobial resistance

The World Health Organisation (2018a) defines AMR as 'the ability of microorganisms (like bacteria, viruses and some parasites) to stop an antimicrobial (such as antibiotics, antivirals and antimalarials) from working against it. As a result, standard treatments become ineffective, infections persist and may spread to others'.

Globally, the focus toward AMR, considered a public health priority, is gathering pace as there is a concentrated effort to decrease antibiotic usage due to increasing resistance making infections harder to treat and the added cost to individuals (increased mortality) and healthcare providers (longer stays and higher costs) (Burchum and Rosenthal, 2019).

Table 9.2 Broad- and narrow-spectrum antibiotics with examples.

Broad-spectrum antibiotics	Narrow-spectrum antibiotics
Effective against a wide variety of microorganisms. Kill variety of organisms. Useful if the cause of infection is unknown. For example, erythromycin, ciprofloxacin and doxycycline.	Effective against only specific microorganisms. Causative organisms are known. For example, vancomycin, clindamycin and older penicillins.

Source: Burchum and Rosenthal (2019), Ashelford, Raynsford and Taylor (2016).

Burchum and Rosenthal (2019) emphasise resistance – that is, bacteria that are no longer sensitive to the antibacterial – comes in two forms: innate and acquired (Xiu and Datta, 2019). Innate resistance occurs naturally or is inborn (Xiu and Datta, 2019). In acquired resistance (happens over time), bacteria grow due to previous exposure (Xiu and Datta, 2019). This type of resistance can develop for many drugs (Burchum and Rosenthal, 2019). Contributing factors to this type of resistance are overuse, underuse and misuse in both healthcare and agricultural disciplines (Barber and Robertson, 2020). This can be evidenced in over- and inappropriate prescribing (WHO, 2018a). An example of a multidrug resistant bacteria is meticillin-resistant *Staphylococcus aureus* (MRSA).

Preventing antimicrobial resistance

The main aim of preventing AMR is to preserve and prolong the effectiveness of known antibiotics and prevent the occurrence and transmission of infections. The World Health Organisation (2018b) sets out action points for individuals, healthcare professionals, health policy makers and the healthcare industry.

The individual's responsibility centres around managing expectations regarding the prescribing of antibiotics and concordance with medication regimens. Furthermore, there is a responsibility to prevent the transmission of infection by using appropriate hand washing, adhering to food preparation hygiene, safer sex practices and updating vaccinations as required.

The focus of the healthcare professional's [HCP] role, specifically the healthcare professional, in preventing AMR is patient education. In frontline clinical skills, such as drug administration or explaining discharge medication, there is a need to explain to the person the action of antibiotics; that is, to target certain bacterial strains. By doing such, this can clarify that antibiotics cannot be prescribed to alleviate discomfort or as an easy remedy/solution. This extends to information about accumulating medication or antibiotics for future use or sharing medications with friends with similar symptoms. When prescribing/administering antibiotics, the healthcare professional should explain that completing the entire course of antibiotics is imperative, even if the patient feels better, as bacterial exposure to antimicrobials can lead to resistance. Additionally, providing further information about taking the medication as prescribed (over the 24-hour period) is required. The aim is to prevent the development of resistant microorganisms by maintaining the serum concentration level. Moreover, promoting healthy behaviour change towards the prevention of spreading infection, by improving measures such as hand washing, promoting the uptake of vaccination programmes, raising awareness of current public health campaigns, reducing unnecessary or inappropriate prescribing, supporting rapid diagnostics, promoting safer sex practices, and actions such as covering one's nose and mouth when sneezing (WHO, 2018a).

In pregnant and breast-feeding women, antibiotic use requires caution by balancing the risks versus benefits, due to fetal or neonatal injury (BMA, 2018). Furthermore, the effectiveness of hormone-based contraceptives is known to be inhibited by certain antibiotic use.

The role of policymakers is to ensure national robust systems to improve infection prevention and control, as well as surveillance of antibiotic resistant infections. WHO (2018b) recommends the healthcare industry funds further research and development of antibiotics, which POST (2017) details as needing to be broad spectrum in nature in order to conquer the numerous microorganism resistance mechanisms.

Clinical consideration 1

Here is a summary of the healthcare professional's role in the principles of good assessment, combating amicrobial resistance and prescribing practice considerations.

- Establish if the person has a history of hepatic and/or renal impairment and allergies, is pregnant or breast-feeding and assess for any contraindications or cautions present in their history specific to antibacterial groups.
- Identify the causative microorganism through microscopy, culture and sensitivity (MC and S).
- Assess the severity of the current illness.

- Determine previous antibacterial therapy.
- Ask about previous adverse/allergic reactions.
- Advise the person to complete the full course of antibiotics, regardless of whether they are feeling better.
- Provide information about taking the course as prescribed to ensure it is completed in full.
- Evaluate the therapeutic effect; for example, improved wellbeing.
- Offer information to the person about not accumulating antibiotics for future use or sharing them with others experiencing similar symptoms.
- Consider concurrent medications and be aware of interaction risk and monitor for potential effects.
- Encourage the person to adopt health-promoting behaviours towards the prevention of infection spreading.
- Educate the person about additional contraceptive precautions, if the prescribed antibiotic is know to reduce effectiveness of these measures.

Source: BMA (2018), NICE (2019), Xiu and Datta (2019).

Antimicrobial stewardship (AMS)

According to the British Society for Antimicrobial Chemotherapy (2017, p. 42) the definition of AMS is 'the right antibiotic, for the right indication (diagnosis), the right patient, at the right time, with the right dose and route, causing the least harm to the patient and future patients'. Furthermore, they argue there is a need to tackle the multifactorial drivers of antibiotic use through adoption of cautious prescribing guidelines driven by AMS overarching goals. These goals include: improving patient outcomes, reducing collateral damage and impact costs. National Institute for Health and Care Excellence (NICE) guidelines (2018) concur that this is about changing prescribing practice to slow AMR and prolong the effectiveness of the current available antibiotics. Alongside this, POST (2017) describes how part of the UK government's five-year strategy is to identify the causative pathogen and prescribe the appropriate antibiotic.

Olans et al. (2018) assert that frontline clinical staff, especially the registered healthcare professional, are an underutilised commodity in the AMR battle. They mapped the daily responsibilities of a registered healthcare professional against AMS components and demonstrated a near congruence between them. They call for a multidisciplinary focused formal AMS educational programme.

Clinical considerations 2

Medication consideration during adulthood

- Poor antimicrobial stewardship: management for antibiotic demand through patient education regarding indications for use, completing the course, non-stockpiling for future use, or sharing of antibiotics with symptomatic people.
- Awareness of drug allergies and emergence of resistant strains.
- Consider use of contraceptive measures in women of reproductive age, whether the prescribed antibiotic is known to be teratogenic and provide relevant patient education.
- Cautions for use in pregnancy: dosage adjustment due to increased maternal hepatic metabolism and glomerular infiltration rate; balance benefits of treatment against risk of foetal harm due to drugs crossing the placental barrier; for example, sulfonamides.

- Caution in lactation as most drugs cross into the breast milk; for example, cause tooth deformities and staining of teeth.
- Interference with hormone-based contraceptives.
- Awareness of renal or hepatic impairment in patient history or associated conditions.

Source: Adapted Burchaum and Rosenthal (2019); Karch (2017).

Antibacterials by action

Dolk et al. (2018) review of antibiotic prescribing in British primary care settings, over a two-year period, provides insights into which antibiotics are used extensively and for which conditions. They conclude that the conditions, most frequently require antibiotics were respiratory and urinary tract infections, with penicillin accounting for 50% of all prescriptions, then macrolides (13%), tetracyclines (12%) and trimethoprim (11%).

Table 9.1 highlights the various classifications of antimicrobials and this next section details the pharmacokinetics of the group or drug; its actions; contradictions and cautions; adverse effects; drug–drug interactions; and nursing considerations. However, some antimicrobials mentioned will not be investigated in this chapter, namely sulfonamides and fluroquinolones. Regardless of which antibiotic group is prescribed, the role the healthcare professional plays in maintaining the principles of antimicrobial stewardship around patient education remains.

Beta-lactams

This antibacterial group houses penicillins, cephalsporins and carbapenams based on their common action of disrupting the bacterial cell wall synthesis (Barber and Robertson, 2020).

Penicillins

Examples of this group of antibacterials, used to treat mild to moderate infections, are penicillin G, flucloxacillin, amoxicillin and piperacillin with tazobactam (Xiu and Datta, 2019). Burchum and Rosenthal (2019) list four classifications of penicillins and explain how they extend from narrow to extended in their spectrum of activity. They are bactericidal in effect (Xiu and Datta, 2019). The main differences between the different penicillins are the spectrum of activity, stability in stomach acid and duration of action (Burchum and Rosenthal, 2019).

Indications (for all penicillins)

These range from middle ear, lung, skin, sexually transmitted infections and can also be used prophylactically before surgical or dental procedures in patients with a history of rheumatic fever (NICE, 2019). Table 9.3 details the four spectrum classifications with examples and indications.

Benzylpenicillin (Penicillin G)

This is indicated for throat infections, pneumonia, otitis media, cellulitis, endocarditis, anthrax (potentially in combination with other antibacterials), meningitis and prophylaxis (Burchum and Rosenthal, 2019; NICE, 2019).

The pharmacokinetics across the penicillin range differ. Benzylpenicillin sodium is the example used here. It is worth noting that Penicillin G (Pen G) is available in four salts: potassium Pen G, procaine Pen G, benzathine Pen G and sodium Pen G (Burchum and Rosenthal, 2019). They differ with regard to route of administration and time course of action (Burchum and Rosenthal, 2019). Table 9.4 below describes its pharmacokinetics.

Table 9.3   Spectrum classifications with examples and indications.

Classification	Examples	Indications
Narrow spectrum: Penicillinase sensitive	Penicillin G (benzylpenicillin sodium)	Effective against aerobic gram-positive, and gram-negative cocci and many anaerobic microbes. Mild to moderate infections.
Narrow spectrum: Penicillinase resistant	Flucloxacillin	Effective in infections caused by penicillin-resistant staphylococci. Used as an adjunct in pneumonia and is effective in ear infections, impetigo, cellulitis, staphylococcal infections, surgical prophylaxis and osteomyelitis
Broad spectrum	Amoxicillin	Effective for upper respiratory infections, urinary tract infections and community acquired pneumonia.
Extended spectrum	Piperacillin with tazobactam	Broad spectrum of activity against a range of both gram-positive and gram-negative bacteria and anaerobes. Used to treat Non MRSA active Septicaemia, hospital-acquired pneumonia, complicated infections involving urinary tract, skin and soft tissues, or acute exacerbations of chronic obstructive pulmonary disease or bronchiectasis. For severe pseudomonas infections, these can be given with an aminoglycoside-synergistic effect.

Source: Modified from Burchaum and Rosenthal (2019); NICE (2019); BMA (2018); Xiu and Datta (2019).

Table 9.4   Pharmacokinetics of benzylpenicillin sodium.

Absorption	Is poorly absorbed in the gastrointestinal tract and best administered by injection – intramuscular (IM) or intravenous (IV) (dependent on variant). Intrathecal injection of benzylpenicillin is not recommended
Distribution	Distributes well to most tissues and fluids. Poor penetration is noted, in the absence of inflammation, to the cerebrospinal fluid, joints and eyes.
Metabolism	Minimal metabolism.
Excretion	Urine (renal).

Source: Wishart et al. (2018); Burchum and Rosenthal (2019); NICE (2019).

Contraindications and cautions (for all penicillins)

Being free from many side effects is the advantage of using penicillin; however, many microorganisms have developed penicillin resistance due to the length of time it has been used (Barber and Robertson, 2020). Contraindications include people with a known immediate allergy to penicillins, cephalosporins and other beta-lactams, or those with a history of atopic allergy (for example, asthma, eczema and hay fever) as they have an increased risk of anaphylaxis (NICE, 2019). Cautious use is recommended in people with renal impairment due to the excretion route. Further cautious use is recommended in pregnancy, due to the potential of the diarrhoeal or superinfection effect and in lactating women, as penicillin enters the breast milk and could result in a superinfection risk for the baby (Karch, 2017).

Benzylpenicillin sodium

In the case of Pen G, there are no known harmful effects in pregnancy, and although Pen G passes into the breast milk, it is deemed safe to use by lactating women (NICE, 2019). Due to renal excretion of Pen G, caution should be exercised in people with renal disease or impairment, as renal failure can result from the accumulation of sodium from injections (NICE, 2019).

Adverse effects (for all penicillins)

Hypersensitivity is the most common adverse effect and can range from rash to anaphylaxis (Xiu and Datta, 2019). Allergy to one type of penicillin may result in allergy to all types, along-side a potential hypersensitivity to other beta-lactam antibiotics (NICE, 2019). Certain blood disorders – leucopoenia or thrombocytopenia – may occur. If administered parenteraly, then pain and inflammation, at the injection site, is possible (Burchum and Rosenthal, 2019).

Diarrhoea is a common adverse effect, especially in oral broad-spectrum penicillin treat-ment, potentially leading to antibiotic-associated colitis (Xiu and Datta 2019; NICE, 2019). Associated with the loss of intestinal flora, further effects are superinfections including yeast infections, nausea, vomiting, abdominal pain, gastritis, glossitis, sore mouth and furry tongue (Burchum and Rosenthal, 2019).

Benzylpenicillin

NICE (2019) highlights fever and the Jarisch–Herxheimer reaction (fever, malaise, sweating and headache) as being common effects, whereas neurotoxicity (seizures, confusion, hallucina-tions) is a rare effect.

Drug–Drug interactions

Some important drug–drug interactions involving penicillin types are listed below; however, this is not an exhaustive list and therefore further reading of, for example, NICE (2019) for indi-vidual antibiotics and further interactions is recommended.

Concurrent parenteral administration of aminoglycosides and penicillins results in inactiva-tion of the former, whereas tetracyclines and penicillins combination can affect the effectiveness of the latter (Burchum and Rosenthal, 2019). Avoidance of combinations is recommended.

Benzylpenicillin

- Methotrexate: increases the risk of toxicity.
- Warfarin: potentially alters the anticoagulant effect.

Flucloxacillin

- Similar interactions to benzylpenicillin regarding anticoagulants and methotrexate.
- Alcohol: can increase the risk of hepatotoxicity.
- Paracetamol: can increase the risk of hepatotoxicity.
- Probenecid: reduces excretion of flucloxacillin.

Amoxicillin

- Similar interactions to benzylpenicillin regarding anticoagulants and methotrexate.
- Allopurinol: increases the risk of a skin rash when taken concurrently.

Piperacillin with tazobactam

- Similar interactions to benzylpenicillin regarding anticoagulants and methotrexate.
- Suxamethonium (and similar type drugs) – the effect can be increased by piperacillin.

(NICE, 2019)

Nursing actions

- Promote principles of good patient assessment, prescribing practice and antimicrobial stewardship through patient education (see Clinical Considerations 1).
- If taking oral doses of penicillin, for example, amoxicillin, these should be taken with a full glass of water one hour before or two hours after meals (antibiotic specific). Certain food stuffs (fruit juice, soft drinks, milk) interfere with certain oral penicillins effectiveness.
- Gastrointestinal discomfort are common effects of penicillins. Educate people on ways to maintain adequate nutrition and hydration.

- Monitor renal function, by assessing intake and output, to prevent injury, for example, in older people, those with known renal impairment, acutely ill or very young.
- Monitor the first and subsequent administration of doses due to allergy risk.
- Advise known penicillin allergy patients to wear appropriate identification.
- Advise the patient to report any signs of an allergic reaction (skin rash, fever, itching, hives, wheezing or swollen joints).
- If concomitant medications include anticoagulants, monitor INR (how long it takes blood to form a clot) and adjust dose as required.
- Consider concurrent medication and be aware of interaction risk and monitor for potential effects.
- Penicillins and aminoglycosides should not be administered in the same intravenous solution as aminoglycosides are inactivated.

Source: Karch, 2017; Burchum and Rosenthal, 2019; NICE, 2019; Barber and Robertson, 2020.   163

Clinical considerations 3

Medication consideration in the older adult

Signs and symptoms of infections can differ in this client group.

Culture and sensitivity are important to establish.

They react more sensitively and with individual variability to the treatment regimens than for younger adults.

Pharmacokinetic changes due to age-related decline of bodily systems requires attention to sites of metabolism (liver/kidney) and excretion (kidney) and may require dose adjustment.

Rate of drug absorption is slower.

More likely to have liver (prolongs drug effect) or renal (non-excretion of drug) impairment.

More likely to experience adverse drug reaction due to body system impairment, polypharmacy, severe illness and pre-existing illness, and drug regimens consisting of high-risk drug–drug interactions.

More susceptible to adverse effects of antimicrobials. Give consideration to hydration and nutritional status alongside safety measures if central nervous system (CNS) side effects are noted.

Consider dose adjustment and lengthen dose intervals in clients with liver or renal impairment, dependence on alcohol or taking concomitant nephrotoxic or hepatotoxic drugs.

Unintentional non-concordance due to forgetfulness, inability to follow instructions, complicated drug regimens, appearance of side effects, inaccessibility to medication due to poor packaging or health inequalities (distance to pharmacy or cost).

Intentional non-concordance due to complicated drug regimen, poor patient education, client feels the drug is not necessary, increased side effects, dosage is too high or poor client–practitioner relationship.

Source: Adapted Burchaum and Rosenthal (2019); Karch (2017).

Cephalosporins

This range of antibacterials have a broad antimicrobial spectrum, acting on gram-negative and gram-positive microorganisms (Xiu and Datta, 2019). The choice of drug is dependent on the type of pathogen. The beta-lactam actions of this group are similar to penicillins (Barber and Robertson, 2020). They are widely used and are mostly bactericidal but can become bacteriostatic, dependent on dose and drug prescribed (Karch, 2017). It is important to note that the rate of cephalosporin-resistant bacteria, conditional on the generation, is on the rise; therefore, discretion over choosing the correct cephalosporin should be exercised (Burchum and Rosenthal, 2019).

There are five generations within this group, each has its own action with regards to antimicrobial spectrum of activity as seen in Table 9.5. There has been progress in three elements of this group of antibiotics as each generation has been developed, these are: 'increasing activity against gram-negative bacteria and anaerobes; increasing resistance to destruction by beta-lactamases and increasing ability to penetrate the cerebrospinal fluid' (Burchum and Rosenthal, 2019, p. 1039).

From all the types of cephalosporins, choosing the drug of choice is dependent on the drug's pharmacokinetics and antimicrobial spectrum. The pharmacokinetics for the generational group of cephalosporins are similar and are presented in Table 9.6.

Indications (for all cephalosporins)

Pneumonia, septicemia, urinary tract infections, biliary tract infections, meningitis and peritonitis. Individual generation's indications are extended beyond the list above, based on duration of action, absorption and target pathogens (BMA, 2018; NICE, 2019).

Cefalexin

This is used against gram-positive and gram-negative bacteria, although is most active against gram-positive bacteria. It is predominantly used in mild to moderate infections; for example, respiratory tract infections, several forms of UTIs, ear infections (paediatrics) and certain skin and skin-structure infections (BMA, 2018; NICE, 2019).

Contraindications and cautions (for all cephalosporins)

A contraindication would be a known allergy to cephalosporins or immediate hypersensitivity to penicillin and other beta-lactams; therefore, they should be avoided in this group of people (Barber and Robertson, 2020). They can be cautiously used in people with mild sensitivity to

Table 9.5 Examples of cephalosporin per generation.

Generation	Cephalosporin	
1st	Cefalexin	Usually used in gram-positive infections and in cases of staphylococci or non-enterococcal streptococci. They have limited success against gram-negative bacteria and do not penetrate the cerebrospinal fluid (CSF).
2nd	Cefuroxime	They act on similar strains of pathogen as the first generation with an improved spectrum of activity against gram-negative bacteria. However, they are known to be less effective against some gram-positive bacteria. They do not penetrate the CSF.
3rd	Cefotaxime	They have a broader spectrum of activity and have a greater effect on certain gram-negative aerobes. They penetrate into the CSF.
4th	Cefepime	Indicated in the treatment of gram-positive and gram-negative bacteria. They penetrate the CSF.
5th	Ceftaroline fosamil	Similar in bactericidal action to third generation drugs; however, this is extended against other gram-positive pathogens which include MRSA and multidrug-resistant *Streptococcus pneumoniae*. Indicated in the treatment of community-acquired pneumonia, complicated skin and soft-tissue infections.

Source: Modified from Burchaum and Rosenthal (2019); NICE (2019).

Table 9.6 Pharmacokinetics of cephalosporins.

Absorption	Each generation has its own set of examples that are well absorbed in the GI tract. The remaining are well absorbed after alternative routes of administration are used; for example, IM injection or intravenously.
Distribution	Widely distributed in the body's tissues; the third-to-fifth-generation – cross the blood–brain barrier when the meninges are inflamed (cefotaxime). They are known to cross the placental barrier and enter into breast milk.
Metabolism	Primarily in the liver.
Excretion	Mainly kidney but some via bile (cefoperazone).

Source: Modified from Karch (2017); Wishart et al. (2018); Burchum and Rosenthal (2019); Barber and Robertson (2020).

penicillin and other beta-lactams (NICE, 2019). Caution in the use of cephalosporins should be exercised in people with hepatic or renal impairment due to the risk of toxicity (NICE, 2019).

In pregnancy and lactation, Karch (2017) highlights that due to limited evidence, the benefits should outweigh the risks of use due to unknown effects on the foetus and infants.

Cefalexin

As with other cephalosporins, caution should be used in those people with chronic renal impairment, previous allergic reactions to penicillin or other cephalosporins, and existing history of blood disorders and concomitant medications (BMA, 2018). NICE (2019) acknowledge the presence of cefalexin in breast milk, but deem it appropriate to use in pregnancy as there are no known harmful effects.

165

Adverse effects (for all cephalosporins)

Generally, this antibacterial group is well tolerated. GI disturbances are the most common adverse effects experienced with cephalosporins; these include, nausea, vomiting and diarrhoea which could develop into pseudomembranous colitis, anorexia, abdominal pain and flatulence (BMA, 2018; NICE, 2019; Barber and Robertson, 2020). A hypersensitivity reaction, inclusive for penicillin sensitive patients, is a possible adverse effect, whereas an uncommon effect is an anaphylactic reaction. Hematologically, blood disorders can occur; for example, ceftriaxone can cause bleeding tendencies by interfering with the metabolism of vitamin K (Burchum and Rosenthal, 2019). Neurologically, dizziness, headache and lethargy are noted effects (NICE, 2019). From a vascular perspective, thrombophlebitis can occur at the IV injection site or pain at the site of an intramuscular injection (Burchum and Rosenthal, 2019). Nephrological toxicity can happen, especially in clients with pre-existing renal impairment for example, the older adult. Rarely, there is also an increased risk of infection and/or superinfections due to normal flora death (Burchum and Rosenthal, 2019).

Cefalexin

It is noted that diarrhoea, hypersensitivity or an allergic reaction are the known adverse effects. Some CNS effects (for example, agitation, hallucinations and confusion) are noted, but their frequency remains unknown. Alongside these, also noted are fatigue, GI discomfort and vaginal discharge (NICE, 2019).

Drug–Drug interactions (for all cephalosporins)

There is an increased risk of nephrotoxicity when cephalosporins and aminoglycosides are administered concurrently (NICE, 2019). Additionally, certain cephalosporins (ceftriaxone) can increase the risk of bleeding if taken concurrently with similar acting drugs, such as anticoagulants, thrombolytics, non-steroidal anti-inflammatory drugs and aspirin (and other antiplatelet drugs) (Burchuim and Rosenthal, 2019).

Probenecid may delay, in some cephalosporins, excretion (via kidneys), which in turn lengthens their effect. A disulfiram-like reaction, although rare, may occur between alcohol and certain cephalosporins (cefazolin and cefotetan), even after the treatment has been completed.

Cefalexin

The risk of nephrotoxicity is increased in numerous concomitant medication administration; for example, colistimethate (antibiotic) – especially if administered intravenously (NICE, 2019).

Nursing actions for cephalosporins

- Promote principles of good patient assessment, prescribing practice and antimicrobial stewardship through patient education (see Clinical Considerations 1).

- Advise the person to take cephalosporins with food if gastric discomfort occurs.
- Offer advice to the person about the signs and symptoms of an allergic reaction: urticaria, rash, itching, hypotension, dyspnea and hives.
- Educate the person about concomitant medications.
- Monitor parenteral administration sites for signs of phlebitis in intravenous administration and pain in IM injections. Inform the person of potentially painful intramuscular injection.
- Educate the person to observe for signs of induration, tenderness and redness after IM injection.
- Advise the person to refrain from alcohol up to 72 hours after treatment completion to prevent a disulfiram-like reaction (flushing, sweating, palpitations dyspnea, syncope, vertigo, blurred vision, hypotension, throbbing headache, chest pain, nausea and vomiting – potentially leading to convulsions, cardiovascular collapse and death).
- Monitor renal function (blood urea and nitrogen and creatinine levels) when clients are taking concomitant aminoglycosides and cephalosporins.
- Offer advice and observe the person regarding symptoms of potential blood loss (bleeding gums, easy bruising) – especially if taking anticoagulant drugs (or similar) concurrently with cephalosporins. If prescribed ceftriaxone, instigate measures to reduce haemorrhage risk. Monitor clotting factors (prothrombin time and/or bleeding time); if required, administer parenteral vitamin K, provide information and monitor for signs and symptoms of bleeding.
- If diarrhoea is experienced, advise the person about maintaining hydration so that lost fluids are replaced. Inform the person about the treatment schedule and adverse effects and monitor them for signs of superinfection.
- If CNS effects occur, implement safety measures inclusive of adequate lighting, side rails on bed, ambulatory assistance, avoid driving and hazardous tasks and changing positions slowly.
- Follow local guidelines and best evidence regarding calcium and ceftriaxone, particularly in neonates, with regards to reconstitution and intravenous administration.

Source: Karch, 2017; BMA, 2018; Burchum and Rosenthal, 2019; NICE, 2019; Barber and Robertson, 2020.

Carbapenams

Examples within this group, whose action is similar to other beta-lactams, are imipenem, meropenem and ertapenem. They have the widest spectrum of activity among the beta-lactams group (Xiu and Datta, 2019). This group is non-MRSA active (NICE, 2019). Burchum and Rosenthal (2019) assert that carbapenams should be used sparingly, which will delay resistance to them. They are bactericidal in action (Karch, 2017).

Imipenem

Normally, this is combined with cilastatin as certain renal enzymes destroy imipenem (NICE, 2019).

Indications

This is a broad-spectrum antibiotic effective against many anaerobic and aerobic gram-negative and gram-positive bacteria, including *Pseudomonas aeruginosa*, severe hospital-acquired septicaemia, intra-abdominal infections, severe infections of lower respiratory tract (pneumonia), urinary tract (complicated), skin, bones, gynaecological and joints, but it is not indicated for CNS infections. Table 9.7 presents the pharmacokinetics of imipenem.

Table 9.7 Pharmacokinetics of imipenem.

Absorption	Is not absorbed by the GI tract; therefore, parenteral administration only.
Distribution	Distributes well to body fluids and tissues and is able to pass into the CSF. It is known to pass into the breast milk but it is unclear if it passes the placental barrier.
Metabolism	Renal.
Excretion	Urine.

Source: Wishart et al. (2018), Burchum and Rosenthal (2019).

Contraindications and cautions

It is contraindicated in people with an immediate hypersensitivity reaction to other beta-lactam antibiotics (NICE, 2019). Further caution is advised in people with CNS disorders or epilepsy and in patients with renal impairment; imipenem should be avoided if the creatine clearance is less than 15 mL/minutes, and should be used with caution in people with known sensitivity to the beta-lactam group of antibacterials (NICE, 2019).

Use of imipenem in pregnancy should be avoided unless the potential benefits outweigh the risks of use (NICE, 2019). When breast-feeding, it is known to enter the breast milk but absorption is said to be unlikely, according to the NICE (2019); however, Karch (2017) states that potentially it could cause serious effects in infants.

Adverse effects (for all carbapenams)

These tend to be like other beta-lactams antibiotics. Common GI tract effects include nausea, vomiting and diarrhoea (Burchum and Rosenthal, 2019). Thrombophlebitis is a potential side effect (NICE, 2019). Rarely, there is a potential for pseudomembranous colitis (Karch, 2017). Further rare effects include the development of superinfections, seizures, hypersensitivity reactions (for example, rashes, pruritus, drug fever), psychiatric disorders and blood disorders (NICE, 2019). Cross sensitivity may occur in patients allergic to penicillins and other beta-lactams (Burchum and Rosenthal, 2019).

Drug–Drug interactions

Imipenam is believed to interact with anti-viral medications. It increases the risk of seizures when given with ganciclovir or valganciclovir. Alongside this, it is said to decrease the concentration of valproate, an anticonvulsant, therefore the risk of breakthrough seizures increases (NICE, 2019; Burchum and Rosenthal, 2019).

Nursing actions

- Promote principles of good patient assessment, prescribing practice and antimicrobial stewardship through patient education (see Clinical Considerations 1).
- Assess for possible cautions or contraindications: known history of renal impairment or allergy to carbapenem and/or other beta-lactam antibiotic, seizure disorder, pregnancy or lactational state and inflammatory bowel disorders.
- If administration of imipenem is required alongside valproate; consider additional anticonvulsant therapy to prevent the occurrence of breakthrough seizures.
- Regular renal function testing is advised, due to the metabolism and excretion route.
- See local guidelines or manufacturer's instructions for specialist instructions regarding dilution, rate of administration and concentration.
- Instruct the person to monitor for signs of side effects and to report if any altered bowel patterns or superinfection symptoms are present.
- Provide instruction about reporting any difficulties associated with hypersensitivity and/or altered bowel patterns.

Source: Karch, 2017; Burchum and Rosenthal, 2019; NICE, 2019; Barber and Robertson, 2020.

Protein synthesis interference

This is a group of antibiotics whereby their action is to interfere with the protein synthesis in the cell. They include: tetracyclines, chloramphenicol, aminoglycosides, macrolides and lincosamides (Xiu and Datta, 2019). An example of each group now follows.

Tetracyclines

Examples in this group of broad-spectrum antibiotics include tetracycline, doxycycline, minocycline and demeclocycline. They have bacteriostatic properties and are effective against gram-positive and gram-negative bacteria (Xiu and Datta, 2019). The effectiveness of

Table 9.8   Pharmacokinetics of tetracycline.

Absorption	Absorption occurs in the GI tract, predominantly administered orally. This is affected by the presence of food or milk, calcium, iron, aluminium, magnesium-containing drugs and other drugs in the stomach.
Distribution	Distributed to most body fluid (poor penetration to the cerebrospinal fluid) and tissue. Is known to cross the placental barrier and enter into breast milk.
Metabolism	Concentrates in the liver.
Excretion	Urine.

Source: Modified from Agwuh and MacGowan (2006); Coppoc (1996b); Burchum and Robertson (2019).

tetracyclines have decreased for several pathogenic microorganisms, due to the growth of resistant microorganisms and overuse (Barber and Robertson, 2020). Table 9.8 details the pharmacokinetics of tetracycline.

Indications (for all tetracyclines)

These are used for chlamydia causing infections, ricksettia, acne, brucella, destructive dental diseases, respiratory and genital mycoplasmal infections, chronic bronchitis and MRSA infection (BMA, 2018; NICE, 2019).

Tetracycline

Tetracycline is often used in skin conditions such as acne vulgaris (NICE, 2019). Additionally, it is effective against chlamydia, rickettsia, mycoplasma (pneumonia), Lyme, disease, rosacea, acne, diabetic diarrhoea in autonomic neuropathy, non-gonococcal urethritis and some genital infections (Burchum and Rosenthal, 2019; NICE, 2019).

Contraindications and cautions (for all tetracyclines)

The contraindications for the use of tetracyclines include those with allergies, pregnant women or lactating mothers, people with significant renal impairment and it is not recommended for administration to children under twelve years (BMA, 2018; Burchum and Rosenthal, 2019; NICE, 2019).

Caution for its use in people with hepatic impairment (various tetracyclines are excreted either renally or hepatically) (NICE, 2019). NICE (2019) extends caution, in the case of all tetracyclines, in people with myasthenia gravis (may increase muscle weakness) and systemic lupus erythematosus (may cause exacerbation).

Tetracycline

Similar to other tetracyclines, the above mentioned cautions and contraindications apply. Moreover, the manufacturer advises to avoid high dose therapy in those with hepatic impairment (NICE, 2019).

Adverse effects (for all tetracyclines)

Gastrointestinal adverse effects include direct irritation to the gastro-intestinal tract causing epigastric burning, nausea, vomiting and diarrhoea (Burchum and Rosenthal, 2019). Oesophageal irritation or ulceration may occur (BMA, 2018). Additional GI symptoms can include abdominal pain, glossitis and dysphagia. Superinfections are also a possibility due to the destruction of the normal gut flora- this could be life threatening (Karch, 2017; Burchum and Rosenthal, 2019). Dermatological effects can be photosensitivity (increases skin sensitivity to ultra violet light), rash formation as well as hypersensitivity reactions (urticaria to anaphylaxis) (Burchum and Rosenthal, 2019). Tetracyclines can cause teeth discolouration in the younger child and for an unborn child, if taken when pregnant, it is the milk (deciduous) teeth which discolour (BMA, 2018; Barber and Robertson, 2020). Less common effects can include haematolytic anaemia, or decreased appetite. Benign intracranial hypertension can happen, evident in headaches and visual disturbances (NICE, 2019; Burchum and Rosenthal, 2019).

Tetracyclines in high doses intravenously has been reported as being hepatotoxic, due to an irritating effect on the liver, especially in pregnant and postpartum women who have pre-existing renal disease (Burchum and Rosenthal, 2019).

Tetracycline

Rarer side effects for tetracycline are agranulocytosis, aplastic anaemia, renal impairment or nephritis (NICE, 2019).

Drug–Drug interactions

Tetracyclines are known to interact with a wide range of medications such as digoxin (monitor levels), iron (decreases tetracycline effectiveness), anti-coagulants (increases their action- monitor INR), retinoids (Vitamin A drugs) (increases risk of benign intracranial hypertension) and finally antacids and milk (interferes with absorption of tetracycline and may reduce effectiveness) (BMA, 2018; NICE, 2019). Hepatotoxicity is a further risk when tetracycline is taken with, for example, atorvastatin or valproate or paracetamol. The ability of tetracyclines to reduce the effectiveness of oral contraceptives is an area of dispute (Karch, 2017; NICE, 2019).

Nursing actions

- Promote principles of good patient assessment, prescribing practice and antimicrobial stewardship through patient education (see Clinical Considerations 1).
- Take on an empty stomach one hour before or two hours after medication or meals.
- Do not take with dairy products, iron preparations, calcium supplements, magnesium-containing laxatives or antacids. If required, leave a minimum of two hours between ingestion of tetracycline and these aforementioned medications.
- Stand/sit upright and drink a full glass of water with each dose – this can prevent oesophageal irritation/ulceration. Do not lie down immediately after taking medication.
- Inform the person that the solution to GI disturbances is taking tetracyclines with meals, but this also affects the absorption rate.
- Do not take before going to bed.
- Advise the client to report any hypersensitivity reaction.
- Encourage the client to report any diarrhoea, due to superinfection risk.
- Inform the client to report any adverse effects, such as other infections (for example, fungal), changes in faeces/urine colour or amount of urine passed, severe cramps, difficulty in breathing, and light sensitive rash/itching, jaundice and headache or visual disturbances.
- Avoid prolonged exposure to sunlight, wear protective clothing and use sunscreen (use SPF 30 and above) on exposed skin and avoid using sunbeds.

Source: Karch, 2017; BMA, 2018; Burchum and Rosenthal, 2019; NICE, 2019; Barber and Robertson, 2020.

Chloramphenicol

This is a broad-spectrum antibiotic, effective against gram-positive and gram-negative bacteria; however, it should be reserved for life-threatening infections when being used systemically (NICE, 2019). It has both bacteriostatic and bactericidal effects (Xiu and Datta, 2019). See Table 9.9 for the pharmacokinetics of chloramphenicol.

Indications

It is used in superficial eye infections (acute bacterial conjunctivitis), bacterial otitis externa and life-threatening infections – particularly *Haemophilus influenzae* and Typhoid fever, as well as meningitis. Topical administration is available for ear and eye infections (BMA, 2018; NICE, 2019).

Table 9.9 Pharmacokinetics of chloramphenicol.

Absorption	Rate of absorption varies according to route. It can be administered via oral, intravenous and topical routes.
Distribution	Distributes well through the body including the CSF. It is known to cross the placental barrier and pass into the breast milk.
Metabolism	Liver.
Excretion	Urine.

Source: Modified from Coppoc (1996a).

Skills in practice

Medication: eye administration

Essential equipment

• Personal protective equipment	• Electronic identity check equipment, where relevant
• Non-sterile powder-free gloves	• Low-linting swabs
• Eye preparation to be administered	• Sterile 0.9% sodium chloride or warm water
• Recording sheet or book as required by law or hospital policy	• Eye drops at room temperature or eye ointment
• Patient's prescription chart, to check dose, route, etc.	

Optional equipment

• Eye swab

Pre-procedure

Action	Rationale
1 Introduce yourself to the patient, explain and discuss the procedure with the patient.	To ensure that the patient understands the procedure and gives their valid consent (NMC, 2018).
2 Ask the patient to explain how their eyes feel, if they are able to.	To gain a baseline understanding of current problems or changes the patient is experiencing.
3 Before administering any prescribed drug, look at the patient's prescription chart and check the following.	To ensure that the correct patient is given the correct drug in the prescribed dose using the appropriate diluent and by the correct route (DH, 2003b; RSP, 2019). To protect the patient from harm (DH, 2003b).
(a) The correct patient is being given the drug	
(b) Drug	
(c) Dose	
(d) Date and time of administration	
(e) Route and method of administration	
(f) Diluent as appropriate	
(g) Validity of prescription	
(h) Signature of prescriber	
(i) The prescription is legible	
If any of these pieces of information are missing, unclear or illegible do not proceed with administration and should consult with the prescriber.	To prevent any errors occurring.

4 Wash hands and apply well-fitting gloves.	To reduce the risk of cross-infection (DH, 2007; Fraise and Bradley, 2009).

Procedure

5 Take the medication and the prescription chart to the patient. Check the patient's identity by asking them to state their full name and date of birth. If the patient is unable to confirm these details, then check the patient identity band against the prescription chart. If an electronic identity check system for the patient and/or medicine identification is in place, then use it in accordance with hospital policy and procedures. Check the patient's allergy status by asking them or by checking the name band.	To ensure that the medication is administered to the correct patient and prevent any errors related to drug allergies (NPSA, 2005).
6 Ask the patient to sit back with their neck slightly hyperextended or lie down.	To ensure a position that allows easy access for medication instillation and to avoid excess running down the patient's cheek (Stollery et al., 2005). Correct positioning minimises drainage of eye medication into the tear duct (Potter and Perry, 2016).
7 If there is any discharge, proceed as for eye swabbing (see Chapter 13 Diagnostic tests). If any crusting or drainage is present around the eye, gently wash away with warm water or 0.9% sodium chloride and a swab. Always wipe clean from inner to outer canthus.	To prevent the introduction of micro-organisms into the lacrimal ducts (Potter and Perry, 2016).
8 Ask the patient to look at the ceiling and carefully pull the skin below the affected eye using a wet swab to expose the conjunctival sac.	To move the sensitive cornea up and away from the conjunctival sac and reduce stimulation of blink reflex (Potter and Perry, 2016).
9 If administering both drops and ointment, administer drops first.	Ointment will leave a film in the eye which may hamper the absorption of medication in drop form (Jevon et al., 2010).
10 *Either:*	
Administer the prescribed number of drops, holding the eye dropper 1–2 cm above the eye. If the patient blinks or closes their eye, repeat the procedure.	To provide even distribution of medication across the eye. Therapeutic effect of drug is obtained only when drops enter conjunctival sac (Potter and Perry, 2016).
Or:	
Apply a thin stream of ointment evenly along the inner edge of lower eyelid on conjunctiva from the nasal corner outwards. If there is excess medication on the eyelid, gently wipe it from inner to outer canthus.	To provide even distribution of medication across the eye and lid margin and reduce the risk of cross-infection, contamination of the tube and trauma to the eye (Fraise and Bradley, 2009; Perry, 2015; Stollery et al., 2005). To avoid excess ointment irritating the surrounding skin (Stollery et al., 2005).
11 Ask the patient to close their eyes and keep them closed for 1–2 minutes.	To help distribute medication (Aldridge, 2010; Potter and Perry, 2016).
12 Explain to the patient that they may have blurred vision for a few minutes after application. Explain that they should refrain from driving or operating machinery until their vision returns to normal.	To ensure the patient understands why they have blurred vision (Aldridge, 2010).

Post-procedure

13 Clean any equipment used and discard all disposable equipment in appropriate containers.	To minimise the risk of infection (DH, 2007; Fraise and Bradley, 2009).
14 Record the administration on appropriate charts.	To maintain accurate records, provide a point of reference in the event of any queries and prevent any duplication of treatment (RSP, 2019).

Source: Barrott et al. (2020). Medicine optimization, procedure guideline 15.8, p 864–865.

Contraindications and cautions

The oral and intravenous administration of chloramphenicol is contraindicated in people with acute porphyria (NICE, 2019). Additionally, avoid prolonged use of chloramphenicol when administering via the otic route and avoid repeated or prolonged courses of treatment when being administered intravenously or orally as this could increase the risk of blood disorders (BMA, 2018). In people with severe renal impairment, intravenous and oral administration of chloramphenicol is best to be avoided; whereas in people with hepatic impairment, the manufacturer's advice is to be cautious with intravenous or oral administration due to the raised bone-marrow depression risk.

In pregnancy, the manufacturers advise to avoid administering intravenously or orally as neonatal grey baby syndrome may occur, especially if used in the third trimester. Similarly, in breast-feeding, avoid use as it may cause bone-marrow toxicity in the infant. Only administer optically if necessary to pregnant or lactating women, as it carries a theoretical risk of bone-marrow toxicity (NICE, 2019).

Adverse effects: dependent on route of administration

A common side effect of all routes of administration is bone-marrow disorders (NICE, 2019). Sore throat, fever and unusual tiredness could indicate signs of blood abnormalities, in any route of administration. When administered systemically (orally or parenterally), due to the severity of potential hematological side effects, chloramphenicol is only used in life-threatening conditions (BMA, 2018).

Most other adverse effects are rare, and these include irritation in the eye and ear from topical administration, circulatory collapse, death, diarrhoea, ototoxicity; nausea and vomiting occur when administered orally. Furthermore, in parenteral use, side effects include depression, headache and fungal superinfection, to name a few (BMA, 2018; NICE, 2019).

Grey baby syndrome in neonates and premature babies, if administered in the third trimester, can occur. This presents with abdominal distension, diarrhoea, vasomotor collapse, hypothermia, flaccidity, pallid cyanosis, abnormal respiratory rate and being ashen in colour (BMA, 2018; Barber and Robertson, 2020; NICE, 2019; Xiu and Datta, 2019).

Drug–Drug interactions

Chloramphenicol is known to increase the effectiveness of certain drug groups, such as oral anti-coagulants, anti-diabetics and phenytoin whereas phenobarbital or rifampicin may reduce the effect of chloramphenicol. It increases the concentration of one immunosuppressant (tacrolimus) and is known to reduce the effectiveness of iron replacement medications (BMA, 2018; NICE, 2019).

Nursing actions

- Promote principles of good patient assessment, prescribing practice and antimicrobial stewardship through patient education (see clinical considerations box 1).
- Monitor plasma concentration, in intravenous and oral administration, in the following groups: the elderly, people with hepatic or renal impairment and children under four years of age.
- Monitor blood cell counts, prior to and periodically throughout the course of treatment, due to the potential for blood abnormalities.
- Consult local guidelines for diluent and administration routes.
- Try to give ear drops at the same time every day, if possible.
- Write the date on the chloramphenicol container when opened and do not keep opened chloramphenicol ear drops for longer than four weeks.
- Do not put cotton wool or ear buds into a child's ear during the treatment.
- Eye drops should be stored in the fridge and should be taken out two hours before use; this prevents stinging.
- Best to stop wearing contact lenses during treatment to avoid irritation.
- Avoid cross infection between eyes through good hand hygiene – provide information.
- Potentially transient eye irritation occurs, so provide instruction about avoiding driving and hazardous work until the effect of chloramphenicol is established. Periodic eye tests may be advisable.

- In concomitant administration of:
  - antidiabetic medication – monitor capillary blood glucose;
  - anticoagulants – check INR;
  - phenytoin – monitor seizure pattern.

Source: Karch, 2017; BMA, 2018; Burchum and Rosenthal, 2019; NICE, 2019; Barber and Robertson, 2020.

Skills in practice

Medication: topical applications

Essential equipment

• Personal protective equipment	• Electronic identity check equipment, where relevant
• Medicine(s) to be administered	• Glass of water
• Recording sheet or book as required by law or hospital policy	• Medicine container (disposable if possible)
• Patient's prescription chart, to check dose, route, etc.	

Pre-procedure

Action	Rationale
1 Introduce yourself to the patient, explain and discuss the procedure with them, and gain their consent to proceed.	To ensure that the patient feels at ease, understands the procedure and gives their valid consent (NMC, 2018).
2 Wash hands with bactericidal soap and water or alcohol-based handrub.	To minimise the risk of cross-infection (DH, 2007; Fraise and Bradley, 2009).
3 Before administering any prescribed drug, check that it is due and has not already been given. Carry out any required assessments, such as pulse, blood pressure and respiration. Check that the information contained in the prescription chart is complete, correct and legible.	To protect the patient from harm (DH, 2003b; NMC, 2018). Assessments are required to ensure the patient is fit enough to receive medication, for example blood pressure check before antihypertensives (Chernecky et al., 2005).
4 Before administering any prescribed drug, look at the patient's prescription chart and check the following.	To ensure that the correct patient is given the correct drug in the prescribed dose using the appropriate diluent and by the correct route (DH, 2003b; RSP, 2019). To protect the patient from harm (DH, 2003b; NMC, 2018).

(a)   The correct patient is being given the drug

(b)   Drug

(c)   Dose

(d)   Date and time of administration

(e)   Route and method of administration

(f)   Diluent as appropriate

(g)   Validity of prescription

(h)   Signature of prescriber

(i)   The prescription is legible

If any of these pieces of information are missing, unclear or illegible, do not proceed with administration and should consult with the prescriber.	To prevent any errors occurring.

Procedure

5 Select the required medication and check the expiry date.	Treatment with medication that is outside the expiry date is dangerous. Drugs deteriorate with storage. The expiry date indicates when a particular drug is no longer pharmacologically efficacious (DH, 2003b; RPS, 2019).
6 Empty the required dose into a medicine container. Avoid touching the preparation.	To minimize the risk of cross-infection. To minimize the risk of harm to the nurse (DH, 2007; Fraise and Bradley, 2009).
7 Take the medication and the prescription chart to the patient. Check the patient's identity by asking them to state their full name and date of birth. If the patient is unable to confirm these details, then check the patient identity band against the prescription chart. If an electronic identity check system for the patient and/or medicine identification is in place, then use it in accordance with hospital policy and procedures. Check the patient's allergy status by asking them or by checking the name band.	To ensure that the medication is administered to the correct patient and prevent any errors related to drug allergies (NPSA, 2005).
8 Evaluate the patient's knowledge of the medication being offered by asking them to tell you what the medication is for and what side-effects to expect. If this knowledge appears to be faulty or incorrect, offer an explanation of the use, action, dose and potential side-effects of the drug or drugs involved.	Patients have a right to information about treatment (NMC, 2018). To ensure that the patient understands the procedure and gives their valid consent (Griffith and Jordan, 2003; NMC, 2018).
9 Assist the patient into a sitting position where possible. A side-lying position may also be used if the patient is unable to sit.	To ease swallowing and prevent aspiration (Chernecky et al., 2005).
10 Administer the drug as prescribed.	To meet legal requirements and adhere to hospital policy (DH, 2003b; NMC, 2018; RPS, 2019).
11 Offer a glass of water, if allowed, assisting the patient where necessary.	To facilitate swallowing of the medication (Chernecky et al., 2005; Jordan et al., 2003).
12 Stay with the patient until they have swallowed all the medication.	To ensure that the medication is taken on time (Chernecky et al., 2005).
Post-procedure	
13 Record the dose given and sign the prescription chart. Also sign in any other place made necessary by legal requirement or hospital policy.	To meet legal requirements and adhere to hospital policy (DH, 2003b; NMC, 2018; RPS, 2019).

Source: Barrott et al. (2020). Medicine optimization, procedure guideline 15.2, p 849–850.

Aminoglycosides

Examples of this antibacterial group, which inhibit protein synthesis, are gentamicin, strepto-mycin, neomycin, tobramycin and amikacin (Xiu and Datta, 2019). They have a broad spectrum of activity and are active against several gram-negative bacteria; for example, aerobic bacilli and certain gram-positive bacteria (NICE, 2019). Bacterial resistance is ever increasing, similar

Table 9.10   Pharmacokinetics of aminoglycosides.

Absorption	Not absorbed in the GI tract. Gentamicin is most commonly administered in parenteral (injectable) preparations but are available as eye and ear preparations. Other aminoglycosides are available in topical preparations.
Distribution	According to Burchum and Rosenthal (2019), distribution tends to be limited to the extracellular fluid and does not cross into the CSF (so not effective in adults with meningitis); however, NICE (2019) lists gentamicin as a possible treatment for meningitis in adults. It has the potential to be fetotoxic (hearing defects with injectable administration) as it crosses the placental barrier. Also enters the breast milk when parenteral routes are used.
Metabolism	Not metabolised.
Excretion	Urine.

Source: Adapted Burchaum and Rosenthal (2019); Karch (2017).

to other antibiotic groups. They are used for severe infection and have a bactericidal effect in the presence of oxygen (Barber and Robertson, 2020).

Burchum and Rosenthal (2019) explain that the pharmacokinetics are similar for all aminoglycosides, see Table 9.10 for the pharmacokinetics of aminoglycosides.

Indications (for all aminoglycosides)

They are indicated in the treatment of severe infections (NICE, 2019).

Gentamicin

It is used for lung, urinary tract, bone, bacterial eye infections, otitis externa infections, joint and wound infections, meningitis, septicemia and peritonitis. As well as for pneumonia in hospitalised patients and for gram-positive bacterial endocarditis in combination with other antibiotics. It is utilised as a surgical prophylaxis (NICE, 2019).

Contraindications and cautions (for all aminoglycosides)

Use of this antibacterial group is contraindicated in the following client groups: those who have experienced previous allergic reaction to aminoglycosides and myasthenia gravis (injectable forms) (NICE, 2019).

Cautious use should be exercised with older people (increased likelihood of adverse effects), those with a pre-existing renal impairment, those with a hearing disorder, Parkinson's disease or other conditions characterised with muscular weakness, those on concomitant ototoxic, nephrotoxic, or neuromuscular blockade agents and dosing (aminoglycosides main adverse effects are dose related) (BMA, 2018; NICE, 2019).

Caution in pregnancy as the usage of injectable aminoglycosides benefits should outweigh the risk to the foetus. There is a possible risk of auditory or vestibular damage if used in the second and third trimesters (NICE, 2019).

Gentamicin

Otic applications of gentamicin is contraindicated in people with perforated ear drums or have patent grommets, unless being used under specialist guidance. Furthermore, prolonged use in ear infections should be avoided. Additionally, advise caution in clients administering concomitantly potentially ototoxic and nephrotoxic (cephalosporins, vancomycin or NSAIDs) drugs and neuromuscular blocking agents (NICE, 2019).

Burchum and Rosenthal (2019) assert in breast-feeding women, gentamicin is potentially safe to use; although there is limited evidence to support this.

Adverse effects (for all aminoglycosides)

This group is known to have severe adverse effects on the ears and kidneys (NICE, 2019). Ototoxicity presents as deafness or balance disruptions (vestibular damage) coming predominantly from injectable routes (Barber and Robertson, 2020). Ototoxicity, mostly irreversible, occurs because of prolonged exposure to excessive trough (that is, lowest level of drug between doses) levels and the risk of toxicity increases due to renal impairment and prolonged excessive dose use (longer than 10 days) (Burchum and Rosenthal, 2019). According to NICE (2019), tinnitus is a common side effect.

Nephrotoxicity presents itself as acute tubular necrosis, a reversible effect of taking aminoglycosides. Nephrotoxicity risk is more common in people with existing renal impairment, older people and those receiving other nephrotoxic drugs (Burchum and Rosenthal, 2019).

Further possible adverse effects are fatal respiratory depression and flaccid paralysis as aminoglycosides can hinder neuromuscular transmission (Burchum and Rosenthal, 2019). As with all antibacterial therapy, hypersensitivity signs such as purpura, rash, itching and urticaria can happen.

Gentamicin

As with all aminoglycosides, it is ototoxic and nephrotoxic. NICE (2019) extend these to include antibiotic-associated colitis, blood disorders, depression, encephalopathy, hallucinations, hepatic reaction, neurotoxicity, peripheral neuropathy, seizure and vestibular damage in parenteral use.

Drug–Drug interactions (for aminoglycosides)

Not all drug interactions are bad; aminoglycosides together with penicillins can be used to increase treatment efficiency. However, they should not be mixed together in the same intravenous solution, as this leads to inactivation of aminoglycosides by the penicillins (Burchum and Rosenthal, 2019).

Ototoxicity and nephrotoxicity generally occur alongside concurrent administration of medications which have ototoxic and nephrotoxic properties respectively (Burchum and Rosenthal, 2019).

Concurrent administration of aminoglycosides with skeletal muscular relaxants, for example pancuronium, increases the risk of respiratory arrest as aminoglycosides potentially intensify the induced neurotransmission blockade (NICE, 2019; Burchum and Rosenthal, 2019).

Gentamicin

Many drugs listed by NICE (2019) illustrate the increased risk of ototoxicity (for example, torsemide), nephrotoxicity (for example, ibuprofen), neuromuscular blocking effects (for example, suxamethonium) and hypocalcemia (for example, alendronate).

Nursing actions

- Promote principles of good patient assessment, prescribing practice and antimicrobial stewardship through patient education (see Clinical Considerations 1).
- Limit parenteral use of aminoglycosides to seven days.
- Dosing should be individualised due to variations in serum levels of aminoglycosides at similar dosage. Individual factors affecting this variation include weight, renal function, age, percentage of body fat, fever, oedema and dehydration.
- Assessment of renal function should occur prior to and during treatment with aminoglycosides. Blood aminoglycosides plasma levels (peaks and troughs) monitoring is dependent on the prescription (dosing) and should be kept within a therapeutic range. Refer to local guidelines for dosing regimens.
- Correct dehydration before commencement of aminoglycosides.
- With intramuscular or intravenous gentamicin administration, doses for obese patients should be calculated using ideal weight for height as this avoids excessive dosage.

- Serum concentration monitoring in parenteral administration of aminoglycosides *must* be determined in older people, obese people, people with cystic fibrosis, those with renal impairment (lengthen dose interval and/or reduce dose) and if high doses are being given. It *should* be monitored in all persons receiving parenteral aminoglycosides. This extends to use in pregnancy: serum levels should be monitored.
- Encourage the person to report signs and symptoms of ototoxicity (tinnitus, persistent headache, high-frequency hearing loss, nausea, unsteadiness, dizziness, vertigo). Discontinue treatment at first two symptoms to prevent further hearing loss.
- Monitor for signs of nephrotoxicity (proteinuria, urinary casts, dilute urine production, increased serum creatinine and blood urea nitrogen). If oliguria or anuria develops, discontinue treatment and report to medical team.
- Monitor renal function, blood urea nitrogen and serum creatine to assess renal injury.
- Monitor intake and output and promote fluid intake unless there is a reason for restrictions.
- Check local guidelines for doses, dilution, route of administration and scheduling of administration.
- Encourage the person to report difficulty in breathing, rashes and itching, severe headache, hearing loss or ringing in ear and changes in urine output.
- Observe people with myasthenia gravis, those receiving skeletal relaxants or general anaesthetics alongside the administration of aminoglycosides due to the risk of respiratory depression, because of neuromuscular blockade. This reversible condition is treated with intravenous calcium gluconate.

Source: Karch, 2017; BMA, 2018; Burchum and Rosenthal, 2019; NICE, 2019; Barber and Robertson, 2020.

Macrolides

This broad-spectrum antibacterial group inhibits bacterial protein synthesis. They have a similar antibacterial spectrum to penicillin (Barber and Robertson, 2020). Examples of this group are erythromycin, azithromycin and clarithromycin. Erythromycin has a bacteriostatic action but can assume bactericidal properties. Table 9.11 describes the pharmacokinetics of erythromycin.

Indications

Macrolides are used in the treatment of respiratory tract infections (pneumonia), gastrointestinal tract (campylobacter enteritis), skin (acne vulgaris) and sexually transmitted infections (Chlamydia) (NICE, 2019). Alongside these, it is the treatment of choice for Legionnaire's Disease and mycoplasmal infection (BMA, 2018). Topical use for acne vulgaris is known alongside prophylactic use in minor skin abrasions. They can be used prophylactically for endocarditis risk, in, for example, dental procedures in high risk valvular heart disease patients who are allergic to penicillin (NICE, 2019).

Table 9.11   Pharmacokinetics of erythromycin.

Absorption	Absorption in GI tract varies due to gastric acid destroying erythromycin in the stomach but is absorbed by the small intestine if placed in an acid-resistant coating. It has three oral variants. It can be administered IV but not IM as this is deemed too painful.
Distribution	Distributes well to the most tissues and bodily fluids and penetration of the CSF is poor. It crosses the placental barrier and is known to enter the breast milk.
Metabolism	Liver.
Excretion	Bile (faeces) and urine (small amounts).

Source: Wishart et al. (2018), Burchum and Rosenthal (2019).

Erythromycin

It is active against the majority of gram-positive bacteria and some gram-negative bacteria and is used as an alternative for people who are allergic to penicillin and related groups (Burchum and Rosenthal, 2019; NICE, 2019). It is used to treat throat infections, whooping cough, middle ear, skin, urinary tract, chest and sexually transmitted infections as well as gastroenteritis (BMA, 2018).

Contraindications and cautions (for all macrolides)

Contraindications would be in those who have a known allergy, as cross-sensitivity is known to occur. Cautious use would be in those who have hepatic impairment as it can alter the metabolism of the drug and renal impairment as it can interfere with the drug excretion (NICE, 2019).

With IV and oral administration of macrolides, there is a risk of electrolyte disturbances, predisposition to QT prolongation and they may exacerbate myasthenia gravis symptoms (NICE, 2019).

Erythromycin

Cautions and contraindications for erythromycin include chronic hepatic impairment, renal impairment, previous allergic reaction to erythromycin and acute porphyria. With systemic use in neonates (less than two weeks of age), there is a risk of developing hypertrophic pyloric stenosis (NICE, 2019). The Joint Formulary (2020b) states in pregnancy, if used, there is no evidenced risk to the foetus and although in breast-feeding erythromycin passes into the breast milk, there should be no adverse effect for the infant (BMA, 2018).

Adverse effects (for all macrolides)

The most common effects are those affecting the GI tract, these being epigastric pain, anorexia, nausea, vomiting and diarrhoea, and rarely, pseudomembranous colitis (NICE 2019; Barber and Robertson 2020). The severity of these can limit the use of this group. Further uncommon effects potentially affect the CNS, for example, drowsiness or emotional lability (anxiety), and a range of hypersensitivity reactions as well as superinfection due to the loss of normal intestinal flora – this is considered to be a rare side effect (NICE, 2019).

Erythromycin

This is considered one of the safest antibiotics available.

In oral administration, this can cause nausea, vomiting and abdominal cramps. Other effects include transient hearing loss (after high dose therapy), rash to anaphylaxis, liver disorders (jaundice) and fever (BMA, 2018). Hypersensitivity and superinfections may occur. There is a small risk of sudden cardiac death due to QT prolongation (Burchum and Rosenthal, 2019). Thrombophlebitis can occur by IV administration of erythromycin due to inflammation of the vein (Barber and Robertson, 2020).

Drug–Drug interactions

Aminophyllin and theophylline (causes hypokalaemia), carbamazepine, digoxin and other some immunosuppressants (plasma levels can increase if taken with macrolides – potentially leading to toxicity) and warfarin (increased risk of bleeding) (BMA 2018; NICE 2019). There is a risk of increased adverse effects with ergotamine (antimigraine) and erythromycin (BMA, 2018). Mizolastine (non-sedating antihistamine) and erythromycin increase the risk of adverse effects on the heart, whereas concomitant use of erythromycin and statins potentially increase the risk of muscle aches and pains (BMA, 2018). The potential for cardiotoxicity is increased when erythromycin is given concurrently with medications which increase the QT interval; for example, amiodarone (NICE, 2019).

Concurrent administration of erythromycin and chloramphenicol or clindamycin is to be avoided as they antagonise each other's antibacterial effects. Erythromycin should not be administered with other macrolides as this can lead to severe effects (Burchum and Rosenthal, 2019).

Furthermore, drugs inhibiting erythromycin metabolism should not be used; these include some calcium channel blockers (verapamil), azole antifungal drugs (ketoconazole) and HIV protease inhibitors (ritonavir) (Burchum and Rosenthal, 2019).

Nursing actions

- Promote principles of good patient assessment, prescribing practice and antimicrobial stewardship through patient education (see Clinical Considerations 1).
- Limit oral course to a maximum of 14 days as the risk of liver damage potentially increases.
- Advise the person to take the medication on an empty stomach, with a full glass of water, one hour before meals or two hours afterwards.
- Offer information to the person about reducing gastrointestinal adverse effects by taking erythromycin with meals. This is dependent on the erythromycin variant prescribed, as some forms can be taken without any considerations to mealtimes.
- Monitor for signs of toxicity if concurrently taking the drugs Theophylline (monitor levels) or Carbamazepine (monitor levels) or warfarin (monitor INR), concomitantly with erythromycin.
- Monitor concurrent medications known to interact, raise serum levels or risk adverse effects.
- Check local guidelines for dilution, dosing and infusion rates for intravenous administration of erythromycin.
- Patient teaching about reporting any adverse effects experienced, especially the GI disturbances surrounding the potential for superinfections (pseudomembranous colitis).
- Monitor liver and renal function.
- Monitor the IV site for pain, swelling and redness.

Source: Karch, 2017; BMA, 2018; Burchum and Rosenthal, 2019; NICE, 2019; Barber and Robertson, 2020.

Lincosamides

Lincosamides and macrolides have similar properties: they inhibit the bacteria's protein synthesis; however, the former is considered more toxic (Xiu and Datta, 2019). Examples of lincosamides are clindamycin and lincomycin.

Clindamycin is a bacteriostatic; however, it can assume bactericidal properties (Burchum and Rosenthal, 2019). It acts on most gram-positive cocci, gram-negative and gram-positive anaerobes and gram-positive aerobes (NICE, 2019). It is used against streptococci and penicillin-resistant staphylococci (Xiu and Datta, 2019). Table 9.12 presents the pharmacokinetics of clindamycin.

Indications

Clindamycin is used for Staphylococcal bone (osteomyelitis) and joint infections as well as meticillin-resistant S.Aureus in bronchiectasis, peritonitis, intra-abdominal sepsis, acne vulgaris and bacterial vaginosis (NICE, 2019).

Table 9.12 Pharmacokinetics of clindamycin.

Absorption	Absorption via the GI tract, so can be administered orally, intramuscularly and intravenously. Topical administration also possible.
Distribution	Distributes well to most body fluids, including bone and synovial fluid and tissues, but not the CSF. It does not cross the blood–brain barrier.
Metabolism	Liver.
Excretion	Urine and bile (faeces).

Source: Wishart et al. (2018), Burchum and Rosenthal (2019).

Contraindications and cautions

When using systemically, exercise caution in middle-aged and older women undergoing surgical procedures as they are the most susceptible group to antibiotic associated colitis (NICE, 2019). Furthermore, avoid in those with acute porphyria (hereditary disorders of haem biosynthesis) as this could induce an acute crisis (NICE, 2019). Additionally, due to the routes of metabolism and excretion, caution is advised in those with renal or hepatic impairment. In people with combined renal and hepatic impairment, the drug can reach toxicity if dosages are not reduced (Burchum and Rosenthal, 2019).

Caution is advised in the first trimester of pregnancy (limited data) and in breast-feeding women as clindamycin is known to enter the breast milk, thus posing a risk of infantile diarrhoea (NICE, 2019). Benefits of clindamycin use should outweigh the risk to foetus or neonate (Karch, 2017). Caution extends in the use of vaginal preparations as clindamycin cream is known to damage latex condoms and diaphragms (NICE, 2019).

Contraindications would include those already with a known diarrhoeal status (NICE, 2019).

Adverse effects

The most extreme effect of clindamycin is antibiotic-associated diarrhoea, which can develop four to six weeks after completing a course of clindamycin (Burchum and Rosenthal, 2019). This is known to occur more frequently with clindamycin than other types of antibiotics (BMA, 2018).

Generally, skin reactions are a common side effect. A common side effect associated with oral use, besides antibiotic-associated diarrhoea, is abdominal pain; whereas an uncommon side effect is nausea and vomiting. Additional effects include pain, abdominal discomfort and vulvovaginal infection (NICE, 2019). Other side effects based on route of application can arise.

Drug–Drug interactions

Clindamycin is known to interact with drugs used in anaesthetic induction and surgery, by increasing their effects. These are: atracurium, cisatracurium, mivacurium, pancuronium, rocuronium, suxamethonium and vecuronium (NICE, 2019).

Nursing actions

- Promote principles of good patient assessment, prescribing practice and antimicrobial stewardship through patient education (see Clinical Considerations box).
- Advise the person to report any bouts of diarrhoea to their healthcare professional due to the potential of clindamycin to cause fatal antibiotic-associated diarrhoea. Discontinue treatment immediately if prolonged, severe or bloody diarrhoea occurs.
- Oral capsules should be swallowed with a glass of water.
- Advise strengthening of contraceptive measures using vaginal preparations.
- If concurrently taking clindamycin and breast-feeding, advise the woman to monitor their child for diarrhoea or candidiasis (both indicate gastrointestinal flora disturbances) or bloody stools (indicates potentially antibiotic associated diarrhoea).
- In longer duration of treatment regimens (10 days or more), monitor liver and renal function (systemic use).
- Monitor liver and renal function in neonates and infants (by systemic use).
- In adults, avoid rapid intravenous administration.
- In children, read clinical information for dilution, rate of administration and diluting agent.

Source: Karch, 2017; BMA, 2018; Burchum and Rosenthal, 2019; NICE, 2019; Barber and Robertson, 2020.

Episode of care

Dora, an 84-year-old woman, was admitted to the ward with a diagnosis of an urinary tract infection. Her initial prescription was trimethoprim 500 mg twice daily, but her symptoms persisted. Her new prescription is amoxicillin 500 mg four times daily. Her past medical history contains vascular dementia, atrial fibrillation, anaemia, folate deficiency and hypertension. She has a known drug allergy to penicillin. Outline the plan of care for this patient within the first 48 hours of admission.

Episode of care

Leo, a 16-year-old male, was admitted to the ward with a diagnosis of upper respiratory tract infection and an acute cough. He has been very unwell over the last few days. His prescription is amoxicillin 500 mg three times a day for five days. His past medical history contains Down syndrome, hypothyroidism, acne vulgaris, hay fever and an iron deficiency anaemia. He has a litre of milk across the day. His current medication is tetracycline, ferrous sulphate and levothyroxine. Highlight the nursing actions required for Leo to ensure his care is safe and evidence based.

Conclusion

This chapter has provided the reader with an overview of the use of antibacterial medication. The role of the healthcare professional is key in preventing the overuse of antibacterial therapy to ensure their sustained usability to protect from emerging resistant pathogens. The healthcare professionals role is paramount, primarily through offering advice and information to those who use health and social care services regarding expectations of antimicrobial therapies and the principles of antimicrobial stewardship.

References

Agwuh, K.N. and MacGowan, A. (2006). Pharmacokinetics and pharmacodynamics of the tetracyclines including glycylcyclines. *Journal of Antimicrobial Chemotherapy* 59 (2): 256–265. doi: 10.1093/jac/dkl224 (accessed 8 August 2019).

Aldridge, M. (2010). Miscellaneous routes of medication administration. In: Jevon, P., Payne, L., Higgins, D. & Endecott, R. (eds) *Medicines Management: A Guide for Nurses*. Hoboken, NJ: John Wiley & Sons, pp. 239–261.

Ashelford, S., Raynsford, J., and Taylor, V. (2016). *Pathophysiology & Pharmacology for Nursing Students*. UK: Sage Publications Ltd.

Barrott, L., Foreman, E., Harchowal, J., et al. (2020). Medicines optimization: ensuring quality and safety in Lister,S., Hofland,J., and Grafton H., (eds). The Royal Marsden Manual of Clinical Nursing Procedures. Chicester, UK. Wiley Blackwell pp. 820–939.

Barber, P. and Robertson, D. (2020). *Essential Pharmacology for Nurses*, Fourthe. Berkshire, UK: Open University Press.

British Medical Association (2008). *New Guide to Medicines & Drugs*, 7e. London, UK: Dorling Kindersley.

British Medical Association (2018). *New guide to Medicines & Drugs*, 10e. London, UK: Dorling Kindersley.

British Society for Antimicrobial Chemotherapy (2017). Antimicrobial stewardship. www.bsac.org.uk/antimicrobialstewardshipebook/BSAC-AntimicrobialStewardship-FromPrinciplestoPractice-eBook.pdf (accessed 16 May 2019).

Burchum, J.R. and Rosenthal, L.D. (2019). *Lehne's Pharmacology for Nursing Care*. Missouri, USA: Elsevier.

Cattini, P. and Kiernam, M. (2020). Infection prevention and control. In: *The Royal Marsden Manual of Clinical Nursing Procedures*. Tenth Professional edition (eds. S. Lister, J. Hofland and H. Grafton), 64–122. West Sussex, UK: Wiley-Blackwell Publishing.

Chernecky, C., Infortuna, H. and Macklin, D. (2005). *Saunders Nursing Survival Guide: Drug Calculations and Drug Administration*, 2nd edn. Philadelphia: W.B. Saunders.

Coppoc G.L. (1996a). Chloramphenicol. http://www.cyto.purdue.edu/cdroms/cyto2/17/chmrx/cap.htm (accessed 8 August 2019).

Coppoc G.L. (1996b) Tetracycline antibiotics. http://www.cyto.purdue.edu/cdroms/cyto2/17/chmrx/tetra.htm (accessed 8 August 2019).

Department of Health (DH) (2003b). *Building a Safer NHS for Patients: Improving Medication Safety*. London.

Department of Health (DH) (2007). *Safer Management of Controlled Drugs: A Guide to Good Practice in Secondary Care (England)*. London.

Dolk, F.C., Pouwels, K.B., and Smith, D.R.M. (2018). Antibiotics in primary care in England: which antibiotics are prescribed and for which conditions? *Journal of Antimicrobial Chemotherapy* 73 (suppl_2): ii2–ii10. https://doi.org/10.1093/jac/dkx504.

Dougherty, L., Lister, S. and West-Oram, A. (2015). Medicines management. In the Royal Marsden Manual of Clinical Nursing Procedures: Student Edition (9th eds).

Fraise, A.P. and Bradley, T. (eds) (2009). *Ayliffe's Control of Healthcare-Associated Infection: A Practical Handbook*, 5th edn. London: Hodder Arnold.

Griffith, R. and Jordan, S. (2003). Administration of medicines part 1: The law and nursing. *Nursing Standard*, 18 (2): 47–53.

Jevon, P., Payne, L., Higgins, D. and Endecott, R. (eds) (2010). *Medicines Management: A Guide for Nurses*. Hoboken, NJ: John Wiley & Sons.

Joint Formulary Committee (2019). *British National Formulary*, 74e. London: BMJ Group and Pharmaceutical Press.

Joint Formulary Committee (2020a). Antibacterial drug choice. https://bnf.nice.org.uk/treatment-summary/antibacterials-principles-of-therapy.html (accessed 28 October 2020).

Joint Formulary Committee (2020b). Erythromycin. https://bnf.nice.org.uk/drug/erythromycin.html#indicationsAndDoses (accessed 28 October 2020).

Jordan, S., Griffiths, H. and Griffith, R. (2003). Administration of medicines part 2: Pharmacology. *Nursing Standard*, 18 (3): 45–54.

Karch, A.M. (2017). *Focusing on Nursing Pharmacology*, 7e. Philadelphia, USA: Wolters Kluwer Publishing.

National Institute for Health and Care Excellence (2018). Antimicrobial stewardship. www.nice.org.uk/guidance/ng15 (accessed 14 September 2019).

National Institute for Health and Care Excellence (2019). Joint Formulary publications. https://www.JointFormulary.org/products/JointFormulary-online/ (accessed 15 September 2019).

Nursing and Midwifery Council (NMC) (2018). *The Code: Professional Standards of Practice and Behaviour for Nurses, Midwives and Nursing Associates*. Available at: https://www.nmc.org.uk/standards/code (accessed 25 November 2020).

NPSA (2005). *Wristbands for Hospital Inpatients Improve Safety* [Safer Practice Notice 11]. London: National Patient Safety Agency.

Olans, R.N., Olans, R.D., and DeMaria, A. Jr. (2018). The critical role of the staff nurse in antimicrobial stewardship- unrecognised, but already there. *Clinical Infectious Diseases* 62: 84–88.

Parliamentary Office of Science and Technology (2017). UK trends in infectious disease. https://researchbriefings.files.parliament.uk/documents/POST-PN-0545/POST-PN-0545.pdf (accessed 14 September 2019).

Perry A.G. (2015). Administration of nonparenteral medications. In: Perry, A.G., Potter, P.A. & Ostendorf, W. (eds) *Nursing Interventions & Clinical Skills*, 6th edn. St Louis, MO: Elsevier, pp. 555–596.

Potter, P. and Perry, A. (2016). *Fundamentals of Nursing*, 9th edn. St Louis, MO: Elsevier.

RPS (2019). *Professional Guidance on the Administration of Medicines in Healthcare Settings*. Available at: https://www.rpharms.com/Portals/0/RPS%20document%20library/Open%20access/Professional%20standards/SSHM%20and%20Admin/Admin%20of%20Meds%20prof%20guidance.pdf?ver=2019-01-23-145026-567 (accessed 25 November 2020).

Stollery, R., Shaw, M. and Lee, A. (2005). *Ophthalmic Nursing*, 3rd edn. Oxford: Blackwell.

World Health Organisation (2018a). Factsheet on antimicrobial resistance. https://www.who.int/antimicrobial-resistance/en (accessed 15 September 2019).

World Health Organisation (2018b). Factsheet on antibiotic resistance. https://www.who.int/en/news-room/fact-sheets/detail/antibiotic-resistance (accessed 14 September 2019)

Xiu, P. and Datta, S. (2019). *Pharmacology*, 5e. London, UK: Elsevier Publishers.

Young, S. and Pitcher, B. (2016). *Medicine Management for Nurses at a Glance*. Chicester, UK: Wiley Blackwell.

Zurlinden, T.J. and Reisfeld, B. (2017). Characterising the effects of race/ethnicity on acetaminophen pharmacokinetics using physiologically based pharmacokinetic modeling. *European Journal of Drug Metabolism and Pharmacokinetics* 42 (1): 143–153.

Further reading

Clayton, B.D., Stock, Y.N., and Cooper, S.E. (2010). *Basic Pharmacology for Nurses*, 15e. Missouri, USA: Mosby Elsevier.

Department of Health and Social Care (2019). Antimicrobial resistance strategic publications. https://www.gov.uk/government/collections/antimicrobial-resistance-amr-information-and-resources

Ha, D., Forte, M.B., Olans, R.D. et al. (2019). A multidisciplinary approach to incorporate bedside nurses into antimicrobial stewardship and infection prevention. *The Joint Commission Journal on Quality and Patient Safety* 45 (5): 600–605.

Kee, J.L., Hayes, E.R., and McCuistion, L.E. (2012). *Pharmacology: A Nursing Process Approach*, 7e. USA: Elsevier.

National Institute for Health and Care Excellence (2019a). Joint formulary. https://JointFormulary.nice.org.uk/.

National Institute for Health and Care Excellence (2019b). NICE guidelines. www.nice.org.uk/guidance.

Peate, I. (2015). Antimicrobial resistance: the nurse's essential role. *British Journal of Nursing* 24 (1): 5.

Pearce, L. (2019). Antimicrobial resistance: how you can make a difference. *Nursing Standard* 34 (5): 53–54.

Redwood, R., Knobloch, M.-J., Pellegrini, D. et al. (2018). Reducing unnecessary culturing: a systems approach to evaluating urine cultures ordering and collection practices among nurses in two acute care settings. *Antimicrobial Resistance and Infection Control* 7 https://doi.org/10.1186/s13756-017-0278-9.

Wilson, A. (2019). Antimicrobial resistance: what can nurses do? *British Journal of Nursing* 28 (1): 16–17.

Wishart D.S., Feunang, Y.D., Guo, A.C., et al. (2018). Drugbank 5.0. https://www.drugbank.ca/about (accessed 1 November 2019).

World Health Organisation (2015). Global action plan on antimicrobial resistance. https://www.who.int/antimicrobial-resistance/publications/global-action-plan/en.

Multiple choice questions

1. What does the term 'bactericidal' mean?
   - (a) Inhibits bacterial growth
   - (b) Destroys bacteria
   - (c) Aids bacterial growth
   - (d) Aids bacterial cell replication
2. Which group of antibacterials does imipenem belong to?
   - (a) Sulfonamides
   - (b) Quinolones
   - (c) Aminoglycosides
   - (d) Beta-lactams
3. Neonatal grey baby syndrome is associated with which antibiotic?
   - (a) Cefalexin
   - (b) Chloramphenicol
   - (c) Ciprofloxacin
   - (d) Co-trimoxazole
4. The action of clindamycin is?
   - (a) Folate interference
   - (b) Bacterial DNA inhibition
   - (c) Protein synthesis interference
   - (d) Disruption of the cell wall
5. Erythromycin is known to increase the levels of which drug?
   - (a) Warfarin
   - (b) Paracetamol
   - (c) Ferrous sulphate
   - (d) Gabapentin

6. Tetracycline is contraindicated in which client group?
   (a) Pregnant women
   (b) Breast-feeding mothers
   (c) People with renal impairment
   (d) All of the above
7. In which group of antibiotics is there a possibility of disulfiram-like reaction occurring if alcohol is consumed alongside the treatment?
   (a) Penicillin
   (b) Aminoglycosides
   (c) Sulfonamides
   (d) Cephalosporins

8. Antibacterials can have _____ effects on people?
   (a) Hepatotoxic
   (b) Nephrotoxic
   (c) Ototoxic
   (d) All of the above
9. Ototoxicity is a known adverse effect of which antibacterial group?
   (a) Aminoglycosides
   (b) Tetracyclines
   (c) Cephalosporins
   (d) Penicillins
10. Concomitant administration of erythromycin and which medication can induce hypokalemia?
    (a) Theophylline
    (b) Ferrous sulphate
    (c) Warfarin
    (d) Ibuprofen
11. Which antibiotic group disrupts the bacteria cellular wall??
    (a) Carbapenems
    (b) Lincosamides
    (c) Chloramphenicol
    (d) Aminoglycosides
12. The term antibacterial is used interchangeably with which other term?
    (a) Antihypertensive
    (b) Antibiotic
    (c) Anti-emetic
    (d) Anticoagulant
13. Which factors can affect the pharmacokinetics of antibiotics?
    (a) Age
    (b) Renal function
    (c) Hepatic function
    (d) All of the above
14. Photosensitivity is a potential adverse effect of which antibiotic group?
    (a) Cephalosporins
    (b) Penicillins
    (c) Carbapenems
    (d) Tetracyclines

15. A main priority of good antimicrobial stewardship is?
   (a) Monitor for tendon damage
   (b) Identify the causative organism
   (c) Monitor hepatic function
   (d) Monitor renal function

Find out more

The following are a list of conditions that are associated with the use of antibiotics. Take some time and write notes about each of the conditions. Think about the medications that may be used in order to treat these conditions and be specific about the pharmacokinetics and pharmacodynamics. Remember to include aspects of patient care. If you are making notes about people you have offered care and support to, you must ensure that you have adhered to the rules of confidentiality. Needs two more

The condition	Your notes
Nausea and vomiting	
Pseudomembranous colitis	
Anaphylaxis	
Tinnitus	
Photosensitivity	

Chapter 10

Medications used in the cardiovascular system

Jan Guerin and Cecilia Mihaila

Aim

This chapter provides the nurse and healthcare worker with cardinal knowledge of cardiovascular system medications prescribed as therapeutic interventions for the management of cardiovascular diseases.

Learning outcomes

By the end of this chapter, the learner should be able to:

1. Explain the basic pathophysiology of the major cardiovascular diseases
2. Discuss the major classes of medications related to the management of cardiovascular disease
3. Describe the major effects of various medications on cardiac and vascular function
4. Explain the important clinical considerations when administering these medications
5. Justify and explain the importance of health education and promotion for the known risk factors for cardiovascular disease

Test your knowledge

1. Do you know what the major cardiovascular diseases are in the world?
2. What classes of cardiovascular medications do you know?
3. Do you think that nurses have a role in health prevention and promotion to address the burden of disease? If yes, what could you do? If no, why do you think so?
4. What do you think are the barriers for patients that result in non-concordance with their medication regimen?
5. Do you know what cardiovascular system medications are used for non-cardiovascular conditions or diseases? How many medications can you name?

Fundamentals of Pharmacology: For Nursing and Healthcare Students, First Edition. Edited by Ian Peate and Barry Hill.
© 2021 John Wiley & Sons Ltd. Published 2021 by John Wiley & Sons Ltd.

Introduction

Cardiovascular diseases, also referred to as heart and circulatory diseases, are reported to be the number one cause of death globally (World Health Organisation, [WHO] 2019). The WHO statistically estimated 17.9 million deaths worldwide in 2016, which are representative of 31% of the total cause for all global deaths. In the United Kingdom (UK) this burden of disease is represented statistically as 7.4 million people (British Heart Foundation [BHF], 2019). Modifiable risk factors (BHF, 2019) are identified as hyperlipidaemia, diabetes mellitus, hypertension, smoking, obesity and physical inactivity; non-modifiable risk factors are age, ethnic background and family history of heart disease. The results from a 21-country study (The Prospective Urban Rural Epidemiology: PURE study) (Rosengren et al., 2019) concluded that further modifiable risk factors exist from a global perspective. These risks include: poor educational attainment (primary education level or less), poor diet, excessive alcohol, high sodium intake, household pollution from solid fuel cooking, ambient air pollution, depression and low grip strength. A group of non-communicable diseases with the potential for early death or lifelong morbidity are classified as:

- ischaemic heart disease
- myocardial infarction
- atrial fibrillation
- heart failure
- cerebrovascular disease
- vascular dementia
- out-of-hospital cardiac arrests.

Diseases not related to lifestyle are congenital heart disease, affecting 1–2% of the total population, along with inherited conditions of hypertrophic cardiomyopathy and familial hyperlipidaemia affecting 620 000 people in UK (BHF, 2019).

The National Health Service (NHS) Long Term Plan for Cardiovascular Disease (2019) high-lights that cardiovascular disease is largely preventable and is the single biggest area where the NHS can save people's lives over the next 10 years. It advocates this with lifestyle changes, along with the combined actions of public health and the NHS working on tobacco and smoking addictions, obesity, food reformulation and alcohol misuse (Public Health England [PHE], 2019).

The burden of cardiovascular disease is more than considerable, and nurses and healthcare workers provide an essential role in caring for people with cardiovascular conditions at many levels within different healthcare clinical settings. Their responsibilities include health education/promotion and safe medicines management with optimisation of patient adherence. In the context of the management of established cardiovascular disease, optimising the function of the failing organs in order to limit morbidity, preventing mortality with an overall aim to improve the quality of life for the person by means of effective medication interventions, sets the stage for this chapter.

Medications used in the management of cardiovascular diseases

It may not be an absolutely achievable goal for every nurse and healthcare worker to be able to learn everything about every medication. Pharmacology is an extensive subject with a potential to create 'information overload', so to be able to master it on all levels expertly becomes a 'mission impossible'. Furthermore, new medications are introduced during not only your period of education but throughout your lifetime as healthcare professionals, making the ongoing need to keep up to date with developments in new medications even more challenging. The most efficient way of learning medications may be by their class, related to the specific body system or related to the pathophysiology of the disease at hand. Knowing normal from abnormal physiology will afford critical analysis and increase your ability to recall what you have learned at any time needed. The British National Formulary (BNF) is a resourceful tool to find specific information that may need to be considered in patients with pre-existing non-cardiac diseases (see Chapter 2 of this book to learn how to use the BNF and other pharmacological reference guides). In the following sections of this chapter, medications will be discussed with reference to known cardiovascular system disease processes.

Atheroma and the hyperlipidaemias

Atherosclerosis is deemed a dominant cause of cardiovascular disease (Frostegard, 2013). It is a degenerative disease in its course and affects the interior walls of the coronary arteries resulting in narrowing as a result of fatty deposits secondary to the accumulation of cholesterol. It is important to note that this same pathophysiological process occurs in other arteries in the body as well, making it a contributory risk factor for diseases such as erectile dysfunction, hypertension, aneurysm rupture, heart failure, peripheral vascular disease, deep vein thrombosis, cerebrovascular accident (stroke) and vascular dementia, to name a few.

When the coronary artery vessel lumen becomes narrowed or occluded, the blood flow reduces or ceases leading to nutrient and oxygen deprivation of the heart muscle (Figure 10.1). Coronary artery disease may be managed with medications and/or medical interventions. However, should the blood vessel become critically narrowed with subsequent rupture of the atheromatous plaque, the patient may sustain an acute myocardial infarction.

Cholesterol is a fat-like waxy substance (lipid), which in natural amounts is not harmful and found in all cells. Cholesterol is essential for good cell health, in that it is a structural component of cell membranes and plays a key role in making hormones, vitamin D, as well as bile acids for a healthy gastrointestinal digestion system. However, an increased circulating level of cholesterol becomes harmful as it journeys through the blood stream in the form of lipoproteins. In order to diagnose this hyperlipidaemia, a specific blood test is used to ascertain the levels of cholesterol and fats in the blood, called a serum lipid profile (Table 10.1).

The aetiology of hyperlipidaemia may be due to a number of factors: i.e., familial/hereditary, diabetes mellitus, kidney disease, hypothyroidism, obesity, smoking and a diet high in

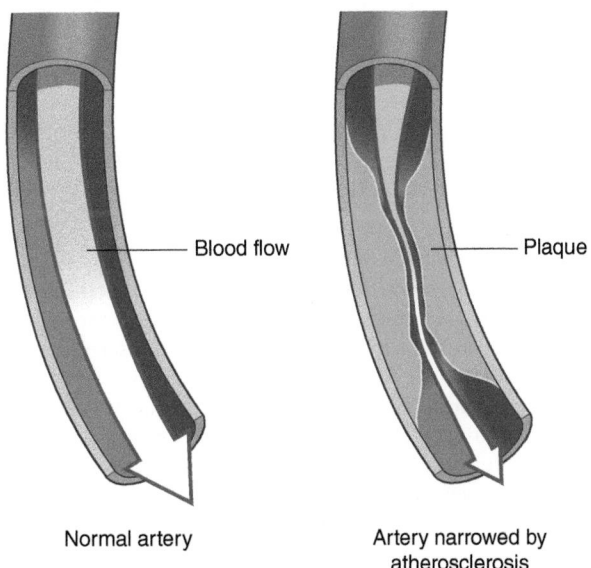

Blood flow   Plaque

Normal artery   Artery narrowed by atherosclerosis

Figure 10.1 Coronary artery disease. Source: Peate and Wild (2nd Ed) Nursing Practice Knowledge.

189

Table 10.1 Healthy cholesterol profile (Department of Health (DH), National Health Service (NHS), 2019).

Normal Serum (Blood) Lipid Levels
Total cholesterol: 5 mmol/L or below
HDL: 1 mmol/L or above
LDL: 3 mmol/L or below
Non-HDL: 4 mmol/L or below
Triglycerides: 2.3 mmol/L or below

Source: Adapted from NHS (2019).

saturated fats and cholesterol. Other causes are related to adverse effects from some medications, such as corticosteroids, thiazide diuretics, beta-blockers, protease inhibitors and estrogen. Further to the above lipid profile risk factors, trans fats, which are artificially manufactured, increase the risk of acute myocardial infarctions and cerebrovascular incidents.

The first line of managing hyperlipidaemia is to identify and manage the medical causes, e.g. hypothyroidism or uncontrolled diabetes mellitus. Further to this, educating patients about the known risk factors as well as offering advice for non-pharmacological interventions to reduce total cholesterol, LDL, triglycerides and increase HDL; these recommendations are found in the National Institute for Health and Care Excellence (NICE) (CG181, 2014). However, when lifestyle changes are not adopted or seen to be ineffective, a medication intervention is prescribed.

Medications used to regulate lipids: Antihyperlipidaemic medications

- Statins: HMG-C0A reductase inhibitors.
- Inhibitors of cholesterol absorption.
- Fibrates.
- Bile-acid-binding resins: cholesterol absorption inhibitors.
- PCSK9 inhibitors.
- Nicotinic acid: Vitamin B3.
- Omega-3 fatty acids.

Statins: HMG-CoA reductase inhibitors
Atorvastatin, Simvastatin, Rosuvastatin, Fluvastatin, Pravastatin

Statins are the first line of lipid-lowering medications prescribed. Statins are a group of medications that lower cholesterol in the blood by interfering with cholesterol synthesis by inhibiting the enzyme hydroxy-methylglutaryl-co-enzyme (HMG-CoA) in the liver, resulting in a depletion in intracellular cholesterol. This causes the cell to seek cholesterol from the intravascular space, thus reducing further circulating cholesterol and LDL. Statins also have the added benefit of improving endothelial function as well as integrity, reducing inflammation and preventing platelet aggregation (Stringer, 2017). These medications have a common mechanism of action; however, the various formulations have different chemistry and pharmacokinetics. In general, statins are rapidly absorbed after oral administration and undergo extensive first-pass metabolism in the gut and liver, thus having a bioavailability of around 14%. Statins are predominantly metabolised by the cytochrome P450 in the liver and eliminated in the bile. Statins have mild side effects that may be myalgia, constipation, diarrhoea, headaches or abdominal pain. Serious adverse effects are hepatotoxicity with subsequent liver failure. In cases of liver impairment or excess alcohol use, NICE (CG181, 2014) recommends pre-serum liver function tests (LFTs) with follow-up tests every three months after starting treatment. A serious adverse effect is rhabdo-myolysis that can damage the kidneys.

Clinical considerations for statins

- Follow up with practice nurse (pn)/general practitioner (GP) to monitor serum cholesterol levels and LFTs as per appointment planning.
- Avoid grapefruit juice.
- Take once daily at bedtime as cholesterol synthesis is most active at nighttime and food intake may affect absorption.
- Keep close observation to recognise the signs of rhabdomyolysis, such as unexplained joint or muscle pain when taking medication.
- Observe for a change in the colour of urine to rose or red. This requires immediate escala-tion to senior staff/PN or GP for prompt attention.
- Note drug interactions occur with diltiazem, erythromycin and serotonin reuptake inhibi-tors (SSRis).
- Contraindicated in pregnancy.

Inhibitors of cholesterol absorption
Ezetimibe

This medication acts by inhibiting dietary and biliary intestinal cholesterol absorption in the small intestine, thus reducing the amount transported back to the liver. The positive outcome is increased clearance of cholesterol from the blood with reduced stores in the liver, resulting in a reduction in total cholesterol, LDL, triglycerides and an increase in HDL. It is taken orally at any time of the day without fasting, is rapidly absorbed, and extensively undergoes enterohe-patic recycling and slow elimination (Kosoglou et al., 2005). The medication has a long half-life of around 22 hours and is mostly eliminated in the faeces with the residual amount in the urine. It may be prescribed for those who are intolerant to statins or if they respond poorly to the recommended statin therapy (Bergheanu et al., 2017). In the latter patient group, this med-ication can be used as an addition to a statins, except in patients with hepatic failure (Vavlukis and Valvlukis, 2018). Common side effects include headaches, rhinorrhoea, sore throat, diarrhoea, gastrointestinal discomfort/disorders and asthenia.

Fibrates
Fenofibrate, Gemfibrozil

Fibrates lower serum triglyceride levels by 30–60%. Their mode of action is reducing the produc-tion of very low density lipoproteins (VLDLs), thus enhancing the clearance of triglycerides from the blood (Joint Formulary Committee, (JFC, 2020). Elevated serum triglycerides are further rec-ognised to increase the risk for cardiovascular disease even in the absence of serum elevated total cholesterol levels. Fibrates may also be prescribed as adjunctive therapy to a diet for those intolerant of or unsuitable to take statins. This medication is well absorbed by the gastrointesti-nal system and elimination is via urine with a small amount via faeces. Side effects are dyspepsia, fatigue, vertigo, with more severe effects being elevation in serum transaminases and pancyto-penia. They may also be prescribed in dual therapy for identified high-risk patients (JFC, 2020). Their use is contraindicated in people with active liver disease, gall bladder disease, severe renal impairment/end stage renal disease and photosensitivity induced by ketoprofen.

A high-risk patient group are those classified as having 'metabolic syndrome' (Table 10.2) requiring this dual therapy approach.

Table 10.2   Criteria for metabolic syndrome. Metabolic syndrome is present if a patient has three or more of the following risk factors.

1. Abdominal obesity: waist circumference:
   >102 cm in men
   >88 cm in women.
2. Hypertension <135/85 mmHg.
3. Elevated serum triglycerides <1.7 mmol/l.
4. Low serum HDL – <1.04 mmol/l in men and <1.30 mmol/l in women.
5. High fasting blood glucose >6.1 mmol/l.

Source: Diabetes (2019).

Clinical considerations for fibrates

- Should be taken about a half an hour before a meal.
- Attend planned follow-up appointments with PN/GP for monitoring of LFTs and renal function.
- The risk for pancytopenia requires attendance of planned appointments for monitoring of full blood count (FBC) to assess mainly haemoglobin, platelet and white cell counts.

Bile-acid-binding resins: Cholesterol absorption inhibitors
Cholestyramine, Colesevelam Hydrochloride

These medications are anion exchange resins (also known as bile-acid sequestrants) that act by binding to negatively charged bile acids in the small intestine. They lower LDL by affording acids to be eliminated via the faeces, so preventing re-entry of cholesterol into the blood stream. The liver then converts further cholesterol into bile acids to be eliminated via the faeces. Resins are not absorbed so the toxicity risk is low. This medication needs to be used in conjunction with a cholesterol-lowering diet so as to achieve 15–20% reduction in serum LDL. Side effects are related to the gastrointestinal system; abdominal discomfort, bloating, constipation and diarrhoea. This medication is contraindicated in those with severe hypertriglyceridaemia and complete biliary obstruction.

Clinical considerations

Bile-acid-binding resins
- Medication is in powder form; dispense into some fruit juice, as it is unpleasant in taste, and take just before a meal.
- Advise to take other medications one hour before or four to six hours after taking this medication as it may interfere with other orally taken medications.

PCSK9 inhibitors
Alirocumab

This is a relatively recent addition to the management of hyperlipidaemia for people who have not responded positively to diet and maximal dosing of other antilipid medications. Its classification is as a human monoclonal antibody that binds to PCSK9 (proprotein convertase subtilisin/kexin type 9); it acts by binding to a pro-protein involved in the regulation of LDL receptors on the liver, upcycling the number of receptors and therefore optimises the clearance of cholesterol from the plasma (Manniello and Pisano, 2016). It is administered by subcutaneous injection and has a half-life of 17–20 days. However, this absorption following a subcutaneous injection occurs within three to seven days. At least three doses are required to be administered every two weeks in order to achieve a steady state for bioavailability (Manniello and Pisano, 2016). Local side effects involve local injection site reactions such as pain, bruising and erythema. Systemic side effects include rhinorrhoea and sore throat.

Alternatives to statins
Nicotinic acid: Vitamin B3
Niacin

NICE (CG181, 2016) does not advocate the use of this medication for the prevention of cardiovascular disease in primary prevention nor in patients with chronic kidney disease with type 1 or type 2 diabetes mellitus. However, patients without the abovementioned risk factors (BHF, 2019) suggest it as one of the alternatives to statins, stating that there is some evidence that it lowers LDL and raises HDL but does not reduce the risk for acute myocardial infarction or stroke. It is only available via prescription due to the 'extreme' dose which may result in adverse side effects. It is taken as an oral preparation of tables/capsules. Niacin works by inhibiting synthesis of cholesterol, therefore reducing levels of total cholesterol, LDL and triglycerides. Side effects related to the high dose are prostaglandin-mediated flushing occurring within the first hour of taking orally. Patient education is to observe for signs of excessive or unexplained bleeding, as long-term use may result in the depletion of vitamin K.

Omega-3 Fatty Acids
Fish Oil

This is a well-known treatment, taken as an oral supplement for the prevention of cardiovascular disease. In a large randomised control study of marine n-3 fatty acids, Manson et al. (2019) found that supplementation with these fatty acids did not lower the incidence of major cardiovascular events.

Medications used in management of hypertension

Hypertension is a condition when the blood pressure (BP) remains chronically elevated above the healthy level (Table 10.3). NICE (CG136, 2019) advocates the following criteria for diagnosis of HPT.

Table 10.3   Criteria for diagnosis of hypertension (NICE CG 136, 2019).

Criteria for diagnosis of hypertension (NICE CG136, 2019)
Stage 1: Clinic BP 140/90 mmHg to 159/99 mmHg and subsequent ABPM daytime average or HBPM average BP ranging from 135/85 mmHg to 149/94 mmHg.
Stage 2: Clinic BP 160/100 mmHg or higher but less than 180/120 mmHg and subsequent ABPM daytime average of HBPM average BP of 150/95 mmHg or higher.
Stage 3 or Severe HPT: Clinic systolic BP of 180 mmHg or higher or clinic diastolic BP of 120 mmHg or higher.

Source: National Institute for Clinical Excellence (NICE) (2019).

Skills in practice

A case of 'white coat syndrome'

It is accepted that many people may present a trend showing a variation in their BP measurements over a 24-hour period. However, a portion of population that may either be normotensive or hypertensive find that their measurements may be considerably higher when obtained by a healthcare professional. This phenomenon is referred to as 'white coat syndrome'. The reason for this may be attributed to the effect of our neuro-endocrine reflex mediated by the sympathetic nervous system. When the person arrives for their appointment, they are already anxious and perhaps overthinking about other illness or worries while having their BP measurement checked (Pioli et al., 2018).

The elevated BP may result in:

- inappropriate initiation of antihypertensive medication;
- inappropriate increase in the dosage of existing medication;
- cancelation or postponement of a planned procedure or treatment.

Recommendations

- Demonstrate the '6 Cs of nursing' from the first moment of interaction with your patient and continue throughout the entire patient journey.
- Demonstrate self-control; do not be impatient with the already anxious patient, demonstrate empathy in your interactions, this will provide reassurance and calm the patient as they will feel understood and safe in your care.
- Ensure your patient is comfortable and confident by orientating to the clinical setting, providing an area map and answering questions/concerns.
- If the patient is a known hypertensive, ensure that their medical team have given them instructions to take their medication on the morning of the procedure.
- If possible, provide an opportunity for patients to meet their named team prior to their procedure and attempt to make appointments with the same team for future follow-up visits.
- If the patients BP is elevated on initial assessment, reassure them and provide an opportunity for their BP to be measured a second time in a quieter environment.
- Follow the recommendations of NICE Guidelines (Table 10.3) for diagnosis of hypertension using ABPM and HBPM to decrease risk of 'white coat syndrome'.

The causes of hypertension may be classified as essential, whereby the specific cause is unknown; it may be due to genetics with shared environmental influences. Bolivar (2013) suggests that environmental/lifestyle factors can include:

- obesity
- excess alcohol intake
- high sodium intake diet
- unmanaged acute/chronic stress
- insulin resistance related to metabolic syndrome.

Secondary hypertension may be due to endocrine diseases such as pheochromocytoma, renal system disorders such as Cushing's syndrome, obstructive sleep apnea and hyper/hypothyroidism. Medications associated with causing secondary hypertension are non-steroidal anti-inflammatory drugs (NSAIDs), steroids, 'diet pills', sympathomimetics, e.g. nasal decongestants, and recreational drugs (Puar et al., 2016).

BP is regarded as an independent risk factor for cardiovascular disease, therefore medication management will be rationalised using QRISK 3 (England) or ASSIGN (Scotland) as a risk scoring system (these risk tools can be found at: https://qrisk.org/three and http://www.assign-score.com/about/beginners/).

Regardless of the aetiology, chronically elevated systemic BP has the potential to result in long-term negative health effects damaging the brain, heart, kidneys, eyes and blood vessels. The rationale for treating hypertension is to reduce the risk of mortality as well as morbidity which leads to the burden of developing a chronic diseased state (Begg, 2016) such as:

- coronary artery disease
- atrial fibrillation
- left ventricular failure
- stroke
- chronic kidney disease
- blindness.

Subsequent pharmacological interventions follow an assessment period with lifestyle changes unless there is evidence of end organ damage or complications associated with the hypertension (NICE, CG136 2019). It is essential for the patient to understand the treatment regimen prescribed in order to be concordant with the medication regimen, as outcomes of the efficacy of the chosen medication/s is reliant on this factor.

Pharmacological approaches are based on manipulating the physiological determinants of BP, this is systemic vascular resistance and/or heart rate along with lifestyle modification for hypertension (NICE, CG136 2019).

Medications used to manage hypertension

- Angiotensin-converting enzyme inhibitors (ACEi).
- Calcium channel blockers (CCBs).
- Diuretics.
- Angiotensin receptor blockers (ARBs).
- Beta blockers (BB).
- Adrenergic blockers (Alpha I).
- Central adrenergic blockers (Alpha 2).
- Vasodilators.
- Centrally acting agents.
- Direct renin inhibitors (DRIs).
- Nitrates.

Angiotensin-converting enzyme inhibitors (ACEi)
Lisinopril, Enalapril, Captopril, Ramipril, Perindopril

These medications act on the renin–angiotensin aldosterone system (RAAS) pathway. ACEis inhibit the conversion of angiotensin I to angiotensin II. This lowers systemic BP due to inhibiting vasoconstriction, aldosterone and less sodium reabsorption. The net result is a reduction in both preload and afterload, thus reducing the work of the heart. Note that, although different types of ACEi exhibit the same mode of action to reduce BP, they may have different chemical structures (JFC, 2020). They are administered orally, binding to plasma and tissue protein, and are eliminated via the kidney. The most significant and potentially fatal adverse effect is angioedema, an induced oedema due to kinin metabolism which may be potentially life-threatening (Kostis et al., 2018). A benefit of ACEi is that they offer renal protection not only in their action in controlling BP but also by reducing proteinuria (Bakris, 2008).

Clinical considerations for ACEi

- A dry, non-productive paroxysmal cough occurs in some people. The patient may decide if they can tolerate it in order to continue with the medication. This can be discussed with the prescriber as there is no treatment to halt this cough.
- Advise patient to be mindful that getting up quickly may provoke dizziness and a fall.
- High risk for renal failure; therefore monitoring, as per PN/GP appointment planning, of renal function in certain groups, i.e. known renal artery stenosis.
- Monitoring, as per PN/GP appointment planning of LFTs.
- Monitoring, as per PN/GP appointment planning for hyperkalaemia in patients with impaired kidney function, or those taking potassium-sparing diuretics or trimethoprim-sulphamethoxazole.
- Advise patient with poor kidney function that adverse effects may be potentiated if they take NSAIDs.
- Contraindicated in patients taking DRis.

Calcium channel blockers (CCBs)
Amlodipine, Felodipine, Nifedipine, Nicardipine
Diltiazem and Verapamil

This group of medications is the most widely used in cardiovascular disease as it has a role in hypertension, angina and tachyarrhythmias (JFC, 2020). CCBs do not all possess the same pharmacodynamics, so it makes it a little more difficult to understand them as they are not a single class of medication. Amlodipine, felodipine, nifedipine and nicardipine are classified as dihydropyridines and their predominant effect is on peripheral vasodilation. Verapamil is a phenylakylamine and along with Diltiazem (benzothiazepine derivative) is classified as a rate-limiting CCB as it affects the sinoatrial and atrioventricular nodes, thus reducing conduction as well as myocardial contractility (JFC, 2020). In general, when administered orally they are well absorbed, however, and have a low and variable bioavailability due to extensive first-pass metabolism. They are all highly protein bound with a high volume of distribution and excretion via the kidneys. Importantly, CCBs that are taken in toxic dosage or in repeated doses cause the hepatic enzymes responsible for their metabolism to become saturated, thus reducing the first-pass effects and thereby increasing absorption of the active medication. Therefore, these medications may be given in the formulation of modified release. The adverse effects for the dihydropyridines are headache and flushing as a result of the peripheral vasodilation. Other adverse effects are on the microcirculation, which usually reduces over time, this is ankle swelling with cool hands and feet (McKeever and Hamilton, 2019). In contrast, the non-dihydropyridines may lead to severe constipation and have a potential to worsen cardiac output along with a symptomatic bradycardia. Two interesting facts: although listed as uncommon side effects in the JFC (2020), long-term treatment with CCBs is associated with gingival hyperplasia which results in problems with mastication, speech and limited access for good oral hygiene. This patient group has an increased vulnerability to bacterial infections, periodontal diseases and dental caries (Umeizudike et al., 2017). Second, a more marked BP reduction occurs in the elderly and those of Afro-Caribbean descent people due to what is termed 'low renin hypertension' (Sahay and Sahay, 2012).

Clinical considerations for CCBs

- Monitor vital signs before administration then at least two hourly, paying attention to sudden changes in systolic blood pressure. Continue to monitor as guided by the prescriber's targeted systolic blood pressure. Record observations on NEWS 2 and escalate drop in systolic blood pressure of <100 mmHg as per escalation action plan.
- Monitor for changes in level of consciousness, dizziness, fatigue and postural hypotension.
- Monitor for hypersensitivity 'angioedema'.
- Routine monitoring as planned by PN/GP/Physician of kidney and LFTs.
- Advise patients to maintain good oral hygiene and visit dentist regularly for check-ups.

Diuretics

There are three main classes of diuretics:

- loop diuretics
- thiazide diuretics
- potassium-sparing diuretics.

Diuretics increase diuresis; sometimes patients refer to these types of medications as 'water-tablets'. These medications alter the way in which the kidney deals with sodium, therefore by excreting more sodium, water follows. Diuretic medications are available in different formulations acting on different segments of the renal tubular system. A patient may be prescribed a combination of two different types for best effect. This 'synergistic effect' may be required as the kidney's nephron system can compensate for altered sodium reabsorption in another portion of the nephron segment (Klabunde, 2017). The best effects of diuretics can be achieved by blocking multiple sites in the nephron.

Loop diuretics
Furosemide, Bumetanide

These diuretics are indicated in chronic heart failure more often than hypertension. They are very efficacious as they act on the thick ascending limb of the loop of Henle and macula dense, where 20–25% of sodium that is filtered through the glomerulus is reabsorbed, making them potent at forcing diuresis. Loop diuretics also contribute to keeping the kidney at optimum functioning as they induce renal synthesis of prostaglandins that promote an increase in renal artery blood flow as well as redistribution of renal cortical blood flow (Klabunde, 2017). Furosemide administered intravenously has a short half-life; however, if taken orally, gastrointestinal absorption is slower than the rate of elimination. About 50% is excreted via the kidneys unchanged and the bioavailability of oral Furosemide is around 60%. Loop diuretics are organic anions that are tightly bound to albumin and volumes of distribution are low except in extreme cases of hypoalbuminaemia. Therefore, the efficacy of loop diuretics on natriuresis is impaired in these situations.

Thiazide diuretics
Hydrochlorothiazide, Chlortalidone, Indapamide

These medications block the sodium-chloride channel in the proximal segment of the distal convoluted tubule, resulting in decreased movement of sodium into the luminal membrane, thus reducing sodium and water movement into this passage. In comparison to loop diuretics, this target area of action leads to less of a diuretic and natriuretic effect, making them less potent. However, chlortalidone and indapamide are deemed to be efficient in meeting therapeutic requirements as a diuretic in the management of hypertension (JFC, 2020).

Clinical considerations for thiazides

- Monitoring as per appointment planning with PN/GP of BP, weight to assess for fluid retention, serum electrolytes and serum lipids.
- Close monitoring of serum potassium (s) K+), especially in patients on several medications.
- Advise patient of foods rich in potassium as they are at a high risk for hypokalaemia.
- Contraindicated in patients with a sulphonamide allergy.

198

Potassium-sparing diuretics

Amiloride Hydrochloride, Triamterene.
Aldosterone Antagonists.
Eplerenone, Spironolactone.

These act on the distal part of the nephron from the late distal tubule to the collecting duct (Horisberger and Glebisch, 1987). Amiloride and Triamterene act on the distal convoluted tubule, blocking epithelial sodium channels and thereby reducing sodium reabsorption and promoting water elimination. JFC (2020) advocates the use of these two diuretics most for management of oedema. In contrast, Eplerenone binds to the mineralocorticoid receptor, thus binding to aldosterone which inhibits sodium reabsorption. Spironolactone is indicated for patients with resistant hypertension and chronic heart failure, whereas Eplerenone is most used in heart failure (JFC, 2020). Diuretics will be discussed further in this chapter. See Table 10.4 that compares common adverse effects of diuretics.

In summary, the use of loop, thiazide and potassium-sparing diuretics is advocated in practice in patients with stage 1–4 hypertension along with a lifestyle changes including a diet

Table 10.4   Comparing common adverse effects of diuretics.

Loop diuretics	Thiazide diuretics	Potassium-sparing	Aldosterone antagonists:
• Hypokalaemia • Hypomagnesemia • Dehydration leading to hypotension • Ototoxicity	• Hypokalaemia • Dehydration leading to hypotension • Hyponatremia • Metabolic alkalosis • Hypercalcemia • Hyperglycaemia in people with diabetes • Hyperuricemia • Hyperlipidaemia	• Hyperkalaemia • GI problems – peptic ulcer	*Spironolactone*: • Hyperkalaemia • Gastrointestinal effects – nausea and vomiting • Electrolyte disturbances • Gynecomastia • Sexual dysfunction – ant androgen activity • Mood changes • Menstrual disturbances *Eplerenone:* • Hirsutism • Acne vulgaris • Female pattern hair loss

reduced in sodium intake. Decisions for which class and dosage depends on the patient's identified clinical needs.

Angiotensin receptor blockers (ARBs)
Losartan, Candersartan, Irbesartan, Olemesartan, Valsartan

ARBs are similar to ACEi in that they may be prescribed not only for hypertension but also heart failure or in the acute care setting post acute myocardial infarction (Klabunde, 2017). ARBs are angiotensin receptor antagonists that block both angiotensin I and II receptors in the blood vessels as well as in other tissues in the heart. The dilation of arteries and veins leads to a fall in BP and reduced preload, as a result of peripheral vasodilatation and reduced workload of the heart as it reduces afterload. Other actions are to block angiotensin II, promoting renal excretion of water and sodium, thus reducing circulating volume. In patients with longstanding hypertension, heart failure or acute myocardial infarction, overwork of the cardiac muscle leads to hypertrophy in order to compensate for the added workload (similar to exercising your arm muscles to make them grow larger). ARBs inhibit this process of compensation of cardiac and vascular remodelling (Hill et al., 2019). This class of medication is classified as low in negative side effects compared with ACEis (Hill et al., 2019).

199

Clinical considerations for ARBs

- Patient monitoring using NEWS 2 due to risk for hypotension.
- Monitoring renal function as clinically indicated.
- Contraindicated in patients concomitantly taking potassium sparing diuretics, ACEis, DRis and NSAIDs due to high risk of hyperkalaemia.

Beta-adrenoceptor antagonists (beta-blockers)

Selective β_1 blockers: cardioselective: Atenolol, Bisoprolol, Metoprolol.
Non-selective: Propanolol, Sotalol, Labetalol, Carvedilol.

Generally, these are classified as either β_1 selective or non-selective. β_1 receptors located in heart tissue cause heart activity and function to mimic the actions of the sympathetic nervous system – 'Fight-or-Flight'. Innervation of the sympathetic nervous system would result in increased heart rate and BP. The β_1 receptors found in the sinoatrial node if blocked would result in a decreased heart rate and β_1 receptors in the myocardium decrease contractility. β_1 receptors are also found in the kidneys and blocking these results in inhibition of the release of renin, and so reduction in BP by interfering with the RAAS. Note that β_2 receptors are found in the lung, skeletal muscle and peripheral blood vessels. The therapeutic purpose of using this class of medication is that it decreases heart rate, cardiac output and BP and thus myocardial oxygen demand. Carvedilol and labetalol have the added action of also inhibiting α_1 receptors, further reducing heart rate and BP, thus making them very effective in the management of hypertension. These medications may be administered orally or parentally with a short half-life. When taken orally, some are water soluble, i.e. atenolol, so eliminated by the kidney; whereas labetalol, metoprolol and propranolol are lipid soluble, requiring liver metabolism for clearance.

Clinical considerations for beta-blockers

- Can induce bronchospasm secondary to β_2 activity.
- Bradycardia may occur.
- Patient may report cold hands and feet: this is due to peripheral vasoconstriction.
- Central nervous system effects: vivid dreams and nightmares especially with the lipid soluble preparations.
- Masking of hypoglycaemia in type I insulin dependent diabetics.
- Postural hypotension could lead to a fall with injury.
- Erectile dysfunction is a high possibility and this may lead to non-concordance with the prescribed drug regimen.

Alpha-adrenergic blockers: Alpha blockers

Prazosin, Doxazosin, Terazocin, Indoramin

This class of medication is also known as sympathetic blocking medications, acting by blocking the α_1 receptors in the smaller arteries and arterioles. In their mode of action, they reduce arterial BP. They are usually prescribed in dual therapy for patients with hypertension that is difficult to treat (JFC, 2020). Common side effects with the use of these medications include:

- dry mouth
- drowsiness
- sedation
- severe orthostatic hypotension.

Alpha blockers are well absorbed when taken orally, they undergo extensive hepatic metabolism and are eliminated via the kidneys. This class of medications are cardio-protective as they also have a good effect on lowering total cholesterol, LDL and triglycerides (Pool, 1991).

Clinical considerations with ARBs

- Close monitoring and observation as per NEWS2 as adverse effects are usually related to the first dose resulting in hypotension with reflex tachycardia.
- Take medication at nighttime.
- Monitoring as clinically indicated for renal function and electrolytes as hyperbola.
- Hyperkalaemia may be a potential problem.

Vasodilators

Hydralazine, Minoxidil

These medications are only used in the management of refractory hypertension in combination with beta-blockers and diuretics (JFC, 2020). Their mechanism of action is directly on the small arteries, arterioles and pre-capillary sphincters with resultant marked reduction in BP. The adverse effect is a fall in BP, which is counterproductive as it results in baroreceptor activation and stimulation of the RAAS and so negates the beneficial effects (JFC, 2020). This class of medication results in 'tolerance'. requiring increases in dosage to achieve the desired effect, and thus may not be reliable and is therefore not commonly used for managing long-term hypertension.

Central acting agents
Clonidine, Methyldopa

Indicated for use in refractory hypertension. The mode of action is via the α_2-adrenoreceptors in the brain stem, thereby inhibiting sympathetic outflow which leads to decline in peripheral vascular resistance (JFC, 2020). Adverse effects of clonidine are sedation and drowsiness, this medication is prescribed in highly agitated patients during ventilator weaning in the critical care setting. Methyldopa causes serious immunological problems such as pyrexia and hepatitis; however, it is justified for use in hypertension in pregnancy in the first or middle trimester as it is safe for the foetus and mother (JFC, 2020).

Direct renin inhibitors (DRIs)
Aliskiren

This is a new class of medication and the only DRI licensed for the treatment of hypertension (Jackson and Bellamy, 2015). It competes with angiotensinogen for access to the active site of renin, by doing this it decreases renin activity by 75% as well as reducing levels of angiotensin I and II. It is administered orally and is poorly absorbed, so requires repeated dosing. Elimination is via the biliary system, giving it a long half-life of 24–40 hours (Jackson and Bellamy, 2015). It is indicated for use in essential hypertension either as mono therapy or concomitantly with ACEi and/or angiotensin II receptor antagonist medication (JFC, 2020).

Nitrates will be discussed in the following section.

Episode of care

Mrs. Java, a 70-year-old lady, was admitted to hospital for management of uncontrolled stage 2 hypertension and hyperlipidaemia. Following her four-day hospital stay with medication interventions she is deemed fit for discharge with the following prescribed medications:

Aspirin 75 mg orally per day.
Ramipril 2.5 mg orally per day.
Indapamide 2.5 mg orally in the morning per day.
Atorvastatin 20 mg orally at nighttime.

Mrs. Java lives independently with support from her children, who live nearby. Her daughter Violet is at her bedside awaiting her discharge. Mrs. Java tells her nurse that she has had a lovely conversation with her doctor and agrees with all the medications that have been prescribed. However, she shares her concerns that she has never had to take medications before and is worried that she will forget what they are for and either forget to take them as prescribed or take them incorrectly. Mrs. Java is very anxious about being able to manage her medications safely on her own. The nurse then has a discussion with Mrs. Java and her daughter and offers the following advice:

- Use a multicompartmental medicine box which can be filled for a seven-day period with the help of your daughter Violet.
- Take your medication at a similar time each day. Perhaps taking your medicine in the morning after brushing your teeth and taking your nighttime medication once you retire to bed.
- Keep a journal to record the medicine you have taken. This will enforce learning the names, doses and times that they need to be taken.
- Offering medications information available at www.bhf.org for more information about the medications.
- Follow-up with visits to PN/GP to monitor BP and heart rate at regular intervals.
- If unsure of medication or feeling unwell, visit the local pharmacist for advice and support.

Medications used in managing ischaemic heart disease

- Nitrates: short and long acting.
- CCBs.
- Beta-blockers.
- Hyperpolarisation-activated cyclic nucleotide-gated (HCN) channel blockers.
- Potassium channel activators.
- Antiplatelet drugs.

Angina pectoris, also known as 'angina of effort', is defined as a symptom of ischaemic heart disease. The pathophysiology is a reduction in coronary artery blood flow (Figure 10.1). In most cases this is secondary to narrowing of the coronary arteries as a result of atherosclerosis secondary to hyperlipidaemia. These narrowed coronary arteries are unable to supply adequate blood flow to meet the increased myocardial oxygen demands required to increase heart rate and cardiac output to complete the task or deal with the event. Angina may be classified as stable, unstable or variant (Prinzmetal's angina).

Skills in practice

A tool for helping in the assessment of the patient with chest pain.

May be used as an assessment tool *prior* to administration of medication and *post* administration of medication to evaluate effectiveness.

Using the PQRST pain assessment approach for angina

P = What *provokes* the pain? What activity were you doing?
Q = Describe the *quality* – Is it burning, dull, pressure, heavy or stabbing?
R = Does the pain *radiate* to any other body part?
S = How *severe* is your pain graded on a pain scale of 1–10?
T = How long in *time* does it last and that makes it worse and what relieves it?

Glyceryl trinitrate (GTN)

The body naturally makes the chemical nitrate called nitric oxide, which causes vasodilatation of veins and arteries. In order for the body to compensate for increased oxygen demands required by the heart during periods such as increased physical activity, vasodilation of the coronary arteries affords an increase in blood flow. In people with coronary artery disease, this demand is not easily achieved due to almost fixed diameters of the vessels from the presence of atheroma. Therefore, this natural ability to increase blood flow is not effective.

Soman and Vijayaraghavan (2017) noted that the therapeutic advantages of nitrates include:

- potent coronary artery vasodilator
- reduces preload
- reduces afterload
- reduces myocardial oxygen demand
- reduces platelet aggregation.

GTN is available in several preparations:

- oral: sublingual tablets, aerosol spray
- skin: transdermal application patches and ointment
- parenteral.

Of special note: nitrate use for many patients on long-acting oral or transdermal patches may rapidly develop tachyphylaxis (tolerance) and therefore will experience a diminished response to successive doses. Patients may be advised to have a 'nitrate free period' every 24 hours (JFC, 2020).

Contraindications for nitrates (JFC, 2020)

- Aortic stenosis.
- Hypotension.
- Hypovolaemia.
- Marked anaemia.
- Mitral stenosis.
- Brain injury with raised intracranial pressure.

203

Sublingual tablets

Administered sublingually, these have a rapid onset within 60 seconds and last for 5–30 minutes (JFC, 2020). Patients with stable angina may choose to use sublingual tablets as required as they may anticipate that doing exercise or a particular activity will provoke their chest pain. They must not be swallowed as GTN will be absorbed by the blood vessels and enter the liver, where it will be broken down rapidly. The first-pass effect results in insufficient amounts of active drug being available to treat the angina episode.

Safe storage and care of medication for patients taking sublingual GTN tablets

- Tablets have a short shelf life and deteriorate as soon as the bottle is opened.
- Date the bottle and discard as per the instructions.
- Withhold hoarding several open bottles.
- Keep the bottle tightly sealed to protect from air.

Metered aerosol GTN spray

This preparation is sprayed under the tongue. This method of absorption is quick and highly effective as the area under the tongue is highly vascular and so efficient in absorbing the drug rapidly. This preparation is commonly used in acute care settings, e.g. urgent care centres (UCC) and accident and emergency departments (ED).

Transdermal patches of GTN

In patients requiring a constant dose of GTN, patches may be prescribed. The impregnated GTN provides a time-released method of dosing.

Clinical considerations

GTN transdermal patches
- If appropriate, shave the area where the pad is to be applied.
- Apply new patch first THEN remove the old patch.
- Avoid touching the patch or getting any adhesive on fingers.
- Avoid placing pad on skin that is irritated or damaged, i.e. scar or in between skin folds.
- Apply patch on upper arms or chest.
- Remove used patch and dispose of it safely as residual medication may harm others or pets.

GTN ointment

This is an ointment preparation which is applied to the skin every three to four hours as required by the patient. This may be applied to the skin of the chest, arm or thigh and then the ointment is covered with a surgical tape.

Parenteral (intravenous) GTN

Administered only in an acute care setting providing continuous BP and ECG monitoring. Indicated for use if the patient is in a serious clinical state, such as unstable angina with impending acute myocardial infarction.

Isosorbide dinitrate and isosorbide mononitrate

These medications are classified as long-acting nitrates used in the management of stable angina. Isosorbide dinitrate orally has low plasma levels as it goes through extensive first-pass hepatic metabolism (70–80%) (Soman and Vijayaraghávan, 2017).

It is converted to its active mononitrate form in the liver and eliminated via the kidneys. Food intake inhibits the absorption. Isosorbide mononitrate has a 100% bioavailability with a half-life of four to six hours. The benefit of this formulation is that is does not undergo hepatic metabolism.

Potassium channel activators

Nicorandil

This medication is indicated as a second-line treatment and prophylaxis for stable angina (JFC, 2020). It works as a potassium channel opener with nitrovasodilator properties acting on arterial and venous beds. Its mechanism is dual action, increasing coronary artery dilation as well reducing preload and afterload (Tarkin, 2018). It is administered in oral preparation, being well absorbed from the gastrointestinal tract with a bioavailability of around 75%. It undergoes extensive hepatic metabolism and is eliminated by the kidneys. Serious side effects are on the skin, mucosa of the gastrointestinal tract and eye ulceration.

Other medications for the management of angina are: CCBs, BB, HCN channel blockers and antiplatelet medications.

Medications used for cardiac arrhythmias

Anti-arrhythmic medications may be required in conditions where the heart muscle may be damaged as a result of ischaemic heart disease or an acute myocardial infarction and therefore is unable to effect a normal rhythm and rate. In health, the electrical conduction system is dependent on neural and endocrine controls, adequate amounts of adenosine triphosphate (ATP), oxygen and electrolytes to maintain normal electrochemical gradients. This then results in nodal and non-nodal action potentials that produce a rhythmical, coordinated, regular rhythm of atrial and ventricular contraction followed by relaxation. In diseased or metabolic states, patients may experience an arrhythmia that may result in negative effects on their circulation and BP, so the patient will need to receive anti-arrhythmic medications to correct the rhythm. See Figure 10.2a and b, depicting the conducting system of the heart.

Disorders of heart rhythm and rate

Explanations of algorithms are beyond the scope of this chapter; please refer to the Resuscitation Council (UK) Peri-arrest arrhythmias (www.resus.org.uk).

(a)

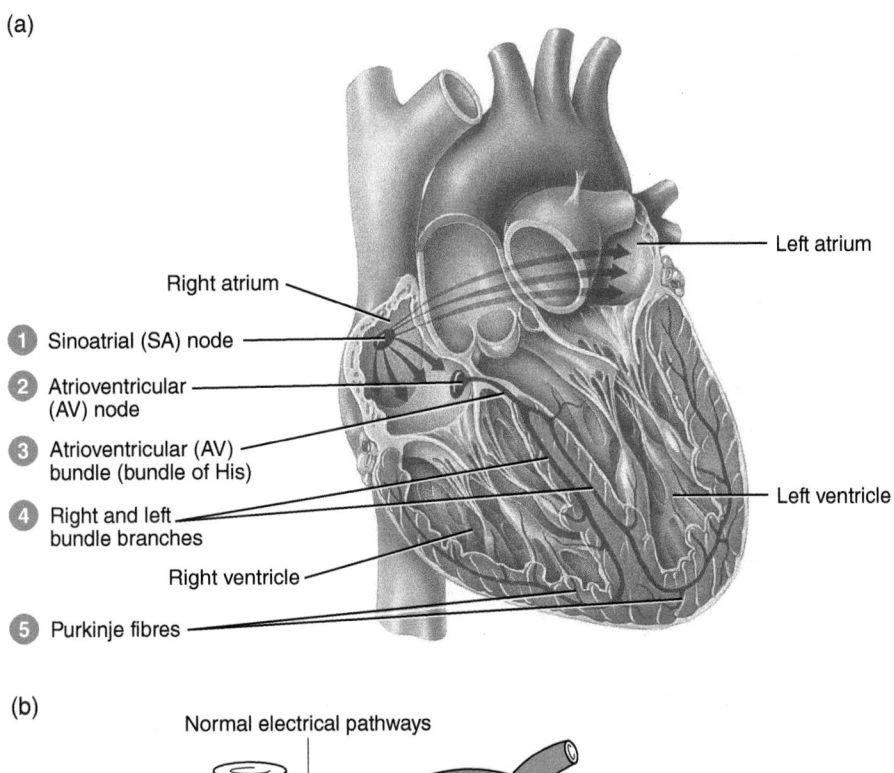

Left atrium

Right atrium

1 Sinoatrial (SA) node

2 Atrioventricular (AV) node

3 Atrioventricular (AV) bundle (bundle of His)

Left ventricle

4 Right and left bundle branches

Right ventricle

5 Purkinje fibres

(b)

Normal electrical pathways

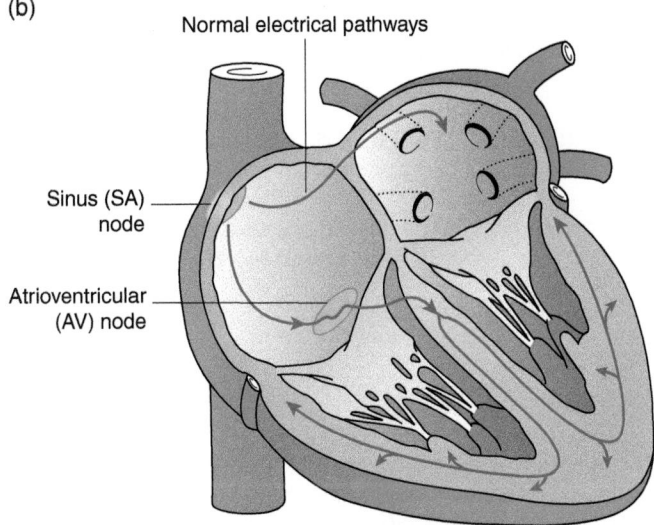

Sinus (SA) node

Atrioventricular (AV) node

Figure 10.2   (a) The conducting system of the heart. (b) Normal electrical conduction. Source: Peate and Nair (2017) (2nd Ed) Fundamentals of A+P.

Atrial fibrillation (AF)

Atrial fibrillation is defined as when the atria beat in an uncoordinated fashion producing an irregularly irregular rhythm. It is potentially a dangerous rhythm as it may lead to emboli being sent into the aorta with subsequent migration up into the cerebral blood vessels, resulting in a stroke. This arrhythmia decreases the cardiac output by as much as 20–25% and in the long term may lead to heart failure.

Amiodarone

Amiodarone is classified as an anti-arrhythmic medication with 'broad spectrum' properties as it is effective for both supra ventricular and ventricular arrhythmias. Amiodarone acts by prolonging the short period before each contraction of the heart during the time when the muscle will not respond to any stimulus (refractory period). It decreases sinoatrial node automaticity, atrioventricular node conduction speed, as well as inhibits ectopic pacemaker automaticity. Intravenous administration requires an infusion via a pump with rate and dose control. Taken orally it undergoes extensive enterohepatic circulation, thus having a poor bioavailability with only about 50% of the dose being absorbed. This medication has a long half-life of about 58 days and is eliminated primarily by hepatic metabolism and biliary excretion. It has a large volume of distribution; it is stored in adipose tissue, muscle, liver, lungs and skin, and thus it may take days of dosing to reach a steady state. Special precautions are to be considered as it contains a high concentration of iodine so may cause both hypothyroidism and thyrotoxicosis. Amiodarone has several drug interactions as it inhibits the action of cytochrome P450 that metabolises medications such as cyclosporine, flecainide, diltiazem, phenytoin and simvastatin, and thus may lead to accumulative effects resulting in potential toxicity.

Clinical considerations

Amiodarone
- Concomitant use with digoxin may lead to a severe bradycardia.
- Monitoring as per appointment planning with PN/GP for blood prothrombin time (PT) and international normalised ratio (INR) if they are also taking warfarin.
- Take the drug with a meal, as this is a lipid soluble drug, thus making absorption better.
- Advise the patient to seek medical attention for any of the following side effects: cough, pyrexia, chills, dyspnoea, epigastric discomfort, chest pain or noted jaundice of their eyes, skin and dark-coloured urine.
- Monitoring as per planned appointment with PN/GP for thyroid function tests.
- Long-term adverse effects are related to pulmonary fibrosis, so six-monthly chest X-rays may also be warranted.

Digoxin

This is a cardiac glycoside, used predominantly in patients with heart failure and AF. It has direct action on the heart to increase contractility and ejection fraction; in doing this, it reduces preload and backward failure of the heart which leads to pulmonary congestion. This medication may be therapeutic in patients with chronic heart failure. It also works indirectly to decrease heart rate via activation of the parasympathetic nervous system via the vagus nerve. Following oral administration, about 70–80% is absorbed in the small intestine affording sufficient bioavailability. It has a half-life of 36 hours and produces no active metabolites. Digoxin is widely distributed in the body and is able to cross the blood–brain barrier. Importantly, digoxin has a low therapeutic index; therefore, it is potentially toxic at a slightly higher plasma concentration (Table 10.5). Digoxin dosage requires adjustment in patients with kidney impairment as it is eliminated via the kidneys. Alternatively, Digitoxin may be used as it has a similar mode of action, exhibits an almost triple half-life and is eliminated via the liver.

Clinical considerations

Digoxin
- Always check the patients pulse prior to administration. Never administer if heart rate is less than 60 beats per minute.
- Potentially toxic, therefore requires monitoring of blood levels to ensure safe therapeutic range is achieved. Normal blood test therapeutic range is between 1–2.6 mmol/l.
- Remember that concomitant diuretic therapy reduces potassium levels.
- Digoxin and potassium compete for the same receptors in the cardiac muscle tissue, so if potassium levels are low, digoxin will bind and thus become more toxic; ensure normal serum potassium levels prior to administration.
- Medication interactions with verapamil, diltiazem and amiodarone.
- Know the signs of overdosage and toxicity.
- Advise the patient that simultaneous food intake slows absorption and meals high in fibre decrease absorption.

Table 10.5   Digoxin overdose and toxicity.

Signs and symptoms	Cause and action
Heart rate less than 60 beats per minute	Excessive effect on the sinoatrial node or conducting system. Dose needs to be omitted and reviewed by medical team.
Nausea which may or may not be associated with vomiting	Stimulation of brain's vomiting centre in the medulla. Escalate concern to senior staff.
Coloured vision – yellow halos	A sign of overdose. Escalate concern to senior staff.
New onset confusion	Seen commonly in the older adult patient. Escalate concern to senior staff.
Ectopic beats on palpation: double beat followed by a pause.	Increased ventricular excitability. May result in a lethal rhythm so dose needs to be omitted. Escalate concern to senior staff.
Complete heart block	Can only be identified on ECG.

Magnesium sulphate

An electrolyte often used in the management of atrial fibrillation. Magnesium is the second most common intracellular cation and possesses electrophysiological effects that reduce ventricular conduction as well as inhibition of early and late depolarisations (Lundin et al., 2015). Myocardial cell action potentials are mediated by $Na+$, $K+$ and $Ca++$ channels and if these are altered it may lead to arrhythmias. The role of magnesium is to regulate the movement of these ions, thus making it anti-arrhythmic in action (Barker, 2016).

Arrhythmias due to conduction defects

Atrioventricular nodal block may result if the bundle of His fails to transmit the electrical impulse from the atria to the ventricles. The rate is slow and results in profound symptomatic hypotension. If left untreated, it may precipitate heart failure, so often requires interventions with medications and or artificial pacing to maintain the rhythm making it adequate for cardiac output. This may be in a clinical scenario, such as post acute myocardial infarction, where a patient may develop a bradycardia with associated hypotension.

Atropine sulphate

It is classified as an antiparasympathetic or anticholinergic medication. Its mode of action is to inhibit parasympathetic innervation and it thus affords pre-existing sympathetic innervation to predominate. The action results in increased heart rate and cardiac output. It is indicated for use in symptomatic bradycardia in the absence of reversible causes. It may only be administered in intravenous or intraosseous routes to a maximum dosage of 3 mg in the adult patient. It is metabolised in the liver and excreted in the urine.

Common side effects of atropine

- Tachycardia.
- Skin flushing due to its action on sweat glands with resultant increase in body temperature.
- Xerostomia due to it blocking action on the parasympathetic system to produce saliva.
- Cycloplegia, which is paralysis of the accommodation reflex of the eye so the patient will have loss of normal vision.
- Disorientation and confusion results from atropine's ability to cross the blood–brain barrier.
- Anhidrosis, especially in high-risk groups of patients such as the older adult.

Medications used in the management of heart failure

Chronic heart failure develops over months or years. It is regarded as a complex clinical syndrome; cardiac output is insufficient to meet metabolic demands. Infarcted heart tissue post acute myocardial infarction does not contribute positively to efficient mechanical pumping action of the heart and the non-infarcted areas of the heart have extra work to do, reducing the heart's overall performance. It readapts to the situation and may either dilate or hypertrophy. The end result of these mechanisms leads to cardiac remodelling, fluid retention, decreased contractility, tachyarrhythmias and decreased cardiac output, known as backward and forward failure of the heart. These compensatory mechanisms are innervation of the RAAS, natriuretic peptide system, sympathomimetic nervous system, parasympathetic activation, vasopressin and other endothelial pathways (Jackson et al., 2000); these form the framework for pharmacological interventions. The clinical picture of cardiac failure is represented in Figure 10.3.

The aetiology of chronic heart failure is most commonly secondary to coronary artery disease, long standing hypertension, or myocardial infarction. Other causes include valvular disease or congenital defects, or infections from bacteria or viruses leading to myocarditis (Zairian and Fonarow, 2016). Further to these, pathologies and non-cardiac conditions such as hyperthyroidism, diabetes and kidney failure compound the problem and worsen the prognosis. In the UK, heart failure is categorised by using the functional classification according to the New York Heart Association (NYHA), American Heart Association (2019).

Pharmacological approaches to managing patients with chronic heart failure are aimed at reducing their risk for death, relieving their symptoms, improving exercise tolerance, as well as reducing incidence of acute exacerbations, e.g. pulmonary oedema (Lainscak et al., 2015).

Medications used in heart failure

1. Controlling excessive fluid: diuretics.
2. Reducing the heart's workload: CCBs, ARBs, ACEi, amiodarone, beta 1 blockers, anticoagulants.
3. Optimising the contractility of the heart: digoxin and nitrates.

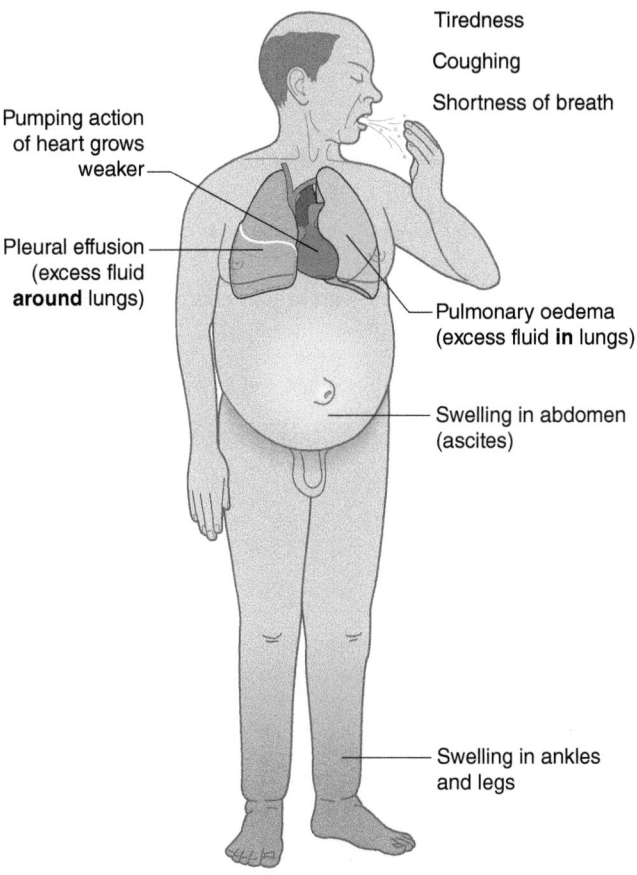

Tiredness

Coughing

Shortness of breath

Pumping action
of heart grows
weaker

Pleural effusion
(excess fluid
around lungs)

Pulmonary oedema
(excess fluid **in** lungs)

Swelling in abdomen
(ascites)

Swelling in ankles
and legs

Figure 10.3 Clinical picture of cardiac failure. Source: Peate and Wild (2018) Nursing Practice Knowledge and Care (2nd Ed).

Controlling Excessive Fluid

Loop diuretics and mineralocorticoid receptors antagonist (MRAs).
Diuretics are prescribed to treat and prevent the symptoms of:

- peripheral oedema
- ascites
- anasarca
- pleural effusion.

The choice of the type of diuretic depends on the clinical needs of the patient. Diuretic therapy is aimed at achieving euvolaemia, this is the patients 'dry weight' (Casu and Merella, 2015). This will maintain a steady reduction in intravascular volume ensuring reduction in preload and afterload, which reduces myocardial workload, improves contractility of the heart, improves cardiac output, as well as reducing the pulmonary/systemic congestion that occurs due to oedema. Recall that heart failure patients have a low cardiac output state due to the secondary ineffective pumping action of the heart that leads to the activation of the RAAS, thus causing increased sodium and water retention by the kidneys as a compensatory mechanism. Furosemide is generally a first-line of diuretic therapy prescribed; however, if the patient becomes resistant and non-responsive, bumetanide or torasemide may be prescribed. Long-term use of loop diuretics leads to structural adaptations in the distal nephron causing non-responsiveness (Sica, 2015). Therefore, these other loop diuretics are more potent, and have a longer half-life and increased bioavailability of around 90%.

Mineralocorticoid receptors antagonist (MRAs)
Spironolactone, Eplerenone

These are potassium-sparing diuretics, with a mechanism of action as aldosterone receptor antagonists. Their action is at the cortical collecting duct to reduce water and sodium absorption. Sodium absorption is minimal, therefore they are not efficacious in their diuretic effect; however, due to their potassium-sparing ability, they may be used in combination with other diuretics (Casu and Merella, 2015). Diuretic therapy in this patient group may lead to major negative adverse effects such as hypotension, electrolyte imbalance and further renal compromise.

Reducing the workload of the heart

Beta blockers.
ACEi.
ARBs.
HCN channel blockers.
MRAs.
Angiotensin receptor neprilysin inhibitors.

Hyperpolarisation-activated cyclic nucleotide-gated (HCN) channel blockers
Ivabradine

This medication blocks the channel responsible for the normal cardiac pacemaker current, which is responsible for regulating the heart rate (Tser and Mazzola, 2015). This provides a reduction in heart rate with a prolonged diastolic time, thus decreasing the workload of the heart. The therapeutic benefit is reduction in arrhythmias, which occur secondary to cardiac hypertrophy (Badu-Boateng and Hammersley, 2018). It is taken in oral preparation, without food and reaches peak concentration in one hour with a bioavailability about 40%. It is bound to plasma on absorption and has a half-life of 11 hours. It is metabolised in the liver and eliminated equally in the urine and faeces.

Clinical considerations

Ivabradine
- Monitor patient for adverse effects such as syncope, vertigo, hypotension, diplopia, erythema, rash and pruritis.
- Closely observe for signs on angioedema.
- *NOTE contraindication for administration in patients with:*
- BP <90/50 mmHg.
- Bradycardia – sick sinus rhythm, third-degree heart block unless they have a pacemaker.
- Medication interactions with Verapamil and Diltiazem.

210

Angiotensin receptor neprilysin inhibitors

Sacubitril

Heart failure exacerbations may be as a the result of the activation of the natriuretic peptide system, which results in an elevated B-type natriuretic peptide (BNP) and N-terminal pro-hormone B-Type natriuretic peptide (NT-pro BNP). Sacubitril is indicated for use in this patient group (Ayalasomayajula et al., 2017). This class of medication is used in patients with a reduced ejection fraction and the mechanism of action is to inhibit neprilysin and angiotensin I and II. It improves contractility and reduces afterload. Its formulation is as a combination product also containing valsartan (ARB). It is administered via oral preparation with rapid plasma concentrations achieved within two hours. It takes up to three days to reach a therapeutic steady-state. The half-life is around 12 hours. It is eliminated via the kidneys and faeces.

Optimising contractility of the heart

Cardiac glycosides: Digoxin.
Nitrates: short and long acting.

Lastly, antiplatelet and anticoagulant medications used in heart failure will be discussed in the following part of this chapter.

Medications that affect haemostasis

In this last section, we will explore the role of medications that act on coagulation, thus preventing thrombosis which is a potential risk factor associated with cardiovascular diseases. A thrombosis is classified as a pathological clot formation that occurs when haemostasis is excessively activated in the absence of any bleeding (Rasche, 2001). In health, people have a well-regulated haemodynamic system that keeps blood free from clots in the vessels while simultaneously providing the important formation of localised clots if there is an injury to the blood vessel. This process of haemostasis is very complex; it is a natural process that occurs in order to stop blood loss when an injury occurs.

However, in non-traumatic injury, such as when the endothelium is injured as a result of disease, for example, atherosclerosis increases the risk of thrombi development. When the barrier of the endothelium becomes dysfunctional, it predisposes the vessel to vascular lesions, vasoconstriction, inflammation, plaque rupture and thrombosis. Therefore, it is viewed as an important prognostic marker for all the cardiovascular events that have been described in the context of pharmacological interventions within this chapter. Barthelmes et al. (2017) further highlight that cardiovascular protective medications, healthy nutrition and lifestyle changes all ameliorate endothelial dysfunction.

Thrombosis may be characterised by the uncontrolled extension of clots that occlude blood vessels as a result of:

- Genetic or acquire hypercoagulability.
- Injury to the endothelium – hyperlipidaemias and hypertension.
- Abnormal blood flow through the vessels – increased turbulence to stasis associated with atherosclerosis, valvular heart disease, arrhythmias and heart failure.

Classes:

- Antiplatelet medications.
- Anticoagulants.
- Thrombolytics.
- Phosphodiesterase inhibitors.

Antiplatelet medications
Aspirin

This medication is classified as a cyclooxygenase inhibitor as it blocks thromboxane A2-dependant platelet aggregation, inhibiting the formation of thrombi (Gale, 2011). It is a weak acid absorbed in the acid environment of the stomach. Most of the absorption from aspirin occurs on the large surface area of the microvilli contained in the ileum. It is metabolised by the esterases of the plasma and mostly in the liver to salicylate. Aspirin is not advocated by either SIGN or NICE for use in primary prevention, but for secondary prevention in the management of patients with established cardiovascular disease (Patrono and Baigent, 2019). It may also be administered as an emergency intervention in unstable angina and acute myocardial infarction. If patients have the risk factor for developing gastrointestinal bleeding, then a proton pump inhibitor will concurrently be prescribed (see Chapter 14). Aspirin is contraindicated in patients with active peptic ulcer disease, bleeding disorders, children under the age of 16 years (risk of Reye's syndrome this is severe liver and or brain damage) and those with haemophilia (JFC, 2020).

Clinical considerations

Aspirin
- Special precautions in existing allergic disease such as asthma.
- Should be taken with a meal to reduce gastrointestinal side effects.
- Note that aspirin is also classed as a NSAID agent.
- May be administered as a rectal suppository in emergency situations.

Clopidogrel, Prasugrel and Ticagrelor

This group of medications are called oral thienopyridines. Their mechanism of action is to block P2Y12 receptors, thereby inhibiting the adenosine diphosphate(ADP-)dependent platelet activation pathways and thus prolonging bleeding time (Damman et al., 2012). They can be prescribed as a monotherapy in patients allergic to aspirin or dual therapy.

Dipyridamole

A phosphodiesterase inhibitor blocking the metabolism and uptake of adenosine by the erythrocytes and vascular endothelial cells, resulting in inhibiting platelet aggregation. It is mostly only prescribed as an adjunct with other anticoagulants for the prophylaxis of thromboembolism associated with prosthetic heart valves, as well as secondary prevention of ischaemic stroke (JFC, 2020).

Glycoprotein 11b/111a inhibitors
Abciximab, Eptifibatide, Tirofiban

These medications inhibit platelet adhesion by binding the glycoprotein IIb/IIIa receptors on the plasma membranes of the platelets. They are indicated and administered intravenously in acute coronary syndromes, i.e. acute myocardial infarction and elective PCI. This class of medications is used in specialised areas only.

Overall clinical considerations for antiplatelet medications:

- Advise patients on self-care: to brush their teeth with a soft toothbrush to limit gum bleeding.
- Shave with an electric razor.
- Avoid contact sports.
- Ensure they inform medical providers that they are taking antiplatelet medications, especially their dentist.
- Always check with PN/GP before taking other medications, e.g. NSAIDs and over-the-counter medications, as well as herbal remedies.

Anticoagulants

Anticoagulants inhibit the formation of clots as well as the extension of the clot size; this is critical in circumstances such as an acute myocardial infarction and also to prevent deep vein thrombosis. Their focus of action is to interfere with the coagulation phase of haemostasis.

Unfractionated heparin.
Low molecular weight heparins (LMWH).
Vitamin K inhibitors: warfarin.
Direct factor Xa inhibitors: apixaban.

Heparin

Heparin is a complex acidic mixture of substances found naturally in the body, contained within the mast cells and basophils needed for normal haemostasis. It has been used for the prevention and management of thrombosis for decades (Thrombosis Advisor for Healthcare Professionals, 2019). Heparin has a major anticoagulant effect in the body occurring from binding to antithrombin III, this leads to prolonging the clotting time and thus preventing clot formation.

Heparin is found in two preparations:

- unfractionated
- LMWH.

Unfractionated heparin binds to antithrombin III (ATIII) causing inactivation of factors IIa and Xa as well as IX, XI, XII and plasmin, thereby preventing extension of existing clots as well as further clotting. The use of intravenous heparin, therefore, will only be in specialised areas of clinical practice.

Low molecular weight fragments of heparin (LMWH)
Fondaparin, Tinzaparin, Dalterapin, Enoxaparin

The mechanism of action of LMWH is to bind to antithrombin III, a protease inhibitor that forms a complex with activated clotting factors (II, IX, X and XI). It is administered as a subcutaneous injection at a dosing interval with almost 90% bioavailability. Therapeutic indications may be for emergent clinical needs, i.e. massive deep vein thrombosis, post acute myocardial infarction or prior to cardioversion. LMWHs are also indicated for use in reducing hospital-acquired deep vein thrombosis or pulmonary embolism (NICE, 2018)

Vitamin K inhibitors
Warfarin

Warfarin is taken in oral preparation on a long-term basis in patients with deep vein thrombosis, atrial fibrillation, prosthetic heart valves or following an acute myocardial infarction (Xu, 2014). Its mechanism of action is to interfere with the synthesis of vitamin K and thereby inhibit the activation of vitamin K-dependent clotting factor (II, VII, IX and X). It has a narrow therapeutic index, so requires regular INR levels to be taken. It is 99% bound to plasma proteins and eliminated by the liver. On oral administration, it has a rapid onset with gastrointestinal complete absorption within 60 minutes. It is prescribed in small daily doses and then adjusted according to the PT and this may take up to seven days. Patients who are taking warfarin need vigilant monitoring as this medication has a long half-life and narrow therapeutic range, it often leads to iatrogenic hospital admissions (Burn and Pirmohamed, 2018).

Clinical considerations

Warfarin
- Most serious adverse effect is haemorrhage.
- Interactions with Aspirin, Cimetidine and Phenytoin.
- Avoid foods high in Vitamin K.
- Avoid herbal supplements.
- Advise to carry an 'Anticoagulant Alert Card'.

Direct-acting oral anticoagulants (DOACs)
Dabigatran, Rivaroxaban, Apixaban, Edoxaban

These medications are regarded as a safer alternative to Warfarin due to their advantage of posing less risk for major bleeding (Burn and Pirmonamad, 2018; Vinogradova et al., 2018). Apixaban directly inhibits factor Xa and thereby decreases clot generation and thrombus formation; furthermore, it inhibits free and clot-bound Xa which inhibit clot growth. It is administered orally and is rapidly absorbed mainly by small intestine, bound by protein, with a bioavailability of 50%, as it is not influenced by food intake. First-pass metabolism is via the gut and liver. Onset of action is three to four hours with a half-life of around 12 hours. Elimination occurs via multiple pathways including metabolism, direct excretion via the intestines, biliary excretion and renal. Different preparations are prescribed for specific clinical conditions and each have special clinical considerations (Table 10.6).

The thrombolytics

Thrombolytics are a group of medications that promote breaking down of the fibrin that binds the clot. This is necessary to re-establish the blood flow in an occluded vessel occurring in diseases such as an acute myocardial infarction; this process is called fibrinolysis and is initiated by the activation of plasminogen to plasmin. Plasmin is then responsible for degrading the fibrin so that the vessel lumen becomes patent (Stringer, 2017). Use of these medications is usually seen in specialised areas such as A&E, CCU or ITU.

Table 10.6   Differences in DOACs indications and clinical considerations.

DOACs	Indications	Clinical Considerations
Apixaban	Thromboprophylaxis for hip or knee replacement surgery Stroke prevention with AF	• May be crushed or added to water to be administered via enteral feeding tubes
Dabigatran	Thromboprophylaxis for hip or knee replacement surgery Stroke prevention with AF	• Large capsules containing tartaric acid to increase solubility of the active ingredient, so need to swallow capsule whole • Keep capsules in aluminium foil to protect from moisture • Not easy for those with poor manual dexterity
Rivaroxaban	Thromboprophylaxis for hip or knee replacement surgery Stroke prevention with AF Treatment of DVT and PE Prevention of recurrent DVT and PE	• May be crushed or added to water to be administered via enteral feeding tubes

Source: British Society for Haematology (2018).

- First generation: Streptokinase, Urokinase.
- Second generation: tissue plasminogen activator (tPA): Alteplase, Reteplase, Tenecteplase.

First generation: Streptokinase

This works by converting all plasminogen to plasmin throughout the plasma resulting in systemic fibrinogenolysis with a marked increased in bleeding (Greenstein, 2009).

Second generation: Tissue plasminogen activator (tPA)
Alteplase, Reteplase, Tenecteplase

This second generation of thrombolytics is designed to selectively activate only the plasminogen that is bound to fibrin.

Medications used in peripheral vascular disease
Phosphodiesterase inhibitors
Cilostazol

Peripheral arterial occlusive disease is caused by either an inflammatory process or atherosclerotic lesions. The stenosis results in limb ischemia due to reduced distal artery blood flow manifesting in intermittent claudication, leaving the person unable to mobilise. Cilostazol, a phosphodiesterase inhibitor, acts as an antiplatelet agent as well as reducing calcium-induced contractions to enhance vasodilation, thus improving peripheral blood flow (JFC, 2020). It is only indicated for use in persons who do not have any pain at rest or peripheral tissue necrosis. It well absorbed taken orally, and has a long half-life of 11–13 hours, It is a protein bound, metabolised extensively in the liver and excreted mainly in the urine (about 70%) with a small percentage in the faeces (30%).

Medications used in cardiac arrest
Oxygen, Adrenaline, Amiodarone

Cardiac arrest is defined as a cessation of normal blood circulation due to the failure of the heart muscle to contract. This may also be called sudden cardiac death (SCD) (Resus Council UK, 2015).

The aetiology of SCD is:

- coronary artery disease
- cardiomyopathies
- valvular heart disease
- Brugada syndrome
- catecholaminergic polymorphic ventricular tachycardia
- congenital heart disease.

As nurses and healthcare workers, you will have undertaken training to establish proficiency in basic life support (BLS). Knowledge of the advanced life support algorithm is an essential skill as every clinical area has emergency equipment and medications to be used in cardiac arrest.

Oxygen

A lack of oxygen is detrimental to the heart and brain as these organs are not able to survive for more than a few minutes. The heart does not adequately store oxygen or substrates due to its high metabolic rate, thus making it totally dependent of a continuous delivery to overt myocardial ischemia. During resuscitation, 100% oxygen is administered to the person via manual ventilations using a bag-valve-mask-reservoir device until a definitive airway is placed in the trachea. Administration of oxygen via manual ventilations during chest compressions is crucial in order to re-oxygenate the myocardium and achieve return of spontaneous circulation (ROSC) (Angelos, 2010).

Adrenaline

Adrenaline is a natural stimulant produced by the adrenal glands becoming activated, and is released in response to sympathetic system innervation; this is the 'Flight – Fight' response. It is indicated in cardiac arrest situations for use in ventricular fibrillation, pulseless ventricular tachycardia and asystole. It may be administered intravenously or intraosseously. Adrenaline is classed as an α_1-adrenoreceptor agonist; when administered during heart compressions, it increases arterial BP which in turn increases coronary artery perfusion and cerebral perfusion pressure with the aim to achieve ROSC (Gough and Nolan, 2018).

Amiodarone

This is indicated for use in a cardiac arrest situation for managing ventricular fibrillation and pulseless ventricular tachycardia, administered intravenously or intraosseously. It is an effective medication terminating the ventricular arrhythmia as well as preventing its recurrence after ROSC (Van Herendael and Dorian, 2010).

Pharmacological interventions: The future

Reflecting on the burden of cardiovascular disease and its associated complications, not only in the UK but worldwide, it is evident that it is ever increasing in its severity as well as incidence – the major causes being mostly related to the lifestyle behaviour described by the WHO (2019). Thus, cardiovascular disease prevention appears to be somewhat inadequate. This may possibly be due to professional non-adherence to guidelines, increasing costs of medications and patients' non-adherence to treatment regimens (Sanz and Fuster, 2012); therefore, it has caused the advent of a new formulation of medication offering a fixed dose combination therapy: these are the 'polypills'. These medications are aimed at primary and secondary prevention of cardiovascular disease in high-risk patient groups (Roshandel et al., 2019). The high-risk population groups living in low-income to middle-income countries – where mortality and morbidity are highest – are the target for this intervention. Some examples are: Aspirin, Enalapril, Atorvastatin and Hydrochlorothiazide. Furthermore, Cimmaruta et al. (2018) emphasise that this approach used as a medication intervention demonstrates increased concordance with concomitant risk factor reductions.

Conclusion

This chapter has provided cardinal knowledge of cardiovascular system pharmacology related to common disease processes. Nurses and healthcare workers are pivotal in their roles in the custodianship as well as administration of medications in their responsibilities in caring for patients, ensuring patients are at the centre of all that is done. Medications management does not simply require only the task of applying the approach of the 'rights of medication administration'; it necessitates a good foundation knowledge of pharmacology. Ensuring patient safety and efficacy of pharmacological interventions involves the integration of pharmacokinetic and pharmacodynamic principles into clinical practice (Durham, 2015). Therefore, it requires critical thinking with the resultant formulation of clinical judgments; this in practice is knowing the person's health problems/needs and ensuring that the medication administered is not only safe but serves these needs. The intention of this chapter was to provide an overview of fundamental knowledge that will create a good basis for the understanding of cardiovascular system medications in order to provide the nurse and healthcare worker with a framework on which to build. The broader picture of this chapter on pharmacology knowledge is that it will also influence patient autonomy, agreement, self-efficacy, concordance and regulation of symptoms of the disease through the provision of evidenced-based considerations, advice and health education. The aim of this chapter is to inspire, motivate and encourage you to further develop in expanding your knowledge, skills, proficiency and confidence in safer medicines management.

References

American Heart Association (AHA) (2019). Classes of heart failure. http://www.heart.org/HEARTORG/ Conditions/HeartFailure/AboutHeartFailure/Classes-of-Heat-Failure_UCM_306328_Article.jsp#. XbBCmC2ZNsM (accessed July 2020).

Angelos, M.G. (2010). The role of oxygen in cardiac arrest resuscitation. *Signa Vitae* 5(S1): 28–31. doi: 10.22514/SV51.092010.6.

Ayalasomayajula, S., Langenickel, T., Pal, P. et al. (2017). Clinical pharmacokinetics of Sacubitril/valsartan (LCZ696): a novel angiotensin receptor-neprilysin inhibitor. *Journal of Clinical Pharmacokinetics* 56 (12): 1461–1478.

ASSIGN. http://www.assign-score.com/about/beginners/ (accessed October 2020)

Badu-Boateng, C. and Hammersley, D. (2018). The therapeutic role of ivabradine in heart failure. *Journal of Therapeutic Advances in Chronic Diseases* 9 (11): 199–207.

Bakris, G.L. (2008). Slowing nephropathy progression: focus on proteinuria reduction. *Clinical Journal of American Society of Nephrologists* 3 (suppl 1): S3–S10. doi: 10.2215/CJN.03250807.

Bakris, G., Waleed, A., and Parati, G. (2019). ACC/AHA versus ESC/ESH on hypertension guidelines *JACC* guideline comparison. *Journal of the American College of Cardiology (JACC)* 73 (23). doi: 10.1016/j. jacc.2019.03.507.

Barker, W.L. (2016). Treating arrhythmias with adjunctive magnesium: identifying future research directions. *European Heart Journal – Cardiovascular Pharmacotherapy* 3 (2): 108–117. https://doi. org/10.1093/ehjcvp/pvw028.

Barthelmes, J., Matthias, P., Nägele, V.L. et al. (2017). Endothelial dysfunction in cardiovascular disease and Flammer syndrome—similarities and differences. *The EPMA Journal* 8 (2): 99–109. doi: 10.1007/ s13167-017-0099-1.

Begg, A. (2016). Top tips: hypertension. Guidelines in practice. Supporting implementation of best practice. www.guidelinesinpractice.co.uk (accessed July 2020).

Bergheanu, S.C., Bodde, M.C., and Jukeman, J.W. (2017). Pathophysiology and treatment of atherosclerosis. Current view and future perspective on lipoprotein modification treatment. *Netherlands Heart Journal* 25 (4): 231–242.

Bolivar, J. (2013). Essential hypertension: an approach to its etiology and neurogenic pathophysiology. *International Journal of Hypertension.* https://doi.org/10.1155/2013/547809 (accessed 9 December 2013).

British Heart Foundation (BHF) (2019). Statistics. www.bhf.org.uk/statistics (accessed July 2020).

British Society for Haematology (2018). DOACs a safe alternative to warfarin. https://b-s-h.org.uk/about-us/news/doacs-a-safe-alternative-to-warfarin/ (accessed July 2020).

Burn, J. and Pirmohamed, M. (2018). Direct oral anticoagulants versus warfarin: is new always better than old? *British Medical Journal Open Heart* 1 (5). http://dx.doi.org/10.1136/openhrt-2017-000712.

Casu, G. and Merella, P. (2015). Diuretic therapy in heart failure – current approaches. *European Cardiology Review* 10 (1): 42–47. https://doi.org/10.15420/ecr.2015.10.01.42.

Cimmaruta, D., Lombardi, N., Borghi, C. et al. (2018). Polypill, hypertension and medication adherence: the solution strategy? *International Journal of Cardiology* 1 (252): 181–186.

Damman, P., Woudstra, P., Kuijit, W.J. et al. (2012). P2Y12 platelet inhibition in clinical practice. *Journal of Thrombosis and Thrombolysis* 33: 143–153.

Diabetes UK (2019). Metabolic syndrome. www.diabetes.co.uk/diabetes-and-metabolic-syndrome.html (accessed July 2020).

Durham, P. (2015). The nurse's role in medication safety. *Nursing2019* 45 (4): 1–4. https://doi.org/10.1097/01.NURSE.0000461850.24153.8b.

Frostegard, J. (2013). Immunity, atherosclerosis and cardiovascular disease. *BMC Medicine* 11: 117. https://doi.org/10.1186/1741-7015-11-117.

Gale, A.J. (2011). Current understanding of hemostasis. HHS Public Access. doi: https://doi.org/10.1177/0192623310389474.

Gough, J.R. and Nolan, J.P. (2018). The role of adrenaline in cardiopulmonary resuscitation. *Critical Care* 22(1): 139. doi: 10.1186/s13054-018-2058-1.

Greenstein, B. (2009). *Troupe's Clinical Pharmacology for Nurses,* 18e. Churchill Livingstone.

Hill, R., Prabhakar, N.V., and Vaidya, N. (2019). Angiotensin II receptor blockers (ARB, ARb). StatPearls. https://www.ncbi.nlm.nih.gov/books/NBK537027 (accessed July 2020).

Horisberger, J.D. and Glebisch, C. (1987). Potassium-sparing diuretics. *Journal of Renal Physiology* 10 (3–4): 198–220.

Jackson, R.E. and Bellamy, M.C. (2015). Antihypertensive drugs. *British Journal of Anaesthesia* 15 (6): 280–285. https://doi.org/10.1093/bjaceaccp/mku061.

Joint Formulary Committee (JFC) (2018). British National Formulary. http://medicinescomplete.com (accessed July 2020).

Joint Formulary Committee (JFC) (2020). *British National Formulary*, 80the. Pharmacy Press.

Klabunde, R.E. (2017). Cardiovascular pharmacology concepts. https://www.cvphysiology.com/Blood%20Pressure/BP001 (accessed July 2020).

Kosoglou, T., Statkevich, P., Johnson-Levonas, A.O. et al. (2005). Ezetimibe: a review of its metabolism, pharmacokinetics and drug interactions. *Journal of Clinical Pharmacokinetics* 44 (5): 467–494.

Kostis, W.J., Shetty, M., Chowdhury, Y.S., and Kostis, J.B. (2018). ACE inhibitor-induced angioedema: a review. *Journal of Current Hypertension Reports* 20 (7): 55. https://doi.org/10.1007/s11906-018-0859-x.

Lainscak, M., Pelliccia, F., Rosano, G. et al. (2015). Safety profile of mineralocorticoid receptor antagonists: spironolactone and eplerenone. *International Journal of Cardiology* 200: 25–29.

Lundin, A., Djarv, J.E., and Hollenberg, P.N. (2015). Drug therapy in cardiac arrest: a review of the literature. *European Heart Journal – Cardiovascular Pharmacotherapy* 2 (1): 54–75. https://doi.org/10.1093/ehjcvp/pvv047.

Manson, J.E., Cook, N.R., Lee, I. et al. (2019). Marine n-3 fatty acids and prevention of cardiovascular disease and cancer. *The New England Journal of Medicine* 380 (1): 23–32.

McKeever, R. and Hamilton, R. (2019). *Calcium Channel Blockers.* StatPearls. https://www.ncbi.nlm.nih.gov/books/NBK482473.

National Institute for Health and Care Excellence (NICE) (2016). Cardiovascular disease: risk assessment and reduction, including lipid modification. Clinical guideline [CG181]. https://www.nice.org.uk/guidance/cg181 (accessed July 2020).

National Institute for Clinical Excellence (NICE) (2018). Clinical guideline [CG89] Venous thromboembolism in over 16s: reducing the risk of hospital-acquired deep vein thrombosis or pulmonary embolism. www.nice.org.uk/guidance/ng89 (accessed July 2020).

National Institute for Clinical Excellence (NICE) (2019). Clinical guideline [CG136] Hypertension in adults: diagnosis and management. www.nice.org.uk/guidance/ng136 (accessed July 2020).

National Institute for Clinical Excellence (NICE) (2014). Clinical guideline [CG181] Cardiovascular disease: risk assessment and reduction, including lipid modification. www.nice.org.uk/guidance/cg181 (accessed July 2020).

NHS (2019). Longterm plan. https://www.england.nhs.uk/long-term-plan (accessed July 2020).

Patrono, C. and Baigent (2019). Role of aspirin in primary prevention of cardiovascular disease. *Journal of Nature Reviews Cardiology* 16 (11): 675–686.

Pioli, M.R., Ritter, A.R.V., Paula de Faria, A., and Modolo, R. (2018). White coat syndrome and its variations: differences and clinical impact. *Integral Blood Pressure Control* 11: 73–79. https://doi.org/10.2147/IBPC.S152761.

Manniello, M. and Pisano, M. (2016). Alirocumab (Praluent): first in the new class of PCSK9 inhibitors. *Pharmacy and Therapeutics* 41 (1): 28.

Pool, J.L. (1991). Effects of doxazosin on serum lipids: a review of the clinical data and molecular basis for altered lipid metabolism. *American Heart Journal* 121 (2): 251–260.

Puar, T.H., Mok, Y., Debajyoti, R. et al. (2016). Secondary hypertension in adults. *Singapore Medical Journal* 57 (5): 228–232.

QRISK 3. https://qrisk.org/three (accessed October 2020).

Public Health England (PHE)(2019). Public health matters. https://publichealthmatters.blog.gov.uk/ (accessed July 2020).

Rasche, H. (2001). Haemostasis and thrombosis: an overview. *European Heart Journal Supplements*.

Resus Council UK (RCUK)(2015). https://www.resus.org.uk/library/2015-resuscitation-guidelines (accessed July 2020).

Rosengren, A., Smyth, A., Rangarajan, S. et al. (2019). Socioeconomic status and risk of cardiovascular disease in 20 low-income, middle-income, and high-income countries: the Prospective Urban Rural Epidemiologic (PURE) study. *The Lancet Global Health* 7 (6): 748–760. https://doi.org/10.1016/S2214-109X(19)30045-2.

Roshandel, G., Khoshnia, M., Poustchi, H. et al. (2019). Effectiveness of polypill for primary and secondary prevention of cardiovascular diseases (Polyran): a pragmatic, cluster-randomised trial. *The Lancet* 394 (10199): 672–683.

Sahay, S. and Sahay, R. (2012). Low renin hypertension. *Indian Journal of Endocrinology and Metabolism* 16 (5): 728–739. https://doi.org/10.4103/2230-8210.100665.

Sanz, G. and Fuster, V. (2012). Maximizing therapeutic envelope for prevention of cardiovascular disease: role of polypill. *The Mount Sinai Journal of Medicine* 79 (6): 683–688.

Sica, D.A. (2015). Mineralocorticoid receptor antagonists for treatment of hypertension and heart failure. *Methodist Debakey Cardiovascular Journal* 11 (4): 235–239.

Soman, B. and Vijayaraghavan, G. (2017). The role of organic nitrates in the optimal medical management of angina. *European Society of Cardiology*. https://www.escardio.org/Journals/E-Journal-of-Cardiology-Practice/Volume-15/The-role-of-organic-nitrates-in-the-optimal-medical-management-of-angina (accessed October 2020).

Stringer, J. (2017). *Basic Concepts in Pharmacology. What You Need to Know for Each Drug Class*, 5e. Mc Graw Hill Education.

Tarkin, M. (2018). Nicorandil and long-acting nitrates: vasodilator therapies for the management of chronic stable angina pectoris. *European Cardiology Review*. 13 (1): 23–28. https://doi.org/10.15420/ecr.2018.9.2.

Thrombosis Adviser For Healthcare Professionals (2019). Heparins. https://www.thrombosisadviser.com/heparins (accessed July 2020).

Tser, S. and Mazzola, N. (2015). Ivabradine (Corlanor) for heart failure: the first selective and specific if inhibitor. *Pharmacy and Therapeutics* 40 (12): 810–814.

Umeizudike, K.A., Olawuyi, A.B., Umeizudike, T.I. et al. (2017). Effect of calcium channel blockers on gingival tissues in hypertensive patients in Lagos, Nigeria: a pilot study. *Journal of Contemporary Clinical Dentistry* 8 (4): 565–570. doi: 10.4103/ccd.ccd_536_17.

Van Herenendael, H. and Dorian, P. (2010). Amiodarone for the treatment and prevention of ventricular fibrillation and ventricular tachycardia. *Vascular Health and Risk Management* 6: 465–472.

Vavlukis, M. and Vavlukis, A. (2018). Adding ezetimibe to statin therapy: latest evidence and clinical implications. *Drugs in Context* 7:212534. doi: 10.7573/dic.212534.

Vinogradova, Y., Coupland, C., Hill, T., and Hippisely-Cox, J. (2018). Risks and benefits of direct oral anticoagulants versus warfarin in a real world setting: cohort study in primary care. *British Medical Journal* 362. https://www.bmj.com/content/362/bmj.k2505.

World Health Organisation (WHO) (2019). Cardiovascular diseases. https://www.who.int/news-room/fact-sheets/detail/cardiovascular-diseases-(cvds) (accessed July 2020).

219

Xu, Haiyan (2014). Antithrombotic therapy for patients with both stable coronary artery disease and atrial fibrillation. https://www.acc.org/latest-in-cardiology/articles/2014/07/18/15/34/antithrombotic-therapy-for-patients-with-both-stable-cad-and-afib (accessed July 2020).

Zairian, B. and Fonarow, G.C. (2016). Epidemiology and aetiology of heart failure. *Nature Reviews Cardiology Journal* 13 (6): 368–378.

Further reading

Bhatnager, P., Wickramasinghe, K., Wilkins, E., and Townsend (2016). Trends in the epidemiology of cardio-vascular disease in the UK. *British Medical Journal* (102): 1945–1952.

Blood Pressure UK (2008). www. http://bloodpressureuk.org (accessed July 2020).

Bray, J. (2018). Updated NICE guideline on FH recommends DNA tests. *The British Journal of Primary Care Nursing* (3). https://www.bjpcn.com/browse/have-you-heard/item/2201-updated-nice-guideline-on-fh-recommends-dna-tests.html.

Catapano, A.L., Graham, I., De Backer, G. et al. (2016). ESC/EAS guidelines for the Management of Dyslipidaemias: the task force for the Management of Dyslipidaemias of the European Society of Cardiology (ESC) and European Atherosclerosis Society (EAS) Developed with the special contribution of the European Association for Cardiovascular Prevention & Rehabilitation (EACPR). *European Heart Journal* (39): 2999. https://doi.org/10.1093/eurheartj/ehw272.

Crossan, C., Dehbi, H., Williams, H. et al. (2018). A protocol for an economic evaluation of a polypill in patients with established or at high risk of cardiovascular disease in a UK NHS setting: RUPEE (NHS) study. *British Medical Journal*. https://bmjopen.bmj.com/content/8/3/e013063.long.

Chan, Y., See, L., Tu, Y. et al. (2018). Efficacy and safety of apixaban, dabigatran, rivaroxaban, and warfarin in Asians with nonvalvular atrial fibrillation. *Journal of the American Heart Association* 7 (8) https://doi.org/10.1161/JAHA.117.008150 (accessed 5 April 2018).

Vecchio, D., Di Maio, M., Noutsias, M. et al. (2019). High prevalence of Proarrhythmic events in patients with history of atrial fibrillation undergoing a rhythm control strategy: a retrospective study. *Journal of Clinical Medicine Research* 11 (5): 345–352.

Ellison, D.H. (2019). Clinical pharmacology in diuretic use. Nephropharmacology for the clinician. *Clinical Journal of the American Society of Nephrology* (8): 1248–1257. https://doi.org/10.2215/CJN.09630818.

Eskandari, D., Zou, D., Grote, L. et al. (2018). Acetazolamide reduces blood pressure and sleep disordered breathing in hypertensive obstructive sleep apnoea patients – a randomized controlled trial. *Journal of Clinical Sleep Medicine* 14 (3): 309–317.

Farkas, J. (2017). Treatment of ACEi-induced angioedema. https://emcrit.org/pulmcrit/treatment-of-acei-induced-angioedema (accessed July 2020).

Ferreira, J.C.B. and Mochly-Rosen, D. (2012). Nitroglycerin use in myocardial infarction patients: risks and benefits. *Circulation Journal* 76 (1): 15–21.

Haass, M. and Kubler, W. (1997). Nicotine and sympathetic neurotransmission. *Journal of Cardiovascular Drugs and Therapy* 10 (6): 657–765.

Hayes, D. (2018). Vaughan Williams classification of antiarrhythmic drugs. *Nursing* 48 (11): 70.

Hebbes, C. and Thompson, J.P. (2018). Drugs acting on the heart. *Anaesthesia & Intensive Care Medicine* 19 (7): 370–374.

Jackson, G., Gibbs, C.R., Davies, M.K., and Lip, G.Y.H. (2000). Pathophysiology. *The British Medical Journal* 320 (7228): 167–170.

King, J. and Lowery, D.R. (2019). *Physiology, Cardiac Output*. StatPearls. https://www.ncbi.nlm.nih.gov/books/NBK470455.

Keller, K.B. and Lemberg, L. (2004). Prinzmetal's angina. *Journal of American Critical Care* 13 (4): 350–354.

Kunti, K. (2005). Metabolic syndrome. *The British Medical Journal* 331 (7526): 1153–1154. https://www.ncbi.nlm.nih.gov/pmc/articles/PMC1285079.

Lamarche, L., Tejpal, A., and Mangin, D. (2018). Self-efficacy for medication management: a systematic review of instruments. *Patient Preference and Adherence*. Dovepress 12: 1279–1287. https://doi.org/10.2147/PPA.S165749 (accessed 20 July 2018).

Lainscak, M., Vitale, C., Seferovic, P. et al. (2016). Pharmacokinetics and pharmacodynamics of cardiovascu-lar drugs in chronic heart failure. *International Journal of Cardiology* 1 (224): 191–198.

NICE Clinical Guideline 43 (2006) and NICE Public Health Guidance 25 (2010): Prevention of cardiovascular disease at population level.

Nicolas, D. and Reed, M. (2019). *Sacubitril/Valsatan*. StatPearls. https://www.ncbi.nlm.nih.gov/books/NBK507904 (accessed July 2020).

Osuna, P.M., Udovcic, M.D., and Sharma, M.D. (2017). Hyperthyroidism and the heart. *Methodist Debakey Cardiovascular Journal* 13 (2): 60–63.

Perazella, M.A. (1997). Hyperkalemia and trimethoprim-sulfamethoxazole: a new problem emerges 25 years later. *Connecticut Medicine* 8: 451–458.

Reiner, Z., Catapano, A.L., De Backer, G. et al. (2011). The Task Force for the management of dyslipidemias of the European Society of Cardiology and European Atherosclerosis Society. *European Heart Journal* 32: 1769–1818.

Tucker, W.D. and Mahajan, K. (2019). *Anatomy*. StatPearls: Blood vessels. https://www.ncbi.nlm.nih.gov/books/NBK470401 (accessed July 2020).

Vincent, J. (2008). Understanding cardiac output. *Critical Care* 12 (4): 174. https://doi.org/10.1186/cc6975 (accessed 22 August 2008).

Vijayalkshmi, K. and Gibson, C.M. (2012). Thrombolytics and myocardial infarction. *Cardiovascular Therapeutics* 30:81–88. https://onlinelibrary.wiley.com/doi/pdf/10.1111/j.1755-5922.2010.00239.x.

Wright, P. and Thomas, M. (2018). Pathophysiology and management of heart failure. *The Pharmaceutical Journal*. https://www.pharmaceutical-journal.com/learning/cpd-article/pathophysiology-and-management-of-heart-failure/20205742.cpdarticle.

Multiple choice questions

Choose the correct answer/s to each question.

1. Which of the following is a contraindication for digoxin administration?
   (a) Heart rate above 80 beats per minute
   (b) Blood pressure of 140/90 mmHg
   (c) Heart rate below 60 beats per minute
   (d) Respiratory rate above 20 beats per minute

2. Mrs. Fastbeat has ventricular ectopics; which of the following medications will be used?
   (a) Digoxin
   (b) Amiodarone
   (c) Adrenaline
   (d) Lidocaine

3. You perform a routine ECG on Mr. Allan. After reviewing it, you decide to call the doctor because Mr. Allan needs an antiarrhythmic. What is the likely ECG rhythm?
   (a) Normal sinus rhythm
   (b) Atrial fibrillation
   (c) Sinus bradycardia
   (d) Sinus tachycardia

4. Beta blocker medications may be contraindicated in which of the following conditions?
   (a) Hypertension
   (b) Atrial fibrillation
   (c) Angina
   (d) Bronchoconstriction

5. Amiodarone:
   (a) Is indicated in cardiac arrest situations
   (b) Is indicated for use in atrial fibrillation
   (c) May be administered orally
   (d) Has an intravenous loading dose of 600 mg

6. When a patient is prescribed thiazides, the nurse and healthcare worker must consider:
   (a) Regular checks of the patient's heart rate
   (b) Regular monitoring for serum electrolytes
   (c) Advise patients to eat foods high in potassium
   (d) Close monitoring of serum potassium

7. A contraindication for nitrates is:
   (a) Hypertension
   (b) Marked anaemia
   (c) Aortic stenosis
   (d) Mitral stenosis

8. Furosemide:
   (a) Is a thiazide diuretic
   (b) Is indicated in chronic heart failure
   (c) Administered intravenously has a longer half-life
   (d) Bioavailability of 60% if taken orally

9. Magnesium:
   (a) Is an electrolyte
   (b) Is a nitrate
   (c) Is used in sinus bradycardia
   (d) Increases ventricular conduction

10. Warfarin (check all that apply):
    (a) Interferes with the synthesis of vitamin K
    (b) May be administered orally
    (c) Dosage is adjusted according to the APTT ratio
    (d) Most serious side effect is flatulence

11. GTN (check all that apply):
    (a) Promotes coronary artery vasoconstriction
    (b) Reduces work of the heart
    (c) Reduces preload
    (d) Reduces after load
    (e) Increases platelet aggregation

12. Side effects of atropine are (check all that apply):
    (a) Bradycardia
    (b) Skin flushing
    (c) Xerostomia
    (d) Cycloplegia
    (e) Loss of hearing

13. Aspirin:
    (a) Is safe to prescribe in patients who have asthma
    (b) Should be taken on an empty stomach for better absorption
    (c) May be administered as a suppository
    (d) Is contraindicated in children under the age of 6 years
    (e) Usual dose is 300 mg orally daily post acute myocardial infarction

14. Alpha-adrenergic blockers (check all that apply):
    (a) Are prescribed for patients with hypertension
    (b) Have side effects that include: dry mouth, drowsiness and sweating
    (c) Can only be administered via intravenous route
    (d) Patient should be advised to take this medication at night time
    (e) Hypokalaemia may be a potential problem
15. Statins (check all that apply):
    (a) When prescribed, advise the patient to avoid grapefruit juice
    (b) Are better absorbed when taken with food
    (c) The patient must follow up with the GP for monitoring cholesterol levels and LFTs
    (d) Side effects may include headaches and blurred vision
    (e) Are safe to use in pregnancy

Chapter 11

Medications and the renal system

Sadie Diamond-Fox and Alexandra Gatehouse

Aim

The aim of this chapter is to provide the reader with an introduction to some of the common renal disease processes that may be encountered within clinical practice, and to explore the pharmacological therapies utilised in their management.

Learning outcomes

After reading this chapter, the reader will:

1. Have gained an understanding of key renal physiology concepts relating to the management of common renal disorders
2. Understand key classes of renal drugs and their pharmacology relating to respiratory conditions, and see how understanding of such is crucial to the promotion of patient safety
3. Understand the side effects of common renal pharmacotherapy and how this should be taken into account when counselling the patient to reach an informed decision regarding their evidence-based care
4. Have gained an understanding of the current evidence base behind key recommendations of pharmacotherapy management of the common renal conditions reviewed in this chapter

Test your knowledge

1. Describe the principle functions of the renal system and its main components.
2. Name four common renal conditions.
3. Discuss the potential risks associated with diabetes.
4. List the common types of drugs used to treat renal disorders.
5. Discuss the role and function of the National Institute of Clinical Excellence (NICE) concerning the management of renal disorders.

Fundamentals of Pharmacology: For Nursing and Healthcare Students, First Edition. Edited by Ian Peate and Barry Hill.
© 2021 John Wiley & Sons Ltd. Published 2021 by John Wiley & Sons Ltd.

Introduction

Renal disease encompasses a wide range of reduced kidney function as a result of an acute or chronic insult and is a general umbrella term that can encompass disease terminology such as acute kidney injury (AKI), chronic kidney disease (CKD) and end-stage renal disease (ESRD). Within the United Kingdom (UK) approximately 1 in 10 of the general population are affected by renal disease, with people from black, Asian and minority ethnic communities five times more likely to experience kidney failure in their lifetime (Kidney Research UK, 2018). Diabetes is the single most common cause of end-stage kidney disease in the UK, with 25% of newly diagnosed patients needing dialysis or transplant due to diabetic-related kidney disease (Kidney Research UK, 2018). Renal disease can affect all age groups, but its prevalence increases with age. The impact upon healthcare services is significant: dialysis requirements in ESRD cost around £30 000 per patient per year. Of those patients in the UK that are fortunate enough to receive a kidney transplant, around £7000 per year is required to fund the NHS services required per patient (Kidney Research UK, 2018). Mortality from the sub-type of renal disease known as AKI show that in-hospital deaths have increased in all age groups from 5107 registered deaths in 2001 (where AKI was either the underlying cause, or a contributory factor toward death) to 12 822 in 2016 (Office for National Statistics, 2018). This chapter will introduce the reader to some of the pertinent anatomy, physiology and pathophysiology of the renal system, along with an introduction to some of the commonly used drug classes and relevant clinical considerations, with case studies used to bring together theory and practice.

Anatomy and physiology of the renal tract

Pharmacotherapy knowledge and understanding is essential in safe medicines management and treatment of complex disease processes, particularly in patients with renal conditions. The following section provides a brief overview of renal physiology, highlighting target sites utilised for the application of appropriate pharmacotherapy.

The main function of the kidneys is maintenance of homoeostasis (physiological stability) through excretory, regulatory and metabolic mechanisms. Waste products of metabolism, for example urea and creatinine, are eliminated via the production and excretion of urine. Fluid, electrolyte and acid–base balance is regulated through filtration, selective absorption and excretion of water, sodium, potassium, phosphate, calcium, hydrogen ions, bicarbonate ions and other substances. In addition, the kidneys have an endocrine function that secretes hormones such as renin (blood pressure regulation) and erythropoietin (red blood cell production). Vitamin D is metabolised, contributing to the regulation of calcium and phosphate, and prostaglandins are synthesised, resulting in renal protection from profound vasoconstriction. There is also renal involvement in glucose homoeostasis, via gluconeogenesis and reabsorption of glucose, which is discussed further in Chapter 4.

The renal system comprises the kidneys, the ureters, the urinary bladder and the urethra. Each kidney receives its blood supply via a renal artery arising from the aorta, and filters approximately 1200 mL of blood per minute which then flows into the renal vein and consequently the inferior vena cava (Nair, 2016). The renal vasculature and juxtaglomerular apparatus is supplied by the sympathetic nervous system. Urine formed by the kidney passes from the collecting duct to the renal pelvis via the papillary duct in the renal pyramid, minor calyx and major calyx. The structure is depicted in Figure 11.1. Peristalsis facilitates the movement of urine along the ureter into the bladder.

The nephrons are the functional units of the kidney and they consist of several segments including: the Bowman's capsule, the glomerulus, the proximal convoluted tubule, the loop of Henle, the distal convoluted tubule (DCT) and the collecting ducts. Figure 11.1 demonstrates the structure of the nephron. The function of the nephron is filtration, selective reabsorption and excretion through various transport processes. Table 11.1 outlines the functions of the segments of the nephron. Each segment presents an opportunity for targeted pharmacotherapy and this will be discussed in subsequent sections of the chapter.

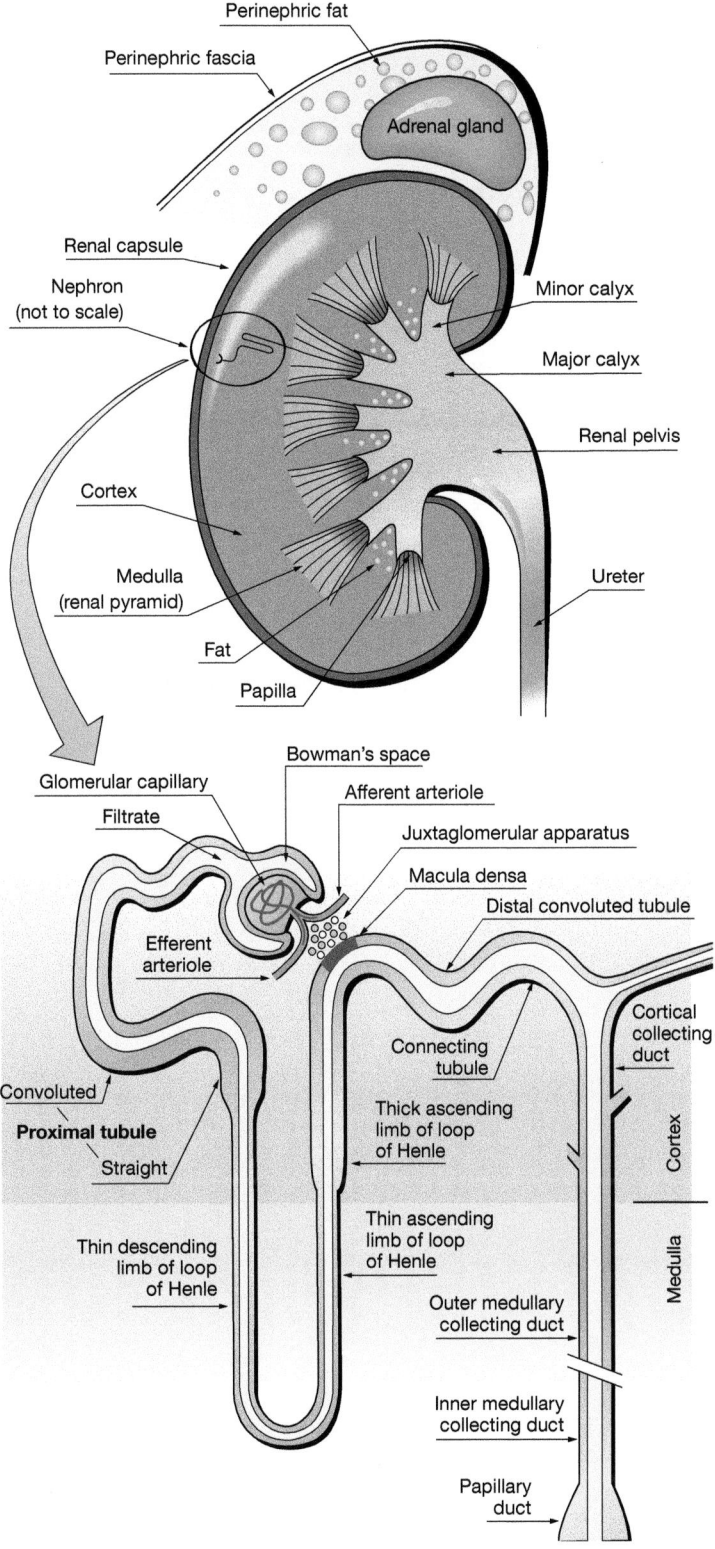

Figure 11.1 The internal structure of the kidney and the nephron.

Table 11.1 Segments of the nephron and their functions.

Segment	Function	Types of cell	Transport Process
Glomerulus and Bowman's Capsule	Filtration of plasma – allows passage o;; • Water • Glucose • Vitamins • Very small plasma proteins • Amino acids • Urea • Ions • Ammonia	• Glomerular capillaries – endothelial cells • Basement membrane – combination of collagen fibres and glycoproteins • Bowman's capsule – podocytes	• Filtration due to high hydrostatic pressure within the afferent and efferent arterioles • Dependent upon molecular size • Glomerular filtration – large fenestrations, passage of all solutes except red blood cells and platelets • Basement membrane – negatively charged, repels negatively charged plasma proteins • Bowman's capsule filtration – filtration slits between foot-like projections of the podocytes
Proximal Convoluted tubule (PCT)	• Accounts for approximately 60–70% of all reabsorption • Includes sodium (Na^+), potassium (K^+), calcium (Ca^{2+}), magnesium (Mg^{2+}), chloride (Cl^-), glucose, phosphate (PO_4^-), urea, water and bicarbonate (HCO_3^-) • Excretion of hydrogen ions (H^+), ammonium ions, creatinine, uric acid and drug metabolites	• Simple cuboidal epithelial cells with microvilli (increased surface area)	• Electrochemical gradient – o Sodium hydrogen (Na^+-H^+) antiporter, sodium reabsorbed into the cells from tubular filtrate • Osmosis – PCT highly permeable to water, water moves into the cells from the tubular filtrate due to the movement of Na^+ • Passive diffusion – of Cl^-, K^+, Ca^{2+} and urea from the tubular filtrate into the cell • Co-transport – glucose, phosphate, amino acids with sodium
Loop of Henle	• Reabsorption of approximately 15% of water, 20–30% of sodium, potassium and chloride, 10–20% of bicarbonate, variable amounts of calcium and magnesium	• Descending limb and thin ascending limb – simple squamous epithelial cells • Thick ascending limb – simple cuboidal to low columnar epithelial cells	• Generation of a concentration gradient through: • Descending loop – impermeable to solute but permeable to water, aquaporins • Thick ascending loop – impermeable to water but permeable to ions – Na^+, K^+, Ca^{2+}, Mg^{2+} o $Na^=$-K^+-Cl^- symporter
Distal Convoluted	• Active reabsorption of 4–8% of sodium and chloride • Secretion of potassium • Selectively reabsorbs water • Regulation of calcium ions • Regulates pH by absorbing bicarbonate and secreting hydrogen ions	• Simple cuboidal epithelial cells	• Sodium channels in principal cells (ENaC) increase reabsorption • Antidiuretic hormone (ADH) causes insertion of water channels (aquaporins) into the membrane • K^+ channels and K^+-Cl^- co-transporter with increased tubular flow contribute to potassium excretion • Parathyroid hormone (PTH) activates Ca^{2+} channels, 1,25-dihydroxycholecalciferol triggers an active Ca^{2+} channel
Collecting ducts	• 2–5% of sodium reabsorption coupled with potassium and hydrogen ion secretion	• Simple cuboidal epithelial cells – principal cells and intercalated cells	• Sodium channels • Hydrogen ion transporter • Aquaporins

Source: Alex Gatehouse.

Common renal conditions

The common pathophysiological processes observed in renal disease include failure to maintain fluid and acid–base balance and electrolyte disturbances, which provide potential targets for pharmacotherapy. Renal disease is vast and complex, and it is beyond the scope of this chapter to discuss all aspects in detail. However, the most common renal conditions that encompass one or more of these processes are explored in the following chapter of this book.

Skills in practice

Urinalysis: reagent strip procedure

Urinalysis using reagent strips is a rapid point-of-care test that is used as one of the primary diagnostic tests for multiple conditions. Urinalysis can aid in the clinical decision-making as to which advanced diagnostic tests are required to investigate for the presence of potential disease.

How to perform urinalysis using reagent strips:

Procedure

3 If taking the specimen from a urinary catheter, it should be collected using an aseptic technique via the catheter side port.

For women, the labia should be separated with cotton wool or a sponge moistened with water, and the vulva should be wiped from the front to the back although disinfectant must never be used. Men should clean the glans penis with soap and water.

4 Obtain a clean specimen of fresh urine from the patient, which is to be analysed within 2 hours from collection. Women should separate the labia. The patient should commence micturition, and when a few millilitres of urine have been passed into the toilet, a container or sterile receptacle should be introduced into the urine stream, and then the remaining urine can pass into the toilet.

5 Check reagent sticks have been stored in accordance with manufacturer's instructions. This is usually a dark dry place in an airtight container.

6 Dip the reagent strip into the urine for no longer than 1 second. The strip should be completely immersed in the urine and then removed immediately. Run edge of strip along the container.

7 Hold the stick at an angle.

8 Wait the required time before reading the strip against the colour chart, usually 60 seconds (see **Action figure 8**).

Post-procedure

9 Dispose of urine sample appropriately in either sluice or toilet. Dispose of urinalysis stick and gloves in correct wastage bin. Ensure cap to urine reagent strips is replaced immediately and closed tightly.

10 Wash and dry hands.

11 Document urinalysis readings and inform medical staff of any abnormal readings.

Renal disease comprises AKI and CKD. An estimated one in five emergency admissions to hospital are for patients with an AKI, and over 3 million people in the UK live with CKD (Kidney Research UK, 2018; Wang et al., 2012). The correct treatment can aid in early detection of renal conditions, effective management of the disease itself and/or diseases that can cause CKD (diabetes and hypertension), help reduce mortality rates, preserve kidney function and minimise further disease progression where possible (NCEPOD, 2009). The renal community leads the 'Think Kidneys' national programs; NHS England and the UK Renal Registry aim to improve the care of patients with or at risk of AKI and improve experiences and outcomes for patients with CKD, part of which includes pharmacological management.

Acute kidney injury (AKI)

AKI is viewed as a spectrum, from mild renal impairment to severe renal failure requiring renal replacement therapy (RRT) (Davies, 2014; Lafayette, 2019). It occurs when the glomerular filtration rate (GFR) falls, leading to a rise in serum creatinine with, or without, a decline in urine output (KDIGO, 2012; O'Callaghan, 2017). Within the UK, AKI is seen in 13–18% of patients admitted to hospital, particularly in older adults, with an incidence of 13–22% in those already hospitalised (NICE, 2013a; Wang et al., 2012). Inpatient mortality due to AKI in the UK varies considerably but is estimated to be 25–30% or more, and in 2009 a national enquiry reported 'good care' in only 50% of those patients who had died as a result of an AKI (NCEPOD, 2009; NICE, 2013a). The need for early recognition, risk assessment, prevention and treatment is paramount.

The aetiology of AKI is classified into pre-renal, intrinsic and post-renal, the causes of which are outlined in Table 11.2. Approximately 50–65% of cases are pre-renal and occur due to impaired renal perfusion, with appropriate physiological responses of glomerular efferent arteriole vasoconstriction and afferent arteriole dilation through sympathetic stimulation, activation of the rennin/angiotensin/aldosterone system and antidiuretic hormone released by the hypothalamus. All of these mechanisms result in maintenance of glomerular filtration, and sodium and water reabsorption in the collecting duct (Lafayette, 2019). However, if this renal hypoperfusion is protracted, the ongoing ischemia leads to injury to the tubular epithelial cells, known as acute tubular necrosis (ATN) (O'Callaghan, 2017).

Intrinsic renal failure describes either primary renal disease or multisystem disease processes that cause structural damage to the glomerulus and/or the renal tubule (Davies, 2014). Due to the complexity and duration of this type of renal failure, full recovery is not assured even with prompt diagnosis and treatment. Drugs, toxins and contrast medium are some potential causes for intrinsic renal failure.

The main cause of post-renal AKI is obstruction, resulting in tubular ischemia and atrophy, secondary to increased tubular pressure (Lafayette, 2019). Pre-renal and post-renal causes of AKI require rapid correction due to the potential for full recovery (Davies, 2014; O'Callaghan, 2017).

According to KDIGO (2012), the definition of AKI includes any of the following:

- An increase in serum creatinine by ≥25.6 μmol/L within 48 hours.
- An increase in serum creatinine to ≥1.5 times baseline, known or presumed within the previous seven days.
- A urine output of <0.5 mL/kg for six hours.

There are several classification systems that may be employed to determine the severity of AKI. Table 11.3 provides a comparison of three severity classification systems.

In 2013, NICE produced criteria for the detection of AKI, taking into consideration all definitions (NICE, 2013a). They include:

- a rise in serum creatinine of 26 μmol/L (0.3 mg/dL) or greater within 48 hours; or
- a 50% or greater rise in serum creatinine known or presumed to have occurred within the past seven days; or
- a fall in urine output to <0.5 mL/kg/h for more than six hours in adults and more than eight hours in children and young people; or

Table 11.2 Pre-renal, intrinsic and post-renal causes of AKI.

	Aetiology
PRE-RENAL	Hypovolemia – • Haemorrhage • Burns • Gastrointestinal losses • Over diuresis • Severe pancreatitis Vasodilatation – • Sepsis • Anaphylaxis Cardiovascular – • Heart failure • Cardiac tamponade • Pulmonary embolism • Myocardial infarction Renovascular disease – • Renal artery stenosis Hepatorenal syndrome
INTRINSIC	Acute tubular necrosis Glomerular nephritis Interstitial nephritis Nephrotoxic drugs – • Non-steroidal anti-inflammatories • Antibiotics • Proton pump inhibitors Hypertension Vasculitis Tubular toxins – • Drugs • Heavy metals • Contrast • Haemoglobin • Myoglobin • Calcium phosphate precipitation
POST-RENAL	Mechanical obstruction – • Tumour • Renal calculi • Blood clot • Prostate hyperplasia • Urinary infection • Urinary retention

Source: Adapted from Lafayette (2019); Davies (2014).

231

- a 25% or greater fall in estimated GFR (eGFR) in children and young people within the past seven days.

The treatment approach to AKI depends upon the aetiology, and interventions include correction of electrolyte and acid–base disturbances, as well as optimisation of fluid status. Clinical Practice Guidelines have been produced for healthcare professionals with regards to the prevention, detection and management of AKI in both the adult and paediatric populations (KDIGO, 2012; NICE, 2013a; UK Renal Registry, 2019). There are no recommended pharmacological treatments specifically for AKI; however, associated complications such as hyperkalaemia and pulmonary oedema may require pharmacotherapy, as discussed later in this chapter.

Table 11.3   AKI severity classifications.

KDIGO severity criteria	RIFLE (Risk, Injury, Failure, Loss of kidney function and End stage kidney disease)	AKIN (Acute Kidney Injury Network)
Stage 1 • Serum creatinine 1.5 to 1.9 times baseline; or • ≥25.6 μmol/L (≥0.3 mg/dL) increase in serum creatinine; or • Urine output <0.5 mL/kg/h body weight for 6–12 hours Stage 2 • Creatinine increased 2.0 to 2.9 times; or • Urine output <0.5 mL/kg/h for 12 hours Stage 3 • Creatinine increased 3.0 times; or • Increase in creatinine to ≥353.6 μmol/L (≥4.0 mg/dL); or • Initiation of renal replacement therapy; or • Urine output <0.3 mL/kg/h for 24 hours OR anuria for 12 hours	Risk • Serum creatinine increased 1.5 times or GFR decrease >25%; or • Urine production of <0.5 mL/kg body weight for 6 hours Injury • Creatinine increased 2.0 times or GFR decrease >50%; or • Urine production of <0.5 mL/kg for 12 hours Failure • Creatinine increased 3.0 times or GFR decrease 75% or creatinine ≥4 mg/dL (acute rise of >0.5 mg/dL); or • Urine output <0.3 mL/kg for 24 hours or anuria for 12 hours Loss • Persistent AKI for more than 4 weeks; complete loss of kidney function End stage renal disease (ESRD) • ESRD (loss >3 months)	Stage 1 • Increase in serum creatinine ≥25.6 μmol/L (≥0.3 mg/dL); or • Increase ≥150–200% from baseline • < 0.5 mL/kg/h for >6 hours Stage 2 • Increase in serum creatinine to >200–300% from baseline • <0.5 mL/kg/h for >12 hours Stage 3 • Increase in serum creatinine to >300% from baseline • <0.3 mL/kg/h for 24 hours or anuria for 12 hours

Source: Bellomo et al. (2004), KDIGO (2012), Mehta et al. (2007).

Chronic kidney disease (CKD)

CKD is defined as an abnormality in kidney function, demonstrated by GFR of less than 60 mL/min per 1.73 m², or markers of kidney damage present for more than three months, with associated health implications (KDIGO, 2013). Worldwide, the estimated prevalence of CKD is 5–15%, with the main causes reported as diabetes, glomerular nephritis, pyelonephritis, polycystic kidney and hypertension (O'Callaghan, 2017; UK Renal Registry, 2019). The risk of developing CKD increases with age due to decline in renal function and increasing prevalence of diseases causing renal impairment (NICE, 2015; O'Callaghan, 2017). There is an increased risk of myocardial infarction or stroke associated with CKD, and premature death is 5–10 times more likely before progression to ESRD (Webster et al., 2017). As CKD progresses, the risk of complications increases, including hypertension, anaemia, sodium and water retention, metabolic acidosis, electrolyte disorders, dyslipidaemia, peripheral neuropathy and nephropathy, malnutrition and mineral bone disease (KDIGO, 2013; NICE, 2019a, b; O'Callaghan, 2017). The increasing frequency and severity of complications associated with CKD results in higher morbidity, mortality and poorer quality of life (Bello et al., 2017).

Detection of CKD is challenging as patients may initially be asymptomatic. It has been recommended that patients should be investigated for CKD if:

- They have risk factors for CKD.
- There is an incidental finding of raised serum creatinine and/or a serum eGFR of less than 60 ml/min/1.73 m², proteinuria, persistent haematuria (after exclusion of a urinary tract infection [UTI]), urine sediment abnormalities.
- There are possible clinical features of CKD.

Source: KDIGO (2012), NICE (2019a), Vassalotti et al. (2016).

Prognosis of CKD by GFR and albuminuria category

Prognosis of CKD by GFR and Albuminuria Categories: KDIGO 2012			Persistent albuminuria categories Description and range		
			A1	**A2**	**A3**
			Normal to mildly increased	Moderately increased	Severely increased
			<30 mg/g <3 mg/mmol	30–300 mg/g 3–30 mg/mmol	>300 mg/g >30 mg/mmol
GFR stages, descriptions and range (ml/min per 1,73m²)	Stage 1 (G1)	Normal or high ≥90			
	Stage 2 (G2)	Mildly decreased 60–90			
	Stage 3 (G3a)	Mildly to moderately decreased 45–59			
	Stage 3 (G3b)	Moderately to severely decreased 30–44			
	Stage 4 (G4)	Severely decreased 15–29			
	Stage 5 (G5)	Kidney failure <15			

Green: low risk (if no other markers of kidney disease, no CKD); Yellow: moderately increased risk; Orange: high risk; Red, very high risk.

Figure 11.2   KDIGO (2012) classification of CKD.

The aim of CKD treatment is to impede decline of renal function and reduce the risk of, or manage, complications. Assessment and investigation may aid identification of the underlying cause and severity of the renal disease. Stratification of severity, as well as local and national guidance, informs healthcare professionals in the care and management of patients with CKD. Figure 11.2 depicts the stages of CKD and its prognosis. Those patients with CKD stage 4 may require referral to renal specialists in addition to specific interventions indicated in stage 3, while stage 5 CKD generally indicates the need for RRT (Davies, 2014).

The national guidance for the early identification and management of CKD in adults in primary and secondary care makes recommendations regarding lifestyle modification, dietary intervention and self-management, in addition to pharmacotherapy (NICE, 2015). Management of blood pressure, mineral and bone disorders, volume status, anaemia, electrolyte disturbance and metabolic acidosis are key to CKD, and some of these targeted pharmacotherapy concepts will be explored later in this chapter.

Diabetic nephropathy

Diabetic renal disease remains the single most common cause of renal failure that requires RRT (UK Renal Registry, 2018). Approximately 40% of Type I and Type II diabetic patients develop diabetic nephropathy, the incidence of which has only recently plateaued and may be attributable to the development of clinical practice guidelines endorsing early diagnosis and prevention (Gross et al., 2005; Haneda et al., 2015). It is less common in Type II diabetic patients of European descent in comparison to African or Asian patients (O'Callaghan, 2017). Diabetic nephropathy may occur as a result of the long-term complications of diabetes mellitus, which causes damage to the structure and function of the kidney (Davies, 2014). When glycaemic control is poor, causing protracted periods of hyperglycaemia, glycosylation of proteins occurs and it is these compounds that cause damage to vascular tissue, significantly increasing the risk of death from cardiovascular disease (Davies, 2014; Gross et al., 2005; Nazar, 2014).

Diabetic nephropathy is categorised according to values of urinary albumin excretion (UAE). Patients with Type I diabetes may have normal UAE for 5–15 years, with an elevated GFR due to hyperfiltration and either normal-sized or hypertrophied kidneys (Nazar, 2014). Microalbuminuria (30–300 mg/24 hours) occurs in 30–50% of patients, and although it does not always progress, 80% do go on to develop overt nephropathy and macroalbuminuria (>300 mg/24 hours) (Nazar, 2014). If Type I diabetes goes undetected, microalbuminuria or proteinuria may be evident on diagnosis (Davies, 2014). The recommendation is that albuminuria is assessed annually in diabetic patients (NICE, 2019a; O'Callaghan, 2017).

The development of diabetic nephropathy is dependent upon specific risk factors, namely hypertension, hyperglycaemia, smoking and dyslipidaemia. The likelihood of developing microalbuminuria and further progression of the disease may be minimised through treatment based upon these risk factors. Evidence supports intensive diabetes management, as aiming to normalise blood glucose levels helps delay the onset of microalbuminuria and progression to proteinuria (Davies, 2014). Proteinuria may be reduced with angiotensin-converting enzyme inhibitors (ACEi) and angiotensin II receptor blockers (ARBs), via down-regulation of nephrin protein levels in the slit pores of the glomerulus (O'Callaghan, 2017). These drugs will also contribute to reduction of hypertension. The pharmacotherapy of diabetes and the cardiovascular system are discussed in the relevant chapters.

Electrolyte disorders

The renal system plays an essential role in maintenance of homoeostasis, controlling fluid, electrolyte and acid–base balance. Renal disease may affect all of these processes, and the aim of the following section is to explore the impact of this and identify how pharmacotherapy may be utilised in management and treatment.

Fluid balance refers to the distribution of body fluid within the intracellular and extracellular (interstitial and intravascular) compartments. Total body volume, and therefore total body water, is regulated within a narrow range, through alteration of sodium and water content (O'Callaghan, 2017; Peate, 2017). Sodium excretion is controlled via the kidneys and regulated by neural and endocrine responses. The sodium–potassium pumps (Na^+–K^+) drive sodium from the tubular cells into the blood, and this creates a lower concentration gradient within the cell. Sodium and water then move from the tubular infiltrate into the cell via various channels or co-transporters, according to the permeability of the cell membrane and the concentration gradient.

Inappropriate renal handling of sodium may occur due to a primary renal problem or due to an abnormality in the volume regulation mechanism. Renal tubulointerstitial disease and Addison's disease (deficiency of the hormone aldosterone) both cause excessive sodium excretion, while primary hyperaldosteronism, renal failure or oedema syndromes (liver disease, congestive heart failure, nephrotic syndrome) result in inadequate sodium excretion (O'Callaghan, 2017). The underlying cause should be identified and treated; however, pharmacotherapy manipulation of renal sodium through the use of diuretics may be useful. This is explored further within this chapter.

Potassium is integral to the maintenance of an electrochemical gradient across the cell membrane, and the ability of nerves and muscle to create an action potential. Hypokalaemia and hyperkalaemia are life-threatening, causing cardiac dysrhythmias and potentially cardiac arrest, and the kidneys and adrenal glands are vital in the maintenance of potassium homoeostasis. Within the nephron, the majority of potassium is reabsorbed prior to the collecting duct, and excretion of potassium occurs in this segment through several mechanisms. The sodium–potassium pumps and the potassium channels in the cell membranes of the collecting duct are affected by the extracellular potassium concentration, the release of aldosterone, the pH, flow rates within the collecting duct, filtrate sodium concentration and intracellular magnesium. Renal tubular acidosis and primary or secondary hyperaldosteronism result in potassium loss and hypokalaemia, while renal failure and hyperaldosteronism cause hyperkalaemia. Life-threatening hyperkalaemia warrants emergency treatment as outlined in the UK Resuscitation Council Guidelines (Soar et al., 2015) and RRT. Pharmacotherapy of longer-term potassium management may include potassium supplementation or potassium-binding agents, both of which are discussed in subsequent sections.

Calcium and phosphate are inextricably linked and are essential to the maintenance of bone density. They are regulated by one of several mechanisms including gut reabsorption, bone reabsorption and renal handling. Calcium is regulated by the thyroid gland, and when levels fall, parathyroid hormone (PTH) stimulates bone reabsorption (release of calcium and phosphate from bone), increases Vitamin D synthesis, increases renal phosphate excretion and increases renal calcium reabsorption. Vitamin D is synthesised within the kidney, increasing phosphate and calcium levels via reabsorption through the gut, bones and renal tubules. In renal failure, bone disease can be caused by Vitamin D deficiency and renal phosphate retention. Due to lack of gut reabsorption and the formation of calcium phosphate deposits (due to hyperphosphataemia), the fall in calcium stimulates PTH, triggering further bone reabsorption and eventually hyperparathyroidism. Pharmacotherapy aims to maintain normal calcium and phosphate levels, preventing hyperparathyroidism, bone pain, poorly mineralised bone and soft tissue deposits as typically seen in CKD.

Acid–base balance, and so pH, is controlled by the respiratory and renal systems. By regulating carbon dioxide (respiratory) and bicarbonate (renal), the pH may be normalised when acidosis or alkalosis occurs. Under normal circumstances, the kidneys excrete excess hydrogen ions (H^+) or acid through increased synthesis of the Na^+–H^+ exchangers or H^+ ATPase pump, reabsorb bicarbonate via the Na^+–HCO_3^- co-transporters and produce more ammonium salts (NH_4^+) for excretion. In renal disease, the kidneys are unable to effectively perform these processes and so metabolic acidosis occurs causing hyperkalaemia, due to H^+ moving into cells and driving K^+ out, with worsening renal bone disease due to the loss of carbonate buffers in an acidic environment. RRT may be used to correct severe metabolic acidosis in both the acute and chronic setting of renal failure. Pharmacotherapy may be utilised to correct the acid–base balance, and this is explored in subsequent sections of this chapter.

Urinary retention and incontinence

There are wide variations in the reported incidence and prevalence of urinary incontinence, but an estimated 14 million, men, women, adolescents and children are living with bladder problems in the UK (Buckley and Lapitan, 2009; Davila, 2018). Lower urinary tract symptoms (LUTSs) affect up to 60% of men, and urinary incontinence affects up to 65% of women (Davila, 2018; NICE, 2010, 2013b).

Micturition is a voluntary process that is regulated by the muscles of the bladder and urethra as well as the nervous system. The bladder fills with urine from the ureters via muscle relaxation (detrusor relaxation) and is prevented from leaving by contraction of the internal and external urethral urinary sphincters. Voluntary nerves control the external sphincter while the parasympathetic nerves control the internal sphincter. Initiation of voiding the bladder is dependent upon the parasympathetic nervous system and relies upon coordination of detrusor contraction and sphincter relaxation. Inhibition of micturition is controlled via the pontine centre in the brain recognising bladder distention. This results in the sympathetic nervous system stimulating β receptors and inhibiting detrusor contraction as well as α receptors causing contraction at the bladder neck and urethra.

The most common LUTS in men is bladder outflow obstruction due to benign prostate hyperplasia. The prevalence of LUTS increases with age, and moderate or severe symptoms are reported in 30% of men in their 50s and 50% of men in their 80s (Allan, 2012). They are further subdivided into voiding, storage and post-micturition symptoms. Other conditions that can cause LUTS include detrusor overactivity or weakness, inflammation of the prostate, UTI, prostate cancer and neurological conditions (NICE, 2010).

Urinary incontinence is the involuntary leakage of urine and can have a profound effect on quality of life, health status, and psychosocial state. It is classified clinically into categories of urgency, stress, mixed, enuresis, continuous and overflow. Table 11.4 outlines the definitions and causes of urinary incontinence. In addition to the causes listed, risk factors include family history and increasing age.

Urgency incontinence is more common in men and the elderly, occurring due to disruption of the process of micturition and inappropriate detrusor activity (Davila, 2018; Nethercliffe, 2012). Stress incontinence is more common in women and tends to be due to weakness of the pelvic floor (with or without sphincter damage) causing intrinsic sphincter deficiency. It is associated with childbirth, age, the menopause, obesity and hysterectomy (Davila, 2018; Nethercliffe, 2012).

Table 11.4   Definitions and causes of urinary incontinence.

Terminology	Definition	Cause
Urgency	Involuntary leakage of urine accompanied or preceded by urgency	• Detrusor overactivity – instability or hyperreflexia 　○ Idiopathic 　○ Secondary to neurological problems – stroke, multiple sclerosis, dementia, spinal cord injury, Parkinson's disease • Inflammation or infection • Alcohol or caffeine • Poor fluid intake • Tumour • Medications • Renal stones • Obstruction
Stress	Involuntary leakage on effort, exertion, sneezing. or coughing	• Weak or incompetent sphincter due to: 　○ Genitourinary prolapse 　○ Childbirth 　○ Obesity 　○ Pregnancy 　○ Pelvic or urological surgery 　○ Trauma • Secondary to neurological problems – stroke, multiple sclerosis, dementia, spinal cord injury, Parkinson's disease • Medications • Connective tissue disorders
Mixed	Presence of urgency and stress	• As for urgency and stress
Enuresis (nocturnal)	Involuntary leakage of urine during sleep	• Detrusor overactivity
Continuous	Leakage of urine is continuous	• Inherited or acquired abnormality • Trauma or surgery
Overflow	Leakage of urine due to an over-distended bladder	• Bladder outflow obstruction – benign prostate hyperplasia • Renal stones • Urethral stricture • Constipation • Previous surgery

Source: BMJ (2018); Nethercliffe (2012).

The National Institute for Clinical Excellence provides the most recent guidance for the management of LURTs in men, and urinary incontinence and pelvic organ prolapse in women, which includes the recommended pharmacotherapy discussed later in this chapter (NICE, 2010, 2019c).

Clinical considerations

Estimating the glomerular filtration rate

Knowledge of GFR is crucial for diagnosis, staging and management of CKD. Accurate GFR may be measured via a marker that is freely filtered, excreted unchanged and not bound to plasma proteins or subject to tubular reabsorption or secretion, all of which would give the filtration rate of functioning nephrons, and therefore renal function. Although 'gold standard', such markers are expensive, time-consuming, labour intensive and unsuitable.

Creatinine may be used to give a simple eGFR, by measuring plasma and urine concentration as well as the urine flow rate per minute. However, despite creatinine being freely filtered by the glomerulus, it is secreted into the renal tubule (potentially over-estimating GFR) and requires 24-hour urine collection, which may not be reliable. GFR may fall to <30 mL/min/1.73 m^2 before creatinine begins to rise due to the renal compensatory systems, delaying early diagnosis of CKD. The National Institute for Health and Care Excellence recommends the use of the Chronic Kidney Disease Epidemiology Collaboration (CKD-EPI) creatinine equation to predict reasonably accurate eGFR taking into account age, sex and ethnicity (NICE, 2019a).

Normal eGFR is >90 mL/min/1.73 m^2 but levels >60 mL/min/1.73 m^2 should be interpreted with caution, as estimates of GFR become less accurate with relatively good renal function. If CKD is suspected, initial investigations should include a serum creatinine, eGFR and measurement of the urinary albumin : creatinine ratio (ACR) (NICE, 2019a). If the eGRF is <60 mL/min/1.73 m^2, the test should be performed two weeks later, and if it remains static, it should be rechecked in three months. An eGFR should always be interpreted with caution in pregnancy, oedema, extremes of muscle mass, malnourishment, protein supplementation or patients of Asian or Chinese origin (NICE, 2019a). In the instance of renal impairment in patients who are elderly or at extremes of muscle mass, the Cockcroft and Gault formula should be used to estimate creatinine clearance (BNF, 2019a). Further information regarding prescribing in renal impairment is available via https://bnf.nice.org.uk/guidance/prescribing-in-renal-impairment.html.

Drug-induced renal damage

The selection of appropriate pharmacotherapy and safe prescribing practice is reliant upon knowledge of pathological disease processes, as well as the pharmacokinetics and pharmacodynamics of the drugs selected to treat the condition in question. As had been explored in the previous section of this chapter, there are a number of sites within the renal system in which pathology can occur that leads to acute or chronic kidney dysfunction. One of the most common and potentially avoidable causes of acute and chronic renal damage is via pharmacotherapy itself. Drugs can cause renal damage in a number of ways, including altered renal blood flow, damage to the nephron, or damage to the interstitial tissues. Figure 11.3 provides a non-exhaustive list of some of the adverse effects that pharmacotherapies can exert upon the kidneys.

It is incredibly important that any healthcare professional involved in the dispensing, administration or otherwise manipulation of pharmacotherapies be aware of the potential adverse effects that drug therapy can have upon the short- and long-term function of the renal system. It is also of utmost importance that these healthcare professionals are aware of how the use of certain drugs in patients with known reduced renal function can give rise to clinical deterioration due to:

- drug toxicity – secondary to reduced renal excretion of a drug or its metabolites;
- increased drug sensitivity;

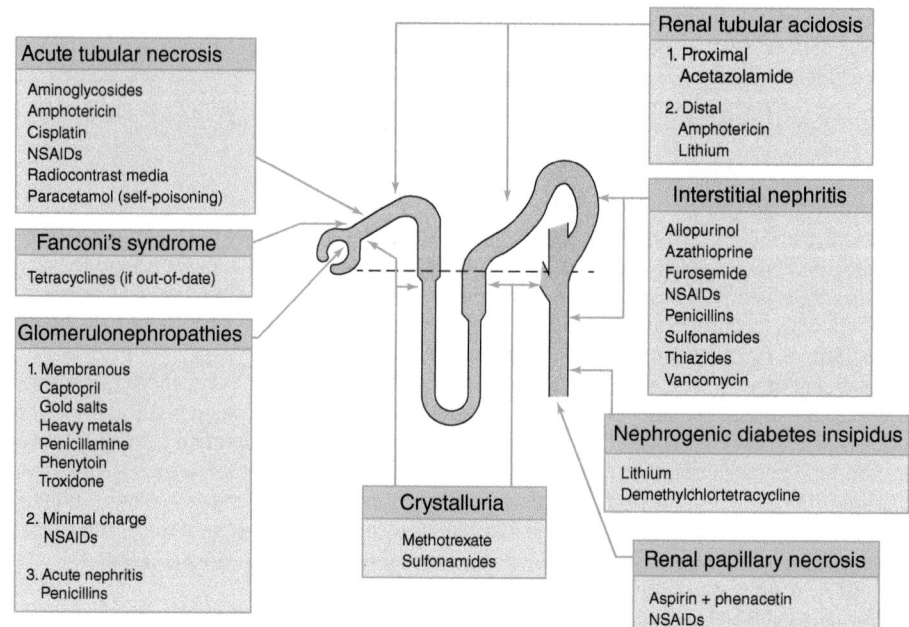

Figure 11.3 The adverse effects of certain drugs upon the kidney. Source: Adapted from Graeme-Smith and Aronson (2002).

- poorly tolerated known side effects of drugs;
- certain drugs are ineffective when renal function is reduced (BNF, 2019a).

The NICE provides very useful guides within the British National Formulary regarding dosage adjustment for impaired renal function, and how to estimate renal function in those patients where a serum creatinine level has been obtained.

Drug classes that act upon the renal system
Overview

Common renal diseases have been discussed earlier in this chapter and the main pathophysiological consequences identified. Drugs that affect the renal system may be classified according to their action, encompassing those used to treat urinary retention (UR) and incontinence, fluid retention, and electrolyte disorders. Another common disorder of the urinary tract, UTI, is not covered with within this chapter and the reader should refer to Chapter 9 – Antibiotics. The following section provides an overview of the classes of renal drugs, the pharmacokinetics and pharmacodynamics of specific examples, and the renal conditions in which they may be utilised. This is outlined in Table 11.5.

Drugs used to treat fluid retention
Overview

Diuretics are used in the treatment of multiple conditions that lead to fluid retention and formation of interstitial oedema, with treatment aiming to increase excretion of sodium chloride and water via the kidneys. Diuretics affect electrolyte and water balance within the

Table 11.5 Common renal drugs.

Drug class	Subclass	Example drug names	Common conditions
Diuretics	Loop diuretic	*Furosemide* *Bumetanide*	• Fluid retention/oedema due to chronic heart failure • Resistant hypertension (not as a first-line agent)
	Thiazides and related diuretics	*Bendroflumethiazide*	• Hypertension (not first-line agent) • Mild to moderate heart failure
		Indapamide	• Hypertension (particularly in diabetic patients)
	Osmotic	*Mannitol*	• Cerebral oedema and raised intraocular pressure
	Potassium-sparing and Aldosterone-antagonists	*Amiloride*	• Oedema (as monotherapy) • Potassium conservation when used as an adjunct to thiazide or loop diuretics for hypertension, congestive heart failure or hepatic ascites
		Spirinolactone	• Oedema • Ascites in cirrhosis of the liver • Nephrotic syndrome • Moderate to severe heart failure (adjunct) • Resistant hypertension (adjunct) • Primary hyperaldosteronism in patients awaiting surgery • Given with thiazide or loop diuretics to preserve serum potassium levels
	Carbonic-anhydrase inhibitors	*Acetazolamide*	• Reduction of intra-ocular pressure • Glaucoma • Epilepsy

(Continued)

Table 11.5 (Continued)

Drug class	Subclass	Example drug names	Common conditions
Electrolyte disorders	Phosphate binders	*Sevelamer* *Lanthanum*	• Control of hyperphosphataemia in patients with chronic renal failure
	Vitamin D supplementation	*Alfacalcidol*	• Patients with severe renal impairment requiring vitamin D therapy • Hypophosphatemic rickets • Persistent hypocalcaemia due to hypoparathyroidism or pseudohypoparathyroidism
		Calcitriol	• Renal osteodystrophy
	Potassium binders	*Calcium polystyrene sulfonate* *Sodium polystyrene sulfonate*	• Hyperkalaemia associated with anuria or severe oliguria, and in dialysis patients
	Potassium supplements	*Sando-K®*	• Potassium depletion
	Bicarbonate supplements	*Sodium Bicarbonate*	• Chronic acidotic states secondary to certain renal disorders
Drugs used to treat urinary retention and incontinence	α_1 receptor antagonists	*Tamsulosin hydrochloride*	• Acute urinary retention • Benign prostatic hyperplasia
		Doxazosin	
	Androgen-synthesis inhibitors	*Finasteride*	• Benign prostatic hyperplasia
	Phosphodiesterase type 5 (PDE5) inhibitors	*Tadalafil*	• Benign prostatic hyperplasia • Erectile dysfunction
	Antimuscarinics	*Oxybutynin hydrochloride*	• Urinary frequency • Urinary urgency • Urinary incontinence • Neurogenic bladder instability • Nocturnal enuresis associated with over-active bladder

Source: Sadie Diamond-Fox.

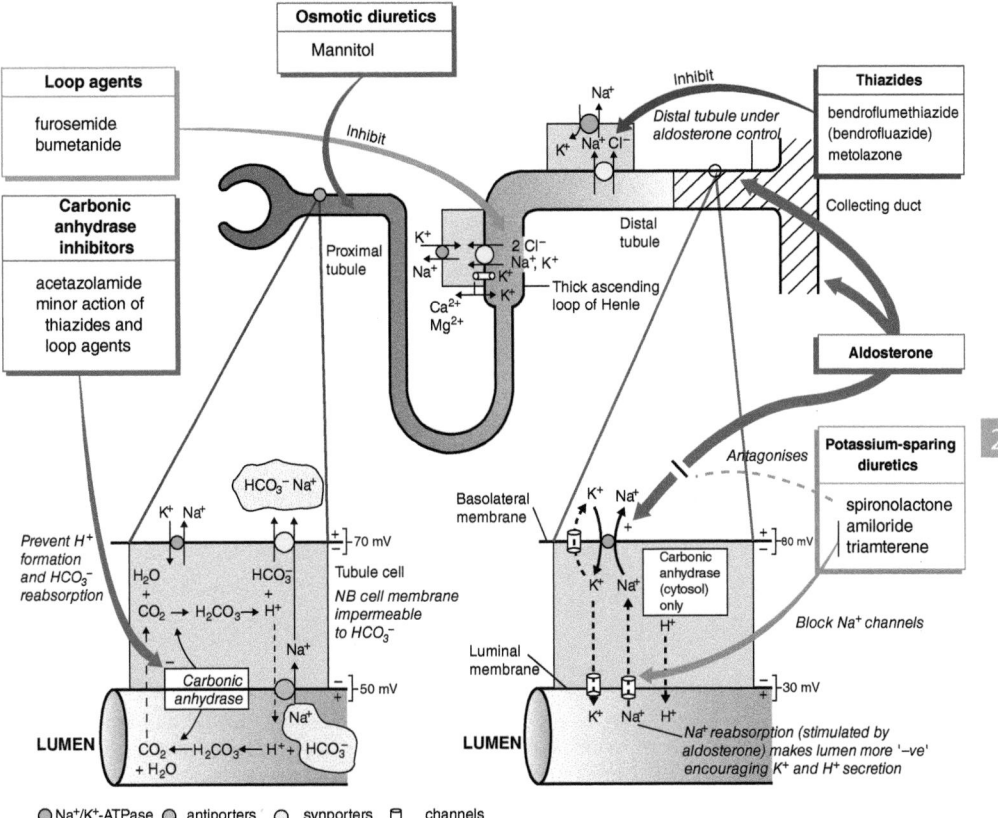

Figure 11.4   Site of diuretic effects upon the nephron. Source: Neal (2016).

nephrons in the kidney via co-transporter pumps, antagonising the effects of aldosterone or inhibiting transport of bicarbonate (see Figure 11.4). The main electrolyte that has a potent diuretic effect when manipulated via pharmacotherapy is sodium – if increased numbers of sodium molecules are excreted (naturesis), then water excretion (diuresis) will follow. There are varying combinations of diuretics that act upon different sites of the nephron that can be co-administered to achieve a synergistic effect, as different segments of the nephron can compensate for altered sodium handling. If multiple sites of the nephron are targeted through various different receptors, then a more potent diuretic effect may be achieved.

Loop diuretics

Loop diuretics, whether taken by the oral or injectable routes, are used to treat many disease processes, a few of which are demonstrated within Table 11.6. As demonstrated within Figure 11.4, loop diuretics act upon the thick ascending limb of the loop of Henle. Prior to reaching the target site, loop diuretics such as furosemide are actively secreted by the proximal tubules into the urine. Here they have a potent diuretic action via the inhibition of the sodium–potassium–chloride co-transporter, or the Na–K–Cl (NKCC2) co-transporter as it is otherwise known. The NKCC2 in normal physiology reabsorbs a high sodium and chloride load, therefore inhibition of this pump via a loop diuretic such as furosemide inhibits sodium and chloride reabsorption. This causes both diuresis and loss of these electrolytes, mainly sodium (naturesis). In addition, potassium secretion is increased under the influence of aldosterone in the DCT, through the exchange of potassium for sodium. This eventually leads to increased potassium excretion and may result in lowered blood serum potassium levels (hypokalaemia).

Table 11.6   Loop diuretics and their related pharmacology.

Medication name	Furosemide	Bumetanide
Mode of action	Inhibition of the sodium–potassium–chloride cotransporter/Na–K–Cl (NKCC2) co-transporter	
Route of administration	Oral, IM or IV	Oral
Indications	**ADULT**	
	• Oedema and resistant oedema • Resistant hypertension	• Oedema and resistant oedema
	CHILD	
	• Oedema in heart failure, renal disease and hepatic disease Pulmonary oedema • Oliguria	• Oedema in heart failure, renal disease and hepatic disease • Pulmonary oedema (severe cases)
Contraindications	• Anuria • Comatose and pre-comatose states associated with liver cirrhosis • Renal failure due to nephrotoxic or hepatotoxic drugs • Severe hypokalaemia • Severe hyponatraemia • Previous anaphylactic reaction	
Precautions	• Can exacerbate diabetes (but hyperglycaemia less likely than with thiazides) • Can exacerbate gout • Hypotension should be corrected before initiation of treatment • Hypovolaemia should be corrected before initiation of treatment • Urinary retention can occur in prostatic hyperplasia • Lower initial doses of diuretics should be used in the elderly because they are particularly susceptible to the side effects. • Dose should then be adjusted according to renal function • Can cause acute urinary retention in children with obstruction of urinary outflow • If there is an enlarged prostate, urinary retention can occur, although this is less likely if small doses and less potent diuretics are used initially; an adequate urinary output should be established before initiating treatment • Hypokalaemia is dangerous in severe cardiovascular disease and in patients also being treated with cardiac glycosides • In hepatic failure, hypokalaemia caused by diuretics can precipitate encephalopathy Pregnancy and Breast-feeding: • Furosemide crosses the placental barrier and should not be given during pregnancy unless there are compelling medical reasons • Furosemide is contraindicated in breast-feeding as it passes into breast milk and may inhibit lactation • Bumetanide should be avoided during the first trimester • Bumetanide has no data on breast-feeding and therefore should not be used in lactating mothers unless essential	
Side effects (Common and Very Common ONLY)	• Dizziness • Electrolyte imbalance • Fatigue • Headache • Metabolic alkalosis • Muscle spasms (secondary to electrolyte disorders) • Nausea	

242

(Continued)

Table 11.6   (Continued)

Medication name	Furosemide	Bumetanide
Interactions	• The dosage of concurrently administered cardiac glycosides, diuretics, antihypertensive agents or other drugs with blood-pressure-lowering potential may require adjustment as a more pronounced fall in blood pressure must be anticipated if given concomitantly with furosemide • The toxic effects of nephrotoxic drugs may be increased by concomitant administration of potent diuretics such as furosemide • Some electrolyte disturbances (e.g. hypokalaemia, hypomagnesemia) may increase the toxicity of certain other drugs (e.g. digitalis preparations [digoxin] and drugs inducing QT interval prolongation syndrome).	• As for furosemide • Should not be administered concurrently with lithium, as diuretics reduce the clearance rate of lithium leading to increased blood-lithium levels with signs of overdose • Should not be given concurrently cephaloridine or amphotericin as it could lead to increased toxic effects
Absorption	• Approximately 65% of the dose is absorbed after oral administration	• Rapidly and almost completely absorbed from the gastrointestinal tract with the bioavailability reported as between 80 and 95%
Distribution	• Furosemide is up to 99% bound to plasma proteins	• 95% bound to plasma proteins • Plasma elimination half-life of 0.75 to 2.6 hours
Metabolism	• Liver and kidney glucuronidation	• Liver • No active metabolites are known
Elimination	• Mainly excreted in the urine, largely unchanged • Also excreted in the bile which significantly increases in renal failure	• ~50% dose excreted unchanged via the kidneys with the remainder excreted via the bile into the faeces

Source: British National Formulary (2019b, c); British National Formulary for Children (2019a, b); Electronic Medicines Compendium (2019a, b).

243

Loop diuretics are highly protein bound to albumin; therefore, during conditions such as extreme hypoalbuminemia or in the presence of another highly protein-bound drug (such as warfarin) the diuretic effect may be less effective due to the impaired delivery of the drug to the kidney. There are some renal conditions in which the co-administration of human albumin solution with a loop diuretic may prove useful, although there is a lack of strong evidence to support this.

Clinical considerations

Monitoring

Patients receiving loop diuretics should undergo regular monitoring of their serum sodium and potassium levels, this is particularly important in the following patient groups:

- The elderly population.
- Patients with impaired renal function and creatinine clearance below 60 mL/min per 1.73 m² body surface area.
- Patients whereby a co-existing disease process exists which may have already caused electrolyte deficiencies (such as liver disease or anorexia nervosa).
- Patients receiving chronic corticosteroid or digoxin therapy. Digoxin has a very narrow therapeutic range and potassium deficiency can trigger or exacerbate the symptoms of digoxin toxicity.

Ototoxicity

Rapid intravenous administration of furosemide can cause tinnitus and permanent hearing loss (ototoxicity). Intravenous administration rates should not usually exceed 4 mg/min, however single doses of up to 80 mg may be administered more rapidly; a lower rate of infusion may be necessary in renal impairment.

Source: British National Formulary (2019b, c), British National Formulary for Children (2019a, b), Electronic Medicines Compendium (2019a, b).

The pharmacokinetics of loop diuretics demonstrate a steep dose–response curve with little diuretic or naturetic effect below a certain threshold/plasma concentration. Once the plasma concentration reaches said threshold, a rapid increase in the response to the administered diuretic is observed. At high plasma concentrations of the drug, a plateau is reached, and further dose increases no longer elicit a therapeutic effect (diuresis). Loop diuretics accumulate in the renal tubules via tubular secretion and it is this urinary concentration that determines the therapeutic threshold, not the serum/blood concentration (Anisman et al., 2019). The effects of both AKI and CKD on the pharmacokinetics and pharmacodynamics of loop diuretics can lead to a reduced diuretic response, including reduced tubular secretion and a blunted response of the NKCC2 co-transporter. Dose adjustment should therefore be taken into consideration.

The following table details some of the pharmacological and clinical date surrounding the prescribing of loop diuretics. It has been composed using the most up-to-date resources at the time of publishing. However, it should only serve as a guide and the latest versions of the British National Formulary and relevant guidelines should be utilised for prescribing in practice within the UK.

Thiazide diuretics

Thiazide diuretics, like loop diuretics, promote both naturesis and diuresis. Administration of thiazide diuretics cause changes in sodium concentrations more distal to the DCT. As demonstrated within Figure 11.4, thiazide diuretics exert their direct effect upon the earliest/proximal portion of the DCT of the nephron, which in normal physiology reabsorbs around 5% of the filtered sodium. Here the thiazides diuretics inhibit the sodium chloride co-transport protein (see Figure 11.5) which is situated on the lumen/tubular side of the cell membrane of the DCT cells; this then inhibits transport of sodium and chloride in to the DCT cells via the luminal membrane and decreases sodium and water passage into the interstitial fluid. Blockage of the sodium chloride co-transport increases the flow of sodium and calcium ions through the sodium/calcium channel on the basolateral membrane. This results in increased calcium reabsorption into the

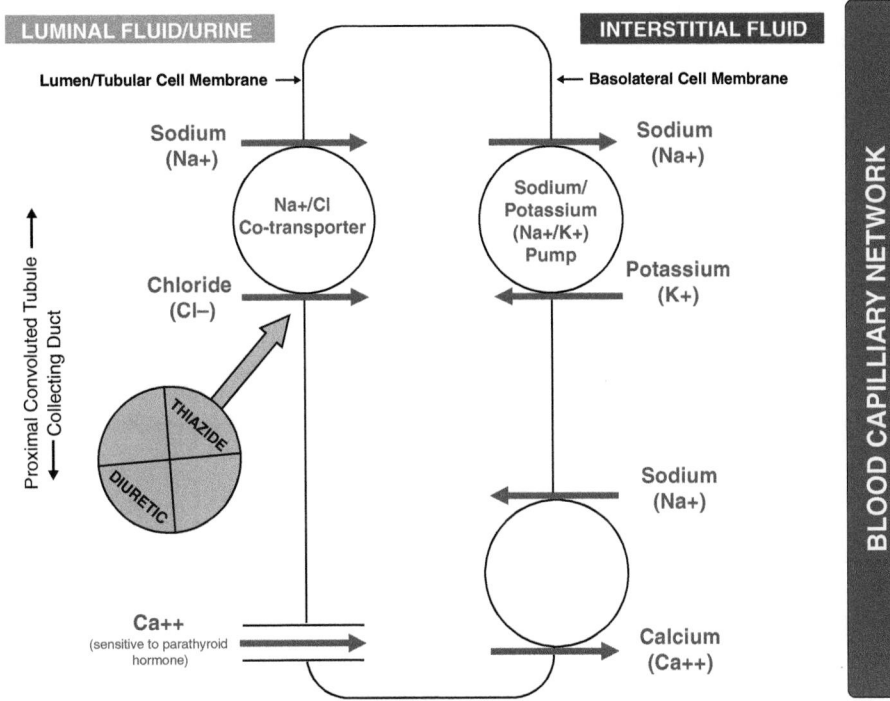

Figure 11.5   Distal convoluted tubule (DCT) cell and thiazide diuretic site of action.
Source: Sadie Diamond-Fox.

interstitium and eventually increased serum calcium levels in exchange for sodium return to the DCT and increased luminal fluid concentrations of sodium. The inhibition of the sodium chloride co-transporter at the more proximal segment of the DCT also results in an increased delivery of sodium load to the distal segments of the DCT and eventually the collecting ducts/tubules (Akbari and Khorasani-Zadeh, 2019). This increased sodium load stimulates sodium exchange with potassium and hydrogen resulting in an increased excretion into the urine and lowered serum levels of potassium and hydrogen, which can result in hypokalaemia and a metabolic alkalosis.

Thiazide diuretics not only aid the mobilisation of oedema, but can also be used to reduce blood pressure. The mechanism of their antihypertensive properties is still debated, however there are various modes of action that have been proposed. First, diuresis induces haemody-namic changes due to volume depletion and a resulting reduction in cardiac output. However, as a result of volume depletion, the activation of the renin–angiotensin–aldosterone system often occurs which can blunt the antihypertensive effects of thiazides. In these causes, the co-administration of an ACEi may be useful to provide a synergistic effect. Direct endothelial or vascular smooth muscle-mediated vasodilation and indirect compensation has also been proposed as a more chronic process which results in antihypertensive effects (Duarte and Cooper DeHoff, 2010).

Table 11.7 details some of the pharmacological and clinical data surrounding the prescrib-ing of two common thiazide diuretics used in current practice.

Osmotic diuretics

Osmotic diuretics are freely filtered by the glomerulus, are minimally reabsorbed by the renal tubules, and have no other pharmacological effects. These diuretics do not affect transporters but are osmotically active particles that generate an osmotic gradient, promoting the movement of

Table 11.7   Thiazide diuretics and their related pharmacology.

Medication name	Bendroflumethiazide
Mode of action	Inhibition of the sodium chloride co-transport protein with the proximal part of the distal convoluted tubule (DCT)
Route of administration	Oral
Indications	**ADULT** • Oedema • Hypertension **CHILD** • Hypertension • Oedema in heart failure, renal disease and hepatic disease • Pulmonary oedema
Contraindications	• Addison's disease • Hypercalcaemia • Hyponatraemia • Refractory hypokalaemia • Symptomatic hyperuricaemia
Cautions	• Diabetes • Gout • Hyperaldosteronism • Malnourishment • Nephrotic syndrome • Systemic lupus erythematosus • Hypokalaemia – dangerous in severe cardiovascular disease and in patients also being treated with cardiac glycosides • Lower initial doses of diuretics should be used in the elderly <u>Pregnancy and Breast-feeding:</u> • Crosses the placenta and its use may be associated with hypokalaemia, increased blood viscosity and reduced placental perfusion, therefore should be avoided • Suppresses lactation • Small amounts pass into breast milk – should be avoided in breast-feeding mothers
Side effects (Common and Very Common ONLY)	• Alkalosis due to hypochloraemia • Constipation • Diarrhoea • Dizziness • Electrolyte imbalance • Headache • Hyperuricaemia • Nausea • Postural hypotension • Urticaria
Interactions	• Antiarrhythmics • Antidepressants • Antidiabetics • Antiepileptics • Antifungals • Antihypertensives • Antipsychotics • Calcium salts • Corticosteroids

(Continued)

Table 11.7   (Continued)

Medication name	Bendroflumethiazide
	• Calcium salts • Cytotoxics • Hormone antagonists • Lithium • Vitamins
Absorption	• Completely absorbed from the gastrointestinal tract • Diuresis is initiated in about 2 hours and lasts for 12–18 hours or longer.
Distribution	• >90% bound to plasma proteins
Metabolism	• Variable degree of hepatic metabolism
Elimination	• ~30% excreted unchanged in urine with the remainder excreted as uncharacterised metabolites

247

Source: British National Formulary (2019d); British National Formulary for Children (2019c); Electronic Medicines Compendium (2019c).

water into the renal tubule. Osmotic diuretics exert their effects in the proximal convoluted tubule, the thin descending loop of Henle and the collecting ducts, as these are the segments that are highly permeable to water.

The majority of filtrate is reabsorbed in the proximal convoluted tubule (60–70%), with the movement of sodium and water into the tubular cells, in addition to other ions and solutes. In the presence of an osmotic diuretic, the concentration gradient increases within the tubule, reducing the movement of sodium and water, producing a diuresis. A significant naturesis is not observed, as the sodium that has not been absorbed is subsequently, in the thick ascending limb of the loop of Henle, the DCT and the collecting duct. As distal flow is increased, the secretion of potassium ions is stimulated in the collecting duct.

An osmotic diuresis also causes increased renal medullary blood flow, which consequently diminishes the normal osmotic gradient created in the thin descending loop of Henle and the medullary collecting ducts. This impairs the movement of water out of the tubule contributing further to the diuretic effect. Mannitol is an osmotic diuretic used in the management of raised intracranial or intraocular pressure as it remains within the extracellular fluid, raising plasma osmolarity, resulting in movement of water from the target tissues (brain, eye) into the circulation. The diuretic effects are subsequently exerted in the kidney. Other uses include prevention of renal injury during major cardiac and vascular surgery as well as promotion of diuresis following renal transplantation, poisoning and in rhabdomyolisis or haemolysis (Shawkat et al., 2012). The following Table 11.8 details the pharmacological data of mannitol.

Potassium-sparing diuretics and aldosterone-antagonists

Plasma potassium concentration is monitored in the adrenal cortex, a rise in which results in the release of aldosterone and, as previously discussed, contributes to the maintenance of potassium homoeostasis. Within the DCT and cortical collecting duct, aldosterone stimulates the reabsorption of sodium via the synthesis of sodium–potassium pumps, in the basolateral membrane, and sodium channels (epithelial sodium channel, ENaC), in the tubular luminal membrane. This creates a negative gradient within the lumen and, as potassium has been driven into the cell via the sodium–potassium pumps, it moves out into the tubular lumen via potassium channels or is co-transported with chloride. Higher flow rates also cause big potassium (BK) channels to open increasing the secretion of potassium. This process is depicted in Figure 11.6.

Potassium-sparing diuretics exert their effects in two ways: either by blocking the sodium channels in the luminal membrane, or by antagonising the effect of aldosterone on the sodium–potassium pumps. Drugs that combine with the sodium channel do so, on a one to

Table 11.8   Osmotic diuretics and their related pharmacology.

Medication name	Mannitol
Mode of action	Freely filtered by the glomerulus and acts as an osmotically active particle in the renal tubule resulting in diuresis
Route of administration	Intravenous
Indications	**ADULT** • Cerebral oedema • Raised intraocular pressure • Oliguria or renal impairment • Elimination of renally excreted toxic substances in poisoning **CHILD** • Cerebral oedema • Peripheral oedema and ascites

Contraindications	• Inhaled
	  ◦ Bronchial hyper-responsiveness to inhaled mannitol
	  ◦ Impaired lung function
	  ◦ Non-CF bronchiectasis
	• Intravenous
	  ◦ Anuria
	  ◦ Intracranial bleeding (except during craniotomy)
	  ◦ Severe cardiac failure
	  ◦ Severe dehydration
	  ◦ Severe pulmonary oedema
	  ◦ Pre-existing plasma hyperosmolarity

Cautions	• Inhalation
	  ◦ Asthma
	  ◦ Haemoptysis
	• Intravenous
	  ◦ Extravasation may cause inflammation and thrombophlebitis
	
	Pregnancy and Breast-feeding:
	• Manufacture advises to avoid unless essential

Side effects
(Common and Very Common ONLY)
	• Cough
	• Headache
	• Vomiting
	• Inhaled
	  ◦ Chest discomfort
	  ◦ Aggravation of condition
	  ◦ Haemoptysis
	  ◦ Respiratory disorders
	  ◦ Throat complaints
	• Intravenous – see BNF as multiple side effects and frequency unknown
	• Pregnancy and Breast-feeding:
	• Manufacturer advises to avoid unless essential

Interactions	• Potentialisation effect with concurrent use of other diuretics • Increased clearance of renally absorbed drugs • Nephrotoxicity of drugs due to fluid imbalance (Ciclosporin, Aminoglycoside) • Potential of neurotoxicity with neurotoxic drugs (Aminoglycoside) • Electrolyte imbalances with drugs that are sensitive to such imbalances
Absorption	• Administered IV
Distribution	• Confined to extracellular fluid

(Continued)

Table 11.8   (Continued)

Medication name	Mannitol
Metabolism	• Minimal liver metabolism
Elimination	• Freely filtered in the glomerulus • Less than 10% reabsorbed • Elimination half-life approximately 2 hours, longer in the presence of renal failure • 80% of the dose is excreted unchanged within 3 hours

Source: British National Formulary (2019e); British National Formulary for Children (2019d); Electronic Medicines Compendium (2019d).

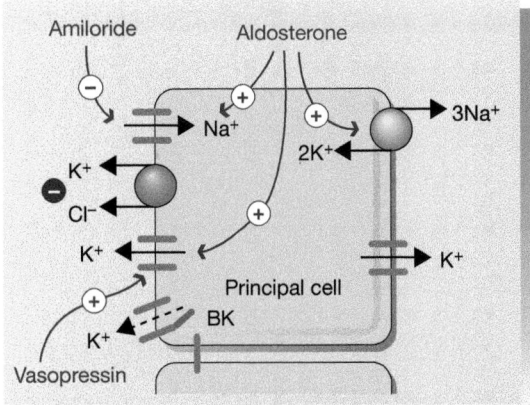

Figure 11.6   The effects of aldosterone on the principal cells. Source: Neal (2016).

one basis, reducing the reabsorption of sodium and the negative lumen gradient, decreasing the excretion of potassium (Neal, 2016). This may occur independently of aldosterone and is therefore associated with hyperkalaemia (Graeme-Smith and Aronson, 2002).

Aldosterone antagonising drugs compete for the aldosterone binding site on the cytoplasmic receptors, reducing the synthesis and insertion of sodium–potassium pumps in the basolateral membrane. Less sodium is reabsorbed and consequently less potassium excreted. Table 11.9 details the commonly used potassium-sparing diuretics and the related pharmacology.

Carbonic-anhydrase inhibitors

Carbonic-anhydrase inhibitors are weak diuretics and rarely used for this purpose (Graeme-Smith and Aronson, 2002; Neal, 2016). Carbonic anhydrase is an enzyme present within the proximal convoluted tubule cells and the tubular lumen where it catalyses the dissociation of water and carbon dioxide into hydrogen ions and bicarbonate ions, and vice versa. Bicarbonate is freely filtered in the glomerulus and the sodium gradient drives the reabsorption of bicarbonate, via a co-transporter, and the secretion of hydrogen ions via the sodium–hydrogen ion exchanger (NHE3) in the proximal convoluted tubule. The secreted hydrogen ions are then recycled in the lumen by carbonic anhydrase. Plasma pH is maintained by the reabsorption of bicarbonate ions. This is demonstrated in Figure 11.7.

Carbonic-anhydrase inhibitors prevent the reaction of hydration of carbon dioxide and the dehydration of bicarbonate resulting in the excretion of bicarbonate, sodium and potassium ions, as well as water, producing a diuresis (Neal, 2016; O'Callaghan, 2017). Table 11.10 details some of the commonly used carbonic-anhydrase inhibitors and the related pharmacology.

Table 11.9 Potassium-sparing diuretics and their related pharmacology.

Medication name	Amiloride	Spironolactone
Mode of action	Blocks sodium channels in the luminal membrane	An aldosterone-antagonist, it competes with aldosterone for the binding site on the cytoplasmic receptor that syntheses basolateral sodium–potassium pumps
Route of administration	Oral	Oral
Indications	• Oedema (monotherapy) • Potassium conservation when used as an adjunct to thiazide or loop diuretics for hypertension or congestive heart failure • Potassium conservation when used as an adjunct to thiazide or loop diuretics for hepatic cirrhosis with ascites • Adjunct to thiazide or loop diuretics for oedema in heart failure and hepatic disease (where potassium conservation desirable)	**ADULT** • Oedema – ascites in cirrhosis of the liver • Malignant ascites • Nephrotic syndrome • Oedema in congestive heart failure • As an adjunct in moderate to severe heart failure • As an adjunct in resistant hypertension • Primary hyperaldosteronism in patients awaiting surgery **CHILD** • Oedema in heart failure and in ascites • Nephrotic syndrome • Reduction of hypokalaemia induced by diuretics or amphotericin
Contraindications	• Addison's disease • Anuria • Hyperkalaemia	• Addison's disease • Anuria • hyperkalaemia
Cautions	• Diabetes mellitus • Elderly Pregnancy and Breast-feeding: • Not to be used to treat gestational diabetes • Manufacturer advises avoidance in breast-feeding	• Acute porphyrias • Elderly Pregnancy and Breast-feeding: • Use only if potential benefit outweighs risk • Metabolites present in breast milk
Side effects (Common and Very Common ONLY)	• See BNF as multiple side effects and frequency unknown	• See BNF as multiple side effects and frequency unknown

Interactions	<ul><li>Risk of hypotension with alcohol, aldesleukin, general anaesthetic, antidepressants, antihypertensives, dopaminergics, muscle relaxants, nitrates and prostaglandins</li><li>Hyponatraemia with antiepileptics and antidiabetic agents</li><li>Increased risk of nephrotoxicity with NSAIDs, lithium</li><li>Risk of hyperkalaemia with NSAIDs, other potassium-sparing diuretics, hormones and other endocrine drugs, immunosuppressants, potassium supplements</li></ul>	<ul><li>Concomitant use with drugs known to cause hyperkalaemia, including co-trimoxazole</li><li>Digoxin – increased digoxin level</li><li>Potentiation of antihypertensive drugs, not routinely used with ACE inhibitors</li><li>NSAIDs may attenuate the diuretic effect</li><li>Reduced vascular response to noradrenaline</li></ul>
Absorption	<ul><li>Incompletely absorbed from the gastrointestinal tract, approximately 50%</li></ul>	<ul><li>Well absorbed orally with bioavailability of >90%</li></ul>
Distribution	<ul><li>Does not bind to plasma proteins</li><li>Apparent volume of distribution greater than body water</li></ul>	<ul><li>Highly plasma protein bound, >90%</li></ul>
Metabolism	<ul><li>It is not metabolised</li></ul>	<ul><li>Metabolised in the liver to active metabolites</li></ul>
Elimination	<ul><li>Excreted in the urine unchanged</li><li>Half-life of approximately 6 hours</li></ul>	<ul><li>Elimination primarily urine, secondarily through biliary excretion in the faeces</li><li>Half-life 1.3 hours, active metabolites 2.8–11.2 hours</li></ul>

Source: British National Formulary 2019f, g; British National Formulary for Children 2019e, f; Electronic Medicines Compendium 2019e, f.

Clinical considerations

Hyperkalaemia and spironolactone

As previously discussed, spironolactone is a competitive aldosterone-antagonist, blocking the effects of aldosterone and producing a diuresis, via increased sodium excretion, with preservation of potassium, through reduced potassium excretion in the distal renal tubule. Hyperkalaemia may occur due to this effect, causing cardiac dysrhythmia and cardiac arrest. Patients with severe renal impairment or pre-existing hyperkalaemia should not be prescribed spironolactone (MHRA, 2016).

Spironolactone is indicated in heart failure and it may be utilised with other pharmacotherapy including ACEi and ARBs, the pharmacology of which is explained in Chapter 10, and side effects include renal dysfunction and hyperkalaemia. Patients being treated with ACEi and ARBs are more likely to have risk factors for developing hyperkalaemia (renal insufficiency and diabetes mellitus) and this in combination with spironolactone significantly increases the likelihood of this occurring.

Within the UK between 1998 and 2015, there were 82 reported cases of abnormal serum potassium, 70 of which were defined as hyperkalaemic, in patients prescribed an ACEi or ARB with spironolactone (MRHA, 2016). There were three fatalities. Initially a landmark trial demonstrated a relative risk reduction in death for patients treated with spironolactone and standard therapy, including an ACEi, with low incidence of hyperkalaemia (Pitt et al., 1999). Following this there was increased reporting of abnormal or increased serum potassium, or hyperkalaemia, with patients prescribed spironolactone and an ACEi or ARB in the UK (MRHA, 2016). Furthermore, a European review has recommended that ACEi and ARB therapy should not be used in combination due to the increased risk of hypotension, impaired renal function and hyperkalaemia (MRHA, 2014).

Source: https://www.gov.uk/drug-safety-update/spironolactone-and-renin-angiotensin-system-drugs-in-heart-failure-risk-of-potentially-fatal-hyperkalaemia.

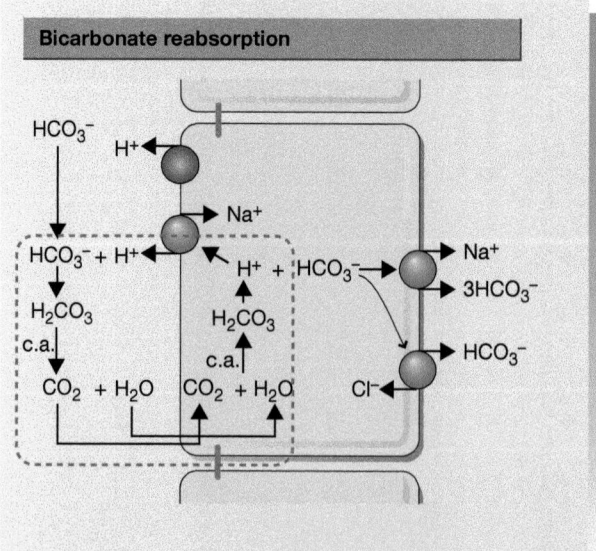

Figure 11.7   The process of bicarbonate reabsorption in the proximal convoluted tubule.
Source: Neal (2016).

Table 11.10 Carbonic-anhydrase inhibitors and their related pharmacology.

Medication name	Acetazolamide
Mode of action	Carbonic-anhydrase inhibitor
Route of administration	Oral
Indications	**ADULT** • Reduction of intraocular pressure in open-angle glaucoma, secondary glaucoma and peri-operatively in angle-closure glaucoma • Glaucoma • Epilepsy **CHILD** • Glaucoma • Epilepsy • Reduction of intraocular pressure in primary and secondary glaucoma (specialist use only) • Raised intracranial pressure
Contraindications	• Adrenocortical insufficiency • Hyperchloraemic acidosis • Hypokalaemia • Hyponatraemia • Long-term administration in chronic angle-closure glaucoma
Cautions	• Diabetes mellitus • Elderly • Impaired alveolar ventilation • Pulmonary obstruction • Renal calculi • Not generally recommended for long-term use Pregnancy and Breast-feeding: • Manufacturer advises against use in pregnancy, particularly the first trimester
Side effects (Common and Very Common ONLY)	• Haemorrhage • Metabolic acidosis • Nephrolithiasis • Abnormal sensation
Interactions	• Potentiation of the effects of folic acid antagonists, hypoglycaemics and anticoagulants • Metabolic acidosis from concurrent administration with aspirin • Modifies metabolism of phenytoin with concomitant use, increases serum levels • Concomitant use with other carbonic-anhydrase inhibitors is not recommended • Enhanced effect of quinidine and duration of amphetamines • May elevate cyclosporine levels, decrease lithium levels and cause renal calculus with co-administration of sodium bicarbonate
Absorption	• Rapid absorption from the gastrointestinal tract • Peak concentration after approximately 2 hours
Distribution	• Plasma half-life of 4 hours • Tightly bound to carbonic anhydrase
Metabolism	• Not metabolised
Elimination	• Excreted unchanged in the urine • Elimination half-life 2–4 hours

Source: British National Formulary (2019h); British National Formulary for Children (2019g); Electronic Medicines Compendium (2019g).

253

Drugs used to treat electrolyte disorders

As already explored earlier within this chapter, electrolyte disorders can occur as a result of altered homoeostasis of the renal system, or as a result of multiple other disease processes (adrenal gland dysfunction, gastrointestinal dysfunction, etc.), or iatrogenic causes such as a result of pharmacotherapy (i.e. potassium depletion due to loop diuretics). This can lead to multiple derangements in serum levels of measured ions and/or vitamins. Due to the delicate nature of ion and vitamin balance within the body and its effect upon all body cells, a derangement out of the normal homoeostatic range can manifest in severe organ dysfunction. The principle treatments of electrolyte disorders involve either replacement or the promotion of excretion of said ions or vitamins. Wherever possible, the primary or underlying cause of the electrolyte and or/vitamin disturbance should be treated to avoid the potential for unnecessary long-term treatment strategies that only mask the underlying problem.

Phosphate binders, calcium supplements and vitamin D supplements

254

Phosphate binders, calcium supplements and vitamin D supplements are commonly used in combination in chronic renal disease due to the altered calcium and phosphate metabolism. This can lead to raised phosphate serum levels (hyperphosphataemia) and lowered serum levels of calcium (hypocalcaemia) and low vitamin D levels, the effects of which and the targets for pharmacotherapy are illustrated in Figure 11.8. Hyperphosphataemia is associated with increased morbidity and mortality among both ESRD patients and in non-CKD patients (Hou et al., 2017; Moon et al., 2019). Secondary hyperparathyroidism can also develop as a result of hyperphosphataemia leading to increased parathormone (PTH) levels. Persistent overproduction of PTH leads to renal osteodystrophy, a defective or abnormal bone development leading to weakness, bone pain and skeletal deformity. There are significant cardiovascular consequences as a result of increased PTH which increase morbidity and mortality rates among this population.

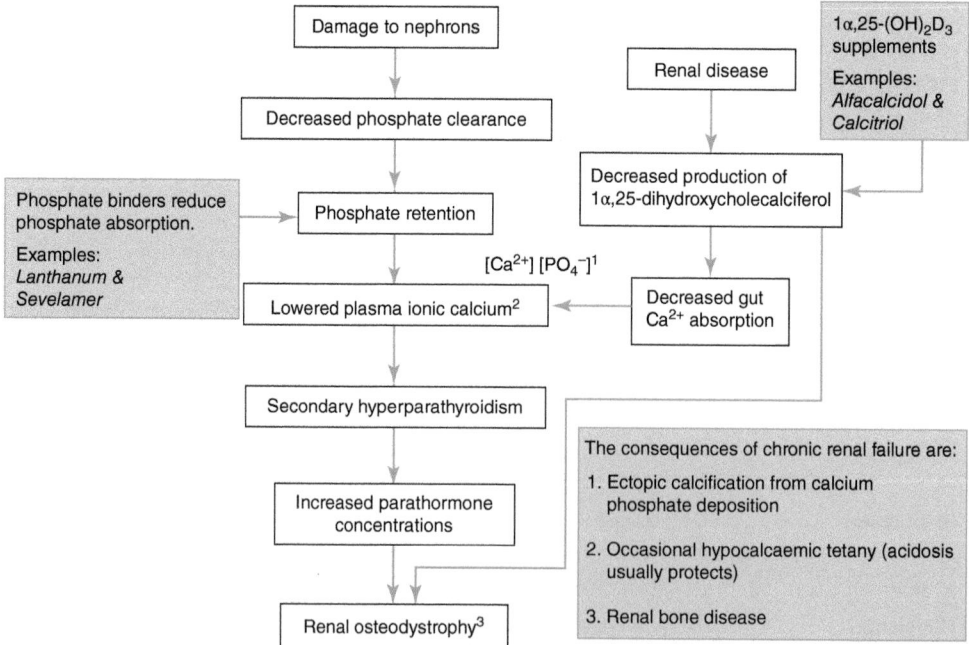

Figure 11.8 The effects of CKD upon phosphate and calcium metabolism. Source: Graeme-Smith and Aronson (2002).

Calcium and calcium phosphate deposits within the cardiovascular system, as a result of increased PTH, cause vascular calcification which mainly effects blood vessels, myocardial tissue and cardiac valves. This can lead to hypertension, myocardial infarction and heart failure (Jablonski and Chonchol, 2013).

Hypocalcaemia due to renal disease is due to two primary causes: phosphate retention and decreased renal production of 1,25 (OH)2 vitamin D. A spectrum of consequences can occur which may be life-threatening (coma, cardiac arrhythmias, seizures, laryngeal stridor) to more chronic, but debilitating (cataracts, extra-skeletal calcification and renal bone disease). Decreased production of 1,25 (OH)2 vitamin D leads to decreased absorption of calcium from the gut, which in turn lowers serum calcium levels. PTH is then secreted from the parathyroid glands in response to lowered serum calcium levels, which can eventually lead to hypertrophy of these glands and other disorders as explored above, as the cycle continues until the underlying cause (decreased vitamin D) is treated.

Phosphate binders, as illustrated in Figure 11.8, inhibit phosphate retention by binding to phosphate within the gut lumen and preventing its absorption. Certain types of phosphate binders, unlike sevelamer and lanthanum, contain calcium which also leads to reduced phosphate retention, but can result in severely raised serum calcium levels which can be life-threatening (Electronic Medicines Compendium, 2019h, i). 1,25 (OH)2 vitamin D supplements are converted rapidly in the liver to 1,25-dihydroxyvitamin D. This is the metabolite of vitamin D which acts as a regulator of calcium and phosphate metabolism. The following Tables 11.11 and 11.12 outline some of the commonly prescribed agents and their pharmacological properties within these drugs classes.

Potassium binders and supplements

Potassium homoeostasis is maintained via the kidneys and the adrenal glands. Potassium binders or supplements may be prescribed depending upon the underlying cause of the potassium imbalance. The causes of hyperkalaemia include drugs (potassium-sparing diuretics, ACEi, ARBs, potassium supplements), acute or chronic renal failure, hypoaldosteronism and any condition resulting in potassium moving out of cells (metabolic acidosis, diabetic ketoacidosis, cell destruction, massive blood transfusion) (Graeme-Smith and Aronson, 2002). Drugs may be down titrated but in cohorts of patients with increased risk factors, such as cardiovascular disease and stroke, outcomes may be poorer with increased risk of mortality (Natale et al., 2018).

Potassium binders are commonly used in chronic renal disease to manage hyperkalaemia associated with anuria, severe oliguria and patients who are dialysis dependent. They are artificial resins containing either sodium or calcium, which is exchanged for potassium in the gastrointestinal tract, and then eliminated in the faeces. Fluid overload, heart failure and hypocalcaemia will dictate the choice of resin. A Cochrane Review is currently being conducted assessing the benefits and harms of potassium binders for treating chronic hyperkalaemia among adults and children with CKD (Natale et al., 2018).

Potassium supplements may be required in conditions causing potassium depletion or hypokalaemia. The causes of which include drugs (diuretics, insulin, corticosteroids, laxatives), gastrointestinal losses (diarrhoea, vomiting), renal losses (diuretic phase of ATN), hyperaldosteronism and malnutrition. Treatment of hypokalaemia should aim to identify and manage the underlying disease or primary causative factor. Mild to moderate hypokalaemia may be treated with oral supplementation. Chloride replacement with potassium depletion is advised, otherwise additional potassium will not be retained due its renal handling (Graeme-Smith and Aronson, 2002). Tables 11.13 and 11.14 outline some of the commonly used potassium binders and potassium supplements.

Bicarbonate supplements

The kidneys control bicarbonate levels contributing to the maintenance of acid–base homoeostasis. Metabolic acidosis occurs due to the loss of bicarbonate or the gain of hydrogen ions. Under normal circumstances, sodium bicarbonate is reabsorbed, via the sodium gradient, and hydrogen ions are secreted in the proximal tubule. In the distal tubule, hydrogen ions either contribute to reabsorption of the remaining bicarbonate or are buffered by phosphate.

Table 11.11 Phosphate binders and their related pharmacology.

Medication name	Sevelamer	Lanthanum
Mode of action	Reduction of phosphate absorption within gut lumen	
Route of administration	Oral	Oral
Indications	**ADULT**	
	• Hyperphosphataemia in patients on haemodialysis or peritoneal dialysis • Hyperphosphataemia in CKD	
	CHILD	
	• Hyperphosphataemia in patients on haemodialysis or peritoneal dialysis • Hyperphosphataemia in CKD	
Contraindications	• Previous anaphylactic reaction to this agent • Bowel obstruction	
Cautions	• Gastrointestinal disorders	• Acute peptic ulcer • Bowel obstruction • Crohn's disease • Ulcerative colitis
	Pregnancy and Breast-feeding: • Manufacturer advises use only if potential benefit outweighs risk	Pregnancy and Breast-feeding: • Manufacturer advises avoid – toxicity in *animal* studies.

Side effects (Common and Very Common ONLY)
- Constipation
- Diarrhoea
- Gastrointestinal discomfort
- Gastrointestinal disorders
- Nausea
- Vomiting

Interactions
- Ciprofloxacin
- Anti-arrhythmic medications
- Antiseizure medications
- Levothyroxine
- Antirejection drugs
- Warfarin
- Proton-pump inhibitors
- Antacids
- Chloroquine
- Hydroxychloroquine
- Ketoconazole

Absorption
- Not absorbed from the gastrointestinal tract
- Minimally absorbed following oral administration

Distribution
- No data
- Extensively bound to plasma proteins (>99.7%)

Metabolism
- No data
- Not metabolised

Elimination
- No data
- Excreted mainly in the faeces

Source: British National Formulary (2019i, j); British National Formulary for Children (2019h, l); Electronic Medicines Compendium (2019h, j).

Table 11.12 Vitamin D supplements and their related pharmacology.

Medication name	Alfacalcidol	Calcitriol
Mode of action	1,25 (OH)2 vitamin D supplementation	
Route of administration	Oral	Oral
Indications		**ADULT**
	• Patients with severe renal impairment requiring vitamin D therapy	• Renal osteodystrophy
	• Hypophosphatemic rickets	• Renal osteodystrophy (in patients with normal or only slightly reduced plasma–calcium concentration)
	• Persistent hypocalcaemia due to hypoparathyroidism or pseudohypoparathyroidism	
	• Prevention of vitamin D deficiency in renal or cholestatic liver disease	
		CHILD
	• Persistent hypocalcaemia due to hypoparathyroidism or pseudohypoparathyroidism	• Vitamin D dependent rickets
	• Prevention of vitamin D deficiency in renal or cholestatic liver disease	• Hypophosphatemic rickets
		• Persistent hypocalcaemia due to hypoparathyroidism
		• Pseudo-hypoparathyroidism (limited data)
Contraindications	• Hypercalcaemia	
	• Metastatic calcification	
Cautions	• Nephrolithiasis	
	• Take care to ensure correct dose in infants	
	Pregnancy and Breast-feeding:	
	• High doses teratogenic in *animals* but therapeutic doses unlikely to be harmful.	
	• Caution with high doses; may cause hypercalcaemia in infant – monitor serum–calcium concentration	

Side effects (Common and Very Common ONLY)	• Abdominal discomfort • Hyperphosphataemia • Rash pustular	• Abdominal pain • Headache • Hypercalcaemia • Hypercalciuria • Nausea • Skin reactions
Interactions	• Thiazide diuretics • Other vitamin D-containing preparations • Anticonvulsants • Magnesium-containing antacids • Aluminium-containing preparations	
Absorption	• Via intestines in a dose-related manner.	• Rapidly absorbed from the intestine
Distribution	• No data	• Mostly bound to a specific vitamin D binding protein • Bound to lipoproteins and albumin in a lesser degree
Metabolism	• No data	• Hydroxylated and oxidised in the kidney and in the liver by a specific cytochrome P450 enzyme
Elimination	• No data	• Excreted in the bile

Source: British National Formulary (2019j, k); British National Formulary for Children (2019h); Electronic Medicines Compendium (2019h, i).

259

Table 11.13   Potassium binders and their related pharmacology.

Medication name	Sodium polystyrene sulfonate	Calcium polystyrene sulfonate
Mode of action	Gastrointestinal potassium-binding resin	
Route of administration	Oral or rectal	
Indications	**ADULT**	
	• Hyperkalaemia associated with anuria or severe oliguria, and in dialysis patients	
	CHILD	
	• Hyperkalaemia associated with anuria or severe oliguria, and in dialysis patients	
Contraindications	• Obstructive bowel disease	• Hyperparathyroidism
	• Reduced gut motility in neonates	• Metastatic carcinoma
	• Hypersensitivity to polystyrene sulfonate resins	• Multiple myeloma
		• Obstructive bowel disease
		• Sarcoidosis
		• Reduced gut motility in neonates
		• Hypersensitivity to polystyrene sulfonate resins
Cautions	• Congestive heart failure	• Children – impact of resin with excessive dosage or
	• Hypertension	inadequate dilution
	• Oedema	
	• Children – hypertension, impact of resin with excessive dosage or inadequate dilution, should only be given to neonates rectally	
	Pregnancy and Breast-feeding:	Pregnancy and Breast-feeding:
	• Manufacturers advise only if potential benefit outweighs risk	• Manufacturers advise only if potential benefit outweighs risk

Side effects (Common and Very Common ONLY)	• Severe hypokalaemia, administration should cease once serum potassium level falls to 5 mmol/L • Electrolyte deficiency – calcium or magnesium • Constipation	• Severe hypokalaemia, administration should cease once serum potassium level falls to 5 mmol/L • Electrolyte deficiency – calcium or magnesium • Constipation
Interactions	• Manufacturers advise to take other drugs 3 hours before or after, with a 6 hour separation considered in gastroparesis • Gastrointestinal stenosis, intestinal ischemia and complications if administered with sorbitol • Binding effect reduced with cation-donating agents • Aluminium hydroxide – intestinal obstruction • Toxic effects of digitalis if hypokalemia occurs • Possible decreased absorption of lithium or levothyroxine	
Absorption	• Not absorbed	
Distribution	• As above	
Metabolism	• As above	
Elimination	• Excreted in the faeces	

Source: British National Formulary (2019m, n); British National Formulary for Children (2019l, m); Electronic Medicines Compendium (2019l, m).

Table 11.14   Potassium supplements and their related pharmacology.

Medication name	Potassium chloride
Mode of action	Potassium supplementation
Route of administration	Oral
Indications	**ADULT** ● Prevention of hypokalaemia (patients with normal diet) **CHILD** ● Prevention of hypokalaemia (patients with normal diet) ● Potassium depletion
Contraindications	● Plasma potassium above 5 mmol/L ● Severe renal impairment ● Inadequately treated Addison's disease
Cautions	● Cardiac disease ● With modified-release preparations – hiatus hernia, history of peptic ulcer, intestinal stricture <u>Pregnancy and Breast-feeding:</u> ● No clinical problems encountered but benefit and risks must be considered in pregnancy
Side effects (Common and Very Common ONLY)	● Hyperkalaemia ● Abdominal cramps ● Diarrhoea ● Gastrointestinal disorders ● Nausea and vomiting
Interactions	● Risk of hyperkalaemia increased with potassium-sparing diuretics and ACEi
Absorption	● Readily absorbed from the gastrointestinal tract
Distribution	● Not applicable
Metabolism	● Not applicable
Elimination	● Excretion of potassium via the distal tubules of the kidney, by the faeces, and a smaller amount in the perspiration

Source: British National Formulary (2019o); British National Formulary for Children (2019n); Electronic Medicines Compendium (2019n).

Bicarbonate loss is caused by gut losses, increased sodium chloride administration and renal bicarbonate loss. Renal tubular acidosis results in the kidneys being either unable to excrete hydrogen ions and reabsorb bicarbonate ions due to disorders of the proximal tubule (rare), or secrete hydrogen ions or absorb sodium ions due to secretory, permeability and voltage defects as well as hypoaldosteronism in the distal tubule (O'Callaghan, 2017). The gain of hydrogen ions occurs in lactic acidosis, ketoacidosis, poisoning and renal failure. Metabolic acidosis becomes more common with advancing CKD. Damage to both the glomerulus and renal tubules significantly reduces the number of functioning nephrons and as CKD progresses ammonia excretion is impaired (less hydrogen ions are excreted), bicarbonate absorption is reduced and there is insufficient production of renal bicarbonate (Adamczak et al., 2018).

The use of oral sodium bicarbonate is recommended for patients with CKD and a GFR of less than 30 ml/min/1.73 m² and a serum–bicarbonate concentration of less than 20 mmol/l (NICE, 2015). A recent systematic review and meta-analysis of randomised controlled trials of oral bicarbonate therapy in non-haemodialysis dependent CKD patients reported a modestly improved GFR, but these results should be interpreted with caution due to the high risk of bias and wide variation in outcomes (Hu et al., 2019). Table 11.15 outlines the commonly used sodium bicarbonate supplement.

Table 11.15 Bicarbonate supplementation and the related pharmacology.

Medication name	Sodium bicarbonate
Mode of action	Bicarbonate supplementation
Route of administration	Oral
Indications	**ADULT** • Alkalinisation of urine, relief of discomfort in mild urinary tract infections • Maintenance of alkaline urine • Chronic acidotic states such as uremic acidosis or renal tubular acidosis **CHILD** • Chronic acidotic states such as uremic acidosis or renal tubular acidosis
Contraindications	• Salt restricted diet • Metabolic or respiratory alkalosis • Hypocalcaemia • Hypochlorydia
Cautions	• May affect stability or absorption of other drugs if administered at the same time, allow 1–2 hours before other oral drug administration • Avoid prolonged use in urinary conditions • Cardiac disease • Elderly • Patients on sodium restricted diet • Respiratory acidosis Pregnancy and Breast-feeding: • Not recommended in pregnancy or women of child-bearing potential not using contraception • Risk to a child who is breast-feeding cannot be excluded
Side effects (Common and Very Common ONLY)	• Abdominal cramps • Burping • Flatulence • Hypokalaemia • Metabolic alkalosis
Interactions	• Corticosteroids • Increases excretion of lithium, aspirin and methotrexate • Decreases excretion of quinidine and ephedrine • May reduce the absorption of antibacterials, antifungals, dipyridamole, phenothiazines, chloroquine, phenytoin and penicillamine
Absorption	• Readily absorbed from the gastrointestinal tract
Distribution	• Present in all body fluids
Metabolism	• Not significantly metabolised
Elimination	• Bicarbonate is absorbed if not involved in gastric acid neutralisation, in the absence of a deficit it is excreted in the urine

Source: British National Formulary (2019p); British National Formulary for Children (2019o); Electronic Medicines Compendium (2019o).

263

Drugs used to treat urinary retention and urinary incontinence

The pathophysiology of both UR and incontinence have already been discussed earlier within this chapter. Building upon this discussion, the pharmacotherapy targets of these conditions are mainly upon the nervous system via adrenergic, muscarinic or phosphodiesterase receptors. These receptors exist throughout the body, each with its own discrete action when either inhibited via a drug antagonist or stimulated via a drug agonist. Many of these drugs are not receptor site specific and may well bind to target receptor sites within other parts of the body, which in particular for receptors of the nervous system, may cause adverse effects on other body systems such as the cardiovascular system (see side effects sections in Tables 11.16 and 11.17). This strengthens the rationale that any practitioner involved in pharmacotherapy management of disease should possess a strong knowledge base of the associated physiological and pharmacological processes that occur to ensure patient safety. Figure 11.9 outlines the main receptors present within the urinary tract that may be manipulated to treat UR and urinary incontinence.

α_1 receptor antagonists

α_1 receptor antagonists may be indicated for the treatment of UR due to benign prostatic hyperplasia (BPH), the most common cause of UR in men. Treatment of UR depends upon the underlying condition and can be classified into acute or chronic, which may require catheterisation, surgical intervention or pharmacological manipulation. Alpha-adrenoceptor blockers such as tamsulosin and doxazosin may be used for both acute and chronic UR (BNF 2019q). Their mode of action is upon the α_1 adrenergic receptor. Like other adrenergic receptors, the α_1 receptors are members of the G protein-coupled receptor group. When an agonist (norepinephrine or adrenaline) binds to this receptor, a conformational change occurs which causes a chain of reactions in which an enzyme (Phospholipase C) activates secondary messengers (PIP, IP3 and DAG). In turn this causes the release of intracellular calcium and stimulation of another enzyme (protein kinase C) to cause the physiological response of smooth muscle contraction. This complex process is illustrated within Figure 11.10. The primary effect of α_1 receptor stimulation upon the bladder causes contraction of smooth muscle at various sites (see Figure 11.9). Blockade of this receptor causes smooth muscle relaxation and in the case of BPH, an increase in urinary flow rate which should help to relieve UR symptoms. Table 11.16 details some of the prescribing considerations for this group of drugs.

Clinical considerations

As we have already explored, adrenergic and muscarinic receptors and phosphodiesterase enzymes exist throughout the body, each with its own discrete action when either inhibited via a drug antagonist or stimulated via a drug agonist (see Table 11.17). Many of these drugs are not receptor site specific and may well bind to receptor sites that were not necessarily intended to be targeted as part of the pharmacotherapy management of a particular disease process. This which may result in deleterious side effects for the patient (see side effects sections in with each drug table). This strengthens the rationale that any practitioner involved in pharmacotherapy management of disease should possess a strong knowledge base of the associated physiological and pharmacological processes that occur to ensure patient safety. The following table explores some of the major adrenergic and muscarinic receptor sites throughout the body and may be used as a quick reference guide when considering pharmacological effects of receptor activation.

Table 11.16 α₁ receptor antagonists for urinary tract disorders and their related pharmacology.

Medication name	Doxazosin	Tamsulosin hydrochloride
Mode of action	α₁ receptor antagonist	
Route of administration	Oral	Oral
Indications	• Benign prostatic hyperplasia • Hypertension	**ADULT** • Benign prostatic hyperplasia **CHILD** • Dysfunctional voiding (administered on expert advice)
Contraindications	• Previous anaphylactic response to agent • History of micturition syncope (in patients with benign prostatic hypertrophy) • History of postural hypotension • Previous anaphylactic response to agent • History of postural hypotension	
Cautions	• Care with initial dose (postural hypotension) • Cataract surgery (risk of intraoperative floppy iris syndrome) • Elderly • Heart failure • Pulmonary oedema due to aortic or mitral stenosis • Concomitant administration with phosphodiesterase-5-inhibitors (due to vasodilatory effects) Pregnancy and Breast-feeding: • No evidence of teratogenicity; manufacturers advise use only when potential benefit outweighs risk • Accumulates in milk in *animal* studies – manufacturer advises avoid	• Cataract surgery (risk of intraoperative floppy iris syndrome) • Concomitant antihypertensives (reduced dosage and specialist supervision may be required) • Elderly Pregnancy and Breast-feeding: • Tamsulosin is not indicated for use in women

(Continued)

Table 11.16 (Continued)

Medication name	Doxazosin	Tamsulosin hydrochloride
Side effects (Common and Very Common ONLY)	• Arrhythmias • Chest pain • Cough • Cystitis • Dizziness • Drowsiness • Dry mouth • Dyspnea • Gastrointestinal discomfort • Headache • Hypotension • Muscle complaints • Nausea • Oedema • Palpitations • Vertigo	• Dizziness • Sexual dysfunction
Interactions	• Concomitant administration with phosphodiesterase-5-inhibitors (due to vasodilatory effects) • Co-administration with a strong CYP 3A4 inhibitor, such as: Clarithromycin, Indinavir, Itraconazole, Ketoconazole, Nefazodone, Nelfinavir, Ritonavir, Saquinavir, Telithromycin or Voriconazole	
Absorption	• Absorbed from the intestine • Approximately two thirds of the dose are bioavailable	• Absorbed from the intestine • Almost completely bioavailable
Distribution	• 98% of doxazosin is protein-bound in plasma	• 99% bound to plasma proteins • Volume of distribution is small (~0.2l/kg)
Metabolism	• After oral administration of doxazosin, the plasma concentrations of the metabolites are low • Extensively metabolised in the liver	• Low first-pass effect, metabolised slowly • Most tamsulosin is present in plasma in the form of unchanged active substance. It is metabolised in the liver
Elimination	• primary pathway for elimination is via CYP 3A4	• Mainly excreted in the urine with about 9% of a dose being present in the form of unchanged active substance

Source: British National Formulary (2019q, r); British National Formulary for Children (2019p, q); Electronic Medicines Compendium (2019p, q).

Table 11.17 Receptors of the autonomic nervous system.

Site	Autonomic nervous system			
	Sympathetic		**Parasympathetic**	
	Receptor	**Action** (when activated)	**Receptor**	**Action** (when activated)
Heart	β_1	→ Rate and contractility	Muscarinic (M_2)	→ Rate and contractility
Blood vessels (vascular smooth muscle)	β_2	Dilatation/ Relaxation	Muscarinic (M3)	Dilatation – Nitric oxide induced
			Muscarinic (M3)	Contraction – Acetylcholine induced
Bronchioles	β_2	Dilatation	Muscarinic (M3)	Contraction/ Constriction
Kidney	β_1	Renin secretion		
Gastrointestinal tract smooth muscle – wall	α_2 and β_2	Dilatation/ Relaxation	Muscarinic	Contraction
Gastrointestinal tract smooth muscle – sphincter	α_1	Contraction	Muscarinic	Relaxation
Bladder smooth muscle – wall (trigone)	α_1	Contraction		
Bladder smooth muscle – detrusor	$\beta_{2\&3}$	Relaxation	Muscarinic (M3)	Contraction
Bladder smooth muscle – sphincter	α_1	Contraction	Muscarinic (M3)	Relaxation
Bladder neck	α_1	Contraction	Muscarinic	Relaxation
Prostate gland	α_1	Contraction		
Urethra	α_1	Contraction		

Source: Chess-Williams (2008), Hedge (2006), Klabunde (2012), Rattu (2015).

267

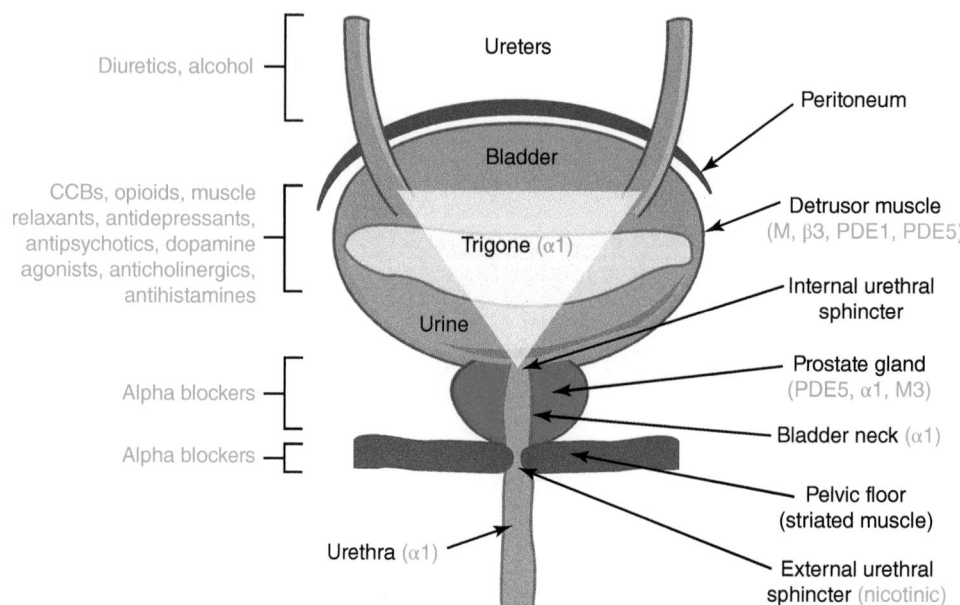

α: alpha-adrenergic; β: beta-adrenergic; CCB: calcium channel blocker; M: muscarinic; PDE: phosphodiesterase; UI: urinary incontinence.

Figure 11.9   Sites of drug action upon urinary tract.

Androgen-synthesis inhibitors

Patients with BPH and a raised prostate-specific antigen (PSA) level and who are deemed at high risk of developing cancer of the prostate, may be offered an androgen-synthesis inhibitor (ASI) along with an α_1 adrenoreceptor blocking agent. BPH is mediated by the testosterone's active metabolite, 5a-dihydrotestosterone. Inhibition of the enzyme (5a-reductase) that converts testosterone into 5a-dihydrotestosterone is the primary site of action for ASIs such as Finasteride.

Phosphodiesterase inhibitors (PDIs), like α_1 receptor blockers, have the potential to exert their effect upon multiple sites of the body. Phosphodiesterase is an enzyme which belongs to a 'superfamily' of enzymes of which there are multiple types that exist within different types of cells within the body. They breakdown chemical bonds involved in the action of second messengers (cyclic guanosine monophosphate [cGMP] and cyclic adenosine monophosphate [cAMP]). Intracellular concentrations of both cGMP and cAMP play an important second messenger role in cellular function depending upon the location of the cell. cAMP is concerned with the regulation of both cardiac and vascular smooth muscle contraction. cAMP is broken down by the cAMP-dependent phosphodiesterase enzyme, type 3 (PDE3). PDE3 inhibition provides a pharmacological target for disorders of the cardiovascular and respiratory system and are explored in more detail within Chapter 10 and Chapter 13 under 'Xanthines'.

cGMP is concerned with the regulation of smooth muscle tone via the nitric oxide (NO)/cGMP pathway which is found within smooth muscle cells of the urinary tract, the corpus cavernosum of the penis, and in vascular smooth muscle. Increased intracellular cGMP levels result in relaxation of the target smooth muscle. It is broken down by the cGMP-dependent phosphodiesterase enzyme, type 5 (PDE5), which when inhibited results in increased intracellular levels of cGMP and therefore increased smooth muscle relaxation via multiple mechanisms. Figure 11.9 details the sites at which PDE5 inhibitors exert their effect upon the urinary tract. Table 11.18 details some of the other pharmacological considerations for both ASIs and PDIs when using these drugs for disorders of the urinary tract.

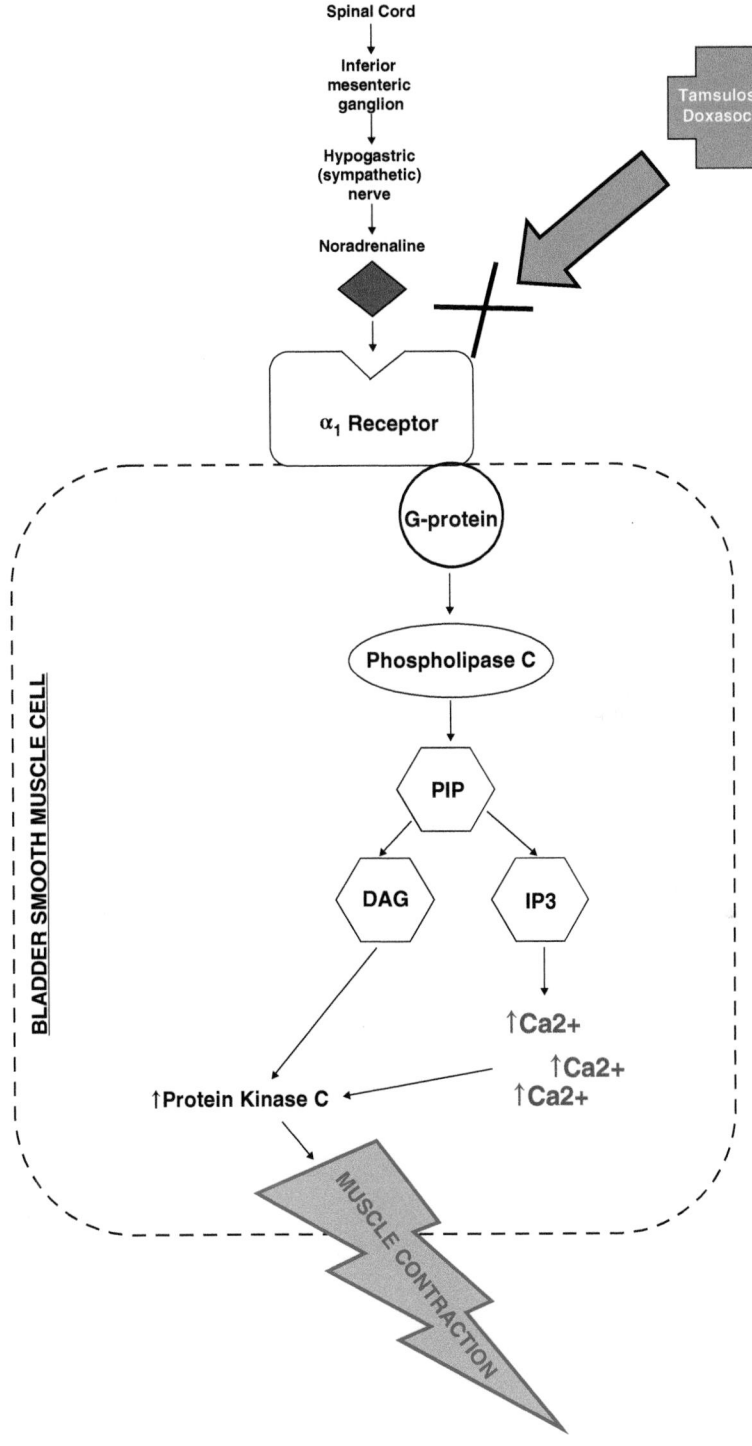

Abbreviations: PIP— phospatidylinositol 4,5-diphosphate; IP3— Inositol trisphosphate; DAG— diacylgycerol; Ca2+ — Calcium;

Figure 11.10 α₁ adrenoreceptor and the site of action of an α₁ antagonist.
Source: Sadie Diamond-Fox

Table 11.18   Androgen-synthesis (5α-reductase) and Phosphodiesterase type 5 (PDE5) inhibitors and their related pharmacology.

Medication name	Finasteride	Tadalafil
Mode of action	Inhibitor of the enzyme 5α-reductase, which metabolises testosterone into the more potent androgen, dihydrotestosterone	PDE5 inhibitor
Route of administration	Oral	Oral
Indications		
	ADULT	
	● Benign prostatic hyperplasia	● Benign prostatic hyperplasia ● Erectile dysfunction ● Pulmonary arterial hypertension
	CHILD	
	● Not licensed	● Not licensed
Contraindications	● Anaphylaxis to previous administration	● Anaphylaxis to previous administration ● Hypotension (avoid if systolic blood pressure below 90 mmHg) ● Heart failure ● Myocardial infarction ● Recent stroke ● Uncontrolled arrhythmias ● Uncontrolled hypertension ● Unstable angina
Cautions	● Obstructive uropathy ● Women of childbearing potential should avoid handling crushed or broken tablets of Finasteride Pregnancy and Breast-feeding: ● Finasteride is not indicated for use in women ● Finasteride is excreted in semen and use of a condom is recommended if sexual partner is pregnant or likely to become pregnant	● Anatomical deformation of the penis ● Aortic and mitral valve disease ● Congestive cardiomyopathy ● Coronary artery disease ● Hereditary degenerative retinal disorders ● Hypotension (avoid if systolic blood pressure below 90 mmHg) ● Left ventricular dysfunction ● Life-threatening arrhythmias ● Pericardial constriction ● Predisposition to priapism ● Pulmonary veno-occlusive disease ● Uncontrolled hypertension Pregnancy and Breast-feeding: ● Manufacturer advises avoid
Side effects (Common and Very Common ONLY)	● Sexual dysfunction ● Cases of male breast cancer have been reported	● Flushing ● Gastrointestinal discomfort ● Headaches ● Myalgia ● Nasal congestion ● Pain

(Continued)

Table 11.18   (Continued)

Medication name	Finasteride	Tadalafil
Interactions	• No drug interactions of clinical importance have been identified	• Antihypertensives • CYP3A4 inducers
Absorption	• Bioavailability of finasteride is approx. 80% • Peak plasma concentrations are reached approx. 2 hours after drug intake • Absorption is complete after 6–8 hours	• Readily absorbed after oral administration • Absolute bioavailability of Tadalafil following oral dosing has not been determined
Distribution	• Binding to plasma proteins is approx. 93%	• 94% bound to proteins
Metabolism	• Metabolised in the liver	• Metabolised in the liver
Elimination	• Approx. 39% excreted in the urine in the form of metabolites. • Approximately 57% is excreted in the faeces	• ~61% excreted in faces • ~36% in urine

Source: British National Formulary (2019s, t); Electronic Medicines Compendium (2019r, s).

Antimuscarinics

Urinary frequency and urge incontinence may be caused by detrusor overactivity. The detrusor muscle is a layer of smooth muscle within the bladder wall and contraction results in voiding of urine, coordinated with relaxation of the sphincter muscles. This muscle is innervated by the parasympathetic nervous system, where release of acetylcholine at muscarinic receptors (M_3 and M_1) results in muscle contraction. Activation of the receptor, via a G protein, stimulates phospholipase C (PLC), cleaving phosphatidylinositol 4, 5-bisphosphate (PIP_2) into two secondary cellular messengers: inositol-1, 4, 5-triphosphate (IP_3) and diacylglycerol (DAG). IP_3 augments the release of calcium ions, producing smooth muscle contraction and hence involuntary micturition. This complex process is outlined in Figure 11.11. Anticholinergics compete with acetylcholine for the muscarinic receptors, reducing detrusor spasm, the number of uninhibited contractions, as well as increasing bladder relaxation and therefore capacity.

Guidance recommends that first-line pharmacotherapy treatment is the use of anticholinergic or antimuscarinic drugs (NICE, 2019c). Table 11.19 outlines the commonly used antimuscarinic agents.

Drugs and dialysis

Patients suffering from acute or chronic renal failure may require the initiation of RRT in the form of haemodialysis, filtration or haemodiafiltration. This is an important consideration when prescribing and monitoring pharmacotherapy in this patient population and the following aspects should be considered:

- *Drug efficacy* – Removal of drugs and their metabolites via dialysis which can reduce their effectiveness.
- *Equipment and mode of RRT* – The type of filter and the size of the pores within the membrane used within the dialysis machine will affect the rate of clearance of the drug by dialysis or filtration. The rate of flow of dialysis and/or filtration fluid will determine the rate at which the drug is cleared. Dialysis or filtration can also result in significant changes in

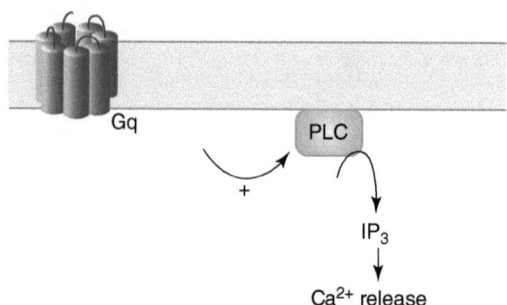

Abbreviations: G_q – G protein; PLC – phospholipase C; IP_3 – inositol-1, 4, 5-triphosphate

Figure 11.11   Muscarinic (M1 and M3) receptor.

serum electrolytes and fluid balance which may alter the drug's effect and the volume of distribution.

- *Molecular weight* – Each drug possesses a molecular weight (measured in Daltons [Da]). The larger the drug's molecular weight, the less quickly it may be cleared by dialysis (depending upon the mode of RRT). Haemodialysis membranes have relatively small pore sizes and will only clear molecules <500 Da, versus haemofilters which have larger pore sizes and can clear larger molecules <5000 Da.
- *Water solubility* – Drugs that possess a low water solubility are poorly dialysed or filtered.
- *Volume of distribution* – May be increased by renal failure (due to fluid retention) and liver failure (due to fluid retention and altered protein binding). Each drug has a specific property that relates to its volume of distribution. Certain drugs (such as paracetamol and lithium) have a low affinity for protein binding and have a relatively low volume of distribution and are therefore easily cleared by dialysis. Drugs that have a large molecular weight (such as amitriptyline) have a high affinity for plasma protein binding (~96% protein bound) and have a large volume of distribution and are very poorly dialyzable.
- *Protein binding* – Drugs that are highly protein bound (mostly to albumin) are poorly cleared by dialysis or filtration. Drug–protein binding varies depending on the drug itself. It is only the unbound drug (free drug) that is pharmacologically active and able to exert its effect upon its target receptor. In patients with renal and liver disease the levels of serum albumin can be significantly lowered, which can significantly elevate the free concentrations of certain drugs. In this case it is particularly important to consider monitoring the free drug levels within the patients' blood, if an assay is available to do so, to prevent toxicity.
- *Route of drug clearance* – If hepatic metabolism is the major metabolic pathway in which a drug is broken down (metabolised), then the rate at which the drug is cleared by dialysis or filtration, in a patient with sufficient hepatic function, may be insufficient to have an effect upon total drug clearance.

Source: Richards et al. (2012), Steddon et al. (2014).

Skills in practice

Estimating glomerular filtration rate and adjusting drug dosages

As already explored within the first Clinical Considerations Box, direct measurement of GFR as marker of overall renal function is practically rather difficult. Using plasma or urinary clearance is considered the best overall index of renal function, but this can be time consuming and is rarely used in everyday practice. Estimations of renal function are therefore derived from either eGFR or creatinine clearance. There are various equations for estimating GFR; however, there is no compelling evidence to support the superiority of any given method (BNF, 2019a). But in order to adjust the dose of renally excreted drugs in response to reduced renal function, it is necessary

Table 11.19 Antimuscarinic drugs and their related pharmacology.

Medication name	Oxybutynin
Mode of action	Competitive antagonist at the muscarinic receptor (M_3 and M_1)
Route of administration	Oral
Indications	**ADULT** • Urinary frequency, urgency and incontinence • Neurogenic bladder instability **CHILD** • Urinary frequency, urgency and incontinence • Neurogenic bladder instability • Nocturnal enuresis associated with over-active bladder
Contraindications	• Gastrointestinal obstruction, intestinal atony, paralytic ileus, pyloric stenosis, severe ulcerative colitis, toxic megacolon • Myasthenia gravis • Severe bladder outflow obstruction, urinary retention
Cautions	• Arrhythmias, cardiac insufficiency, cardiac surgery, conditions characterised by tachycardia, congestive heart failure, coronary artery disease, hypertension • Diarrhoea, gastroesophageal reflux disease, hiatus hernia with reflux esophagitis, ulcerative colitis • Autonomic neuropathy • Hyperthyroidism • Individuals susceptible to angle-closure glaucoma • Pyrexia • Hypersensitivity to oxybutynin or any component Pregnancy and Breast-feeding: • Manufacturers advise avoidance unless necessary
Side effects(Common and Very Common ONLY)	• For all systemic antimuscarinics, see BNF for multiple side effects • Diarrhoea • Dry eye • Acute porphyrias
Interactions	• Care should be taken with administration of other antimuscarinics due to potentiation of effects • Anticholinergic activity of oxybutynin is increased with concurrent use of other anticholinergic antiparkinsonian products, antihistamines, antipsychotics, quinidine, digitalis, tricyclic antidepressants, atropine and related compounds • Oxybutynin may affect the absorption of other drugs • It is metabolised by cytochrome P450 isoenzyme CYP3A4, hence concomitant use with a CYP3A4 inhibitor can inhibit metabolism of oxybutynin and increase exposure • May antagonise the effects of prokinetics • Concomitant administration with cholinesterase inhibitors may result in reduced cholinesterase inhibitor efficacy
Absorption	• Poorly absorbed from the gastrointestinal tract • Peak plasma level reached between 0.5 to 1 hour after administration
Distribution	• Highly bound to plasma proteins
Metabolism	• Metabolised in the liver and intestinal wall
Elimination	• Elimination half-life is biexponential – first phase 40 minutes and the second 2–3 hours • Excreted in the faeces and urine but primarily metabolised in the liver

Source: British National Formulary (2019u); British National Formulary for Children (2019r); Electronic Medicines Compendium (2019t).

273

to make a quantitative estimate of the GFR of the patient. The majority of NHS laboratories now routinely report renal function in adults based on eGFR and this alongside an understanding of a drugs pharmacokinetics should be used to ensure safe prescribing in patients with reduced renal function and those receiving RRT.

The CKD-EPI equation (Levey et al., 2009) is the recommended method for estimating GFR and calculating drug doses in *most* patients with renal impairment (BNF, 2019a). This calculation utilises serum creatinine, age, sex and race as clinical variables to determine eGFR and is recommended by the National Institute of Clinical Excellence (2015) as being the calculation upon which clinical laboratories should be basing measurements of eGFR. The following equation can be used to manually calculate eGFR using the CKD-EPI formula:

$$eGFR \ (ml/min/1.73 \ m^2) = 141 \times min(S_{Cr}/K, 1)\alpha \times max(S_{Cr}/K, 1)^{-1.209} \times 0.993^{Age}$$
$$[\times 1.018 \ if \ female] \ [\times 1.159 \ if \ black]$$

- S_{Cr} = serum creatinine in mg/dl;
- K = 0.7 for females and 0.9 for males;
- α = −0.329 for females and − 0.411 for males;
- $min(S_{Cr}/K, 1)$ indicates the minimum of S_{Cr}/K or 1;
- $max(S_{Cr}/K, 1)$ indicates the maximum of S_{Cr}/K or 1.

Alternatively, the National Institute of Diabetes and Digestive and Kidney Diseases (2019) provide a useful online tool for use in both the adult and paediatric populations which can be adjusted for both conventional units (creatinine measured in mg/dl) or International System (SI) of units (creatinine measured in μmol/L) – https://www.niddk.nih.gov/health-information/communication-programs/nkdep/laboratory-evaluation.

The Renal Drug Database https://renaldrugdatabase.com provides healthcare professionals with easily accessible information on adjusting drug dosages depending upon baseline renal function and types of RRT that may be used. These guides should be used alongside the most up-to-date version of the British National Formulary to ensure safe prescribing practice in this patient group.

Episode of care: Diabetic nephropathy

Mrs. Dixon

Mrs. Dixon is a 52-year-old female who works full time as a teaching assistant. She is married and has two daughters in their 20s. She enjoys walking her dog every day and is a non-smoker. Mrs. Dixon refers to herself as regular social drinker and enjoys a glass of wine with her evening meal. She was diagnosed with Type II diabetes mellitus five years ago and has recently been reviewed by the diabetic practice nurse at her local GP Practice. Mrs. Dixon attends for an appointment at the diabetic clinic at her local general practitioner (GP) surgery for a review and the results of her recent blood tests.

Mrs. Dixons medical notes indicate that she was diagnosed with Type II diabetes seven years ago and hypertension three years ago. According to the diabetic practice nurse's notes, Mrs. Dixon's Type II diabetes is normally well controlled but her blood glucose was 12 mmol/L and so a Haemoglobin A1c (HbA1c) test was performed. She freely admits that her diet has been poor following a recent family bereavement and she feels anxious due to her family history and diagnosis of diabetic nephropathy. Mrs. Dixon reports leg cramps over the last few weeks. Her blood pressure was documented as 124/65. Her previous eGFR, a year ago, was 59 mL/min/1.73 m² with an ACR of 3.5 mg/mmol. This categorises her as having CKD stage 3a according to the KDIGO guidelines (2013).

Mrs. Dixon's prescribed medications include:

- Lisinopril 20 mg once a day.
- Carvedilol 12 mg twice a day.
- Gliptizide 5 mg daily.
- Atorvastatin 20 mg once a day.
- Aspirin 75 mg daily.

On review of her medications, Mrs. Dixon reports that she regularly takes all of the prescribed drugs and does not report any side effects. The most recent blood results are noted as:

- An HbA1c of 64 with a blood glucose of 10.5.
- A eGFR 55 mL/min/1.73 m^2 with a ACR of 5 mg/mmol.
- A serum potassium of 4.3 mmol/L.

This case presents many opportunities for improving management of Mrs. Dixon's CKD and diabetes, reducing morbidity and mortality and preventing further decline in renal function. Mrs. Dixon appears to have suboptimal control of her diabetes which has potentially led to worsening of her renal function. The diabetic practice nurse identified that Mrs. Dixon's diet was poor and gave her advice on healthy lifestyle measures including a healthy diet and reducing her alcohol intake.

In the management of Mrs. Dixon's type II diabetes and CKD, there are several key themes that may be addressed including self-management, monitoring and pharmacological management. The recommendations made will largely relate to the National Institute for Health and Care Excellence clinical guidelines *Early identification and management of chronic kidney disease in adults in primary and secondary care* (NICE, 2015) and the CKD Work Group publication *KDIGO 2012 Clinical practice guideline for the evaluation and management of chronic kidney disease* (KDIGO, 2013).

Supported self-management

- It has been identified that CKD is associated with reduced quality of life and co-exists with other long-term conditions such as diabetes. Currently, there is a significant lack of evidence for self-management support in CKD but it is acknowledged that patients may benefit from education and support.
- Mrs. Dixon has already been given advice by the diabetic practice nurse with regards to healthy lifestyle and given and NHS leaflet with regards to CKD (available on the www. patient.info website). She could also be advised to contact a national charity Kidney Care UK which has a support helpline and further information (website available at www. kidneycareuk.org).
- Mrs. Dixon may also be given advice with regards to the risk of AKI in the context of CKD with acute, severe illness.
- As Mrs. Dixon has suffered a recent bereavement and reports anxiety, she should be assessed for general anxiety disorder and as well as potentially a biopsychosocial assessment.

Monitoring

- Renal function should be checked by measurement of serum creatinine, eGFR and ACR with consideration given to the acceleration of the progression of CKD. Mrs. Dixon is graded as

Stage 3a as her eGFR remains in this category, with no evidence of acceleration as her GFR has only decreased by $4\,mL/min/1.73\,m^2$. Despite an increase in ACR from normal or mildly increased to moderately increased, Mrs. Dixon's eGFR requires repeating annually unless she has any health problems during the subsequent year.

- A full blood count is only indicated if the patient is CKD stage 3b-5 or develops symptoms indicative of anaemia. Mrs. Dixon does not report any clinical symptoms.
- Serum calcium, phosphate, vitamin D levels and PTH test are indicated in patients with CKD stage 4-5 to rule out renal metabolic and bone disorder. Mrs. Dixon reports leg cramps which may indicate low calcium levels. These tests are indicated in stages 1–3 CKD if there is a clinical suspicion of bone disease.

Pharmacotherapy

- Management of hypertension:
  Blood pressure management in CKD reduces disease progression and cardiovascular risk. For patients with diabetes, the recommended blood pressure targets are a systolic <130 mmHg and a diastolic of <80 mmHg, both of which will reduce the risk of adverse outcomes. Mrs. Dixon's blood pressure is well controlled on her current medication and does not require any adjustment.
- Diabetes management:
  Blood glucose should be optimised to prevent or delay microvascular complications of diabetes including deterioration in renal function. Mrs. Dixons HbA1c is 64, suggesting that her Type II diabetes is currently not well controlled. Normal is <42 mmol/mol. Mrs. Dixon has stated her diet has been poor and if improved this may reduce her HbA1c. The dose of gliptizide should be increased to 10 mg daily and advice regarding diet, lifestyle and adherence to drug treatment reinforced. Mrs. Dixon should be given another appointment to see the diabetic practice nurse in three months' time.

- Lipid lowering therapy and anti-platelet therapy – Mrs. Dixon is currently prescribed a statin and aspirin.
- Mrs. Dixon should be offered annual influenza and pneumococcal immunisations
- She should be counselled with regards to over-the-counter medications and avoidance of non-steroidal anti-inflammatory drugs (NSAIDs), herbal remedies and use protein supplements with caution.

Conclusion

As a student healthcare practitioner, you will undoubtedly be involved in the care of a number of patients with one or multiple types of renal disorder. These disorders can be very complex and have the potential to have detrimental effects on a patient's activities of daily living. The causes of renal disorders can be multifactorial and often are interlinked with other co-morbidities, such as cardiovascular disease and diabetes. The incidence of AKI continues to rise despite multiple public health campaigns and NHS initiatives. As such, it is crucial that the healthcare professionals involved in supporting this patient group to manage their acute and chronic disease process have a sound understanding of the pathophysiological, pharmacological and evidence base that underpins the promotion of safe and effective care.

References

Adamczak, M., Masajtis-Zagajewska, A., Mazanowska, O. et al. (2018). *Diagnosis and treatment of metabolic acidosis in patients with chronic kidney disease – position statement of the Working Group of the Polish Society of Nephrology*. https://www.karger.com/Article/Pdf/490475 (accessed September 2019).

Akbari, P. and Khorasani-Zadeh, A. (2019). *Stat Pearls. Thiazide diuretics*. https://www.ncbi.nlm.nih.gov/books/NBK532918 (accessed September 2019).

Allan, J. (2012). Bladder Outflow obstruction. In: *ABC of Urology*, 3e (eds. C. Dawson and J. Nethercliffe), 9–13. West Sussex: Wiley Blackwell.

Anisman, S., Erickson, S., and Morden, N. (2019). *How to prescribe loop diuretics in oedema*. https://www.bmj.com/content/364/bmj.l359?hwoasp=authn%3A1569172103%3A4058629%3A1467218820%3A0%3A0%3ABxWwOYLM8njlrRWgakDdKQ%3D%3D (accessed September 2019).

Bello, A.K., Alrukhaimi, M., Ashuntantang, G.E. et al. (2017). Complications of chronic kidney disease: current state, knowledge gaps, and strategy for action. *Kidney International Supplement* **7** (2): 122–129.

Bellomo, R., Ronco, C., Kellum, J.A. et al. (2004). *Acute renal failure – definition, outcome measures, animal models, fluid therapy and information technology needs: the Second International Consensus Conference of the Acute Dialysis Quality Initiative (ADQI) Group*. https://ccforum.biomedcentral.com/articles/10.1186/cc2872 (accessed September 2019).

BNF: British National Formulary (2019a). *Prescribing in renal impairment*. https://bnf.nice.org.uk/guidance/prescribing-in-renal-impairment.html (accessed September 2019).

British National Formulary (2019b). *Furosemide*. https://bnf.nice.org.uk/drug/furosemide.html (accessed September 2019).

British National Formulary (2019c). *Bumetanide*. https://bnf.nice.org.uk/drug/bumetanide.html#indicationsAndDoses (accessed September 2019).

British National Formulary (2019d). *Bendroflumethiazide*. https://bnf.nice.org.uk/drug/bendroflumethiazide.html (accessed September 2019).

British National Formulary (2019e). *Mannitol*. https://bnf.nice.org.uk/drug/mannitol.html (accessed September 2019).

British National Formulary (2019f). *Amiloride hydrochloride*. https://bnf.nice.org.uk/drug/amiloride-hydrochloride.html (accessed September 2019).

British National Formulary (2019g). *Spironolactone*. https://bnf.nice.org.uk/drug/spironolactone.html (accessed September 2019).

British National Formulary (2019h). *Acetazolamide*. https://bnf.nice.org.uk/drug/acetazolamide.html (accessed September 2019).

British National Formulary (2019i). *Sevelamer*. https://bnf.nice.org.uk/drug/sevelamer.html (accessed September 2019).

British National Formulary (2019j). *Lanthanum*. https://bnf.nice.org.uk/drug/lanthanum.html (accessed September 2019).

British National Formulary (2019k). *Alfacalcidol*. https://bnfc.nice.org.uk/drug/alfacalcidol.html (accessed September 2019).

British National Formulary (2019l). *Calcitriol*. https://bnfc.nice.org.uk/drug/calcitriol.html (accessed September 2019).

British National Formulary (2019m). *Sodium polystyrene sulfonate*. https://bnf.nice.org.uk/drug/sodium-polystyrene-sulfonate.html (accessed September 2019).

British National Formulary (2019n). *Calcium polystyrene sulfonate*. https://bnf.nice.org.uk/drug/calcium-polystyrene-sulfonate.html (accessed September 2019).

British National Formulary (2019o). *Potassium chloride*. https://bnf.nice.org.uk/drug/potassium-chloride.html (accessed September 2019).

British National Formulary (2019p). *Sodium bicarbonate*. https://bnf.nice.org.uk/drug/sodium-bicarbonate.html (accessed September 2019).

British National Formulary (2019q). Doxazosin. https://bnfc.nice.org.uk/drug/doxazosin.html (accessed September 2019).

British National Formulary (2019r). Tamsulosin. https://bnfc.nice.org.uk/drug/tamsulosin-hydrochloride.html (accessed September 2019).

British National Formulary (2019s). *Finasteride*. https://bnf.nice.org.uk/drug/finasteride.html (accessed September 2019).

British National Formulary (2019t). *Tadalafil*. https://bnf.nice.org.uk/drug/tadalafil.html (accessed September 2019).

British National Formulary (2019u). *Oxybutynin*. https://bnf.nice.org.uk/drug/oxybutynin-hydrochloride.html (accessed September 2019).

British National Formulary for Children (2019a). *Furosemide*. https://bnfc.nice.org.uk/drug/furosemide.html (accessed September 2019).

British National Formulary for Children (2019b). *Bumetanide*. https://bnfc.nice.org.uk/drug/bumetanide.html (accessed September 2019).

British National Formulary for Children (2019c). *Bendroflumethiazide.* https://bnfc.nice.org.uk/drug/bendroflumethiazide.html (accessed September 2019).

British National Formulary for Children (2019d). *Mannitol.* https://bnfc.nice.org.uk/drug/mannitol.html (accessed September 2019).

British National Formulary for Children (2019e). *Amiloride.* https://bnfc.nice.org.uk/drug/amiloride-hydrochloride.html (accessed September 2019).

British National Formulary for Children (2019f). *Spironolactone.* https://bnfc.nice.org.uk/drug/spironolactone.html (accessed September 2019).

British National Formulary for Children (2019g). *Acetazolamide.* https://bnfc.nice.org.uk/drug/acetazolamide.html (accessed September 2019).

British National Formulary for Children (2019h). *Sevelamer.* https://bnfc.nice.org.uk/drug/sevelamer.html (accessed September 2019).

British National Formulary for Children (2019i). *Lanthanum.* https://bnfc.nice.org.uk/drug/lanthanum.html (accessed September 2019).

British National Formulary for Children (2019j). *Alfacalcidol.* https://bnfc.nice.org.uk/drug/alfacalcidol.html (accessed September 2019).

British National Formulary for Children (2019k). *Calcitriol.* https://bnfc.nice.org.uk/drug/calcitriol.html (accessed September 2019).

British National Formulary for Children (2019l). *Sodium polystyrene sulfonate.* https://bnfc.nice.org.uk/drug/sodium-polystyrene-sulfonate.html (accessed September 2019).

British National Formulary for Children (2019m). *Calcium polystyrene sulfonate.* https://bnfc.nice.org.uk/drug/calcium-polystyrene-sulfonate.html (accessed September 2019).

British National Formulary for Children (2019n) *Potassium chloride.* https://bnfc.nice.org.uk/drug/potassium-chloride.html (accessed September 2019).

British National Formulary for Children (2019o). *Sodium bicarbonate.* https://bnfc.nice.org.uk/drug/sodium-bicarbonate.html (accessed September 2019).

British National Formulary for Children (2019p). *Doxazosin.* https://bnfc.nice.org.uk/drug/doxazosin.html (accessed September 2019).

British National Formulary for Children (2019q). *Tamsulosin.* https://bnfc.nice.org.uk/drug/tamsulosin-hydrochloride.html (accessed September 2019).

British National Formulary for Children (2019r). *Oxybutynin.* https://bnfc.nice.org.uk/drug/oxybutynin-hydrochloride.html (accessed September 2019).

Buckley, B.S. and Lapitan, M.C. (2009). *Prevalence of urinary and faecal incontinence and nocturnal enuresis and attitudes to treatment and hel-seeking amongst a community-based representative sample of adults in the United Kingdom.* https://onlinelibrary.wiley.com/doi/10.1111/j.1742-1241.2008.01974.x (accessed September 2019).

Chess-Williams, R. (2008). *Muscarinic receptors of the urinary bladder: detrusor, urothelial and prejunctional.* https://onlinelibrary.wiley.com/doi/full/10.1046/j.1474-8673.2002.00258.x (accessed September 2019).

Davies, A. (2014). Acute Kidney injury. In: *Renal Nursing*, 4e (ed. N. Thomas), 97–115. Hoboken, USA: Wiley.

Davila, G.W. (2018).*British Medical Journal Best Practice Guidance. Urinary incontinence in women.* https://bestpractice.bmj.com/topics/en-gb/169/pdf/169.pdf (accessed September 2019).

Duarte, J.D. and Cooper DeHoff, R.M. (2010). *Mechanisms for blood pressure lowering and metabolic effects of thiazide and thiazide-like diuretics.* https://www.ncbi.nlm.nih.gov/pmc/articles/PMC2904515/#!po=10.0000 (accessed September 2019).

Electronic Medicines Compendium (2019a). *Furosemide.* www.medicines.org.uk/emc/product/6012/smpc (accessed September 2019).

Electronic Medicines Compendium (2019b). *Bumetanide.* www.medicines.org.uk/emc/product/2542/smpc (accessed September 2019).

Electronic Medicines Compendium (2019c).*Bendoflumethiazide.* www.medicines.org.uk/emc/product/5727/smpc (accessed September 2019).

Electronic Medicines Compendium (2019d). *Mannitol.* www.medicines.org.uk/emc/product/1839/smpc (accessed September 2019).

Electronic Medicines Compendium (2019e). *Amiloride.* www.medicines.org.uk/emc/product/4986/smpc (accessed September 2019).

Electronic Medicines Compendium (2019f). *Spironolactone.* www.medicines.org.uk/emc/product/5121/smpc (accessed September 2019).

Electronic Medicines Compendium (2019g). *Acetazolamide.* www.medicines.org.uk/emc/product/2785/smpc (accessed September 2019).

Electronic Medicines Compendium (2019h). *Sevelamer hydrochloride.* www.medicines.org.uk/emc/product/207/smpc (accessed September 2019).

Electronic Medicines Compendium (2019i). *Lanthanum.* www.medicines.org.uk/emc/product/7494/smpc (accessed September 2019).

Electronic Medicines Compendium (2019j). *Alfacalcidol.* www.medicines.org.uk/emc/product/5516/smpc (accessed September 2019).

Electronic Medicines Compendium (2019k). *Calcitriol.* www.medicines.org.uk/emc/search?q=%22calcitriol%22 (accessed September 2019).

Electronic Medicines Compendium (2019l). *Sodium polystyrene sulfonate.* www.medicines.org.uk/emc/product/1461 (accessed September 2019).

Electronic Medicines Compendium (2019m). *Calcium resonium.* www.medicines.org.uk/emc/product/1439 (accessed September 2019).

Electronic Medicines Compendium (2019n). *Sando K.* www.medicines.org.uk/emc/product/959 (accessed September 2019).

Electronic Medicines Compendium (2019o). *Sodium bicarbonate.* www.medicines.org.uk/emc/product/10531/smpc (accessed September 2019).

Electronic Medicines Compendium (2019p). *Doxazosin.* www.medicines.org.uk/emc/search?q=Doxazosin (accessed September 2019).

Electronic Medicines Compendium (2019q). *Tamsulosin.* https://www.medicines.org.uk/emc/product/507/smpc (accessed July 2020).

Electronic Medicines Compendium (2019r). *Finasteride.* https://www.medicines.org.uk/emc/product/6044/smpc (accessed July 2020).

Electronic Medicines Compendium (2019s). *Tadalafil.* https://www.medicines.org.uk/emc/product/7431/smpc (accessed July 2020).

Electronic Medicines Compendium (2019t). *Oxybutynin.* https://www.medicines.org.uk/emc/product/11246/smpc (accessed July 2020).

Graeme-Smith, D.G. and Aronson, J.K. (2002). *Oxford Textbook of Clinical Pharmacology and Drug Therapy*, 3e. Oxford: Oxford University Press.

Gross, J.L., de Azevedo, M.J., Silverio, S.P. et al. (2005). Diabetic nephropathy: diagnosis, prevention and treatment. *Diabetes Care* **28** (1): 164–176.

Haneda, M., Utsunomiya, K., Koya, D., et al. (2015). *A new classification of diabetic nephropathy 2014: a report from Joint Committee on Diabetic Nephropathy.* https://onlinelibrary.wiley.com/doi/full/10.1111/jdi.12319 (accessed September 2019).

Hedge, S.S. (2006). *Muscarinic receptors in the bladder: from basic research to therapeutics.* https://www.ncbi.nlm.nih.gov/pmc/articles/PMC1751492 (accessed September 2019).

Hou Y., Li, X., Sun, L. et al. (2017). *Phosphorus and mortality risk in end-stage renal disease: A meta-analysis.* https://pubmed.ncbi.nlm.nih.gov/28903022/ (accessed July 2020).

Hu, M.K., Witham, M.D., and Soiza, R.L. (2019). *Oral bicarbonate in non-haemodialysis dependent chronic kidney disease patients: a meta-analysis of randomised controlled trials.* https://www.mdpi.com/2077-0383/8/2/208/htm (accessed September 2019).

Jablonski, K.L. and Chonchol, M. (2013). *Vascular calcification in end-stage renal disease.* https://www.ncbi.nlm.nih.gov/pmc/articles/PMC3813300/#!po=30.0000 (accessed September 2019).

Kidney Disease Improving Global Outcomes (2012). KDIGO clinical practice guideline for acute Kidney injury. *Kidney International Supplement Vol* **2**: 1–138.

Kidney Disease Improving Global Outcomes (2013). KDIGO clinical practice guideline for acute kidney injury. *Kidney International Supplement* **3**: 1–150.

Kidney Research UK (2018). *Annual report and financial statements.* https://kidneyresearchuk.org/wp-content/uploads/2019/04/KR11606-Annual-Report-2017-18_web_single-2.pdf (accessed July 2020).

Klabunde, E. (2012). *Cardiovascular Physiology Concepts*, 2e. Philadelphia: Lippincott Williams and Wilkinson.

Lafayette, R.A. (2019). *British Medical Journal Best Practice Guidance. Acute kidney injury.* https://bestpractice.bmj.com/topics/en-gb/83/pdf/83.pdf (accessed September 2019).

Levey, A.S., Stevens, L.A. Schmid, C.H., et al. (2009). *A new equation to estimate glomerular filtration rate.* https://www.ncbi.nlm.nih.gov/pmc/articles/PMC2763564 (accessed September 2019).

Mehta, R., Kellum, J., Shah, S., et al. (2007). *Acute Kidney Injury Network: Report of an initiative to improve outcomes in acute kidney injury.* https://ccforum.biomedcentral.com/articles/10.1186/cc5713 (accessed September 2019).

MHRA: Medicines and Healthcare Products Regulatory Agency Drug Safety Update (2014). *Combination use of medicines from different classes of rennin-angiotensin system blocking agents: risk of hyperkalaemia,*

279

hypotension, and impaired renal function – new warnings. https://www.gov.uk/drug-safety-update/
combination-use-of-medicines-from-different-classes-of-renin-angiotensin-system-blocking-agents-
risk-of-hyperkalaemia-hypotension-and-impaired-renal-function-new-warnings (accessed September
2019).

MHRA: Medicines and Healthcare Products Regulatory Drug Safety Update (2016). *Spironolactone and rennin-angiotensin system drugs in heart failure: risk of potentially fatal hyperkalaemia.* https://www.gov.
uk/drug-safety-update/spironolactone-and-renin-angiotensin-system-drugs-in-heart-failure-risk-of-
potentially-fatal-hyperkalaemia (accessed September 2019).

Moon, H., Chin, H.J., Joo, K.W. et al. (2019). *Hyperphosphatemia and risks of acute kidney injury, end-stage
renal disease, and mortality in hospitalized patients.* https://bmcnephrol.biomedcentral.com/
articles/10.1186/s12882-019-1556-y (accessed September 2019).

Nair, M. (2016). The renal system. In: *Fundamentals of Anatomy and Physiology: For Nursing and Healthcare
Students*, 2e (eds. I. Peate and M. Nair). New York: Wiley.

Natale, P., Palmer, S.C., Ruospo, M. et al. (2018). *Potassium binders for chronic hyperkalaemia in people with
chronic kidney disease.* https://www.cochranelibrary.com/cdsr/doi/10.1002/14651858.CD013165/full
(accessed September 2019).

National Confidential Enquiry into Patient Outcome and Death (NCEPOD) (2009). *Adding insult to injury. A review
of the care of patient who dies in hospital with a primary diagnosis of acute kidney injury (acute renal failure).*
www.ncepod.org.uk/2009report1/Downloads/AKI_report.pdf (accessed September 2019).

National Institute of Clinical Excellence (2010). *Lower urinary symptoms in men: management. (CG97)*. www.
nice.org.uk/Guidance/CG97 (accessed September 2019).

National Institute of Clinical Excellence (2013a). *Acute kidney injury: prevention, detection and management.
(CG169)*. www.nice.org.uk/guidance/cg169 (accessed September 2019).

National Institute of Clinical Excellence (2013b). *Lower urinary tract symptoms in men. (QS45)*. www.nice.
org.uk/Guidance/QS45 (accessed September 2019).

National Institute of Clinical Excellence (2015). *Chronic kidney disease in adults: assessment and management.* https://www.nice.org.uk/guidance/cg182 (accessed July 2020).

National Institute of Clinical Excellence (2019a). *Chronic kidney disease.* https://cks.nice.org.uk/chronic-
kidney-disease#!topicSummary (accessed September 2019).

National Institute of Clinical Excellence (2019b). *Hypertension in adults: diagnosis and management.* www.
nice.org.uk/guidance/ng136 (accessed September 2019).

National Institute of Clinical Excellence (2019c). *Urinary incontinence and pelvic organ prolapsed in women:
management.* www.nice.org.uk/guidance/ng123 (accessed September 2019).

National Institute of Diabetes and Digestive and Kidney Diseases (2019). *Laboratory evaluation.* https://
www.niddk.nih.gov/health-information/communication-programs/nkdep/laboratory-evaluation
(accessed September 2019).

Nazar, C.M.J. (2014). Diabetic nephropathy; principles of diagnosis and treatment of diabetic kidney disease. *Journal of Nephropharmacology* **3** (1): 15–20.

Neal, M.J. (2016). *Medical Pharmacology at a Glance*, 8e. West Sussex: Wiley.

Nethercliffe, J. (2012). Urinary incontinence. In: *ABC of Urology*, 3e (eds. C. Dawson and J. Nethercliffe), 14–
18. West Sussex: Wiley Blackwell.

O'Callaghan, C. (2017). *The Renal System at a Glance*, 4e. West Sussex: Wiley.

Office for National Statistics (2018). *Deaths that were caused by 'Acute Kidney Injury', by place of death and broad
age group, England and Wales, registered 2001 to 2016.* www.ons.gov.uk/peoplepopulationandcommunity/
birthsdeathsandmarriages/deaths/adhocs/007984deathsthatwerecausedbyacutekidneyinjurybypla
ceofdeathandbroadagegroupenglandandwalesregistered2001to2016 (accessed September 2019).

Peate, I. (ed.) (2017). Fluid and electrolyte balance and associated disorders. In: *Fundamentals of Applied
Pathophysiology: An Essential Guide for Nursing and Healthcare Students*, 506–533. Hoboken: Wiley.

Pitt, B., Zannad, F., Remme, W.J. et al. (1999). *The effect of spironolactone on morbidity and mortality in
patients with severe heart failure.* https://www.nejm.org/doi/10.1056/NEJM199909023411001?url_
ver=Z39.88-2003&rfr_id=ori%3Arid%3Acrossref.org&rfr_dat=cr_pub%3Dwww.ncbi.nlm.nih.gov
(accessed July 2020).

Rattu. M. (2015). *Pharmacists' role in managing male urinary incontinence.* https://www.uspharmacist.com/
article/pharmacists-role-in-managing-male-urinary-incontinence (accessed September 2019).

Richards, D., Aronson, J., Reynolds, D.J., and Coleman, J. (2012). *Oxford Handbook of Practical Drug Therapy*,
2e. Oxford: Oxford University Press.

Shawkat, H., Westwood, M., and Mortimer, A. (2012). Mannitol: a review of its clinical uses. *Continuing
Education in Anaesthetics Critical Care and Pain* **12** (2): 82–85.

Soar, J., Deakin, C., Lockey, A. et al. (2015). *Resuscitation Guidelines 2015 Adult Life Support*. London: Resuscitation Council UK.

Steddon, S., Ashman, N., Chesser, A., and Cunningham, J. (2014). *Oxford Handbook of Nephrology and Hypertension*, 2e. Oxford: Oxford University Press.

UK Renal Registry (2018). *20th Annual Report of the Renal Association*. https://www.renalreg.org/wp-content/uploads/2018/06/20th-Annual-Report_web_book.pdf (accessed September 2019).

UK Renal Registry (2019). *UK Renal Registry 21st Annual Report*. https://www.renalreg.org/wp-content/uploads/2019/05/21st_UKRR_Annual_Report.pdf (accessed September 2019).

Vassalotti, J.A., Centor, R., Turner, B.J. et al. (2016). *Practical approach to detection and management of chronic kidney disease for the primary care clinician*. https://www.ncbi.nlm.nih.gov/pmc/articles/PMC6184972/ (accessed July 2020).

Wang H.E., Munter, P., Chertow, G.M. et al. (2012). *Acute kidney injury and mortality in hospitalized patients*. https://www.ncbi.nlm.nih.gov/pmc/articles/PMC3362180/ (accessed July 2020).

Webster, A.C., Nagler, E.V., Morton, R.L. et al. (2017). Chronic kidney disease. *Lancet* **389** (10075): 1238–1252.

Further reading

KDIGO Guidelines
https://kdigo.org/guidelines
KDIGO is *the* global non-profit organisation developing and implementing evidence-based clinical practice guidelines in kidney disease. KDIGO guidelines are created, reviewed, published and implemented following a rigorous scientific process.

National Institute of Clinical Excellence (NICE) Guidelines
www.nice.org.uk
NICE provides national guidance and advice to improve health and social care. They provide a number of guidelines concerning all aspects of healthcare delivery. Their aim is to improve health and social care through evidence-based guidance.

Multiple choice questions

1. Diabetes is the single most common cause of end-stage kidney disease in the UK and accounts for ... of new patients needing dialysis or transplant due to diabetic-related kidney disease?
   (a) 25%
   (b) 30%
   (c) 45%
   (d) 10%

2. One of the most common and potentially avoidable causes of acute and chronic renal damage is via pharmacotherapy. Which of the following drugs has potentially the most adverse effects upon multiple sites of the nephron?
   (a) Phenytoin
   (b) Penicillin
   (c) NSAIDs
   (d) Lithium

3. Loop diuretics exert their effect upon which part of the nephron?
   (a) Proximal convoluted tubule
   (b) Collecting
   (c) Loop of Henle
   (d) Glomerulus

4. Furosemide has a potent diuretic effect via the inhibition of which of the following?
   (a) Sodium–potassium–chloride cotransporter, or the Na-K-Cl (NKCC2)
   (b) Phophodiasterase type 5
   (c) Sodium–potassium ATPase pump
   (d) Aldosterone antagonism

5. Secondary hyperparathyroidism can lead to which of the following?
   (a) Hypercalcaemia
   (b) Hyperphosphataemia
   (c) High vitamin D levels
   (d) Diabetes

6. Androgen-synthesis inhibitors inhibits which of the following processes?
   (a) The breakdown of cyclic adenosine monophosphate (cAMP])
   (b) The nitric oxide (NO)/cyclic guanosine monophosphate (cGMP) pathway
   (c) The stimulation of phospholipase C (PLC)
   (d) The enzyme 5a-reductase that converts testosterone in to 5a-dihydrotestosterone

7. The molecular weight of drugs is measured in …
   (a) Daltons (Da)
   (b) International System of Units (SI)
   (c) Grams (g)
   (d) Creatinine clearance

8. Which of the following is NOT a function of the kidney?
   (a) Removal of the waste product of metabolism, including urea and creatinine
   (b) Fluid balance via selective absorption of sodium and water
   (c) Regulation of potassium via the secretion of aldosterone
   (d) Glucose homoeostasis via gluconeogenesis and reabsorption of glucose

9. Which segment of the nephron is critical in the excretion of potassium ions?
   (a) Proximal convoluted tubule
   (b) Collecting duct
   (c) Thick ascending loop of Henle
   (d) Thin descending loop of Henle

10. Which of these conditions is NOT a cause of AKI?
    (a) Hypovolaemia
    (b) Sepsis
    (c) Renal artery stenosis
    (d) Glomerular nephritis

11. Which of the following is NOT one of the criteria used to define AKI?
    (a) A rise in serum creatinine of 26 μmol/L (0.3 mg/dL) or greater within 48 hours
    (b) A 20% or greater rise in serum creatinine known or presumed to have occurred within the past seven days
    (c) A fall in urine output to <0.5 mL/kg/h for more than six hours in adults and more than eight hours in children and young people
    (d) A 25% or greater fall in estimated GFR in children and young people within the past seven days

12. How many stages of CKD are there in the KDIGO classification?
    (a) 7
    (b) 6
    (c) 5
    (d) 4

13. Which of the following definitions indicates microalbuminuria?
    (a) ACR 2 mg/mmol
    (b) ACR 38 mg/mmol
    (c) ACR 12 mg/mmol
    (d) ACR 58 mg/mmol
14. Which of the following is NOT a classification of urinary incontinence?
    (a) Overactive
    (b) Urgency
    (c) Stress
    (d) Overflow
15. One of the potassium-sparing diuretics, spironolactone, exerts its effects by the following mechanisms?
    (a) By blocking the sodium channels in the luminal membrane
    (b) Competes for the aldosterone binding site on cytoplasmic receptors
    (c) Inhibits the sodium–potassium–chloride co-transporter
    (d) Inhibits the enzymic action of carbonic anhydrase

Find out more

The following are a list of conditions that are associated with people who have renal disorders. Take some time and write notes about each of the conditions. Think about the medications that may be used in order to treat these conditions and be specific about the pharmacokinetics and pharmacodynamics. Remember to include aspects of patient care. If you are making notes about people you have offered care and support to, you must ensure that you have adhered to the rules of confidentiality.

The condition	Your notes
Metabolic acidosis	
Renal tubular acidosis	
Diabetes Type II	
Addison's disease	
Hyperparathyroidism	

Chapter 12

Medications and diabetes mellitus

Anne Phillips

Aim

The aim of this chapter is to provide the reader with an introduction to the medication types used with people with diabetes mellitus and to explain the importance of person-centred care and appropriateness of medication choice.

Learning outcomes

After reading this chapter, the reader will be able to:

1. Discuss the importance of person-centred care in diabetes care
2. Appreciate the importance of understanding the pharmacology associated with the medicines used in glycaemic control in diabetes
3. Understand treatment optimisation and respecting individual choice of medication regimens for optimal delivery and person-centred safety
4. Recognise the importance of 'The Right insulin, Right dose, Right way, Right time' for all insulin administration regimens

Test your knowledge

1. Before you read this chapter, jot down what you think you already know about diabetes.
2. Name all the types of diabetes you know.
3. What does medicine safety mean in diabetes care?
4. Which age groups are affected by which type of diabetes?
5. Do you consider diabetes to be a current health concern in the UK; if so why; if not, why?

Fundamentals of Pharmacology: For Nursing and Healthcare Students, First Edition. Edited by Ian Peate and Barry Hill.
© 2021 John Wiley & Sons Ltd. Published 2021 by John Wiley & Sons Ltd.

Introduction

The prevalence of diabetes is increasing across all age groups as a result of population growth, an aging society, urbanisation and more effective diabetes screening. There are many different types of diabetes and sub-types and it is important to recognise which type of diabetes people you care for are diagnosed with. Diabetes UK (2019a) recognise that 90% of people with diabetes have type 2, about 8% have type 1 and about 2% have rarer forms of diabetes. The number of people diagnosed with diabetes has more than doubled in the previous 20 years and about 1 in 15 people have diabetes in the UK; this compares to the estimate of 1 in 11 people being diagnosed with diabetes globally as reported by the International Diabetes Federation (IDF, 2017). Diabetes therefore is a global public health challenge with prevalence rates that are increasing alarmingly (IDF, 2017).

However, in the UK about 1 million people have type 2 diabetes but have not yet been diagnosed, and nearly 10 million people in the UK are considered to be at high risk of developing type 2 diabetes as their HbA1c test results are within 42–47 mmols/mol (Diabetes UK, 2019a). The diagnostic marker for a diagnosis of type 2 diabetes is an HbA1c of 48 mmols/mol in accordance with World Health Organisation diagnostic criteria (WHO, 2011). This chapter, with the help of two case studies, will discuss the use of oral antidiabetic agents and also insulin in a person-centred way to enable people to learn how to self-manage their diabetes.

HbA1c

Glycosylated haemoglobin, known as HbA1c, is a blood test used to assess diabetes. It is reported as mmols/mol and sometimes you will still hear practitioners or individuals refer to their HbA1c as a percentage as this is how HbA1c used to be reported until 2011. In 2011, HbA1c levels were standardised and reported as mmols/mol values also known as the IFCC (International Federation of Clinical Chemistry) units. Glucose in the blood stream binds onto proteins and whatever the level of blood glucose is when the red blood cells are manufactured in the bone marrow, then that percentage of glucose binds onto those red blood cells for their life span, which is usually 120 days. This is a continuous process and the HbA1c measures the amount of glucose bound onto a selection of older, middle aged and new red blood cells. As the average red blood cells last 120 days, the HbA1c test most accurately reflects the individuals' diabetes control for the past six to eight weeks. Everyone has an HbA1c level, but in diabetes care it is an important marker for how well someone's diabetes is controlled and whether the individual is at risk of preventable complications occurring if their HbA1c is too high (hyperglycaemia) or hypoglycaemia if their HbA1c is too low. In practice, HbA1c is measured six monthly in adults and three monthly in children and young people to assess their need for insulin to enable them to grow fully.

Blood glucose measurements

In people without diabetes blood glucose measurements are fairly stable and vary little. Normal blood glucose levels in people without diabetes range between 3.5–6.5 mmols/L (DeFronzo et al., 2015). Blood glucose measurements are lower before eating – known as pre-prandial – and slightly higher after eating – known as post-prandial. In the UK, blood glucose measurements are measured as mmols/L but in the US and across Europe they are measured in mg/dl. Blood glucose measurements should **not** be referred to as a BM as this is inaccurate and incorrect. BM stands for the previous Boehringer Mannheim, which was the pharmaceutical manufacturer of the first available blood glucose monitoring sticks in the mid-1980s. This manufacturer is no longer in existence and therefore it is much more accurate and safer to say 'BGM' for blood glucose monitoring. The NMC (2018) requires all nurses to practise safely, so using the correct terminology helps to protect patient safety.

Normal blood glucose ranges and aims in diabetes care as advocated by National Institute for Health and Care Excellence (NICE) (2012) are illustrated in Box 12.1.

Box 12.1   Normal blood glucose levels for the majority of healthy people

- Between 4.0 and 5.4 mmol/L when fasting.
- Up to 7.8 mmol/L two hours after eating.
- Normal range is 3.5–6.5 mmols/L.

(Source: NICE PH38, 2012)

For people with diabetes, blood glucose level targets are as follows:

- Pre-prandial (before meals): 4–7 mmol/L for people with type 1 or type 2 diabetes.
- Post prandial (after meals): under 9 mmol/L for people with type 1 diabetes and under 8.5 mmol/L for people with type 2 diabetes (NICE PH38, 2012).

Diagnosis and signs and symptoms
Type 1 diabetes

The symptoms of type 1 diabetes come on very quickly and require urgent treatment. Type 1 diabetes is an autoimmune condition and consistent hyperglycaemia (high blood glucose levels) can lead, if untreated or unrecognised, to a condition called diabetic ketoacidosis (DKA). This is a medical emergency and happens when a severe lack of insulin means the individual's body cannot use the glucose in the blood stream available for fuel. The person's body needs energy, so breaks down its fat stores, stored as triglycerides, and these are converted in the liver to ketones. Ketones, despite being an alternative fuel source, enter the blood stream but cannot enter the cells without the presence of insulin. Ketones build up in the blood stream and are poisonous chemicals which cause the person's blood to become acidic.

DKA can kill, so individuals must be referred immediately for medical help and treatment must follow the Joint British Diabetes Societies for Inpatient Care (JBDS-IP, 2013) DKA guidelines and protocol for fluid replacement in adults with DKA (JBDS-IP, 2018) within all NHS trusts. JBDS (2020) have also published a really useful document that details the medical management of people arriving in hospitals as acute emergencies – it is a really worthwhile read and highlights how clear procedures and policy can save the lives of people with diabetes admitted as acute emergencies into hospitals in the UK. Children and young people aged under 18 years have separate guidelines for DKA management published by the British Society of Paediatric Endocrinology and Diabetes (BSPED, 2015).

The UK campaign of 4Ts by Diabetes UK – toilet, thirsty, thinner, tired – highlighted the symptoms of type 1 diabetes for the public and healthcare professionals aiming to promote awareness earlier and enable more effective and timely diagnosis before DKA occurs.

Type 2 diabetes

The symptoms of type 2 diabetes are more subtle and as such are often blamed on other issues such as ageing. Insulin is produced in two waves from the beta cells when a person has eaten food and their blood glucose levels start to raise post-prandially. In type 2 diabetes, the second wave of insulin release is lost, so blood glucose levels can rise quite high and can begin to cause damage through glucose glycosylating (sticking) onto proteins in the eyes, nerves and kidneys – this is how the complications of diabetes can occur (Phillips, 2017). Furthermore, Diabetes UK (2019a) recognise that 6 out of 10 people diagnosed with type 2 diabetes experienced no symptoms. In type 2 diabetes the person's beta cells do produce insulin, but the insulin release can be sluggish and blood glucose levels rise in the blood stream. Also, insulin resistance can

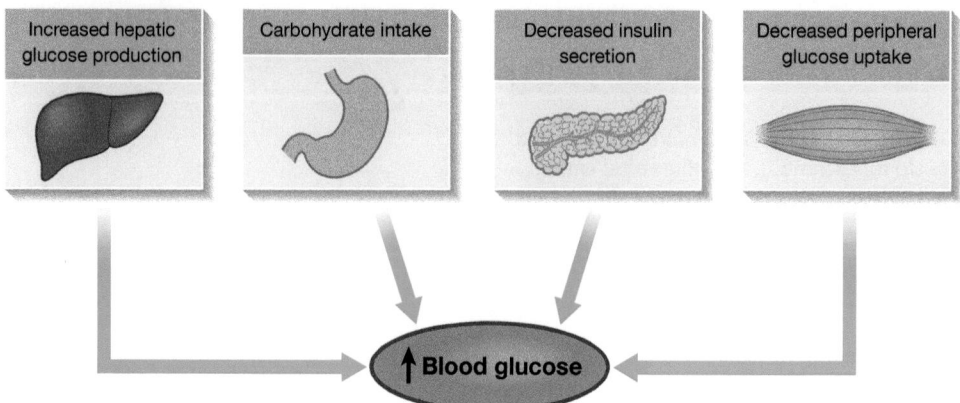

| Increased hepatic glucose production | Carbohydrate intake | Decreased insulin secretion | Decreased peripheral glucose uptake |

↑ Blood glucose

Figure 12.1 Pathophysiology related to abnormal glucose metabolism in type 2 diabetes.
Source: Nair and Peate, Pathophysiology for nurses at a glance.

occur so people produce enough insulin but there is resistance on the cellular wall to allow the glucose to enter the cell for growth, repair or energy (Defronzo et al., 2015). There is only one medication on the market that works directly on the insulin receptor sites on the cell wall and this is Metformin (which will be discussed later in this chapter). The longer people's blood glucose levels are too high, the more at risk they are of microvascular and microvascular complications occurring; one in three people will have complications from their diabetes when they are diagnosed with type 2 diabetes (Defronzo et al., 2015; Diabetes UK, 2019a).

Type 2 diabetes is known as a cardiovascular condition as it shares an association with obesity, hypertension, dyslipidaemia and the tendency for thrombosis. Obesity is responsible for 80–85% risk of developing type 2 diabetes and more than 50% of all cases of type 2 diabetes can be prevented or delayed (NICE PH38, 2012); public awareness is therefore essential. People diagnosed with type 2 diabetes can have a substantially reduced quality of life and increased morbidity and mortality.

Figure 12.1 provides an overview of the pathophysiology related to abnormal glucose metabolism in type 2 diabetes.

Being at risk

Diabetes UK, The University of Leicester and The University Hospitals of Leicester NHS Trust (2019) suggests that along with the 10 million estimated to be at 'high risk' a further 12.3 million people are currently at 'risk' of type 2 diabetes in the UK, with people from a South Asian or All Black background being two to four times more likely to develop type 2 diabetes than White people. The NHS Diabetes Prevention Programme (NDPP, 2019) with NHS England and Public Health England encourages people to reduce their risk, with tailored support to help them lose weight and be more physically active. The NDPP is active across the UK in aiming to prevent type 2 diabetes in populations at risk. Being at increased risk is when an individual's HbA1c is 42–47 mmols/mol. The diagnostic level of type 2 diabetes occurs at HbA1c of 48 mmols/mol, as illustrated in Box 12.2.

However, once diagnosed, individual HbA1c levels will be agreed with each person accordingly, reflecting their personal circumstances, safety and knowledge, and to reduce their risk of hypoglycaemia – this will be discussed later in this chapter.

Importance of glycaemic control

There is a clear causal relationship between glycaemic control, blood pressure control and lipid control in type 2 diabetes. In this chapter, medications to help glycaemic control will be discussed.

In both type 1 and type 2 diabetes, sub-optimal glycaemic control increases the risk of preventable microvascular disease. The landmark Diabetes Control and Complications Trial

Box 12.2   HbA1c levels used to detect diabetes

Normal: Below 42 mmol/mol.

High risk of diabetes: 42–47 mmol/mol.

Diabetes: 48 mmol/mol.

Source: WHO, Global Criteria (2016)

(DCCT) in the US in 1993 for people with type 1 diabetes and the United Kingdom Prospective Diabetes Study (UKPDS, 1998) both established epidemiological analysis underpinning the sustained relationship between the risks for microvascular disease and hyperglycaemia. For every percentage point decrease in HbA1c, these landmark trials reported a 35% reduction in the risk of microvascular complications, a 25% reduction in diabetes-related deaths and a 7% reduction in all-cause mortality, with an 18% reduction in combined non-fatal and fatal myocardial infarctions. Furthermore, the UKPDS (1998) conclusively demonstrated that intensive control of blood pressure in type 2 diabetes significantly contributed to the reduction of preventable microvascular complications (Stratton et al., 2000). A 10 year follow-up study of the UKPDS data demonstrated a longer term legacy effect of a continued reduction in microvascular risk, and emergent risk reductions for myocardial infarction and death from any cause were observed during 10 years of post-trial follow-up (Holman et al., 2008).

Davies et al. (2018) on behalf of the American Diabetes Association (ADA) and the European Association for the Study of Diabetes (EASD) published the latest guidance in the management of medications for people with type 2 diabetes. This followed the very helpful previous guidance published by Inzucchi et al. (2015). The focus of this latest guidance is on evidence-based approaches, person-centred care and supporting person-centred choice. This is helpful and clearly defines working in partnership with individuals, respecting their choices and supporting their decision-making about different treatment options and regimens. This underpins diabetes care, as if the regimen is too burdensome to manage, it can cause people to experience an often overwhelming treatment burden and a lower quality of life (Garcia et al., 2019). Regimens need to be tailored around each individual respecting their needs and abilities to manage their diabetes regimen and also their ability to monitor and escalate or de-escalate treatment accordingly depending on changes in individual circumstances. This supports the guidance published by NICE (2015) which further advocated HbA1c thresholds being relaxed when individuals age to reduce the risk of hypoglycaemia (discussed later in this chapter) and the treatment burden.

Individual assessment

Despite all the guidelines and treatment algorithms available, perhaps the most important aspect of diabetes care is partnership working. Practitioners need to ensure each individual has the necessary tools and resources to understand their diabetes and their treatment options. Their choices should also be supported and their access to person-centred education extenuated via either structured education programmes or digital resources (NHS England, 2019b). Therefore, the aims of care along – with the biochemical markers – can be to enable people to feel that they can manage their diabetes and not experience diabetes-related emotional distress, which can be overwhelming. Wright and Phillips (2017) suggested a skills and desired outcomes method using a staged consultation approach with people with diabetes. This is demonstrated in Table 12.1.

Table 12.1   Skills and desired outcomes of a staged

Stage	Skills	Outcomes
'Listening to the story'	Demonstrate listening Follow the person's concerns Demonstrate empathy Initiate discussion of the person's concerns	To establish joint understanding of the problem
'Creating a different future'	Demonstrate empathy and identify strengths Demonstrate confidence in a potential for change Encourage critical thinking and goal setting Provide health information	To establish a partnership to achieve goals
'Taking action'	Encourage and support action Demonstrate commitment to the plan(s) Review, monitor and evaluate progress Encourage reflection on action	To support action toward achieving and supporting goals

Source: Wright and Phillips (2017).

Treatment guidelines

There are three principal treatment approaches in both type 1 and type 2 diabetes. These are:

- To prevent glycose excursions with hypo- or hyperglycaemia and to maintain glycaemic control to prevent hypo- and hyperglycaemia. This is undertaken with support and education regarding healthy eating, weight loss advice as required and engagement in physical activity.
- To maintain a level of glycaemic control appropriate to the individuals' age, duration of diabetes, existing complications, lifestyle, occupation, knowledge, understanding of diabetes, and cognitive abilities on a day-to-day basis using age-appropriate care approaches.
- To prevent, or treat if existing, any long-term micro- and macro-vascular complications of diabetes.

Types of antidiabetes medications

The commonly used antidiabetes drugs in addition to insulin therapy are: Biguanides, Sulfonylureas, Thiazolidinediones, Incretins, GLP-1 receptor agonists, DPP-4 inhibitors and SGLT-2 inhibitors.

Treatment approaches in type 2 diabetes

Targets from NICE (2015) and for the ADA and EASD (Davies et al., 2018) are as follows.

Individuals aged over 18 years who are newly diagnosed with type 2 diabetes will be seen by a practice nurse who has been educated in diabetes care. Baseline assessments are undertaken to screen for potential complications present at diagnosis. The UKPDS (1998) and the 10-year follow-up study of the UKPDS (Holman et al., 2008) both highlighted the increased incidence of macro- and microvascular complications of type 2 diabetes being present at diagnosis. Baseline assessments include: blood pressure to assess for hypertension, lipid profile to assess for dyslipidaemia, urea and electrolyte assessment to determine kidney function, HbA1c to assess glycaemic control and need for oral hypoglycaemic agents.

Thyroid function tests are also indicated as thyroid disease is more common in people with both type 1 and type 2 diabetes (Biondi et al., 2019). A liver profile is required; however, an abnormal result does not always indicate non-alcoholic fatty liver disease (NAFLD), but can indicate insulin resistance. A follow-up with a liver ultrasound is required as NAFLD is closely linked with increasing risks of cardiovascular disease (Goedeke et al., 2019). A full-blood count would be required to assess for signs of vitamin B_{12} deficiency anaemia, iron deficiency anaemia; bleeding or clotting disorders; and infection or inflammation. Iron deficiency anaemia can cause abnormalities in HbA1c levels, so detecting and treating anaemia is important (Sodi et al., 2018). Testing frustosamine (a glycated protein) as an alternative to HbA1c can be appropriate if individuals do present with iron deficiency anaemia (Sodi et al., 2018).

Further baseline assessments of foot sensation to assess for neuropathy, urinalysis to detect for microalbuminuria and early nephropathy, Body Mass Index and weight, (depending on the individuals muscular phenotype where BMI measurements will be misleading due to the weight of muscle), and a referral for annual retinal screening assessment and recall will be made.

The practice nurse will discuss the individual's diagnosis and support their thoughts and feelings toward the same to help effective emotional adjustment to having type 2 diabetes (Wright and Phillips, 2017). Alongside referral for educational opportunities for individuals, there can be a structured class or the use of digital resources, depending on each individual's requirements. This is essential as people should be encouraged to learn about their diabetes to gain confidence and increase understanding. NHS Right Care identified the need to improve uptake to structured education for people with diabetes within 12 months of diagnosis as a 'national opportunity' to better manage diabetes. However, the National Diabetes Audit (NDA) of 2016–17 found that in 2015, while 77.3% of people newly diagnosed with type 2 diabetes were offered structured education, only 7.4% attended, which means that out of more than 200 000 newly diagnosed people with type 2 diabetes, fewer than 15 000 attended health education programmes. The reasons for non-attendance are multifactorial and complex.

Grumitt et al. (2018) suggested that in view of the massive gap between referral and attendance to structured diabetes education, there are questions about the ability of face-to-face programmes to meet the needs of those they are seeking to attract. Consequently, other forms of education, including digital resources and multilingual resources, are becoming available in England and are supported by NHS England (2019a).

Oral medications

Biguanides (Metformin)

Metformin is generally the most widely used first-line treatment in type 2 diabetes (NICE, 2015). Its main effects are to suppress glucose production in the liver and enhance insulin sensitivity in muscle tissues. Metformin is not metabolised but is excreted via the kidneys; it works on the insulin receptor site at the cell wall and aims to make the receptor 'more receptive' to allow glucose into cells for growth, repair and energy. Metformin decreases HbA1c levels by 1–2%, and the plasma glucose level will start to decrease within three to five days of commencement. It usually takes one to two weeks to achieve its maximum effect (Jennings and Aye, 2017), so treatment escalation should be paced accordingly.

Metformin is initiated at 500 mg once daily always taken with or after meals. The maximum daily dose of 1000 mg twice daily is reported to have maximal benefit (Jennings and Aye, 2017). Side effects include gastrointestinal effects such as diarrhoea and/or nausea and vomiting; the patient should be advised to administer Metformin with or after meals, as this can help to minimise these potential side effects. The main risk of Metformin is lactic acidosis, although this is rare; for those with limited liver or kidney function, they should be advised to stop their Metformin before any procedures using contrast dyes 48 hours before the procedure (Baerlocher et al., 2013).

As Metformin works on the insulin receptor sites, it cannot cause hypoglycaemia. Individuals generally do not need to blood glucose monitor when taking Metformin, unless they have been advised to look for trend data in relation to food intake (Grumitt et al., 2018).

As Metformin is excreted by the kidneys, it should not be commenced or continued if an individual's creatinine levels are >130 mmols/L or if the estimated glomerular filtration (eGFR) rate of the kidneys is declining <45 mL/min/1.73 m^2 in accordance with NICE (2015) guidance.

Clinical consideration

Metformin must always be taken with or after food so please ensure that when administering Metformin, the person is advised to take this medicine with their meal or just afterwards. This helps ameliorate any gastrointestinal side effects such as bloating, flatulence or diarrhoea that Metformin can cause in some people, especially if taken on an empty stomach or pre meal.

Other second-line treatment choices

This will depend on the individual's situation, age, employment and needs and will be managed in agreement with each individual and discussion with their diabetes team, usually in general practice. Encouragement with healthy eating advice and engagement with some physical activity will be supported and target setting encouraged also using the Diabetes UK Information Prescriptions (2019b), which offer agreed targets in relation to person-centred goals, such as weight loss or walking more as examples. Second-line drugs of choice are presented in Table 12.2.

HbA1c target aims

HbA1c targets must be individualised to each person and their individual circumstances. For adults (age over 18 years) on a medication associated with hypoglycaemia, support the person to aim for an HbA1c level of 53 mmol/mol in accordance with NICE (2015) and the ADA/EASD Guidance (Davies et al. 2018). In adults with type 2 diabetes, if HbA1c levels are not adequately managed by Metformin and rise to 58 mmol/mol or higher, the person should be offered support and more tailored advice about healthy eating, and perhaps referred to a community diabetes dietitian, if available. Also discuss human factors which can influence each individual's diabetes control, these include lifestyle choices and understanding and concordance with prescribed medication.

Clinical consideration

It is worth always checking when a person's normal day starts and ends, as if the individual is a shift worker, or works nights, then their meal patterns and sleeping patterns will be variable and, as such, their medication times will need individual adjustment with the prescriber and in consultation with the individual who this concerns with the aim to optimise the medication's effect and to avoid missing any doses.

Support the person to aim for an HbA1c level of 53 mmol/mol; Davies et al. (2018) recommend the introduction of a second-line treatment, the choices of which are outlined Table 12.2.

Consideration should be given to relaxing the target HbA1c level on a case-by-case basis, with particular consideration for people who are older or frail, for adults with type 2 diabetes in accordance with guidance in Figure 12.1. In particular, relax the HbA1c target in people who are unlikely to achieve longer-term risk-reduction benefits; for example, people with a reduced life expectancy, or people diagnosed with dementia where hypoglycaemia and their risk of falls is accentuated, or lack of appetite and their need for safety is paramount over the tight glycaemic control (Forbes et al., 2018).

A relaxation of HbA1c targets is also recommended in people for whom tight blood glucose control poses a high risk of the consequences of hypoglycaemia; for example, people who are at risk of falling, people who live alone, people who have impaired awareness of hypoglycaemia and people who drive or operate machinery as part of their job. Additionally, individual assessment is vital as intensive management would not be appropriate, for example, for people with significant co-morbidities.

Table 12.2 Choice of second agents in treatment people with type 2 diabetes post Metformin.

Medication type	Sodium-glucose Cotransporter-2 (SGLT2) Inhibitors	Glucagon-Like Peptide-1 (GLP1) Receptor Agonists	Dipeptidyl Peptidase-4 (DPP-4) Inhibitors	Sulfonylureas	Thiazolidinediones
Medication names	Canagliflozin Dapagliflozin Empagliflozin Ertugliflozin	Dulaglutide Exenatide Liraglutide Lixisenatide Semaglutide	Alogliptin Linagliptin Saxagliptin Sitagliptin Vildagliptin	Gliclazide Glimepiride Glipizide	Pioglitazone
Mode of action	Insulin-independent, inhibits renal glucose from re-absorption by blocking SGLT2 transporter	Stimulates glucose-dependent insulin release from the pancreas	Increases incretin (GLP1) levels by blocking DPP-4 enzyme which inactivates GLP1	Stimulates insulin secretion from pancreatic beta-cells	Insulin-dependent, reduces hepatic and peripheral insulin resistance at molecular level
Route of administration	Oral	Injectable	Oral	Oral	Oral
Risk of hypoglycaemia	Low	Low	Low	High	Low
Impact on weight	Weight loss	Weight loss	Weight neutral	Weight gain	Weight gain
Precautions and side effects	UTIs, euglycaemic DKA even if Blood glucose is normal – check ketones. Avoid using in people with active diabetes related foot disease.	GI side effects common. Possible increased risk of pancreatitis	GI disturbance. Possible increase in pancreatitis	All users should have access to self-blood glucose monitoring, especially drivers in view of hypoglycaemia risk. Avoid in frailty.	Contradicted in heart failure. Increases fracture risk. Use with caution in macular edema.

(Continued)

Table 12.2 (Continued)

Medication type	Sodium-glucose Cotransporter-2 (SGLT2) Inhibitors	Glucagon-Like Peptide-1 (GLP1) Receptor Agonists	Dipeptidil Peptidase-4 (DPP-4) Inhibitors	Sulfonylureas	Thiazolidinediones
Interactions	Rifampin, Phenytoin, phenobarbital, ritonavir (Norvir) increase the removal of canagliflozin from the body. Canagliflozin increases blood levels and the effect of digoxin.	Increased risk of hypoglycaemia when a GLP-1 agonist is used with a sulfonylurea or insulin. As GLP1s work by delaying gastric emptying, they can modify the absorption of some drugs. This is not normally clinically significant but an increase in INR ratios have been reported when using warfarin.	Saxagliptin concentration is affected by CYP3A4 inhibitors and inducers, and angiotensin-converting inhibitors increase the risk of bradykinin-induced angioedema.	Sulfonylurea-induced hypoglycaemia is worsened by co-administration with azole antifungals, clarithromycin, verapamil, angiotensin-converting inhibitors, DPP-4 s and GLP-1 agonists.	Can cause dose-related fluid retention which may lead to or exacerbate congestive heart failure.
Absorption	Liver and kidneys	With GLP1 receptors in the digestive system	Small intestine	Small intestine	Small intestine
Distribution	Kidneys	Systematic circulation	Binds to target proteins in plasma and peripheral tissues	Systemic circulation	Binds to plasma proteins
Metabolism	Hepatic and renal	Across the tissues by oxidation	Increase incretin levels (GLP-1 and GIP), which inhibit glucagon release, which increases insulin secretion, decreases gastric emptying and decreases blood glucose levels.	Hepatic	Hepatic
Elimination	Via urine	Via urine and faeces	Via urine	Via urine	Via urine

Source: Davies et al. (2018).

Self-blood glucose monitoring in type 2 diabetes

There has been much debate about whether people with type 2 diabetes should self-blood glucose monitor or not. The general advice from NICE (2015) is that people with type 2 diabetes do not need to self-blood glucose monitor (SMBG) unless the person is on oral medication that may increase their risk of hypoglycaemia, such as a sulfonylurea like gliclazide, or there is evidence of hypoglycaemia, or if the individual drives or is driving or operating machinery, or if the person is pregnant or is planning to become pregnant.

Analysing trend data to assess glucose control by SMBG can highlight the effect of dietary intake, and therefore education about SMBG can be highly beneficial to people not taking medication that can cause hypoglycaemia; however, currently this initiative cannot be funded on prescription (Grumitt et al. 2018). Instructions for each blood glucose monitoring device will be with the device and also available online on the device's manufacturing webpages.

Skills in practice

How to self-blood glucose monitor:

* Advise the person to wash their hands.
* Undertake a finger prick to obtain a blood sample on the side of the finger, avoiding the tip. Massage the finger to obtain the blood sample required.
* Check the blood glucose test strips are in-date.
* Instructions for the use of each blood glucose monitoring device will be with the device and also available online on the device's manufacturer's webpages.
* Record the result, and if the result is not within the range expected for the individual concerned, then report this to the nurse in charge and record your actions.
* Wash hands and dispose safely of any used equipment.

Insulin

Insulin is used by all people with type 1 diabetes and some people with type 2 diabetes. The main role of insulin is glucose metabolism. Insulin is a peptide hormone produced in the β cells in the islets of Langerhans in the pancreas (see Figure 12.2).

Insulin regulates the metabolism of carbohydrates and fats by promoting the absorption of glucose from the blood to the skeletal muscles and fat tissue by causing fat to be stored rather than used as energy. Insulin also inhibits the production of glucose by the liver. Insulin is made up of 51 amino acids arranged as a two-chain molecule connected by two disulphide bridges: A chain 21 amino acids, B chain 30 amino acids (see Figure 12.3). When insulin is made synthetically, the amino acid chains are altered, thereby creating different insulins with different duration of action to be made available (see Table 12.3).

The National Patient Safety Agency (2017) and NICE (2019) have published guidelines about insulin safety and administration to reduce unnecessary errors and promote patient safety. The NPSA (2017) and NICE (2019) both promote Six Steps in Insulin Safety:

1. The Right Insulin
2. The Right Dose
3. The Right Way
4. The Right Time
5. Hypoglycaemia
6. Sick Day Advice.

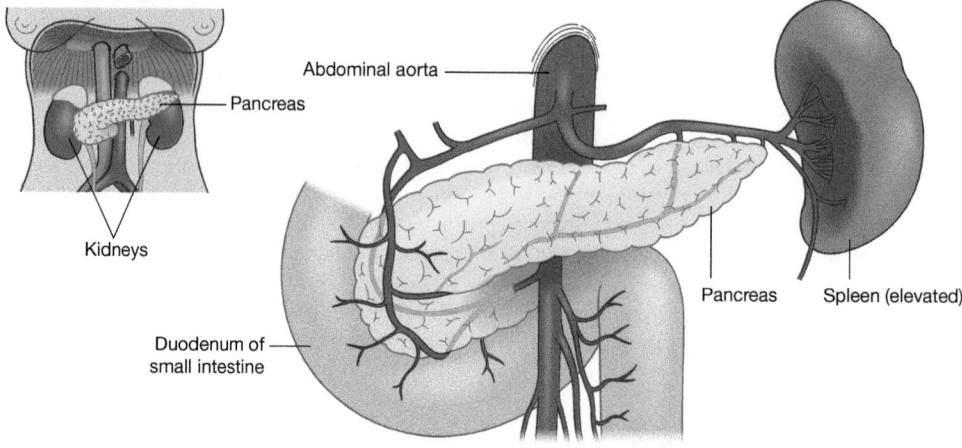

Figure 12.2   The pancreas. Source: Peate and Wild, Nursing Practice Knowledge.

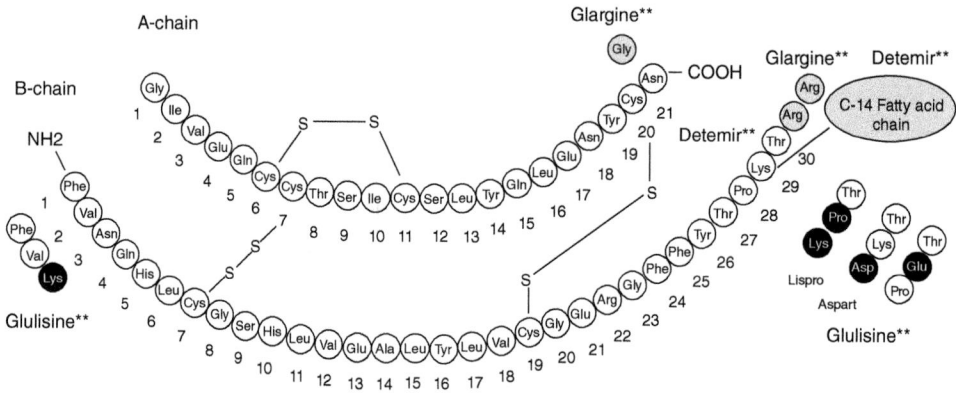

Figure 12.3   Insulin – a two-chain molecule. Source: Peate and Wild, Nursing Practice Knowledge.

The right insulin

There are over 20 different types of insulin on prescription; checking with the individual and re-checking their prescription is vital to avoid unnecessary insulin errors in administration of the wrong insulin type. Teaching people the name and details of their own insulin prescription is also vital to avoid errors in prescribing or dispensing from community or hospital pharmacists (Cousins et al., 2019). Insulin treatment improves quality of life in many people with type 2 diabetes and saves the lives of people with type 1 diabetes. Insulin is used to lower blood glucose levels and replaces the Insulin no longer being produced by the individual from their β cells in their Islets of Langerhans.

Diabetes UK (2017a, b) have published guidance to help nurses avoid unnecessary insulin errors occurring in hospitals. These are important guidelines for nurses to refer to before they dispense insulin to people.

The right dose

Insulin comes in vials for use with insulin syringes and pumps, in cartridges for insulin pens or pre-filled pens. Each should be clearly labelled with the name of the insulin. People using insulin are advised to keep a record of the number of units of insulin they are taking. There are different designs of insulin cartridge, so not all cartridges can be used in all insulin pens. If the individual uses cartridges, the nurse must know what is the correct pen to use: consult the British National Formulary (BNF) (see Chapter 2) and seek advice from the Diabetes Specialist Team, as different pens offer different dosing options and visual displays to suit different users and their prescribed regimens. Always consult the BNF and also the manufacturer's information leaflet for advice.

Clinical considerations

Insulin can be kept at room temperature for up to 28 days and needs to be kept away from heat sources such as radiators or window sills.

The expiry date of all insulin in vials or cartridges must be checked prior to use. Insulin in use does not need to be kept in a fridge and in a ward environment is best left with the person it is prescribed for to enable them to continue self-administrating their insulin. All insulin prescribed should be labelled with the individual's name.

Insulin straight from the fridge can make injections sting and be painful.

297

Pre-filled pens should contain the individual's prescribed insulin. If insulin that is prescribed uses the letter 'U' after the dose needed – instead of writing the word 'units' in full – the 'U' could be mistaken for an '0' (NPSA, 2017). This can lead to a risk of overdose of insulin, for example 60 units instead of 6 units. If administrating insulin to an individual, always ask the registered nurse to double-check the dose to ensure accuracy and avoid an insulin administration error; a student nurse must always administer medication under supervision. There is a national insulin safety week each May in the UK to try to reduce errors in insulin administration and also the Association of British Clinical Diabetologists (ABCD) and Joint British Diabetes Societies (JBDS) Guidelines (2018) regarding insulin administration and safety which are available free to access and download.

Clinical considerations

For advice on how safely to administer insulin and the correct size pen needle to choose, please see these national and international guidelines for insulin administration:

'Injection Technique Matters (ITM) – Best Practice in Diabetes Care' (Training, Research and Education for Nurses in Diabetes [TREND-UK], 2018)

Available via: https://trend-uk.org/injection-technique-matters

The International Forum for Injection Technique (FIT Forum, 2019)

Available via: http://fit4diabetes.com/united-kingdom.

The nurse must always ensure that they are also adhering to local policy and procedure at all times, which will be also based on these guidelines.

The right way

Insulin should be injected subcutaneously at a 90° angle without a pinch up using a 4 mm needle. Guidance about injection technique, safe sites to inject insulin into and how to teach individuals how to self-administer their own insulin are available by both 'Injection Technique Matters (ITM) – Best Practice in Diabetes Care' (Training, Research and Education for Nurses in Diabetes [TREND-UK], 2018) and also The International Forum for Injection Technique (FIT Forum, 2019). These sites offer free downloadable educational resources for both practitioners and also people with diabetes to access.

Many people with type 1 diabetes now use insulin pumps – please seek advice from the individual and leave them to self-manage their insulin pump. If unwell as an inpatient, then seek advice from the local diabetes specialist inpatient nursing team in your hospital trust.

Clinical consideration

Disposal of sharps

Many people who have diabetes need to use sharps; for example, insulin syringes, insulin pen needles, fingertip lancing devices, insulin pump infusion sets and continuous glucose monitoring and flash sensors to treat and manage their condition.

It is essential that these sharps are disposed of safely in order to minimise the risk of accidental injury or the transmission of infectious diseases.

Sharps disposal should be as easy as possible so as to encourage and enable responsible behaviour and take into account the preferences of people with diabetes.

All people with diabetes, according Diabetes UK (2018), who use sharps should have access to:

- Sharps containers that are appropriate to their individual needs and are free of charge.
- A free sharps collection service from their home or agreed alternative location that is provided by their local authority or another appropriate body.
- Alternative means of disposing of sharps locally which are free and convenient and take account of the individual's circumstances.
- Accurate and easy to find information regarding local collection/disposal arrangements for sharps – this should be available on every local authority website and also via the 'request clinical waste collection' page on the gov.uk website.

The right time

Individuals using insulin will be taking different types and doses at different times depending on their prescribed and agreed regimen. Some people will have just once a day background long-acting insulin, some people will take it twice daily, known as BD insulin usually in pre-mixed insulin (see Table 12.3), others will have three times a day insulin, and the majority of people with type 1 diabetes will be prescribed multidose insulin (MDI) self-administered four or five times daily in accordance with NICE (2016) guidance.

Some people need to take insulin with or just after food; others up to 40 minutes before; and some at bedtime. Please ask the individual concerned when they take their insulin, and especially if admitted to hospital and are well enough, please leave their insulin with the individual concerned so that they can self-manage their diabetes – this is really important if an insulin pump is used. Local policy and procedure has to be adhered to with regards to self-management of medication and advice from the diabetes team is recommended for individuals to enable them to continue to self-manage.

Flash glucose testing

People with type 1 diabetes who meet the NHS England (2019a) nationally agreed criteria have access to and use flash glucose testing. This was also agreed in the NHS Long Term Plan (NHS England, 2019b) and flash glucose technology is being used in Scotland, Ireland, Eire and Wales also. This national arrangement facilitates access and safe education to allow more people with type 1 diabetes to use life-changing glucose testing technology. The flash glucose reader sits on the person's upper arm and has a sensor inserted into the interstitial fluid. The sensor reads the interstitial glucose fluid level continuously, so it is generally about five minutes behind what the individual's blood glucose level is at the same time. The individual scans their sensor with either a handset or their smart phone to obtain their glucose reading. Education and support for interpreting and using flash glucose sensing is available nationally via the ABCD DTN Freestyle Libre Education Forum (2019).

Table 12.3 Insulin regimens and names of insulins in use in the UK

Insulin Type	Insulin names	Duration of action	Administration	Solution type	Available as
Rapid	Apidra (Glulisine) Humalog (Human Lispro)	15 minutes from injection – Peak action occurs 13– hours – duration of action can be up to 5 hours	• Immediately prior to, with or after meals • Dose should be omitted if the patient not eating • Can be used for corrective doses	Clear	Vial, cartridge, disposable pen
	Novorapid (Inulin Aspart) Fiasp (Insulin Aspart)	4 minutes from injection – duration up to 5 hours	Used as mealtime insulins in multi-dose injection regimens		
Short	Actrapid Humulin S Insuman Rapid	Acts 30–60 minutes from injection – Peak action 2–4 hours – duration of action can be up to 8 hours	Actrapid used for IV insulin infusions in hospitals	Clear	Vial, cartridge
Intermediate	Humulin I Insulatard Insuman Basal	90 minutes from injection – Peak action 4–8 hours – duration of action can be up to 14 hours	• Administer 30 minutes prior to food or bed • Continue with IV insulin Used in multi-dose injection regimens	Cloudy	Vial, cartridge, disposable pen

(Continued)

Table 12.3 (Continued)

Insulin Type	Insulin names	Duration of action	Administration	Solution type	Available as
Long acting	Lantus (Glargine)	30 minutes from injection – no peak of action – action time 16–24 hours	This medication must be administered with an hour of prescription time Do not omit the dose if nil by mouth	Clear	Vial, cartridge, disposable pen
	Levermir (Detemir)		Continue with IV insulin		
	Abasaglar (Glargine Biosimilar)		Used in multi-dose injection regimens or once a day regimen along with oral medication		Solostar disposable pen
	Tourjeo				
Ultra long (once daily insulin)	Tresiba 100 (Insulin degludec)	2 hours from injection – 36 hours	Has to be administered with an hour of prescription time Do not omit the dose if nil by mouth Continue with IV insulin The dose should only be titrated every 3 days	Clear (if cloudy do not use)	Disposable pen
Mixed insulin	Humalog Mix 25	Mixed insulins are made up of a percentage of rapid acting and intermediate acting insulins – the amount of rapid acting is noted within the name of the insulin; therefore, Humalog 25 has 25%, Novorapid 30 has 30%, Humalog 50 has 50%	Administer immediately before, with or after food.	Has to be mixed before injecting Using 10 rolls between the hands to mix the clear and cloudy parts of mixed insulins	Cartridge, vial, disposable pen
	Novomix 30		This medication is usually prescribed twice or three times per day		
	Humalog Mix 50				Cartridge, disposable pen

Mixed insulin Human	Humulin M3	30 minutes before food or evening meal	Has to be mixed before injecting Using a 10 shake or 10 rolls between the hands to mix both clear and cloudy parts of mixed insulins	Vial, cartridge, disposable pen
	Insuman Comb 25			
	Mixed insulins are made up of a percentage of rapid acting and intermediate acting insulins – the amount of rapid acting is noted within the name of the insulin; therefore, Humulin M3 has 30% and Insuman Comb has 25%			
High strength insulins	Tresiba 200 (Degludec)	2 hours from injection – 36 hours	See duration of action for specific insulin details	Clear	Disposable pen
	Humalog 200 (insulin lispro)	15 minutes from injection to 5 hours		Disposable pen
		30 minutes from injection – 24 hours		
	Toujeo 300 (Glargine)	2 hours from injection – 36 hours		Disposable pen
	Xultophy (insulin degludec/ liraglutide)			Disposable pen

301

Source: Adapted from BNF (2019).

Hypoglycaemia

Insulin and some oral hypoglycaemic agents (see Tables 12.2 and 12.3) can cause hypoglycae-mia. This is of particular concern while people using insulin are inpatients due to changes in their normal regimens, different dietary intake, different meal and medication timings, differ-ent physical activity engagement and inter-concurrent illness. Everyone using insulin or taking an oral medication which can cause hypoglycaemia should be, if possible, self-blood glucose testing. Hypos are considered to be when blood glucose levels fall below 4 mmols/L. However, the UK Government Driving and Vehicle Licensing Agency (DVLA) (2019) advise people using insulin to only drive with their blood glucose at 5 mmols/L or over.

Depending on the type of insulin or medication taken, hypoglycaemia, also known as a hypo, can occur quickly or slowly, and the signs and symptoms of hypos also can alter depend-ing on the speed of the hypo occurring.

Signs and symptoms of hypoglycaemia include:

- pallor
- sweating heavily (diaphoresis)
- confusion
- anxiety
- trembling and shaking
- tingling of the lips
- hunger
- palpitations
- dizziness
- changes in electrocardiograph (ECG).

See Figure 12.4 for some signs and symptoms of hypoglycaemia.

Sometimes people experience no symptoms, so they do not recognise if they are hypo, and therefore are experiencing hypo unawareness. These individuals **must** be referred to a Diabetes Specialist Team at their local Trust. This is especially important in terms of safety for people who are using insulin and perhaps living in the community, residential care, or in detention or prison or are in shelters. Safety is paramount and avoiding hypoglycaemia with

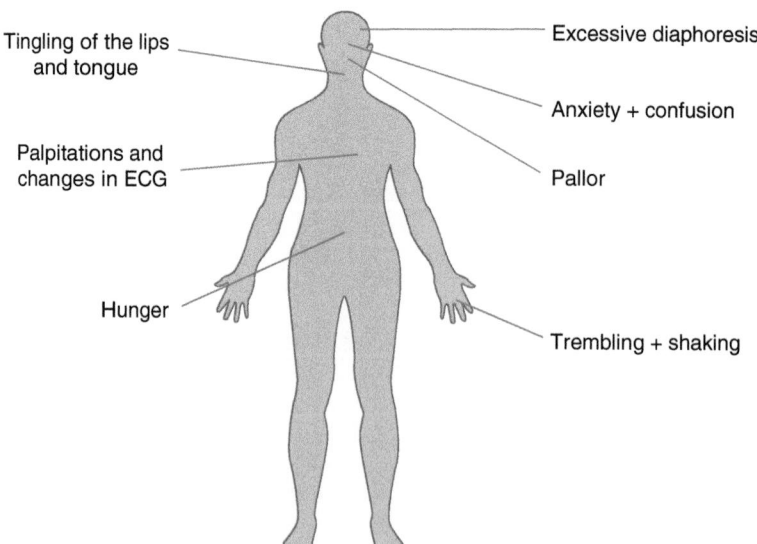

Figure 12.4   Some signs and symptoms of hypoglycaemia.

people who have hypo awareness is a key aim of care. Paramedics who are called to attend to people who are hypoglycaemic have to report their visit and make a referral to the local diabetes teams as part of a national hypo awareness campaign (Duncan et al., 2018).

People are advised to try to avoid hypos by not missing meals and eating regularly, taking their insulin at the recommended times and doses, if they drive testing before driving and every two hours if taking a long journey (DVLA, 2019), keeping within the recommended alcohol limits and avoiding drinking on an empty stomach, and always carrying some quick acting glucose with them and their blood glucose meter.

Older adults with type 2 diabetes using a sulfonylurea drug or insulin can be particularly prone to recurrent hypoglycaemia (Freeman, 2019) and as such need careful review and relaxation of their glycaemic targets to avoid hypoglycaemia. Often signs of hypoglycaemia in older adults are non-specific (sweating, dizziness, confusion, visual disturbances) and Freeman (2019) suggests that they can be mistaken for neurological symptoms or dementia. In older adults, consequences of hypoglycaemia can include acute and long-term cognitive changes, cardiac arrhythmias and myocardial infarction, serious falls, frailty and death. Hypos in older people with type 2 diabetes often result in inpatient stays, which come at a high personal and financial cost.

Clinical considerations

Treatment of hypoglycaemia
Hypoglycaemia occurs when a person with diabetes blood glucose level is below 4 mmols/L.

If a person shows signs of hypoglycaemia, e.g. hungry, shaking, sweating and pale, dizzy, palpitations, confused, 'feels low':

- CHECK BLOOD GLUCOSE LEVEL.
- If above 4 mmol/L, give small carbohydrate snack.
  If blood glucose less than 4 mmol/L:
  Conscious patient

- Immediately give 4–5 glucotabs, 6–8 jelly babies, or 2 tubes glucogel, or 120 mL fruit juice or full sugar coke.
- Check blood glucose after 10–15 minutes; if still below 4 mmols/L, repeat treatment up to three times. Then consider intravenous (IV) 10% glucose at 100 mL/hour (and discuss with doctors if an inpatient)
  Naso-gastric or percutaneous endoscopic gastrostomy fed patients
  50–70 mL forti-juice via tube
  For unconscious patient or nil by mouth

- Protect airway.
- Alert doctor on call if an inpatient; if in the community, call the paramedic service.
- DO NOT give oral fluid.
- Place in recovery position.
- Evaluate for other causes of unconsciousness.
- Stop any IV insulin temporarily.

If established IV access give:

- 10% glucose 150–20 mL over 15 minutes.
  - Can be repeated three times if necessary.

- OR give 1 mg glucagon IM.
  - (If not nil by mouth or severe hepatic disease.)

Document all actions taken when treating someone hypoglycaemic. Always practise according to your local protocols and if in hospital, use the hypo boxes with the protocol in the hypo box lid available in every NHS ward.

Glucagon

This hormone is made in the α cells in the islets of Langerhans in the pancreas. Glucagon works in partnership with insulin and fatty acids to prevent blood glucose levels falling too low in people without diabetes. In people with diabetes, glucagon is used to treat low blood glucose levels and is injected intramuscularly. It works by releasing glucose stored as glycogen in the liver. This triggers blood glucose levels to rise again. As discussed in the treatment of hypoglycaemia earlier, glucagon is only used if the individual is unable to swallow and is unconscious. It is stored in hypo boxes and is also available on prescription for use at home or in the community. Glucagon is also used by paramedics. Figure 12.5 illustrates how insulin and glucagon work in harmony in people without diabetes.

Pancreatic β cells produce insulin to lower blood glucose levels.

Pancreatic α cells produce glucagon to raise blood glucose levels.

Sick day advice

For people with type 1 and type 2 diabetes, being unwell can cause extra challenges. Illness and infections, as well as other forms of stress, will raise blood glucose levels. As part of the body's defence mechanism for fighting illness and infection, more glucose is released into the blood stream. This happens even if people are not eating or eating less than usual.

People who do not have diabetes just produce more insulin to cope. When hyperglycaemia occurs, it causes people to feel thirsty and need to urinate more, this may also lead to dehydration. The symptoms of hyperglycaemia can add to those of the original illness or infection and make it much worse. Dehydration is made worse when individuals are pyrexial or are vomiting. In some cases, hyperglycaemia can become so uncontrolled that there may be a need for hospital admission.

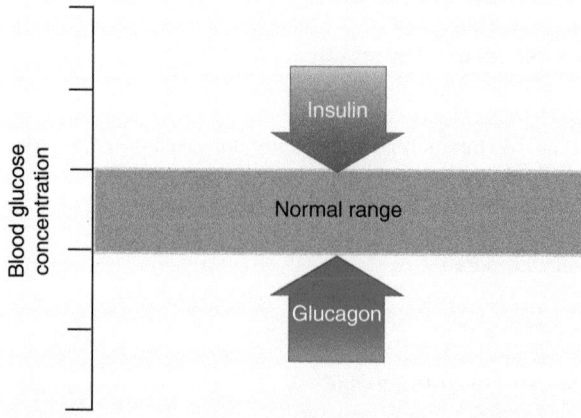

Figure 12.5   How insulin and glucagon work to maintain blood glucose levels.

Box 12.3   Blood ketone test results with people with type 1 diabetes

- Lower than 0.6 mmol/L is a normal reading.
- 0.6–1.5 mmol/L means the person is at a slightly increased risk of DKA and should test their blood ketone levels again in two hours.
- 1.6–2.9 mmol/L means the individual is at an increased risk of DKA and should contact their diabetes team, if in hospital, or their GP if at home.
- 3 mmol/L or over means the person is at very high risk of DKA and should seek medical help immediately.
- If blood ketone testing is not available, then a urine ketone test of 2++ means there is a high chance the individual is developing or has DKA.

With type 1 diabetes, the person should be advised to test either their blood for ketones or their urine if their blood glucose meter cannot test for blood ketones, and if the ketone levels are rising then seek medical help as they are at risk of DKA. People with type 1 diabetes are at serious risk of DKA if their blood ketone level is rising, or if they have 2++ ketones in their urine. Box 12.3 indicates levels of blood ketone test results and the significance of each.

People with type 2 diabetes are advised to seek medical help when they are unwell as they also can deteriorate very quickly. They might need to be admitted to hospital sooner with a condition known as hyperglycaemic hyperosmolar state (HHS), which is a serious metabolic complication of type 2 diabetes. HHS is manifested by marked elevation of blood glucose, hyperosmolality and little or no ketosis, and the mortality rate from HHS is high (Willix et al., 2019).

Episode of care: Type 2 diabetes

Mrs. Singh

Mrs. Singh, a 72-year-old lady, is a retired housewife; she lives with her husband at home.

Mrs. Singh has type 2 diabetes, which was diagnosed four years ago. Her HbA1c is 50 mmols/mol and she is prescribed Metformin 1000 mg twice daily and gliclazide 160 mg twice daily. Mrs. Singh is an active member of her local community and she visits lonely, housebound neighbours and cooks for them and offers them company.

Mrs. Singh was found wandering in town with her shopping bags and appeared disorientated and pale. An ambulance was called, and she was taken to the emergency department where her blood glucose level was 2.8 mmols/L. She was hypoglycaemic and had cardiac rhythm changes in her ECG. Due to the ECG changes it was noted that Mrs. Singh had experienced a silent myocardial infarction (MI) during the hypoglycaemic episode.

Her low blood glucose was treated with intravenous glucose and Mrs. Singh was admitted to the medical assessment unit. The nursing and medical team re-assessed Mrs. Singh and in view of her HbA1c level and this episode of hypoglycaemia, they stopped her oral gliclazide due to the risk of unrecognised hypos and her silent MI. They discussed with Mrs. Singh their decision-making and she was in full agreement with this. She was referred back to her GP team and discharged home on 1000 mg Metformin twice daily and follow-up was arranged in the nurse-led medical cardiac clinic.

Type 2 diabetes is a cardiovascular disease and affects increasingly more older adults due to the declining function of β cells as we age. When a diagnosis of type 2 diabetes is made, 50% cell function of β cell activity has already been lost (UKPDS, 1995). Therefore, treatment of insulin resistance, which causes toxicity to the remaining β cells, is a target aim in type 2 diabetes to try to reduce insulin resistance and Metformin is the initial drug of choice (Davies et al., 2018).

Due to Mrs. Singh's age, and her diagnosis, her ability to maintain a safe environment is the major concern in her care. Hypoglycaemia needs to be avoided, so removing the drug which caused her low blood glucose was the right decision. Mrs. Singh's HbA1c was tightly controlled at 50 mmols/mol and in accordance with both NICE (2015) and Davies et al. (2018); relaxation of Mrs. Singh's HbA1c to 53 mmols/mol is the most appropriate and safe treatment option for her.

Macro- and micro-complications of type 2 diabetes can occur pre-diagnosis of type 2 diabetes (Abdelhafiz et al., 2015). In Mrs. Singh's case, neuropathic complications were present, and this masked her MI. ECG changes in hypoglycaemia are common (Frier et al., 2011), and silent MI is also more common in people who experience ischemic heart disease and can often be missed and attributed to indigestion or fatigue (Harrar, 2016).

An important aspect of Mrs. Singh's discharge will be supporting her adjustment to having experienced this unexpected hypoglycaemic event, which could leave her vulnerable and experiencing emotional distress. As a result of this, careful support and referral to her GP surgery for follow-up and any further risk factor reduction was required. Talking through Mrs. Singh's medication upon discharge, and ensuring she understands her new regimen, may help to increase her knowledge; this is an important aspect of high-quality nursing care.

Episode of care: Type 1 diabetes

Matt Jennings

Matt is a 10-year-old boy with Down's syndrome and type 1 diabetes. Matt lives at home with his parents and younger sister and has a specialist care worker for school and his social activities called Carrie.

Matt has a developing understanding of his type 1 diabetes and is just beginning to perform his own injections with support from his family – and also Carrie at school. Matt is on a MDI regime and he recently started using flash glucose technology to scan his glucose levels. Matt really likes his flash sensor as he found repeated finger pricks painful and often resisted these.

Matts HbA1c is 54 mmols/mol and he has maintained this level of control for some time with minimal episodes of hypoglycaemia or hyperglycaemia.

Matt is going on a residential weekend sports trip away with Carrie his support worker and his classmates from his school. Matt's parents are understandably worried as he has never been away overnight from home before and has not been on any school trips overnight either. Carrie is a calm and a reassuring presence and is supporting Matt's parents to allay their fears.

Matt, his parents, and Carrie met with Matt's diabetes specialist nurse (DSN) to discuss and plan the weekend. Matt will be engaging in many new activities, including some soft wall climbing, swimming and a fun-fair during the weekend. Matt's DSN discusses with Matt whether he can tell her if he knows if he is going hypo – to see if he can identify potential hypoglycaemia. Matt is learning about his diabetes and is growing in confidence, but does need support with his glucose readings to understand what he needs to do if he is going hypo.

Matt really is an active young person and loves to try new activities, so in agreement with his parents and Matt, his DSN agrees a plan of care for his glucose targets and also adjusts his MDI injections both to prevent hypoglycaemia but also to ensure he has enough insulin to keep him active and feeling well. The target glucose regime is agreed for 6–10 mmols/L for the residential weekend. Matt, his parents, and Carrie are happy with this and Matt is very excited to be going to the weekend with his friends.

The weekend goes really well, and Matt takes part in all activities and also wins several awards during weekend; he returns home with renewed spirit and self-belief. Carrie reports he self-administered all his own injections also.

An important aspect of Matt's care is promoting his knowledge, engagement and independence in his diabetes. Also supporting his parents as Matt grows into a young man and begins to transition into adulthood. People with Down's syndrome can be supported really well in their diabetes self-management and key support workers are a valuable resource in supporting and enabling this in practice too.

Conclusion

As a student healthcare practitioner you will meet many people living with diabetes within your practice. You will have a significant impact on those people you have the privilege to care for, and because of this an understanding of their experience of diabetes, knowing which type of diabetes they have, and also listening to their experiences of their diabetes are essential skills. Language Matters was published by NHS England (2018) and is essential guidance for all practitioners working alongside people experiencing diabetes to ensure our approach, the type of language we use, the accuracy of information we give and the need for a welcoming and non-judgemental attitude is fundamental in diabetes care. The nurse should have a wide understanding of the large range of medications people with diabetes are prescribed, and know to follow the six steps for insulin safety with people receiving insulin therapy. With regards to oral medications, the knowledge that people will have individualised regimens and the various resources that are available as demonstrated within this chapter will help you to further your knowledge, an essential aspect of safe clinical practice. Referral to your local diabetes specialist team, either in primary or secondary care, is always an additional resource for further information.

References

ABCD DTN UK (2019). *Freestyle Libre Education Forum*. https://abcd.care/dtn/education (accessed 19 June 2019).

Abdelhafiz, A., Rodríguez-Mañas, L., Morley, J., and Sinclair, A. (2015). Hypoglycaemia in older people – a less well recognized risk factor for frailty. *Aging and Disease* **6** (2): 156–167. https://doi.org/10.14336/AD.2014.0330.

Baerlocher, M.O., Asch, M., and Myers, A. (2013). Metformin and intravenous contrast. *Canadian Medical Association Journal* **185** (1): E78. doi: 10.1503/cmaj.090550.

Biondi, B., Kahaly, G., and Robertson, R. (2019). Thyroid dysfunction and diabetes mellitus: two closely associated disorders. *Endocrine Reviews* **40** (3): 789–824. https://doi.org/10.1210/er.2018-00163.

BNF (2019). *BNF 78*. https://www.bnf.org/.

British Society for Paediatric Endocrinology and Diabetes (2015). *BSPED recommended guideline for the management of children and young people under the age of 18 years with diabetic ketoacidosis*. www.bsped.org.uk/media/1629/bsped-dka-aug15_.pdf (accessed 3 June 2019).

Cousins, D., Crompton, A., Gell, J., and Hooley, J. (2019). The top ten prescribing errors in practice and how to avoid them. *The Pharmaceutical Journal, BMC Medical Informatics and Decision Making* **17** (1): 84.

Davies, M.J., D'Alessio, D.A., Fradkin, J., et al. (2018). Management of hyperglycaemia in type 2 diabetes, a consensus report by the American Diabetes Association (ADA) and the European Association for the Study of Diabetes (EASD). *Diabetes Care* **41** (12): 2669–2701. doi: 10.2337/dci18-0033.

DeFronzo, R., Ferrannini, E., Zimmet, P., and Alberti, G. (2015). *International Textbook of Diabetes Mellitus*, 4e. Oxford:UK: Wiley.

Diabetes UK (2017a). *Improving insulin safety in hospitals*. https://www.diabetes.org.uk/resources-s3/2017-10/InsulinSafety.pdf (accessed 24 June 2019).

Diabetes UK (2017b). *Improve the management of inpatients on insulin*. www.diabetes.org.uk/resources-s3/2017-10/Improve%20the%20management%20of%20inpatients%20on%20insulin%20final_0.pdf (accessed 24 May 2019).

Diabetes UK (2018). *Safe disposal of sharps used by people with diabetes* www.diabetes.org.uk/resources-s3/2018-12/Safe%20disposal%20of%20sharps%20used%20by%20people%20with%20diabetes%20December2018.pdf?_ga=2.206579219.1064135126.1544635527-1362513958.1522313951 (accessed 12 July 2019).

Diabetes UK (2019a). *Us, diabetes and a lot of facts and stats.* www.diabetes.org.uk/resources-s3/2019-02/1362B_Facts%20and%20stats%20Update%20Jan%202019_LOW%20RES_EXTERNAL.pdf (accessed 03 June 2019).

Diabetes UK (2019b). Information prescriptions. www.diabetes.org.uk/professionals/resources/resources-to-improve-your-clinical-practice/information-prescriptions-qa (accessed 18 June 2019).

Diabetes UK, The University of Leicester, and The University Hospital of Leicester NHS Trust (2019) *Type 2 diabetes: know your risk online assessment*, https://riskscore.diabetes.org.uk/start (accessed 3 June 2019).

Duncan, E., Fitzpatrick, D., Ikegwuonu, T. et al. (2018). Role and prevalence of impaired awareness of hypoglycaemia in ambulance service attendances to people who have had a severe hypoglycaemic emergency: a mixed-methods study. *BMJ Open* **8**: e019522. https://doi.org/10.1136/bmjopen-2017-019522.

DVLA (2019). *DVLA rules for a Group 1 driving licence.* https://www.diabetes.org.uk/guide-to-diabetes/life-with-diabetes/driving/driving-licence (accessed October 2020).

FIT Forum for Injection Technique (2019). http://fit4diabetes.com/united-kingdom (accessed 19 June 2019).

Forbes, A., Murrells, T., Mulnier, H., and Sinclair, A. (2018). Mean HbA1c, HbA1c variability, and mortality in people with diabetes aged 70 years and older: a retrospective cohort study. *Lancet Diabetes Endocrinol* **6**: 476–486.

Freeman, J. (2019). Management of hypoglycaemia in older adults with type 2 diabetes. *Postgraduate Medicine* https://www.tandfonline.com/doi/full/10.1080/00325481.2019.1578590.

Frier, B., Schernthaner, G., and Heller, S. (2011). Hypoglycaemia and cardiovascular risks. *Diabetes Care* **34** (Supplement 2): S132–S137. https://doi.org/10.2337/dc11-s220.

Garcia, A., Bose, E., Zuniga, J., and Zhang, W. (2019). Mexican Americans' diabetes symptom prevalence, burden, and clusters. *Applied Nursing Research* **46**: 37–42. https://doi.org/10.1016/j.apnr.2019.02.002.

Goedeke, L., Perry, R., and Shulman, G. (2019). Emerging pharmacological targets for the treatment of non-alcoholic fatty liver disease, insulin resistance and type 2 diabetes. *Annual Review of Pharmacology and Toxicology* **59**: 65–87. https://doi.org/10.1146/annurev-pharmtox-010716-104727.

GpNotebook (2019). *What next after metformin?* www.gpnotebook.co.uk/simplepage.cfm?ID=x20181130 17470437326&linkID=79998&cook=yes (accessed 4 July 2019).

Grumitt, J., Barnard, K., Beckwith, A., et al. (2018). *White Paper: Current Challenges in Diabetes Care and How to Address Them.* https://idealdiabetes.com/publications/ (accessed 17 June 2019).

Harrar, S. (2016). *Silent heart attacks and type 2 diabetes.* https://www.endocrineweb.com/news/diabetes/21656-silent-heart-attacks-type-2-diabetes (accessed 24 June 2019).

Holman, R., Paul, S., Bethel, M. Matthews, D., and Neil, A., (2008). 10-year follow-up of intensive glucose control in type 2 diabetes. *New England Journal of Medicine* **359**: 1577–1589. https://doi.org/10.1056/NEJMoa0806470.

International Diabetes Federation (2017). *Diabetes Atlas 8th Atla*, https://www.diabetesatlas.org (accessed 4 June 2019).

Inzucchi, S., Bergenstal, R., Buse, J. Diamant, M., Ferrannini, E., Nauck, M., Peters, A., Tsapas, A., Wender, R., and Matthews, D. (2015). Management of hyperglycaemia in type 2 diabetes, 2015: a patient-centred approach: update to a position statement of the American Diabetes Association and the European Association for the Study of Diabetes. *Diabetes Care* **38** (1): 140–149. https://doi.org/10.2337/dc14-2441.

Ismail-Beigi, F., Moghissi, E., Tiktin, M., Hirsch, I., Inzucchi, S., and Genuth, S. (2011). Individualizing glycaemic targets in type 2 diabetes mellitus: implications of recent clinical trials. *Annals of Internal Medicine* **154** (8): 554–559. https://doi.org/10.7326/0003-4819-154-8-201104190-00007.

Jennings, P. and Myint, A. (2017). Anti-diabetic treatment options. In: *Principals of Diabetes Care: Evidence-based management for health professionals* (ed. A. Phillips). UK: Quay Books.

Joint British Diabetes Societies for Inpatient Care (2018). *Intravenous insulin prescription and fluid protocol for diabetic ketoacidosis*, https://abcd.care/sites/abcd.care/files/resources/2018_addition_DKA_IPC_Pathway.pdf (accessed 3 June 2019).

Joint British Diabetes Societies Inpatient Care Group (2013). *The Management of Diabetic Ketoacidosis in Adults*, Second Edition Update. https://abcd.care/sites/abcd.care/files/resources/2013_09_JBDS_IP_DKA_Adults_Revised.pdf (accessed 3 June 2019).

308

Joint British Diabetes Societies Inpatient Care Group (2020). *Diabetes at the front door*. February 2020. https://abcd.care/sites/abcd.care/files/site_uploads/JBDS_Diabetes_Front_Door.pdf (accessed August 2020).

National Diabetes Audit Report (2018). 1: *Care processes and treatment targets* https://digital.nhs.uk/data-and-information/publications/statistical/national-diabetes-audit/report-1--care-processes-and-treatment-targets-2018-19-short-report (accessed 17 June 2019).

NHS Diabetes Prevention Programme (NHS DPP) (2019). https://www.england.nhs.uk/diabetes/diabetes-prevention (accessed 3 June 2019).

NHS England (2018). *Language matters: language and diabetes*, https://www.england.nhs.uk/publication/language-matters-language-and-diabetes (accessed 25 June 2019).

NHS England (2019a). *New NHS online support for Type 2 diabetes*. https://www.england.nhs.uk/2019/05/online-diabetes-support (accessed 17 June 2019).

NHS England (2019b). *Flash glucose monitoring: national arrangements for funding of relevant diabetes patients*. https://www.england.nhs.uk/publication/flash-glucose-monitoring-national-arrangements-for-funding-of-relevant-diabetes-patients/ (accessed 19 June 2019).

National Patient Safety Agency (2017). *National patient safety agency, learning from patient safety incidents*. https://improvement.nhs.uk/resources/learning-from-patient-safety-incidents/ (accessed August 2020).

NHS Plan Long Term Health Plan (2019). NHS England long term health plan. https://www.england.nhs.uk/long-term-plan (accessed 19 June 2019).

NICE (2012). *PH38 Type 2 diabetes: prevention in people at high risk*. www.nice.org.uk/guidance/ph38/resources/type-2-diabetes-prevention-in-people-at-high-risk-pdf-1996304192197 (accessed 24 June 2019).

NICE (2015). *Type 2 diabetes in adults: management, NG28*. https://www.nice.org.uk/Guidance/NG28 (accessed August 2020).

NICE (2016). *NG17 Type 1 diabetes in adults: diagnosis and management*. www.nice.org.uk/guidance/ng17 (accessed 19 June 2019).

NICE (2019). *KTT20 Safer insulin prescribing*. www.nice.org.uk/advice/ktt20/chapter/Evidence-context (accessed 19 June 2019).

NMC (2018). *The Code: Professional standards of practice and behaviour for nurses, midwives and nursing associates*, www.nmc.org.uk/standards/code (accessed 4 June 2019).

Phillips, A. (2017). *Principals of Diabetes Care: Evidence-based management for health professionals*. UK: Quay Books.

Sodi, R., McKay, K., Dampetla, S., and Pappachan, J. (2018). Monitoring glycaemic control in patients with diabetes mellitus. *BMJ* **363**: k4723. https://doi.org/10.1136/bmj.k4723.

Stratton, I., Adler, A., Neil, H. et al. (2000). Association of glycaemia control with microvascular and microvascular complications of type 2 diabetes (UKPDS 35): prospective observational study. *BMJ* **321** (7258): 405–412.

The Diabetes Control and Complications Trial Research Group (1993). The effect of intensive treatment of diabetes on the development and progression of long-term complications in insulin dependent diabetes mellitus. *New England Journal of Medicine* **329** (14): 977–986.

TREND (2018). *Injection technique matters*. https://trend-uk.org/injection-technique-matters (accessed 19 June 2019).

UK Prospective Diabetes Study (UKPDS) Group (1998). Intensive blood glucose control with sulphonylureas or insulin compared with conventional treatment and risk of complications in patients with type 2 diabetes, (UKPDS 33). *Lancet* **352** (9131): 837–853.

UK Prospective Diabetes Study (UKPDS) (1995). Overview of 6 years' therapy of type II diabetes: a progressive disease. *Diabetes* **44**: 1249–1258. https://doi.org/10.2337/diab.44.11.1249.

Willix, C., Griffiths, E., and Singleton, S. (2019). Hyperglycaemic presentations in type 2 diabetes. *Australian Journal of General Practice* **48** (5): 263–267. doi: 10.31128/AJGP-12-18-4785.

World Health Organisation (WHO) (2011). *Use of glycated haemoglobin (HbA1c) in the diagnosis of diabetes mellitus*. www.diabetes.org.uk/resources-s3/2017-09/hba1c_diagnosis.1111.pdf (accessed 3 May 2019).

World Health Organisation (WHO) (2016). *Global Report on Diabetes*. https://apps.who.int/iris/bitstream/handle/10665/204871/9789241565257_eng.pdf;jsessionid=31F38B29ACC2A7992F50B81D23FAC34B?sequence=1 (accessed August 2020).

Wright J, Phillips A (2017) *Psychological support for people with diabetes*, Chapter 14 in Phillips A Principals of Diabetes Care: evidence-based management for health professionals, Quay Books: London.

Further reading

Diabetes UK
Putting Feet First
https://diabetes-resources-production.s3-eu-west-1.amazonaws.com/diabetes-storage/2017-08/0997C_
    PFF%20Pathway%20resource%20update_A4%20v2.pdf.
Public Health England
The inequalities of homelessness – how can we stop homeless people dying young?
https://publichealthmatters.blog.gov.uk/2018/02/09/the-inequalities-of-homelessness-how-can-we-stop-them-
    dying-young.
DESMOND
What does the DESMOND Programme currently offer?
There are six self management education modules available:

- DESMOND Newly Diagnosed
- DESMOND Foundation (for those with established diabetes)
- DESMOND BME Culturally Adaptation
- DESMOND Walking Away from Diabetes (for those at high risk of developing type 2 diabetes)
- Going Forward with Diabetes (the follow-on for those that have attended DESMOND Newly Diagnosed
  or Foundation)
- Let's Prevent Diabetes

https://www.desmond-project.org.uk.

Multiple choice questions

1. How many people diagnosed with diabetes have type 2?
   - (a) 60%
   - (b) 80%
   - (c) 90%
   - (d) 95%
2. Is diabetes prevalence across the world
   - (a) Rising in low- and middle-income countries?
   - (b) Rising in high income countries?
   - (c) Falling in high income countries?
   - (d) A & B
3. How long is it, on average, between developing type 2 diabetes and actually being diagnosed?
   - (a) Less than 6 weeks
   - (b) 6–10 weeks
   - (c) Up to 7 years
   - (d) 1–2 years
4. What is the major cause of death among people with type 2 diabetes?
   - (a) Renal failure
   - (b) Anaemia
   - (c) Heart disease
   - (d) Complications of foot problems
5. Can hypoglycaemia occur in both type 1 and type 2 diabetes?
   - (a) No, only type 1
   - (b) Type 1 and type 2 if treated with either insulin or sulfonylurea type medications
   - (c) Yes in both types of diabetes and people should be aware of this
   - (d) A and B

6. Type 1 diabetes accounts for approximately what percentage of all people with diabetes?
   (a) <1%
   (b) 8%
   (c) 30–40%
   (d) 50%
7. Treatment for type 1 diabetes is initially:
   (a) Diet and exercise alone
   (b) To wait and see if symptoms resolve
   (c) Commencement of oral hypoglycaemic agents and blood glucose monitoring
   (d) Insulin therapy and blood glucose monitoring
8. Treatment for type 2 diabetes is initially:
   (a) Diet and increase exercise where appropriate, and possible tablet therapy
   (b) Wait and see if symptoms resolve
   (c) Commencement of pioglitazone and blood glucose monitoring
   (d) Insulin therapy

9. A diagnosis of type 1 diabetes in someone of 35 years who is only slightly overweight is likely to be suspected if there is
   (a) Lack of family history of type 2 diabetes
   (b) Presence of ketones
   (c) Acute nature of symptoms of hyperglycaemia with weight loss
   (d) All of the above
10. Type 1 diabetes is on the increase
    (a) a. True
    (b) b. False
11. Type 2 diabetes should be considered
    (a) A serious cardiovascular risk disease
    (b) A mild condition or 'touch of sugar'
    (c) A serious condition only when the individual commences insulin
    (d) A serious condition only when cardiovascular risk factors are present
12. Type 2 diabetes is seen in children
    (a) Only if misdiagnosed
    (b) Never
    (c) Increasingly
    (d) Less often than previously
13. Presence of high levels of ketones are significant because
    (a) They indicate how high blood glucose levels are
    (b) They can cause pear-drop smelling breath
    (c) In moderate or large amounts, they are acidic and toxic
    (d) They should only be present during infection
14. When type 2 diabetes is treated by insulin, it becomes type 1 diabetes
    (a) a. True
    (b) b. False
15. Metformin is a very effective drug in type 2 diabetes because
    (a) It does not cause weight gain
    (b) It does not cause hypoglycaemia
    (c) It has a cardio-protective effect in the overweight person with type 2 diabetes
    (d) All of the above

Find out more

The following are a list of conditions that are associated with people who have type 1 and type 2 diabetes. Take some time and write notes about each of the conditions. Think about the medications that may be used in order to treat these conditions and be specific about the pharmacokinetics and pharmacodynamics. Remember to include aspects of patient care. If you are making notes about people you have offered care and support to, you must ensure that you have adhered to the rules of confidentiality.

The condition	Your notes
Hyperglycaemia	
Diabetic ketoacidosis	
Hypoglycaemia	
High HbA1c	
Diabetes-related distress	

Chapter 13

Medications and the respiratory system

Sadie Diamond-Fox and Alexandra Gatehouse

Aim

The aim of this chapter is to provide the reader with an introduction to some of the common respiratory disease processes that may be encountered within clinical practice, and to explore the pharmacological therapies utilised in their management.

Learning outcomes

After reading this chapter, the reader will:

- Have gained an understanding of key respiratory physiology concepts relating to the management of common respiratory disorders
- Understand key classes of respiratory drugs and their pharmacology relating to respiratory conditions, and how understanding of such is crucial to the promotion of patient safety
- Understand the side effects of common respiratory pharmacotherapy and how to acknowledge and respect that this should be taken into account when counselling the patient to reach an informed decision regarding their evidence-based care
- Have gained an understanding of the current evidence base behind key recommendations of pharmacotherapy management of common respiratory conditions reviewed in this chapter

Test your knowledge

1. Describe the principle functions of the respiratory system and its main components.
2. Name four common respiratory conditions.
3. Discuss the potential risks associated with smoking.
4. List the common types of drugs used to treat respiratory disorders.
5. Discuss the role and function of the National Institute of Clinical Excellence (NICE) concerning the management of respiratory disorders.

Fundamentals of Pharmacology: For Nursing and Healthcare Students, First Edition. Edited by Ian Peate and Barry Hill.
© 2021 John Wiley & Sons Ltd. Published 2021 by John Wiley & Sons Ltd.

Introduction

Respiratory disease encompasses a wide range of conditions including asthma, chronic obstructive pulmonary disease (COPD), pneumonia, lung cancer, bronchiectasis and interstitial lung disease. Within the United Kingdom (UK) approximately one in five people are affected by respiratory disease, with around 550 000 new diagnoses each year (BLF, 2016; PHE, 2015). It is one of the UK's biggest causes of death, the highest mortality rates of which include lung cancer, COPD and pneumonia (BLF, 2016). Respiratory disease is less common in children than adults, and causes of death include perinatal conditions, congenital respiratory conditions, pneumonia and acute lower respiratory tract infections (LRTI) (BLF, 2016). Mortality rates are affected by a number of factors including social deprivation, smoking, air pollution, occupational hazards and poor housing (BLF, 2016; PHE, 2015).

The impact upon healthcare services is significant. According to national statistics, hospital admissions due to respiratory disease have risen threefold, accounting for 8% of all admissions and 10% of all bed days (BLF, 2016; PHE, 2015). This is particularly apparent in winter months with 80% more respiratory disease admissions contributing to winter pressures (BLF, 2017). Of those patients requiring admission for an exacerbation of COPD, approximately a third have not previously been diagnosed (Bastin et al., 2010).

The National Health Service (NHS) Long Term Plan's (NHS, 2019) aims are to address healthcare costs, hospital admissions due to respiratory disease and contributing risk factors, through investment in improved diagnosis, treatment and support for patients with respiratory disease. Public Health England have set out core principles for healthcare professionals treating respiratory disease, including interventions at a population, community, family and individual level (PHE, 2015).

Anatomy and physiology of the respiratory tract

Pharmacotherapy can be the cornerstone of treatment for multiple disease processes, particularly for those with long-term respiratory conditions. In order to practice safe medicines management, the healthcare professional is required to possess an understanding of the core pharmacological concepts including the interaction between chemical and physiological processes. The following section provides a brief introduction to some of the core concepts concerning respiratory physiology, and the target sites to which pharmacotherapy may be applied in order to treat various pathophysiological disease processes.

The main function of the respiratory system is to facilitate gaseous exchange of oxygen and carbon dioxide via internal (cellular level) and external (alveolar and capillary level) respiration. This highly complex system may be sub-divided into anatomical and functional sections, each with their own unique function. Anatomically, the respiratory system is commonly divided into two major sections: the upper respiratory tract (URT) and the lower respiratory tract (LRT), divided by the vocal cords which lie within the larynx (Figure 13.1). The URT encompasses the nose, pharynx and the portion of the larynx above the vocal cords. The LRT includes the lower portion of the larynx (below the vocal cords), the trachea, the left and right bronchus and the airway divisions that follow (Figures 13.2–13.4) and the left and right lung. A network of blood vessels, lymph nodes and nerves enter each of the lungs via a structure called the hilum. Within this structure lies the pulmonary nerve plexus: a congregation of both parasympathetic and sympathetic motor nerve fibres and visceral sensory fibres, which eventually innervate muscle fibres, glands and blood vessels.

Stimulation of the parasympathetic motor nerve fibres primarily results in bronchoconstriction. In contrast, the sympathetic motor fibres aid in the regulation of bronchodilation (see Figure 13.5). Sympathetic and parasympathetic innervation of the lungs plays a vital role in the development of various respiratory disorders and provides multiple target sites for pharmacotherapy, both of which are explored later within this chapter.

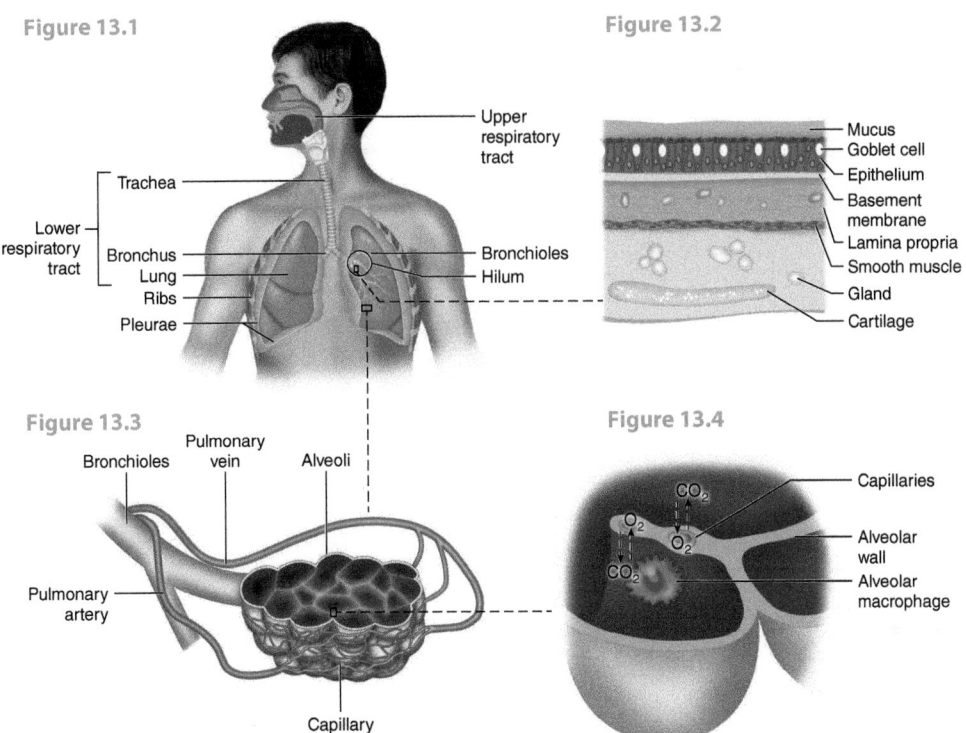

Figure 13.1

Figure 13.2

Figure 13.3

Figure 13.4

Figure 13.1   Macroscopic overview of upper and lower respiratory tract.
Figure 13.2   Magnification of a section through a bronchial wall showing the cellular organisation.
Figure 13.3   Anatomy of an alveolar sack showing the surrounding capillary network.
Figure 13.4   Detailed view through an alveolar wall.

Functionally, the respiratory system is divided into the conducting zone and the respiratory zone, as demonstrated in Table 13.1. The main function of the conducting zone is to allow for the transportation of gases in and out of the lungs, while the respiratory zone is involved in the exchange of oxygen and carbon dioxide with the blood. Both zones possess unique properties which aid in the protection of the respiratory tract from toxic or infectious substances that may affect the delicate homeostatic balance of this particular body system.

There are a number of cell types providing various target sites for pharmacotherapy that exist within the conducting and respiratory zones, the location and functions of which are detailed within Figure 13.2 and Table 13.1.

Common respiratory conditions

Bronchoconstriction, inflammation and loss of lung elasticity are some of the most common processes that result in respiratory compromise, all of which provide potential targets of manipulation with pharmacological therapy. The most common chronic respiratory diseases that can encompass one or multiple of these processes are explored in the following section of this chapter.

A large-scale national project concerning UK respiratory disease epidemiology estimated that around 12 million people, nearly one in five of the population, have received a lung disease diagnosis at some point in their lives (Snell et al., 2016). Respiratory disease accounts for a significant number of acute admissions to hospital year-on-year. The NHS Long Term Plan (2019) highlights several areas in which healthcare professionals can improve the treatment and support of people with respiratory disease, a large proportion of which include pharmacological management of these common conditions.

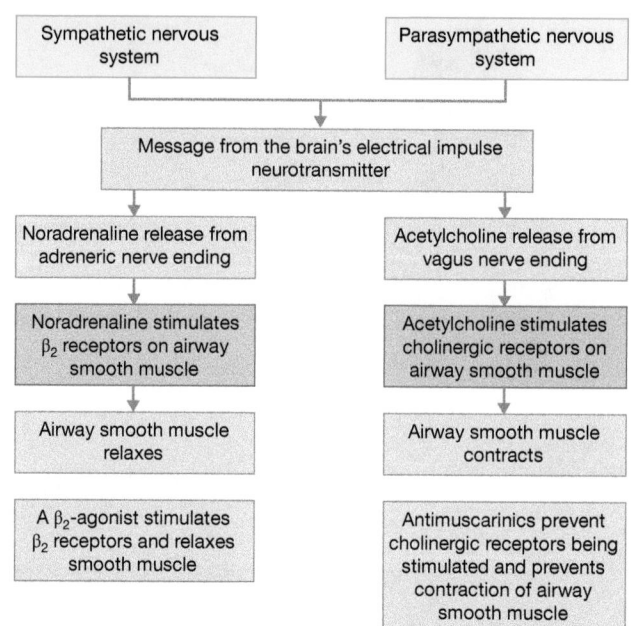

Figure 13.5   Nervous system control of respiratory airways.

Asthma

Asthma is a very common long-term respiratory disorder that can affect both the paediatric and adult populations. Recent statistics released by Asthma UK (2018) suggest that 5.4 million UK residents have asthma, with three people dying every day from an asthma attack – two-thirds of which could be preventable. National data from 2001 to 2015 has shown that despite advances in asthma treatments there have been no significant improvements in the number of asthma-related deaths within the UK, particularly over the winter months when asthma exacerbations can be common (Office for National Statistics, 2018).

Patients often present with recurrent episodes of chest tightness, wheezing, shortness of breath and/or coughing. This disease process is complex with multiple genetic and environ-mental factors that have been identified as the trigger for the two major elements of the pathophysiological development: inflammation and airway hyper-responsiveness (Ibrahim and Choong See, 2018). An initial trigger (cold air, smoke, allergens, infection, etc.) results in a cascade of complex immune and neuronal responses including the activation of inflammatory cells such as mast cells, macrophages, eosinophils and neutrophils, and smooth muscle cells, which ultimately results in a potentially deathly triad of airway constriction, airway narrowing, and obstruction (see Figure 13.6). It has been proposed that the triad of symptoms in the asthma patient may all be inextricably linked to the nervous system (Canning et al., 2012). As we have already explored earlier in this chapter, the human airways are innervated by auto-nomic nerves of both the sympathetic and parasympathetic nervous system. There is some suggestion that there is an imbalance of neuronal control in the airways of the asthmatic patient (see Figure 13.7). Prolonged activation of the inflammatory cascade in this chronic condition eventually leads to adverse changes to the cellular make-up of the respiratory tract in a process known as *remodelling*. The ciliated epithelial cells become ineffective, there is thickening of the epithelial basement membrane, and an increased number of goblet and smooth muscle cells (hypertrophy).

As demonstrated in Figure 13.7, a classic feature of asthma is airflow resistance in expiration. In order to define the initial probability of a diagnosis of asthma, its severity, and/or the pres-ence of an exacerbation, current guidance suggests the use of sequential peak expiratory flow

Table 13.1 Types of cells which reside within the respiratory tract.

	Structure	Airway generation	Smooth muscle	Main cell types	Function
CONDUCTING ZONE	Trachea	0	Arranged in spiral bundles of muscle fibres	Ciliated epithelial cells	• Line the respiratory tract until the level of the alveolar sacs • Provide protection and secretion • Form the mucociliary escalator which consists of fine hair-like projections called cilia which beat continuously to move the mucus secreted by goblet cells and submucosal glands towards the mouth to either be expelled or swallowed
				Goblet cells	• Secrete mucus, a highly viscous fluid which contain proteins called mucins • Aid in protection of respiratory tract in unison with the ciliated cells by trapping particulate material and potential pathogens that enter the respiratory tract
				Basal cells	• Able to differentiate into other cell types (mainly epithelial) such as to aid in the protection of the airways in times of injury
				Serous cells Mucus gland cells	• Produce a watery solution containing bacteria-fighting (bactericidal) proteins
	Primary bronchi	1	Arranged in spiral bundles of muscle fibres	Ciliated cells, goblet cells, basal cells and serous cells	See above
	Secondary bronchi	2			
	Tertiary bronchi	3			
	Small bronchi	4			
	Bronchioles	5			
	Terminal bronchioles	6–16		Basal and ciliated cells	See above
				Clara cells	• Non-ciliated and non-mucus producing secretory cells • Secrete special proteins which play a role in homeostasis and repair of the respiratory tract

(Continued)

Table 13.1 (Continued)

	Structure	Airway generation	Smooth muscle	Main cell types	Function
RESPIRATORY ZONE	**Respiratory bronchioles**	17–19	Bundles of fibres	Basal, ciliated and clara cells	*See above*
				Alveolar type I cells	• Form the majority of the alveolar surface • Involved in the process of gas exchange • Integral to the maintenance of a selective permeability barrier within the alveolus
				Alveolar type II cells	• Highly metabolic • Produce surfactant which reduces surface tension • Have the ability to differentiate in to type I alveolar cells which aids in alveolar repair after injury
	Alveolar sacs	23	Bundles of fibres	Alveolar type I and type II cells	*See above*
				Alveolar macrophage	• Part of the respiratory tracts innate immune system • A type of phagocyte which helps to protect the respiratory tract from infectious, toxic or allergic substances

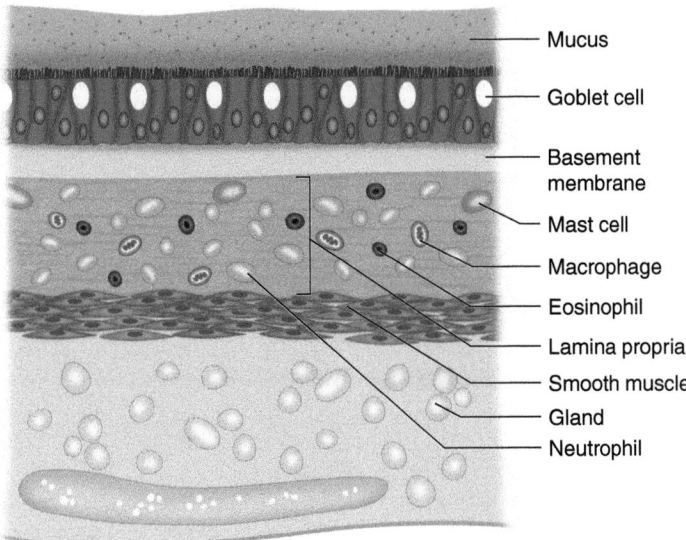

Figure 13.6   Structure of bronchial tissue during an asthma exacerbation. Source: From Anotomy and Physiology, retrived from https://opentextbc.ca/anatomyandphysiology/front-matter/about-this-book/. Public domain.

rate (PEFR) (BTS/SIGN, 2019). PEFR is a simple non-invasive measure of the highest flow achieved on forced expiration from a position of maximum lung inflation, expressed in litres per minute (L/min) (Miller et al., 2005). The standard scale for measuring PEFR in both adults and children has been the ISO standard EN23747 since 2004. The previous Wright–McKerrow scale should no longer be used within the UK and all PEFR metres issued by healthcare professionals should comply with the ISO standard EN23747. Both scales utilise patient age and height, and indicate a predicted value based upon a normal range for these values. However, there is a significant difference in the predicted normal values between Wright–McKerrow

Airway Constriction
- Increased airway smooth muscle (ASM) cell activation causes increased airway tone & airways to narrow (bronchospasm)
- Bronchospasm may result in airway collapse
- Amount of ASM is increased (hypertrophy)
- Increased ASM leads to further activation of inflammatory cascade

Airway Narrowing
- Complex interaction of inflammatory cells, mediators, and other cells and tissues in the airway occurs leading to inflammation
- Increased inflammation leads to increased ASM constriction
- Disrupted air flow = airflow resistance in expiration

Asthma

Airway Obstruction
- Goblet cells & Submucosal glands produce excess mucins = excess mucous secretion in to airways
- Goblet cell numbers increased (hypertrophy)
- Evidence to suggest that certain mucin gene alterations occur in asthma leading to increased viscosity of mucous
- Unsuccessful mucous clearance leads to mucous 'plugging' due to ineffective ciliated epithelial cells and dysfunction of the mucociliary escalator

Figure 13.7   Pathophysiological triad of asthma.

scale and EN23747, hence why the practitioner and patient measuring PEFR should be cogni-
zant of the metre that is in use. The severity and subsequent nature of the management of
asthma can then be quantified by using the PEFR value and current best-evidence severity
scales, such as those proposed by the National Institute of Clinical Excellence (2019a).

Skills in practice

Measuring peak expiratory flow:
1. Ensure peak flow metre is compliant with EU Scale/ISO standard EN 23747.
2. Ask the patient to find a comfortable position, either sitting or standing.
3. Reset the peak flow metre so the pointer is pushed back to the first line of the scale – this is
   usually 60.
4. Ask the patient to hold the peak flow metre so it's horizontal and make sure that fingers are
   not obstructing the measurement scale.
5. Ask the patient to breathe in as deeply as they can and place their lips tightly around the
   mouthpiece.
6. Ask the patient to breathe out as quickly and as hard as they can.
7. When they have finished breathing out, make a note of the reading.
8. This should be repeated three times, and the highest of the three measurements should be
   recorded as the peak flow score.
9. Predicted peak flow scores can then be plotted against a PEFR chart appropriate for the
   patient's age (see Figure 13.8).

   Note: Normal or baseline lung function in an asthmatic patient would be >80% predicted
   PEFR for their age and height, or > 80% of their best PEFR during a time of 'stable' respiratory
   health.
10. Offer additional resources which may aid in self-management of asthma, such as the use of
    a peak flow diary and asthma action plan, available via https://www.asthma.org.uk/advice/
    resources.

Source: National Health Service (2018).

The pharmacological management of asthma involves a step-wise approach (see
Figure 13.9) which aims to address the symptoms previously explored. Joint guidance produced by the British Thoracic Society and The Scottish Intercollegiate Guidelines Network
(2019) provides the latest guidance for UK healthcare professionals on the management of
asthma in both the adult and pediatric populations. Some of the pharmacological targets
mentioned within the guideline are later explored within this chapter, and include classes of
drugs such as bronchodilators, corticosteroids, leukotriene receptor agonists, and expecto-
rants and decongestants.

Chronic obstructive pulmonary disease (COPD)

COPD is a treatable, but largely preventable, disease for which no curative treatment currently
exists. COPD is the second most common respiratory disease in the UK population, second
only to asthma (Snell et al., 2016). Results of the British Lung Foundation's 'Respiratory health
of the nation' project revealed that an estimated 1.2 million people are living with a COPD
diagnosis in the UK. The most current data from the Office of National Statistics (2018) identifies a similar trend to that of asthma-related deaths. Previous research into this disease course
has identified that up to two-thirds of people with COPD remain undiagnosed (British Lung
Foundation, 2019), meaning that the current epidemiological data may be grossly underesti-
mating the extent of this disease within the UK.

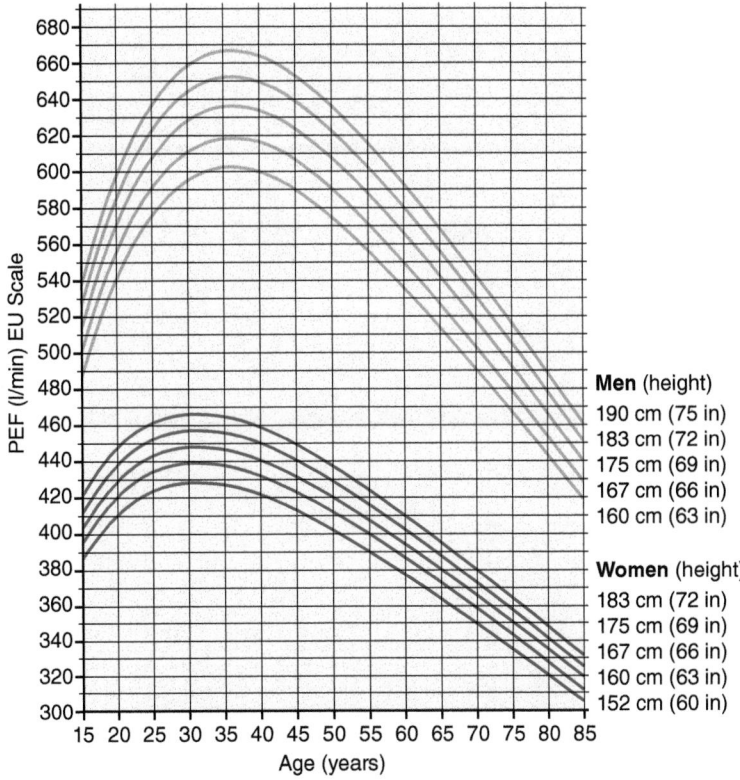

Figure 13.8 Normal peak expiratory flow rate measurements for age 15 years and above. Source: Clement Clarke International.

321

Unlike asthma, COPD is characterised by airflow obstruction which is not fully reversible. Patients may present with a multitude of symptoms which develop as a result of the complex underlying heart–lung interactions involved in the disease course: breathlessness (particularly on exertion), raised cyanosis, wheeze, increased sputum (which may/may not be infective) production, peripheral oedema and raised jugular venous pressures. The main risk factor for the development of COPD is long-term exposure to tobacco smoke; however, exposure to certain types of dust or chemicals may also trigger to disease process.

COPD is an umbrella term which encompasses chronic bronchitis in which there is long-term inflammation of the airways, and emphysema in which there is damage to the alveoli (see Figure 13.10). The main components of these processes are due to goblet cell hyperplasia, enlarged submucosal glands, ciliary dysfunction and/or loss of lung elastic recoil due to destruction of the alveoli. These processes result in the airflow limitation classically observed in COPD and can result in airflow obstruction which in turn causes hyperinflation of the lungs. In advanced disease, gas exchange abnormalities can occur, which coupled with destruction of the pulmonary capillary bed can result in hypoxia and eventually a condition called pulmonary hypertension, which can have devastating effects.

According to the NICE, a patient must meet three distinct criteria to fulfil the diagnosis of COPD:

1. Age older than 35 years.
2. Presence of a risk factor, for example current smoker, history of smoking, or occupational exposure to chemicals or dust.
3. Typical symptoms, such as exertional breathlessness, chronic cough, wheeze, regular sputum production, recurrent chest infection.

Source: NICE (2019b).

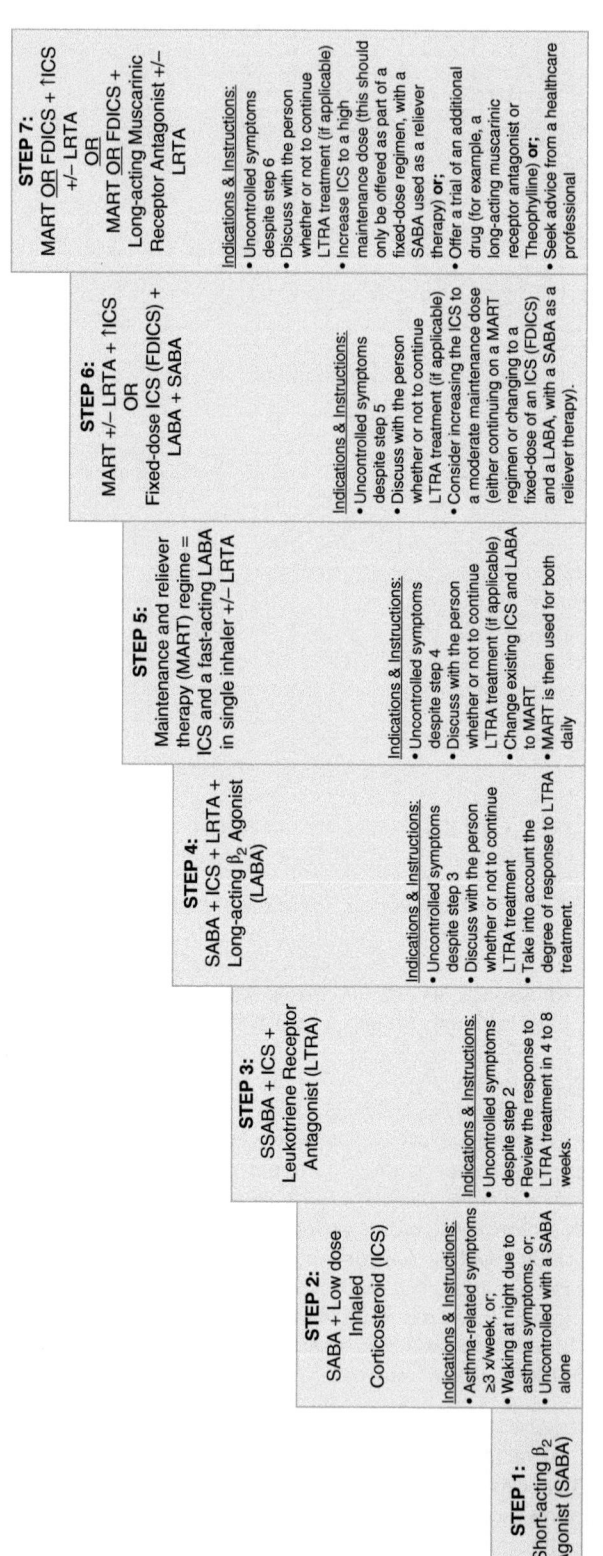

Figure 13.9 Pharmacological treatment pathway of asthma for adults aged 17 and over.

Source: BTS/SIGN (2019); NICE (2017a).

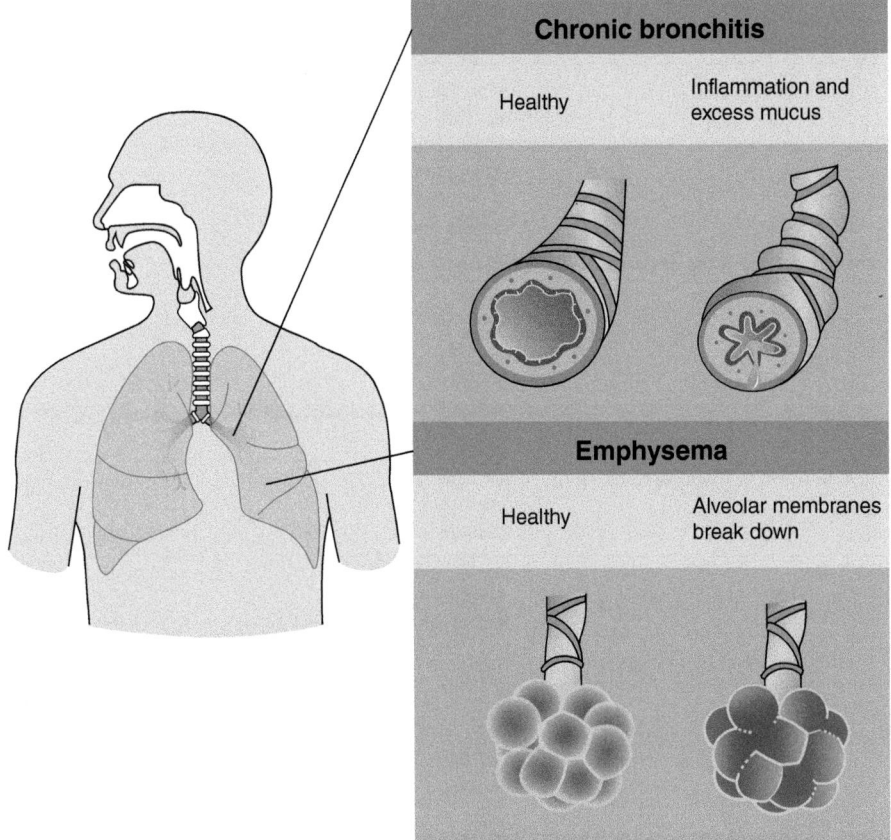

Figure 13.10 Chronic obstructive pulmonary disease. Source: Based on Preston & Kelly, 2017. Respiratory Nursing at a Glance. Page 92. John Wiley & Sons 2017.

The pharmacological management of COPD involves similar treatments to those used in asthma. The 2019 provides the latest guidance for UK healthcare professionals on the management of COPD, of which the recommended pharmacological treatments are explored later in this chapter.

Bronchiectasis

Bronchiectasis is a chronic inflammatory disease of the airways which results in destruction of the elastic and muscular components of the bronchial wall. It can affect both adults and children and is associated with a number of underlying and concurrent diseases. A large study by Qunit et al. (2016) showed the incidence and prevalence of this disease within the UK to be increasing, especially among women and the older adult (>70 years) population. However, it is important to acknowledge that this may be due to improvements in diagnosis. A degree of overlap-syndrome exists between COPD and bronchiectasis, which has only more recently started to be acknowledged within healthcare literature (Hurst et al., 2015).

Bronchiectasis has a number of causes which can be split into several different categories (O'Donnell, 2018), as detailed in Table 13.2. Chronic inflammation of the airways ensues as a result of the host's response to one of more of these causes. A cycle of events (see Figure 13.11) eventually leads to damage to the basement membrane and epithelial surface of the bronchi, destruction of ciliated cells, goblet cell hyperplasia and hypertrophy. This in turn leads to mucous hypersecretion and accumulation within the airways, which provides a perfect environment for bacterial growth and subsequent chronic infection. As is the case with COPD,

Table 13.2   The causes of bronchiectasis by category.

Category	Cause
Post-infectious	• Prior childhood respiratory infections due to viruses (i.e. measles, influenza, pertussis) • Prior infections bacteria (i.e. *Mycobacteria*) • Exaggerated immune response to exposure to inhaled mold (i.e. *Aspergillus fumigatus*) • Chronic bronchiolitis as a child
Deficiencies of the immune system	• Human Immunodeficiency Virus (HIV) and Acquired Immune Deficiency Syndrome (AIDS) • Antibody deficiency (immunoglobulin deficiency)
Genetic	• Cystic fibrosis • Deficiencies of the respiratory cilia (ciliary dyskinesia) • Deficiencies of enzymes which inhibit damage to proteins within the lungs (α_1 antitrypsin enzyme deficiency)
Aspiration or inhalation injury	• Damage to the respiratory tract from the inhalation of oral or gastroesophageal contents • Damage to the respiratory tract or lung tissue from heat, smoke or chemical irritants
Connective tissue disorders	• Chronic disorders in which the body's own immune system attacks itself (rheumatoid arthritis and Sjogren's disease)
Inflammatory bowel diseases	• Chronic inflammation of the digestive tract (ulcerative colitis and Crohn's disease)
Obstruction within the bronchi	• Foreign bodies • Narrowing of the airways (stenosis) • Tumour
Idiopathic	• Cause is unknown (accounts for 7–50% of cases)

Source: O'Donnell (2018).

patients can present with a number of symptoms as a result of the complex inflammatory process, which can eventually result in similar complex underlying heart–lung interactions.

The pharmacological management of bronchiectasis involves similar treatments to those used in COPD. The British Thoracic Society (Hill et al., 2019) provides the latest guidance for UK healthcare professionals on the management of this condition, which is explored later in this chapter.

Cystic fibrosis

Cystic fibrosis (CF) is a genetic multisystem disease which primarily affects the respiratory, reproductive, and gastrointestinal systems, and has severe consequences on life expectancy. Key epidemiological data provided by the UK Cystic Fibrosis Registry shows that there were 10 509 patients living with a diagnosis of CF in the year 2018 (Cystic Fibrosis Trust, 2018). This data also showed that the median age of diagnosis was two months while the median age of death was 32 years, the most common cause of which being respiratory disease.

CF is the result of a gene mutation which results in dysfunction of the cystic fibrosis trans-membrane conductance regulator (CFTR) protein. The CFTR protein is found within epithelial cells lining the lungs, intestines, pancreatic ducts, sweat glands and reproductive organs. It usually maintains the balance of salt and water within the epithelial cells. Dysfunctions of this protein within the lungs cause the mucus within the airways to become dehydrated and therefore more viscous, which in turn results in flattening of the cilia on the surface of the cili-ated epithelial cells and severe impairment of the mucociliary escalator. This eventually causes mucus retention, chronic infection and inflammation which then leads to structural changes within the lung (bronchiectasis).

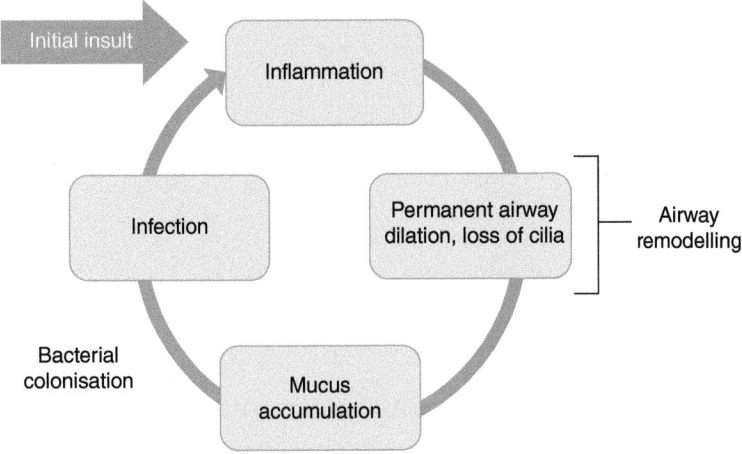

Figure 13.11   The pathophysiological cycle of bronchiectasis as originally proposed by Cole (1986). Source: Adapted from Maselli et al. (2017).

The National Institute for Clinical Excellence (2017a) provides the latest guidance for UK healthcare professionals on the management of this condition, also explored later within this chapter.

Classes of respiratory drugs
Overview
The purpose of pharmacotherapy is to utilise an understanding of the effects of drugs and how these may be applied in the effective treatment of diseases (Ritter et al., 2012). The selection of appropriate pharmacotherapy relies upon knowledge of pathological disease processes, as well as the pharmacokinetics and pharmacodynamics of the drugs selected. Common respiratory diseases have been discussed within this chapter and the main pathophysiological consequences identified, namely: hypoxemia, bronchoconstriction, bronchial mucosal inflammation and bronchial mucus hypersecretion. Respiratory drugs may be classified according to their oxygenation, bronchodilation, anti-inflammatory, immune modulation, or mucolytic effects. The following section provides an overview of the classes of respiratory drugs, the pharmacokinetics and pharmacodynamics of specific examples, and the respiratory conditions in which they may be utilised. This is outlined in Table 13.3.

Oxygen therapy
Oxygen is one of the most common drugs used within the healthcare setting for medical emergencies (Hiley et al., 2019; O'Driscoll et al., 2017). The aim is to correct hypoxemia (low blood oxygen content PaO_2), in order to prevent subsequent tissue hypoxia, organ dysfunction, and in severe circumstances, death. The British Thoracic Society (2017) has produced a guideline for the use of oxygen in adults in healthcare and emergency settings with recommendations for administration, targeted saturation, monitoring and weaning (O'Driscoll et al., 2017).

Critically ill patients or those with serious illness resulting in hypoxemia require immediate oxygen therapy (see Table 13.4). These can include obstetric and perioperative emergencies, and common neonatal conditions such as birth asphyxia and respiratory distress syndrome (World Health Organisation [WHO], 2016). Oxygen therapy will only correct hypoxemia; therefore, diagnosis and treatment of the underlying cause requires timely assessment and investigation (Hiley et al., 2019; O'Driscoll et al., 2017).

Table 13.3 Common respiratory drugs.

Drug class	Sub-class	Example drug names	Common conditions	Relevant guidelines
Oxygen			Any respiratory disorder resulting in low oxygen saturations requiring oxygen supplementation (see specific guidance for targets)	• British Thoracic Society (2017) • British Thoracic Society (2019) • British Thoracic Society and Scottish Intercollegiate Guidelines Network (2019) • British Thoracic Society (2018) • British Thoracic Society (2019)
Bronchodilators	Short-acting β_2 adrenergic receptor agonists (SABA)	*Salbutamol* *Terbutaline*	Asthma COPD Bronchiectasis	
	Long-acting β_2 adrenergic receptor agonists (LABA)	*Salmeterol* *Formoterol*	Asthma COPD	
	Muscarinic receptor antagonists	*Ipratropium* *Tiotropium*	Asthma COPD	
	Xanthines	*Theophylline* *Aminophylline*	Asthma COPD	
Corticosteroids	Inhaled corticosteroids	*Beclometasone* *Budesonide, Fluticasone*	Asthma Bronchiectasis (only if concurrent asthma or COPD is present) COPD	
	Oral corticosteroids	*Prednisolone*	Asthma Bronchiectasis (only if concurrent asthma or COPD is present) COPD	
Immune modulators and Cromones	Mast cell stabilisers	*Sodium cromoglicate* *Nedocromil sodium*	Asthma	
	Leukotriene receptor antagonists	*Montelukast*	Asthma	
Mucolytics		*Carbocisteine* *Acetylcysteine*	Bronchiectasis (non-CF related) COPD	
		Dornase alfa	CF	

Table 13.4   Severity of illness and clinical conditions requiring oxygen therapy in adults.

Severity of illness	Conditions
Critical illness requiring high levels of supplemental oxygen	• Cardiac arrest • Sepsis • Shock • Major trauma • Anaphylaxis • Drowning • Status epilepticus • Major head injury • Major pulmonary haemorrhage • Carbon monoxide poisoning
Serious illness requiring moderate levels of supplemental oxygen in the presence of hypoxemia	• Acute hypoxemia – unknown cause • Acute asthma • Pneumonia • Lung cancer • Interstitial lung disease • Pneumothorax • Pleural effusions • Pulmonary embolism • Acute heart failure • Severe anaemia • Post-operative breathlessness
Conditions requiring monitoring, oxygen therapy only in the presence of hypoxemia	• Myocardial infarction and acute coronary syndrome • Stroke • Hyperventilation or dysfunctional breathing • Poisoning or drug overdose • Metabolic and renal disorders • Acute and subacute neurological and muscular conditions • Pregnancy and obstetric emergencies
COPD or conditions requiring low-dose (controlled) oxygen	• COPD • CF • Neuromuscular disease, neurological condition and chest wall deformity • Morbid obesity

Source: Adapted from O'Driscoll et al. (2017).

Pulse oximetry measures the percentage of oxygenated haemoglobin in the blood (SpO_2) (Preston and Kelly, 2016; WHO, 2016). It can be used alongside clinical examination and assessment to identify hypoxic patients (low tissue oxygenation), allowing implementation and monitoring of oxygen therapy (Preston and Kelly, 2016). Guidelines state that pulse oximetry should be available in all clinical settings where oxygen therapy is used, and documented alongside the oxygen delivery device and inspired oxygen (FiO_2) (O'Driscoll et al., 2017). Clinical staff must be trained in their use and have awareness of its limitations in order to minimise inaccuracies (Preston and Kelly, 2016). The advantages and disadvantages are outlined in Table 13.5.

Hypoxemia is the result of low blood oxygen content (PaO_2), which is measured invasively by an arterial blood gas, with a normal range of 12–14.6 kilopascals (kPa) (O'Driscoll et al., 2017). An arterial blood gas is indicated for an unexpected or inappropriate fall in oxygen saturation level to <94% in a patient breathing air or oxygen, or a fall of ≥3% in a previously stable chronically hypoxemic state (O'Driscoll et al., 2017). Hypoxemic hypoxia or type I respiratory failure is defined as an SpO_2 level < 90% or a PaO_2 level < 8 kPa. Pulse oximetry provides no information regarding arterial carbon dioxide and hence ventilator

Table 13.5 Comparison of advantages and disadvantages of pulse oximetry.

Advantages

- Non-invasive
- Simple
- Allows continuous or intermittent monitoring
- Gives two readings – oxygen saturations and pulse rate
- Immediate results
- Portable – used in clinical or domicillary settings
- Inexpensive

Disadvantages

- Inaccurate readings due to:
    - Poor peripheral circulation – vasoconstriction or cold environment
    - Low blood pressure due to hypovolemic shock, low cardiac output or cardiac arrhythmia
    - Motion artifact – shivering, movement
    - Carbon monoxide poisoning – over estimation of oxygen saturation
    - Ambient light interference – bright light
    - Broken or dirty probe sensor
    - Nail varnish or pigmentation
- Not a measure of arterial oxygen content of blood
- Margin of error greater at lower SpO_2
- No indication of ventilation – respiratory rate, tidal volume, arterial carbon dioxide content
- Oxygen saturations may still be normal in the presence of anaemia

Source: Preston and Kelly (2016); WHO (2011).

efficiency (WHO, 2016). Normal range of arterial carbon dioxide ($PaCO_2$) is 4.6–6.1 kPa, if above this range the patient is deemed to have hypercapnic or type II respiratory failure (O'Driscoll et al., 2017).

Oxygen is a drug and must be prescribed according to a targeted oxygen saturation range either on a paper or electronic drug chart (BNF, 2019; O'Driscoll et al., 2017). Ideally this should occur on hospital admission, but the absence of a prescription does not prohibit oxygen therapy in an emergency situation. Normal oxygen saturation levels are 94–98%, however this can be affected by pre-existing co-morbidities and age (Hiley et al., 2019; O'Driscoll et al., 2017).

In emergency situations, adult and pediatric critically ill patients require immediate high concentration oxygen therapy at a rate of 15 L/min via a reservoir mask, until pulse oximetry is available (O'Driscoll et al., 2017; Soar et al., 2015). Any adult or child with an SpO_2 level < 90% requires oxygen therapy, with the exception of children with chronic hypoxemia secondary to congenital heart disease (WHO, 2016). The recommended targeted range is 94–98% for most patients (Hiley et al., 2019; Preston and Kelly, 2016) but there are groups of patients (such as those with severe COPD) for whom this target could be detrimental, and recent evidence has suggested may suffer potential harm and increased mortality from hyperoxemia (high levels of oxygen) (Chu et al., 2018; Hiley et al., 2019).

Patients at risk of type II or hypercapnic respiratory failure require a lower target oxygen saturation of 88–92% (O'Driscoll et al., 2017; Preston and Kelly, 2016). This group of patients includes those with moderate or severe COPD and other risk factors such as neuromuscular disorders, severe bronchiectasis, advanced CF, chest wall deformities and morbid obesity (BNF, 2019). These patients may be identified with oxygen alert cards or wristbands (Hiley et al., 2019).

Hyperoxemia is beneficial in specific clinical situations such as carbon monoxide and cyanide poisoning, spontaneous pneumothorax, cluster headaches and sickle cell crisis (O'Driscoll et al., 2017; Siemieniuk et al., 2018). However, there are both physiological and clinical risks of hyperoxemia as outlined in Table 13.6. A clinical practice guideline for oxygen therapy in acutely ill adult medical patients recommends maintaining saturation levels ≤96%, and no

Table 13.6   Physiological and clinical risks of hyperoxemia.

Physiological Risks

- Decreased ventilation with worsening ventilation/perfusion matching
- Absorption atelectasis
- Vasoconstriction of coronary and cerebral arteries, reducing blood flow
- Decreased cardiac output
- Tissue damage from oxygen free radicals
- Increased systemic vascular resistance

Clinical Risks

- Worsening or increased risk of type II respiratory failure
- Failure to recognise clinical deterioration
- Increased mortality – post cardiac arrest, stroke and myocardial infarction

Source: O'Driscoll et al. (2017).

oxygen therapy in the case of acute myocardial infarction or stroke patients with $SpO_2 \geq 92\%$. These groups should have target saturations of 90–92% (Siemieniuk et al., 2018). In the first few hours of life, neonates' SpO_2 levels should be no higher than 95% to reduce the risk of eye damage (WHO, 2016).

Oxygen supplies exist in the form of cylinders or are piped in within the hospital setting, and as oxygen concentrators or cylinders within the domiciliary setting. Selection of interface depends upon the cause of hypoxia as well as pre-existing and current medical conditions (Preston and Kelly, 2016). The devices are outlined in Table 13.7 and Figures 13.12–13.15. Oxygen therapy may also be delivered via non-invasive ventilation or invasive ventilation, but it is beyond the scope of this book to include these devices.

Following high concentration oxygen therapy in an emergency situation, once stability and saturations are obtained the appropriate delivery device should be applied according to target saturations (Hiley et al., 2019). Arterial blood gases will provide additional information regarding the risk of type II respiratory failure.

Administration and titration of oxygen should be performed by clinical staff that appropriately trained to detect and manage complications (WHO, 2016). The flow chart below (Figure 13.16) demonstrates a stepwise approach to titrating therapy according to targeted saturations (O'Driscoll et al., 2017). Oxygen saturation levels should be observed for 5–15 minutes after commencing therapy or increasing concentration and be rechecked after an hour, then four hourly (O'Driscoll et al., 2017; WHO, 2016). Monitoring of oxygen therapy is an element of the physiological track and trigger system, the National Early Warning Score (NEWS) and any acute deterioration warrants a prompt medical review (O'Driscoll et al., 2017; Preston and Kelly, 2016). Stable patients may have observations performed four times a day, and oxygen therapy may be discontinued once the patient is stable with saturation levels within target range, but should be monitored for five minutes following cessation and rechecked after one hour (O'Driscoll et al., 2017; WHO, 2016).

Table 13.7   Oxygen therapy devices.

High concentration oxygen device

- Non-rebreathe or reservoir mask.
  - At 15 L/min it delivers approximately 60–90% oxygen
  - Used in emergency situations therefore short-term use
  - For patients where type II respiratory failure is unlikely
  - Reservoir bag needs to be filled with oxygen prior to application
  - Figure 13.12 depicts a non-rebreathe mask

(Continued)

Table 13.7   (Continued)

Medium concentration device

- Simple facemask
  - Flow rates of 5–10 L/min delivers approximately 40–60% oxygen, dependent upon patient's respiratory pattern
  - Not suitable for patients with type II respiratory failure due to flow rates of <5 L/min resulting in rebreathing build up of exhaled carbon dioxide
  - Short-term use
  - Figure 13.13 depicts a simple facemask

Fixed performance (controlled) device

- Venturi mask
  - Gives an accurate concentration of oxygen with less dependence on the flow rate
  - Minimum flow rates of 2 L, 4 L, 6 L, 8 L, 10 L, 12 L deliver 24% (blue), 28% (white), 35% (yellow), 40% (red) and 60% (green) oxygen
  - 24% and 28% commonly used with patients at risk of type II respiratory failure
  - Deliver low and medium concentration oxygen
  - Figure 13.14 depicts the venturi valves used in fixed performance devices

Nasal cannulae

- Flow rates of 0.5–4 L/min deliver approximately 24–40% oxygen, dependent upon patient's breathing pattern
- Infants and children <5 years 0.5–1 L/min neonates, 1–2 L/min for infants, 1–4 L/min for older children
- Deliver low and medium concentration oxygen
- Comfortable and well tolerated in paediatrics and adults
- Can be worn while eating and drinking
- No risk of rebreathing carbon dioxide
- Not recommended for patients with unstable type II respiratory failure
- Flow rates above 4 L/min may cause mucosal irritation
- Not appropriate if nasal passages severely congested or blocked
- Figure 13.15 depicts nasal cannulae

High-flow humidified nasal cannulae

- Flow rates of 10–70 L/min deliver 21–100% oxygen
- Deliver medium and high concentration oxygen
- Comfortable and well tolerated by paediatrics and adults
- Airway humidification improving secretion clearance
- Dynamic positive airway pressure making inspiration easier, increasing lung aeration and reducing dead space (improved clearance of carbon dioxide)

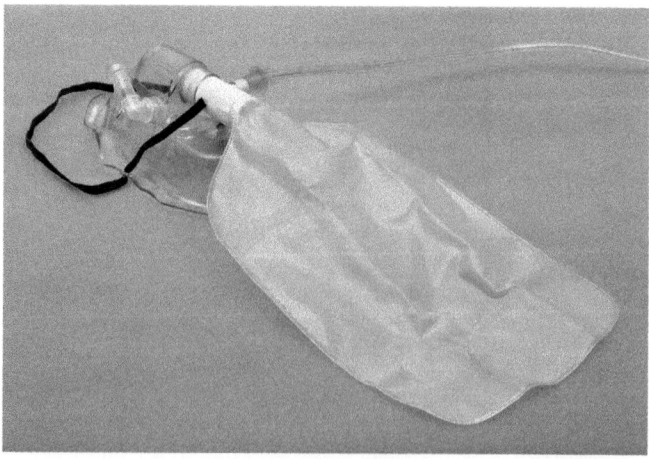

Figure 13.12   Non-rebreathe mask. Source: Pictures taken from the Royal Marsden Handbook of Nursing Procedures, 9e. Dougherty & Lister (2015). pp 436–437. © 2015, John Wiley & Sons.

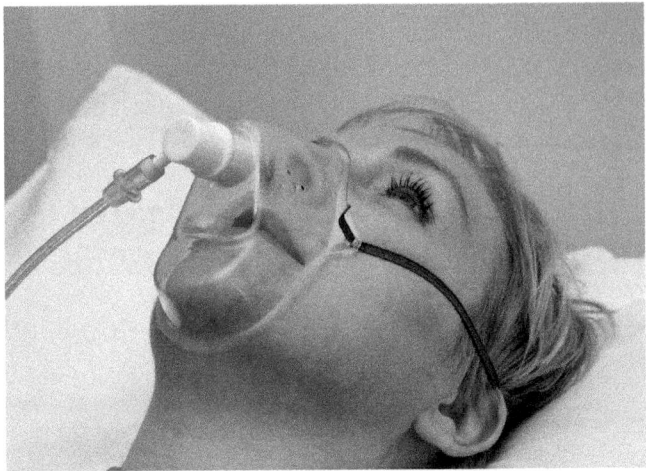

Figure 13.13 Simple facemask. Source: Pictures taken from the Royal Marsden Handbook of Nursing Procedures, 9e. Dougherty & Lister (2015). pp 436–437. © 2015, John Wiley & Sons.

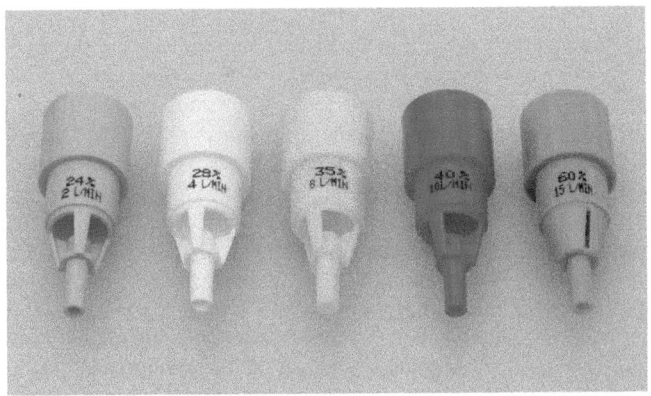

Figure 13.14 Venturi valves. Source: Pictures taken from the Royal Marsden Handbook of Nursing Procedures, 9e. Dougherty & Lister (2015). pp 436–437. © 2015, John Wiley & Sons.

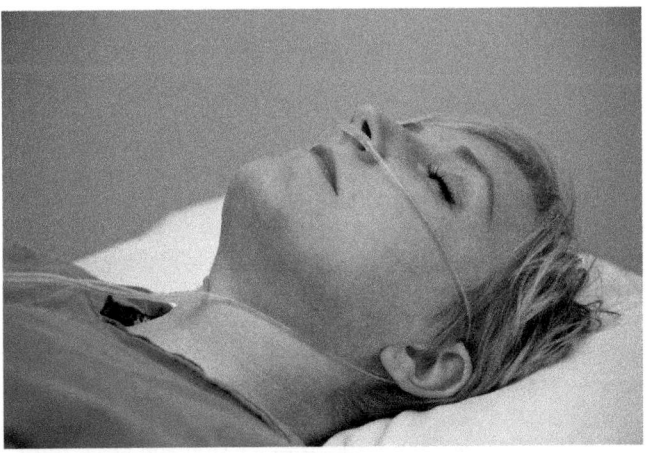

Figure 13.15 Nasal cannulae. Source: Pictures taken from the Royal Marsden Handbook of Nursing Procedures, 9e. Dougherty & Lister (2015). pp 436–437. © 2015, John Wiley & Sons.

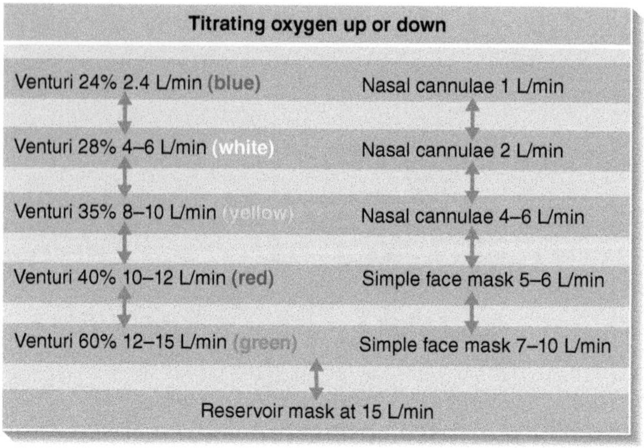

Titrating oxygen up or down	
Venturi 24% 2.4 L/min (blue)	Nasal cannulae 1 L/min
Venturi 28% 4–6 L/min (white)	Nasal cannulae 2 L/min
Venturi 35% 8–10 L/min (yellow)	Nasal cannulae 4–6 L/min
Venturi 40% 10–12 L/min (red)	Simple face mask 5–6 L/min
Venturi 60% 12–15 L/min (green)	Simple face mask 7–10 L/min
Reservoir mask at 15 L/min	

Figure 13.16   Flow chart for titration of oxygen therapy.

Bronchodilators

Bronchodilators are drugs primarily administered via inhalation to treat asthma, COPD and bronchiectasis. Oral and intravenous preparations are available but do not exert a direct, targeted affect and may have more adverse systemic effects. Bronchoconstriction is one of the pathophysiological disease processes and is caused by several mechanisms. Within the bronchial smooth muscle are both parasympathetic (muscarininc [M_3]) and sympathetic receptors (beta-adrenoceptor [β_2]) which when stimulated, result in contraction or dilatation respectively. Increased cholinergic (parasympathic) and decreased adrenergic (sympathetic) drive occurs due to an imbalance in nervous innervation in asthma, causing bronchoconstriction (Graeme-Smith and Aronson, 2002). The release of inflammatory mediators mainly from mast cells within the bronchial wall has a direct bronchoconstrictive effect in asthma, COPD and bronchiectasis. Bronchodilators are classified into four groups: short acting β_2 adrenergic receptor agonists (SABA), long acting β_2 adrenergic receptor agonists (LABA), short and long acting muscarinic receptor antagonists (SAMA, LAMA) and xanthines. The tables within each subsection detail examples of various commonly used bronchodilator agents. The drugs included are not exclusive and the information has been compiled from the most up-to-date resources at the time of publishing. The most recent version of the British National Formulary and relevant national guidelines should be consulted for UK prescribing.

β_2 adrenoceptor agonists

Stimulation of β_2 adrenoceptors results in a guanine nucleotide-binding (G_s) protein increasing cyclic adenosine monophosphate (cAMP) intracellular concentration. Myosin light chain kinase (MLCK) normally phosphorylates myosin in smooth muscle, causing contraction. However, inhibition of this enzyme, via cAMP, leads to relaxation and therefore bronchodilation. This complex process is demonstrated in Figure 13.17.

The release of inflammatory mediators from mast cells within the bronchial wall is dependent upon the influx of calcium ions (Ca^{2+}). However, when intracellular cAMP concentration is increased, the cell membranes permeability to Ca^{2+} is reduced. Therefore, β_2 adrenoceptor agonists may lessen the inflammatory response (Neal, 2015).

Short acting β_2 adrenoceptor agonists (SABA)

The onset of action of SABAs is within 5–15 minutes, with duration of action approximately four hours (e.g. salbutamol and Terbutaline sulphate) (Preston and Kelly, 2016). They are recommended as reliever therapy for wheeze, breathlessness, exercise limitation and symptomatic asthma (BTS/SIGN, 2019; NICE, 2017b). Good asthma control does not usually require SABAs

Clinical considerations

Oxygen safety

Oxygen is typically provided to the patient in cylinders, piped within the hospital or via oxygen concentrator within the domiciliary setting.

- Cylinders come in a variety of sizes containing differing amounts of compressed oxygen held under high pressure. They may be used to allow the patient to mobilise while on oxygen, so are ideal for transporting dependent patients within or outside the hospital setting. Oxygen cylinders must be stored in an upright, secure position to prevent the risk of injury from a pressurised system and should be kept away from heat sources due to the risk of explosion. Oxygen supports combustion and should not be used in close proximity to flammable materials or liquids such as alcohol, oil, or grease, or be used near a source of ignition such as smoking, electrical equipment or synthetic fabrics (may cause static electric discharge) due to the risk of burns. All cylinders should be colour coded, labelled and checked prior to administration to the patient in order to prevent inadvertent administration of an incorrect gas (BCGA, 2018). The amount of oxygen in the cylinder should always be checked prior to use, in addition to ensuring that the valve is open, as a recent patient safety alert highlighted risk of death and severe harm from failure to obtain and continue flow from oxygen cylinders (NHS Improvement, 2018a).
- Piped oxygen and air may be found within the hospital setting and carries a significantly reduced risk of running out compared with individual cylinders. Following several incidences of accidental administration of air instead of oxygen, and a subsequent stage three national alert in 2016 regarding the risk of severe harm or death, this was deemed a Never Event in 2018 (NHS Improvement, 2016, 2018b). The latest guidance recommends removal of air flowmetres from wall sockets, a designated air outlet cover when not in use, and a labelled, movable flap fitted to the air flowmetre (O'Driscoll et al., 2017).
- Oxygen concentrators are used primarily within the domiciliary setting for patients requiring long-term oxygen therapy. The device may be portable or piped and concentrates oxygen from a gas supply (usually room air), allowing oxygen flow rates up to 8 L/min (Hardinge et al., 2015). As with oxygen cylinders, there is risk of burns if used with flammable materials or near sources of ignition; for example, smoking.

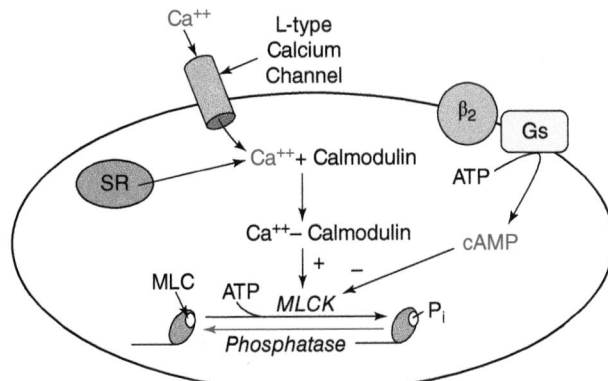

Abbreviations: ATP— Adenosine triphosphate; B2—Beta2 receptor; Ca++ - Calcium; Gs –g protein; MLC—Myosin Light Chain; MLCK—Myosin Light Chain Kinase; Pi—Myosin Phosphorylation

Figure 13.17 β_2 adrenoceptor.

333

and increasing use of them requires urgent assessment, indicating either exacerbation or inadequate management (BTS/SIGN, 2019). Oral and intravenous preparations are available for patients who are unable to reliably use inhaled therapy. Table 13.8 gives examples of short-acting β_2 adrenoceptor agonists and the related pharmacology.

Table 13.8   Short-acting β_2 adrenoceptor agonists and their related pharmacology.

Medication name	Salbutamol	Terbutaline sulphate
Mode of action	Stimulates the β_2 adrenoceptor causing bronchodilation and reduced release of inflammatory mediators.	
Route of administration	Inhaled (maybe nebulised at different doses), oral, SC, IM, IV	Inhaled (may be nebulised at different doses), oral, SC, IM, IV
Indications	**ADULTS**	

	• Asthma (other conditions associated with reversible airway obstruction):
	  ○ Acute – moderate, severe or life-threatening
	  ○ Chronic
	• Prophylaxis of allergen- or exercise-induced bronchospasm
	Note: inhaled route preferred over oral route
		• Asthma (other conditions associated with reversible airway obstruction):
		  ○ Moderate, severe or life-threatening
		Note: inhaled route preferred over oral route

	CHILDREN	

	• Asthma
	  ○ Acute
	  ○ Moderate, severe or life-threatening acute asthma
	  ○ Chronic
	• Exacerbation of reversible airways obstruction, prophylaxis of allergen- or exercise-induced bronchospasm
	Note: inhaled route preferred over oral route
		• Asthma
		  ○ Acute asthma
		  ○ Moderate, severe or life-threatening acute asthma
		  ○ Exacerbation of reversible airways obstruction, prophylaxis of allergen- or exercise-induced bronchospasm
		Note: inhaled route preferred over oral route

Contraindications	<u>Selective β2 adrenoceptor agonists:</u> • Severe pre-eclampsia Hypersensitivity to salbutamol or lactose monohydrate	
Cautions	• Arrhythmias, cardiac insufficiency, myocardial ischemia, hypertrophic obstructive cardiomyopathy, hypertension • Diabetes (risk of hyperglycemia and ketoacidosis) • Hyperthyroidism • Hypokalaemia – potentially serious in severe asthma as concomitant treatment may potentiate this effect and hypoxia • Susceptibility to QT-interval prolongation <u>Pregnancy:</u> • Continue asthma medication regularly to maintain control <u>Breast-feeding:</u> • Inhaled drugs taken as normal. Oral or IV: careful consideration as excreted in breast milk	

(Continued)

334

Table 13.8   (Continued)

Medication name	Salbutamol	Terbutaline sulphate
Side effects (Common or very common ONLY)	For all β2 adrenoceptor agonists: • Arrhythmias • Dizziness • Headache • Hypokalaemia • Nausea • Palpitations • Tremor Salbutamol: • Muscle cramps	For all β2 adrenoceptor agonists: • Arrhythmias • Dizziness • Headache • Hypokalaemia • Nausea • Palpitations • Tremor Terbutaline sulphate: • Muscle cramps • Hypotension
Interactions	• Concomitant administration with non-selective β-blocking drugs not recommended • Additional adrenergic drugs in addition to salbutamol may have deleterious cardiovascular effects • Hypokalaemia with xanthines, corticosteroids and potassium-excreting diuretics • Increases risk of digoxin toxicity when given together • Tricyclic antidepressants and monoamine oxidase inhibitors with Terbutaline may potentiate cardiovascular effects	
Absorption	• Oral administration well absorbed, peak plasma concentrations 1–4 hours	• Pulmonary bioavailability is approximately 16%, peak plasma concentration achieved about 1.3 hours • Oral: 14–15% absorbed if patient fasted
Distribution	• Approximately 10–25% distributed to the lung, rapidly seen in the circulation • Major proportion retained in the delivery device or in the oropharynx and is swallowed and absorbed from the GI tract	• Acts topically within the airways • Approximately 25% protein binding
Metabolism	• Undergoes considerable first-pass metabolism	• Oral dosing: partially metabolised in the liver, main metabolite: sulphate conjugate
Elimination	• Plasma concentrations of inhaled salbutamol are considerably lower than oral doses • Rapidly excreted in urine (~80% within 24 hour) and faeces • Half-life is 2.7–5.5 hours	• SC administration: 90% excreted in urine, 60% unchanged • Half-life 16–20 hours

Source: British National Formulary (2019a), b; British National Formulary for Children (2019a, b); Electronic Medicines Compendium (2019a, b).

Long acting β₂ adrenoceptor agonists (LABA)

The onset of action of LABAs is 3–20 minutes, with duration of action lasting 12–24 hours (e.g. salmeterol and formeterol) (Preston and Kelly, 2016). Add-on therapy may be indicated for patients with asthma where inhaled corticosteroids (ICS) are not providing adequate control. Despite research, there is no absolute threshold for introduction of add-on therapy. LABAs are first choice in adults, are not licensed for children under the age of four and are equivocal to leukotriene receptor antagonists in children (BTS/SIGN, 2019). They must not be prescribed without regular ICS, due to an increased risk of asthma mortality, and combination inhalers will negate this risk in addition to potentially improving adherence (BTS/SIGN, 2019; Nelson et al., 2006). LABA and ICS maybe considered for COPD patients who remain breathless and have exacerbations despite using a SABA where there are asthmatic features and clinical suggestion of steroid responsiveness (NICE, 2018). Table 13.9 gives examples of LABAs and the relevant pharmacology.

Table 13.9   Long-acting β_2 adrenoceptor agents and their related pharmacology.

Medication name	Salmeterol	Formoterol
Mode of action	Stimulates the β_2 adrenoceptor causing bronchodilation and reduced release of inflammatory mediators.	
Route of administration	Inhaled	Inhaled
Indications	**ADULTS**	
	<ul><li>Reversible airways obstruction, nocturnal asthma, prevention of exercise-induced bronchospasm in patients requiring long-term bronchodilator therapy, chronic asthma only in patients who regularly use an ICS</li><li>COPD</li></ul>	
	CHILDREN	
	Reversible airways obstruction, nocturnal asthma, prevention of exercise-induced bronchospasm in patients requiring long-term bronchodilator therapy, chronic asthma only in patients who regularly use an ICS	
Contraindications	<ul><li>Severe pre-eclampsia</li><li>Hypersensitivity to salbutamol or lactose monohydrate</li></ul>	
Cautions	<ul><li>Arrhythmias, cardiac insufficiency, myocardial ischemia, hypertrophic obstructive cardiomyopathy, hypertension</li><li>Diabetes (risk of hyperglycemia and ketoacidosis)</li><li>Hyperthyroidism</li><li>Hypokalaemia – potentially serious in severe asthma as concomitant treatment may potentiate this effect and hypoxia</li><li>Susceptibility to QT-interval prolongation</li></ul> Pregnancy: <ul><li>Salmeterol – Precautionary measure to avoid salmeterol during pregnancy</li><li>Formeterol – Consider administration at all stages of pregnancy if poor asthma control</li></ul> Breast-feeding: <ul><li>Formeterol – Unknown if passes to breast milk, should only be considered if maternal benefits outweigh risks to the child</li><li>Salmeterol – Excreted in breast milk therefore risk–benefit to mother and child must be considered</li></ul>	
Side effects	For all β2 adrenoceptor agonists: <ul><li>Arrhythmias</li><li>Dizziness</li><li>Headache</li><li>Hypokalaemia (with high doses)</li><li>Nausea</li><li>Palpitations</li><li>Tremor</li></ul>Salmeterol: <ul><li>Muscle cramps</li></ul>	For all β2 adrenoceptor agonists: <ul><li>Arrhythmias</li><li>Dizziness</li><li>Headache</li><li>Hypokalaemia</li><li>Nausea</li><li>Palpitations</li><li>Tremor</li></ul>Terbutaline sulphate: <ul><li>Hypotension</li><li>Muscle spasms</li></ul>

(Continued)

Table 13.9   (Continued)

Medication name	Salmeterol	Formoterol
Interactions	• Concomitant administration with non-selective β-blocking drugs not recommended • Hypokalaemia with xanthines, corticosteroids and potassium excreting diuretics • Potent cytochrome P450 3A4 (CYP3A4) inhibitors, namely ketoconazole, administered with salmeterol may significantly increase plasma concentration increasing the incidence of systemic effects, e.g. palpitations, prolongation of QTc interval	• Theoretical risk that administration with other QTc prolonging drugs there is an increased risk of ventricular arrhythmines e.g. antihistamines, antiarrhythmics, erythromycin and tricyclic antidepressants • Levodopa, levothyroxine, oxytocin, and alcohol may reduce cardiac tolerance • Titration of dose if administered with other β_2 agonists due to additive desirable and undesirable effects • Hypokalaemia with xanthines, corticosteroids, and potassium-excreting diuretics • Concomitant administration with non-selective β-blocking drugs not recommended
Absorption	• Acts locally in the lung, plasma levels are not predictive of therapeutic effects due to low plasma concentrations at therapeutic doses	• Approximately 80% swallowed and absorbed from the gastrointestinal tract • Rapid and extensive absorption: post inhalation peak plasma concentration achieved after 5 minutes, oral dose peak plasma concentration is achieved after 30–60 minutes
Distribution	• Plasma protein binding 96%	• Plasma protein binding 61–64%
Metabolism	• Metabolised in the liver via CYP3A4	• Metabolised in the liver via direct glucuronidation and O-demethylation

Elimination	• Excreted in the faeces (60%) and urine (25%)
	• Half-life elimination 5.5 hours
	• Duration of action 12 hours
		• Biphasic elimination:
		  • Children 5–12 years: urine 6% unchanged drug, 7–9% direct glucuronide metabolites
		  • Adults: 2–10% unchanged drug, 15–18% direct glucuronide metabolites
		• Duration of action >12 hours

Source: British National Formulary (2019c, d); British National Formulary for Children (2019c, d); Electronic Medicines Compendium (2019c, d).

Muscarinic receptor antagonists

Bronchospasm may occur due to stimulation of the parasympathetic nervous system. Acetylcholine, a neurotransmitter, is released from nerve endings and activates muscarinic receptors (M_3) on the bronchial smooth muscle cells. Activation of the receptor, via a G protein (G_q), stimulates phospholipase C (PLC) cleaving phosphatidylinositol 4, 5-bisphosphate (PIP_2) into two secondary cellular messengers: inositol-1, 4, 5-triphosphate (IP_3) and diacylglycerol (DAG). IP_3 augments the release of calcium ions producing smooth muscle contraction and hence bronchoconstriction. This complex process is outlined in Figure 13.18. M_3 receptors are

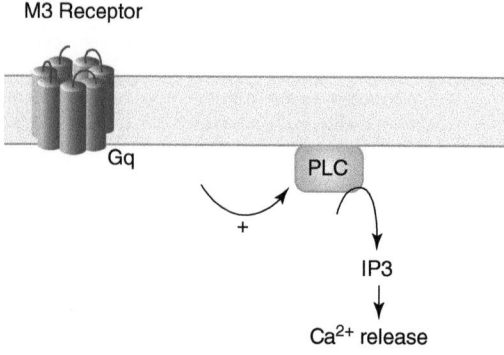

Abbreviations: G_g – G protein; PLC – phospholipase C;
IP_3- inositol-1, 4, 5-triphosphate

Figure 13.18   Muscarinic (M_3) receptor. Source: Based on Neal (2016) Medical Pharmacology at a Glance. 8th ed. Section 14. Wiley & Sons for part (a).

also located in bronchial glands, stimulation of which results in mucus secretion. Muscarinic antagonists compete with acetylcholine blocking the M_3 receptor, reducing bronchoconstriction and bronchial mucus secretion.

Short acting muscarinic antagonists (SAMA)

The onset of action of SAMAs are 30–60 minutes with duration of action 3–6 hours (e.g. ipratropium bromide) (Preston and Kelly, 2016). SAMAs may be used as reliever therapy for infrequent short-lived wheeze in asthma and empirically to alleviate breathlessness and exercise limitation in COPD (BTS/SIGN, 2019; NICE, 2018). Significantly greater bronchodilatation occurs with nebulised ipratropium bromide and a SABA in comparison to SABA alone in life-threatening asthma, reducing duration of admission and increasing rate of recovery (BTS/SIGN, 2019).

Long acting muscarinic antagonists (LAMA)

The onset of action of LAMAs is approximately 30 minutes, with a duration of action of 12–36 hours (e.g. tiotropium bromide) (Preston and Kelly, 2016). Inadequate control of asthma on recommended initial reliever, preventer or add-on therapies requires specialist care. Tiotropium bromide is considered a specialist therapy and in addition to an ICS and LABA, evidence suggests fewer exacerbations, improved lung function and asthma control with fewer non-serious adverse events (BTS/SIGN, 2019). LAMA and LABA may be offered to patients with COPD who do not have features suggestive of asthma or steroid responsiveness but remain breathless, adversely impacting their quality of life, and have severe exacerbations or two moderate exacerbations every a year (NICE, 2018). Table 13.10 gives examples of SAMAs and LAMAs and the relevant pharmacology.

Xanthines

As previously discussed, stimulation of β_2 adrenoceptors via β_2 agonists leads to a rise in intracellular cAMP, resulting in bronchodilation and a reduction in inflammatory mediator release. However, there is an alternative mechanism which creates the same effects without receptor stimulation. Phosphodiesterase is an enzyme that breaks down cAMP under normal circumstances, and if this is inhibited cAMP concentration will increase. Xanthines are phosphodiesterase type 3 and 4 inhibitors, which have similar effects to β_2 agonists as demonstrated in Figure 13.19.

There are two main xanthines used in the management of asthma and COPD: Theophylline and aminophylline. In children who are unable to use inhalers, oral Theophylline may be an appropriate alternative (Neal, 2015). Onset of action of Theophylline is approximately 1–2 hours with duration of action being up to 12 hours for sustained-release preparations. Theophylline may be offered to COPD

Table 13.10   Muscarinic antagonist agents and their related pharmacology.

Medication name	Ipratropium bromide	Tiotropium
Mode of action	Compete with acetylcholine for the M_3 receptor, acting as an antagonist, causing bronchodilation and reduced bronchial mucous secretion.	
Route of administration	Inhaled (may be nebulised at different doses)	Inhaled
Indications	**ADULTS**	
	• Reversible airways obstruction, particularly in COPD • Acute bronchospasm • Severe or life-threatening acute asthma	• Maintenance treatment of chronic obstructive pulmonary disease • Maintenance treatment of COPD, severe asthma (add-on to ICS [at least 800 mcg budesonide daily or equivalent] and at least 1 controller in patients who have suffered one or more severe exacerbations in the last year) **Note: different inhalers have varying dosages in the capsules, the delivered dose is 10 mcg**
	CHILDREN	
	• Reversible airways obstruction • Acute bronchospasm • Severe or life-threatening acute asthma	• Severe asthma (add-on to ICS (over 400 mcg budesonide daily or equivalent) and 1 controller, or ICS (200–400 mcg budesonide daily or equivalent) and 2 controllers, in patients who have suffered one or more severe exacerbations in the last year) • Severe asthma (add-on to ICS (over 800 mcg budesonide daily or equivalent) and 1 controller, or ICS (400–800 mcg budesonide daily or equivalent) and 2 controllers, in patients who have suffered one or more severe exacerbations in the last year)
Contraindications	Hypersensitivity to atropine or its derivatives	
Cautions	For all inhaled muscarinic antagonists: • Bladder outflow obstruction • Paradoxical bronchospasm • Prostate hyperplasia • Susceptibility to angle-closure glaucoma Pregnancy: Only to be used if potential benefit outweighs risk Breast-feeding: Only to be used if potential benefit outweighs risk	For all inhaled muscarinic antagonists: • Bladder outflow obstruction • Paradoxical bronchospasm • Prostate hyperplasia • Susceptibility to angle-closure glaucoma For tiotropium: • Arrhythmia (unstable, life-threatening, or requiring intervention in the previous 12 months) • Heart failure (admission to hospital in the previous 12 months with moderate to severe heart failure) • Myocardial infarction in the previous 6 months

339

(Continued)

Table 13.10   (Continued)

Medication name	Ipratropium bromide	Tiotropium
		• Plasma concentration increases with decreased renal function (moderate to severe renal impairment) tiotropium should only be used if benefits outweigh the risks Pregnancy: Manufacturer advises to avoid use Breast-feeding: Manufacturer advises to avoid use
Side effects (Common and very common ONLY)	For all inhaled muscarinic antagonists: • Arrhythmias • Dizziness • Cough • Dry mouth • Headache • Nausea Ipratropium bromide: • Gastrointestinal motility disorder • Throat complaints	For all inhaled muscarinic antagonists: • Arrhythmias • Dizziness • Cough • Dry mouth • Headache • Nausea Tiotropium: • Gastrointestinal disorders • Increased risk of infection • Taste altered
Interactions	• Concomitant administration with other anticholinergic drugs is not recommended • The risk of acute glaucoma in patients with a history of narrow-angle glaucoma may be increased with nebulised ipratropium bromide and β_2 agonists	• Concomitant administration with other anticholinergic drugs is not recommended
Absorption	• 10–30% deposited in the lungs and rapidly absorbed • The remainder is swallowed but gastrointestinal absorption is negligible	• Approximately 20% deposited in the lungs, with 19.5% bioavailability • The remainder is swallowed but gastrointestinal absorption is negligible
Distribution	• Minimally bound to plasma protein <20% • Systemic bioavailability: oral 2%, inhaled 7–28%	• Plasma protein binding approximately 72%
Metabolism	• After inhalation approximately 60% of the available dose is metabolised in the liver by hydrolysis (41%) and conjugation (36%)	• Minimally metabolised by the liver
Elimination	• Approximately 40% is excreted via the kidneys, less than 10% via bile and faeces • Half-life elimination is 3.2 hours	• Urinary excretion is 7% of the unchanged drug over 24 hours, the remainder (non-absorbed) is eliminated in faeces • Half-life elimination 27–45 hours

Source: British National Formulary (2019e, f); British National Formulary for Children (2019e, f); Electronic Medicines Compendium (2019e, f).

patients who have had trials of SABAs, SAMAs, LABAs and LAMAs, or who are unable to use inhaled therapy (NICE, 2018). Aminophylline is an intravenous preparation, a compound of Theophylline and ethylenediamine which improves its solubility. It may be used for acute exacerbations of asthma and COPD. Table 13.11 gives examples of common xanthines and the related pharmacology.

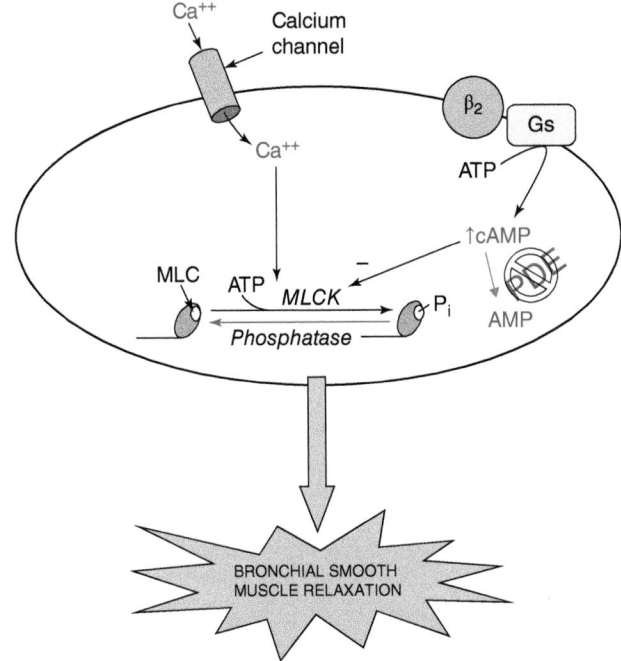

Abbreviations: AMP—Adenosine Monophosphate; ATP— Adenosine triphosphate; B2—Beta2 receptor; Ca++ - Calcium; Gs –g protein; MLC—Myosin Light Chain; MLCK—Myosin Light Chain Kinase; PDE—Phosphodiesterase; Pi—Myosin Phosphorylation

Figure 13.19 β_2 adrenoceptor and the site of action of Xanthines (PDE inhibitors).

Table 13.11 Xanthine agents and their related pharmacology.

Medication name	Theophylline	Aminophyline
Mode of action	A phosphodiasterase inhibitor which prevents the breakdown of intracellular cAMP, by phosphodiasterase, resulting in bronchodilation and reduced mucus secretion.	
Route of administration	Oral	IV or oral
Dosage Guidelines		**ADULTS**
	• Reversible airways obstruction, severe acute asthma, chronic asthma	• Severe acute asthma • Severe acute exacerbation of COPD • Reversible airway obstruction
		CHILDREN
	• Chronic asthma: • Modified-release medicine – dose depends upon brand of oral medication	• Severe acute asthma • Chronic asthma

(Continued)

341

Table 13.11   (Continued)

Medication name	Theophylline	Aminophyline
Contraindications	• Hypersensitivity to xanthines or excipients (hydroxyethylcellulose, povidone, cetostearyl alcohol, magrogol, talc, magnesium stearate) • Patients with porphyria • Concomitant administration with ephedrine in <6 years • Contraindicated in <6 months	• Hypersensitivity to ethylenediamine (added to Theophylline to produce aminophylline) • Concurrent use with other xanthines is contraindicated due to the risk of toxicity • Allergies to caffeine, theobromine, • Patients with acute porphyria • IV aminophylline in children <6 months is not recommended
Cautions	• Cardiac arrhythmias or other cardiac disease • Elderly • Epilepsy • Fever • Hypertension • Hyperthyroidism • Peptic ulcer • Risk of hypokalaemia – particularly with β_2 agonists, Theophylline derivatives, corticosteroids, diuretics and by hypoxia Pregnancy: Only to be used if potential benefit outweighs risk Breast-feeding: Only to be used if potential benefit outweighs risk	• Arrhythmias following rapid IV injection • Cardiac arrhythmias or other cardiac disease • Elderly • Epilepsy • Fever • Hypertension • Hyperthyroidism • Peptic ulcer • Risk of hypokalaemia – particularly with β_2 agonists, Theophylline derivatives, corticosteroids, diuretics and by hypoxia Pregnancy: Only to be used if potential benefit outweighs risk Breast-feeding: Only to be used if potential benefit outweighs risk
Side effects	• Anxiety • Arrhythmias • Diarrhoea • Dizziness • Gastrointestinal discomfort • Gastroesophageal reflux disease • Headache • Hyperuricemia • Nausea • Palpitations • Seizure • Skin reactions • Sleep disorders • Tremor • Urinary disorders • Vomiting	Aminophylline: • Headache • Nausea • Palpitations • Seizure (more common if IV injection too rapid) • Abdominal pain • Anxiety • Confusion, delirium, dizziness, insomnia, mania • Electrolyte imbalance • Gastrointestinal haemorrhage or reflux disease • Diarrhoea, vomiting • Hyperthermia • Hypotension, tachycardia • Hyperventilation • Metabolic disorder • Pain • Skin reactions • Vertigo, visual impairment
Interactions	• Smoking and alcohol can increase Theophylline clearance, increased doses may be required	• Smoking and alcohol can increase Theophylline clearance, increased doses may be required

342

Table 13.11   (Continued)

Medication name	Theophylline	Aminophyline
	• Theophylline clearance is also increased by: aminogluthethimide, carbemazepine, isoprenaline, Phenytoin, rifampicin, ritonavir, sulfinpyrazone, barbiturates and St. John's Wort • Theophylline clearance is reduced by: aciclovir, allopurinol, carbimazole, cimetidine, clarithromycin, diltiazem, Disulfiram, erythromycin, fluconazole, interferon, isoniazid, methotrexate, mexiletine, nizatidine, pentoxifylline, propafenone, propanolol, thiabendazole, verapamil and oral contraceptives • May interact with some quinolone antibiotics including ciprofloxacin • Viral infections, liver disease and heart failure also reduce Theophylline clearance • Reduced seizure threshold with concomitant use of ketamine **Note: Theophylline has a narrow therapeutic index of 5–20 mcg/mL, above this level there are associated toxic effects. Plasma Theophylline concentration should be measured 5 days after commencing oral treatment and 3 days following dose adjustment, or 4–6 hours following an oral dose of modified release preparation**	• Theophylline clearance is also increased by: aminogluthethimide, antiepileptics (carbemazepine, Phenytoin), isoprenaline, rifampicin, ritonavir, sulfinpyrazone and barbiturates • Theophylline clearance is reduced by: fluvoxamine, allopurinol, cimetidine, macrolide antibiotics (clarithromycin, erythromycin), calcium channel blockers (diltiazem, verapamil), Disulfiram, fluconazole, interferon, isoniazid, methotrexate, mexiletine, propafenone, propanolol, thiabendazole, tacrine, thyroid hormones, St. John's Wort, Zafirlukast and oral contraceptives • Other interactions: lithium, benzodiazepines, quinolones, general anesthetics, pancuronium, sympathomimetics, β_2 agonists, beta blockers, cardiac glycosides, adenosine, leukotriene anatagonists, doxapram and Regadenoson **Note: Theophylline has a narrow therapeutic index of 5–20 mcg/mL, above this level there are associated toxic effects. Plasma Theophylline concentration should be checked if administering IV aminophylline 4–6 hours after commencing treatment**
Absorption	• Oral administration – efficiently absorbed with 100% bioavailability • Peak concentrations at approximately 5 hours • Effective plasma concentration 5–12 mcg/ml	• IV preparation
Distribution	• Approximately 60% bound to plasma proteins, distributed through all body compartments	• Plasma protein binding approximately 60%, decreased to about 40% in neonates and adults with hepatic disease
Metabolism	• Metabolised in the liver	• Metabolised by the liver
Elimination	• Mainly excreted in the urine, approximately 10% is excreted unchanged • Mean elimination half-life is approximately 7 hours	• Mainly excreted in the urine, approximately 10% is excreted unchanged • Half-life elimination variable due to inter-individual variation

Source: British National Formulary (2019g, h); British National Formulary for Children (2019g, h); Electronic Medicines Compendium (2019g, h).

343

Corticosteroids

Corticosteroids (also known as glucocorticosteroids, glucocorticoids or steroids), whether taken by the oral or inhaled route, are used to treat many respiratory disease processes, a few of which are demonstrated within Table 13.12. The human body has its own (endogenous/internal) glucocorticosteroids in the form of cortisol, which is produced within the cortex of the adrenal gland as part of a negative-feedback loop and is vital to maintaining homeostasis. Cortisol is released at the end of a pathway of neural and hormonal responses involving the hypothalamic–pituitary–adrenal axis (HPA axis), and is released in increased levels in response to a stimulus/stressor (infection, trauma or disease) as part of the 'fight or flight' response (see Figure 13.24). These pathways can become exhausted, especially in chronic disease states, requiring the administration of an external (exogenous) form of glucocorticosteroids in order to mimic the effects of the naturally occurring endogenous steroid-hormone, cortisol. When administered exogenously, the pharmacological dose of corticosteroids exceeds the normal endogenous dose within a 24-hour period, in order to produce the desired anti-inflammatory effect. This is known as a 'supraphysiologic dose' and can result in a number of undesirable effects.

Another class of steroid hormones known as mineralocorticoids (aldosterone) also exist in both endogenous and exogenous/synthetic forms (fludrocortisone) and help control salt

Clinical considerations

Inhalation therapy is the cornerstone of treatment for COPD, asthma and bronchiectasis. Bronchodilators and corticosteroids may be delivered via aerosol inhalers, dry powder inhalers or nebulisers. An understanding of these devices is essential to ensure effective and safe delivery of the inhaled drug. Techniques for the use of these devices are outlined in the Skills for Practice box later in this chapter.

- Aerosol inhalers – a metered dose inhaler (MDI) delivers the drug in the form of a spray, mist or fine powder from a small, pressurised aerosol can. The drug is often suspended in a propellant. The valve dispenses a fixed volume and therefore metered dose of the drug. Poor co-ordination between administration of the drug and deep inhalation may be eliminated with the use of a spacer, improving lung deposition and preventing side effects of high-dose inhaled steroids (Dougherty and Lister, 2015; Preston and Kelly, 2016). This reduces the speed of dose delivery and the cold effect, due to the propellant at the back of the throat. A breath actuated MDI will administer the drug without compression of the aerosol can. Figures 13.20 and 13.21 depict a MDI and spacer.
- Dry powder inhaler – the drug is delivered in the form of a powder either from a capsule or from within the inhaler. It is breath actuated and requires sufficient breath inhalation for activation but may also trigger a cough reflex. Multi-dose DPIs all have individual priming techniques where priming occurs either by opening the cover, sliding a lever, pushing a button or twisting the base (Preston and Kelly, 2016). Figure 13.22 depicts a dry powder inhaler.
- Nebulisers – oxygen or air is driven through a solution of a drug resulting in a fine mist which is inhaled either via a face mask or mouthpiece. Nebulisers allow administration of higher dosages of drugs in comparison to standard inhalers, due to the generation of smaller particles, and require no co-ordination which is beneficial to those patients who are critically ill or who have poor manual dexterity (Dougherty and Lister, 2015; Preston and Kelly, 2016). Dose delivered is variable due to deposition of the drug within the equipment, breathing pattern and particle size generated. Figure 13.23 depicts a nebuliser.

Table 13.12 Corticosteroid agents and their related pharmacology.

Medication name	Prednisolone	Beclometasone dipropionate	Budesonide	Fluticasone
Mode of action	Exerts predominantly glucocorticoid effects with minimal mineralocorticoid effects.			
Route of administration	Oral	Inhaled	Inhaled (may also be nebulised at differing doses)	Inhaled (may also be nebulised at differing doses)
Indications	• Acute exacerbation of COPD • Mild to life-threatening acute asthma • Prophylaxis of asthma **CHILDREN** • Acute exacerbation of COPD • Mild to life-threatening acute asthma • Prophylaxis of asthma	**ADULTS**		
Contraindications	• Previous anaphylactic reaction • Avoid live virus vaccines in those receiving immunosuppressive doses (post-transplant patients, etc.)	• Previous anaphylactic reaction		
Precautions	Pregnancy and Breast-feeding: • Benefit of treatment with corticosteroids during pregnancy outweighs the risk • Additional corticosteroid cover is required during labour • Appears in small amounts in breast milk, however doses ≤40 mg daily are unlikely to cause systemic effects in the infant Prolonged treatment: (Generally ≥40 mg daily for >7 days in adults, ≥2 mg/kg daily for 1 week or ≥1 mg/kg daily for 1 month in children + likelihood disease relapse will occur) • Abrupt withdrawal can lead to acute adrenal insufficiency, hypotension or death	Important prescribing information: Beclometasone dipropionate inhalers (Qvar® and Clenil Modulite®) are **not** interchangeable and should be prescribed by brand name and dose-adjusted as per the BNF Pregnancy and Breast-feeding: Inhaled drugs for asthma, COPD and bronchiectasis can be taken as normal during pregnancy		

(Continued)

Table 13.12 (Continued)

Medication name	Prednisolone	Beclometasone dipropionate	Budesonide	Fluticasone
Side effects	• Psychiatric and psychotic reactions, behavioural disturbances, irritability, anxiety, sleep disturbances and cognitive dysfunction • Increased susceptibility to infection and opportunistic infections • Increased blood glucose levels	• **Paradoxical bronchospasm** – may be prevented by inhalation of a short-acting β_2 agonist beforehand • Headache • Oral thrush/candidiasis – can be reduced by using a spacer device • Pneumonia (in patients with COPD) • Taste alterations • Voice alteration		
Interactions	• Live vaccines • Antacids (magnesium or aluminum containing agents) • Antibacterials – rifampicin and isoniazid • Anticoagulants – Warfarin • Antiepileptics – carbamazepine, phenobarbital, Phenytoin and primidone effect corticosteroids • Antifungals – amphotericin and ketoconazole • Cytotoxics – methotrexate • Contraceptives • Non-steroidal anti-inflammatory drugs – aspirin and Indomethacin • Sympathomimetics – high doses of bambuterol, fenoteral, formoterol, ritodrine, salbutamol, salmeterol and Terbutaline	• General interactions are unlikely • Possibility of systemic effects with concomitant use of **strong** CYP3A inhibitors (e.g. ritonavir, cobicistat, itraconazole, ketoconazole) – increases systemic exposure to budesonide		
Absorption	• Rapidly absorbed after oral administration • Reaches peak plasma concentrations after 1–3 hours • Biological half-life lasts several hours	• Systemic absorption of unchanged beclomethasone dipropionate (BDP) occurs through the lungs • Negligible oral absorption of the swallowed dose • Prior to absorption there is extensive conversion of BDP to its active metabolite B-17-MP. • The systemic absorption arises from both lung (36%) and oral absorption of the swallowed dose (26%).	• Most of budesonide delivered to the lungs is systemically absorbed	• Systemic absorption occurs mainly through the lungs • Absorption is initially rapid then prolonged

Distribution	• Dose-dependant: Increase in dose leads to an increase in volume of distribution and plasma clearance • Degree of plasma protein binding determines the distribution and clearance of free, pharmacologically active drug, therefore reduced doses may be required in patients with hypoalbuminemia	• Tissue distribution is higher for active metabolite B-17-MP • Plasma protein binding is high (87%)	• Volume of distribution of approximately 3 L/kg. • Plasma protein binding averages 85–90%	
Metabolism	• Primarily in the liver to a biologically inactive compound • Crosses the placenta, however 88% of is inactivated	• Cleared very rapidly from the systemic circulation by metabolism mediated via enzymes that are found in most tissues	• Rapidly and extensively metabolised in liver to two major metabolites	• Rapidly and extensively metabolised in liver
Elimination	• Excreted in the urine	• Excreted in urine and faeces	• Excreted in urine and faeces	• Excreted mostly in faeces, some in urine

Source: British National Formulary (2019i, j, k, l), British National Formulary for Children (2019i, j, k, l); Electronic Medicines Compendium (2019i, j, k, l).

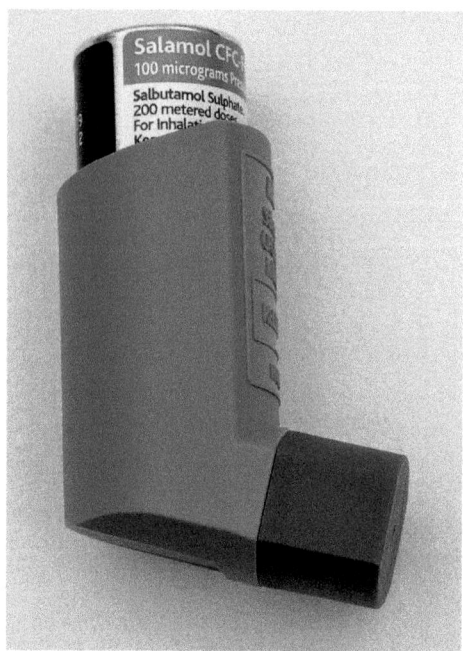

Figure 13.20   Metered dose Inhaler. Source: Pictures taken from the Royal Marsden Handbook of Nursing Procedures, 9e. Dougherty & Lister (2015). pp 708–709. © 2015, John Wiley & Sons.

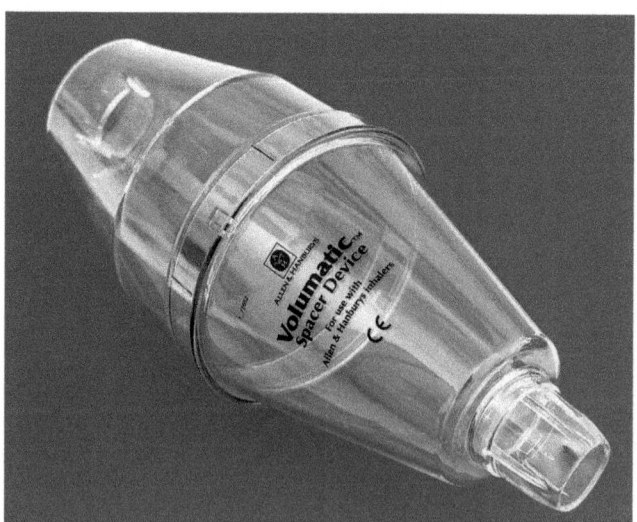

Figure 13.21   Spacer. Source: Pictures taken from the Royal Marsden Handbook of Nursing Procedures, 9e. Dougherty & Lister (2015). pp 708–709. © 2015, John Wiley & Sons.

and water homeostasis (osmoregulation). Some drugs used to mimic or inhibit mineralocorticoids also have glucocorticoid effects; however, the drug therapies used in respiratory disorders concerned with this chapter have minimal to no effect upon mineralocorticoid activity. Such drugs are mainly used in the treatment of cardiovascular or renal diseases (please see Chapters 10 and 11).

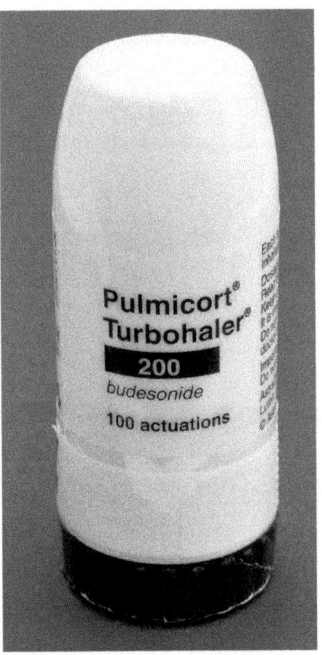

Figure 13.22   Dry powder inhaler. Source: Pictures taken from the Royal Marsden Handbook of Nursing Procedures, 9e. Dougherty & Lister (2015). pp 708–709. © 2015, John Wiley & Sons.

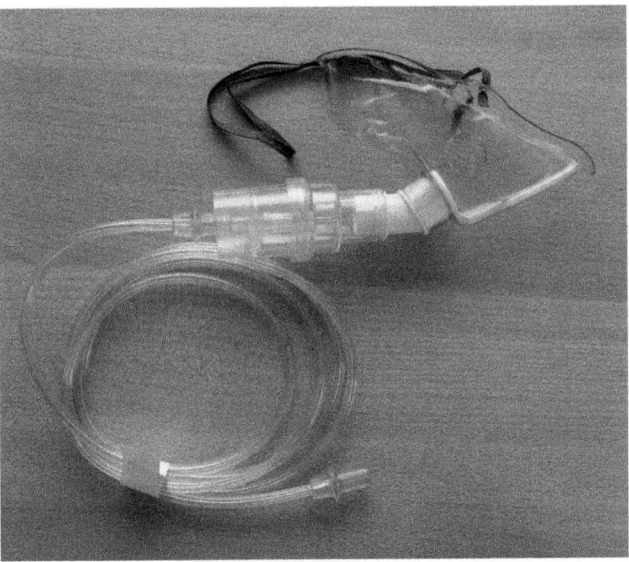

Figure 13.23   Nebuliser. Source: Pictures taken from the Royal Marsden Handbook of Nursing Procedures, 9e. Dougherty & Lister (2015). pp 708–709. © 2015, John Wiley & Sons.

Corticosteroids affect numerous steps in the inflammatory pathway, which can be induced by trauma, infection or disease to name a few. They have multiple applications in treating inflammation of the respiratory tract as their predominant effect is upon the inflammatory cells, in turn inhibiting the mobilisation of pro-inflammatory cells into the respiratory tract via a process called chemotaxis. The pharmacological effect of corticosteroids is exerted upon the

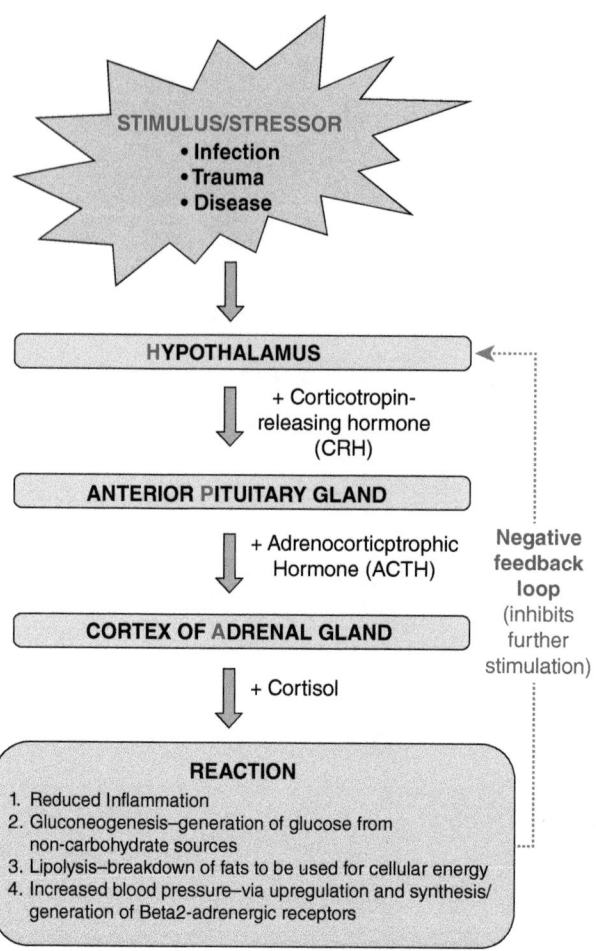

Figure 13.24   The hypothalamic–pituitary–adrenal (HPA) axis.

nucleus of the inflammatory cells (macrophages, eosinophils, lymphocytes, mast cells) and the structural cells of the respiratory tract (epithelial, endothelial, goblet and smooth muscle cells). Corticosteroids diffuse across the cell membrane of their target cells into the cytoplasm and bind to a cytoplasmic glucocorticoid receptor (CGR), where it then forms a drug–receptor complex (glucocorticoid–CGR complex) and activates said receptor. This drug–receptor complex then enters (translocates) into the cell's nucleus, where it stimulates the synthesis of anti-inflammatory gene proteins and inhibits synthesis of inflammatory gene proteins. Figure 13.25 shows this complex process in further detail.

A. Glucocorticoid enters cell via cell membrane into cell cytoplasm where cytoplasmic glucocorticoid receptor (CGR) receptor resides.
B. Glucocorticoid and CGR bind to make drug-receptor (CGRD) complex which crosses into cell nucleus.
C. CGRD complex binds to region of steroid-responsive genes. This interaction either switches gene transcription on or off.
D. Effect of different gene transcriptions has various effects throughout the body.

Skills in practice

Administration of an inhaled medication via a metered dose inhaler (MDI):

1. Explain and discuss the procedure with the patient.
2. Ask the patient to find a comfortable position in an upright position in the bed or sitting in a chair.
3. Prior to administering the drug, the following checks must be conducted:
   - correct patient
   - drug
   - dose
   - administration time, date, route and method
   - prescription.
4. Remove the mouthpiece cover from the inhaler and shake the device for two to three seconds.
5. Without a spacer device:
   Ask the patient to take a deep breath and exhale fully, open mouth, and place the mouthpiece with the opening towards the back of the throat, closing the lips tightly.
   With a spacer device:
   Insert the MDI into the appropriate end of the spacer device. Ask the patient to exhale and grip the spacer mouthpiece with their teeth and lips, holding the inhaler.
6. Ask the patient to tip their head back slightly, inhaling slowly and deeply for approximately two to three seconds while depressing the canister completely.
7. Ask the patient to hold their breath for approximately 10 seconds and remove the MDI from the mouth if a spacer is not being used. The patient should exhale through pursed lips. If a spacer is being used, the patient should take 4–5 deep breaths, through the mouth only, prior to removing the mouthpiece.
8. Ask the patient to wait 20–30 seconds between inhalations, if it is the same medication, or 2–5 minutes if it is a different medication. The bronchodilator should always be given before the inhaled corticosteroid.
   Note: for capsule DPIs a capsule containing the drug needs to be place inside the inhaler chamber and pierced as the manufacturer's instructions. The inhalation technique needs to be quick and deep with a good seal around the mouthpiece, holding the breath for 5–10 seconds. If any powder is left the inhalation technique should be repeated.
9. Ask the patient to rinse out their mouth with water for approximately two minutes if the medication is a steroid.
10. Record the administration in the appropriate documentation.

Source: Dougherty and Lister (2015).

The following table details some of the cornerstones of treatment for the respiratory diseases previously discussed in this chapter. It has been composed using the most up-to-date resources at the time of publishing. However, it should only serve as a guide and the latest versions of the British National Formulary and relevant guidelines should be utilised for prescribing in practice within the UK.

Immune modulators

The process of inflammation characterised in many of the respiratory disorders explored within this chapter involves multiple immunological reactions that affect the airway epithelium. Immune modulating agents are used to target certain parts of these immunological chain of reactions, to

Skills in practice

Administration of an inhaled medication via a nebuliser:

1. Explain and discuss the procedure with the patient.
2. Either ask the patient to find a comfortable position in the bed or chair, or position the patient in an upright position if possible.
3. Prior to administering the drug, the following checks must be conducted:
   - correct patient
   - drug
   - dose
   - administration time, date, route and method
   - prescription.
4. Only one drug should be administered at a time unless otherwise specified.
5. Assemble the nebuliser equipment as the manufacturer's instructions.
6. Measure the liquid medication with a syringe, adding a diluent as required and place in the nebuliser.
7. Attach the nebuliser, with either a face mask or mouthpiece interface, to piped oxygen or air via to tubing, as prescribed. If the patient has a clinical need for oxygen therapy, the nebulised drug should be given with oxygen. Pulse oximetry should be applied and monitored for the duration of the nebuliser. For hypercapnic or acidotic patients, medical air should be used to administer the nebuliser.
8. Apply the face mask or ask the patient to place the mouthpiece between their lips.
9. Ask the patient to take a slow deep breath, pause briefly and exhale.
10. Turn on the piped medical air or oxygen to a minimum rate of 6–8 L, sufficient flow to form a mist.
11. Ask the patient to continue to breathe as in step 10 until the nebuliser is complete. Approximately 0.5 mL will remain in the chamber.
12. The duration of optimal nebulisation of 4 mL is approximately 10 minutes.
13. Following the nebuliser, reapply appropriate and prescribed oxygen therapy.
14. Record the administration in the appropriate documentation.

Source: Dougherty and Lister (2015)

either aid in the prevention or treatment of the pathophysiological process of respiratory diseases. They do this by binding and inhibiting/antagonising sites within the airways that pro-inflammatory signalling molecules (eicosanoids) would usually bind to. These eicosanoids are released from immune cells (mast cells and eosinophils) and would usually result in bronchoconstriction, mucous secretion, vascular permeability, and further immune cell recruitment (chemotaxis). By antagonising these binding sites, the above processes can be inhibited. These agents are used as preventative treatments versus those used in acute exacerbations of disease.

Mast cell stabilisers

Mast cells have been identified as playing an important role in the development of allergies, asthma, COPD, respiratory infections and pulmonary fibrosis due to their pro-inflammatory and pro-fibrotic activity (Erjefält, 2014). Mast cells belong to a large group of cells under the umbrella term 'immune cells' and are present within most tissues of the human body, existing densely within the airways. They are key players in the inflammatory response, mounting a rapid and profound reaction to pathogens and other stimulants through the release of special granules containing various substances that affect the inflammatory cascade (see Figure 13.26). The pharmacological action of mast cell stabilisers upon this process has been disputed in recent decades; however, their mechanism of

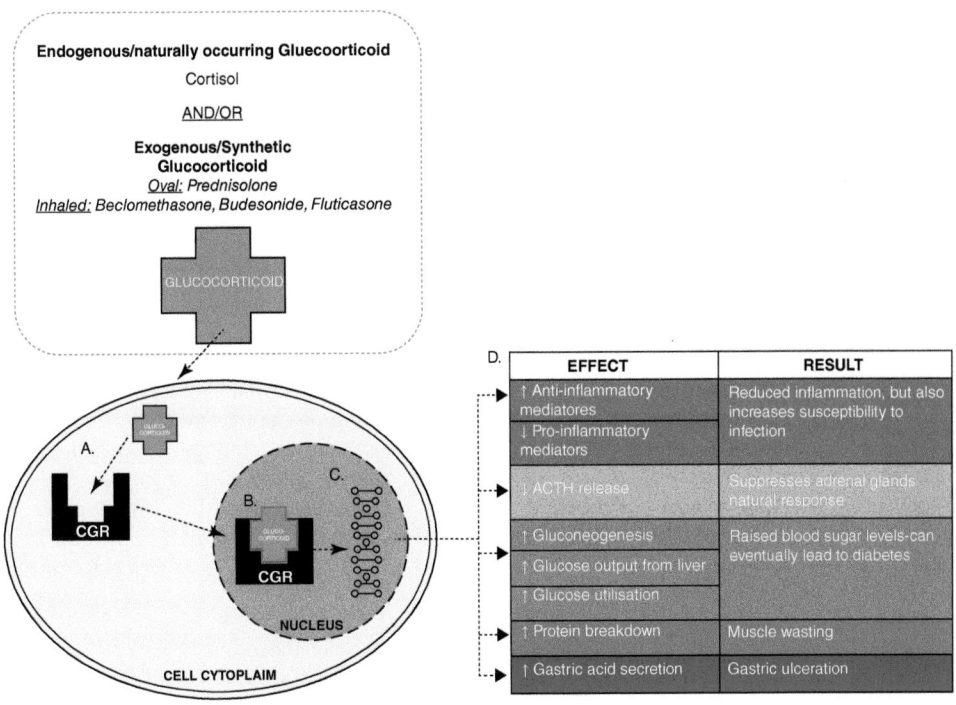

Figure 13.25   The pharmacological effect of glucocorticoids.

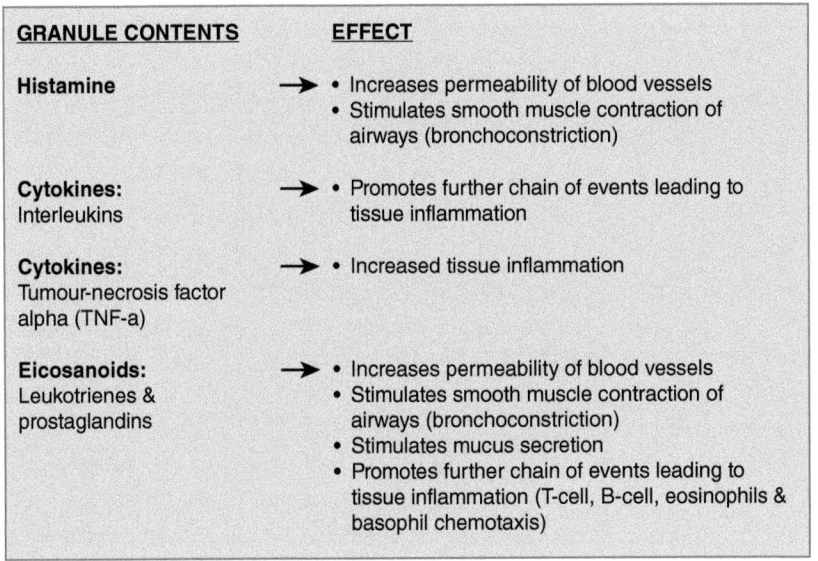

Figure 13.26   Mast cell granule contents and their effects.

Clinical considerations

Patients on long-term corticosteroid treatment (>2 week course) should carry a **Steroid Treatment Card** along with a patient information leaflet that gives guidance on minimising risk and provides details of prescriber, drug, dosage and duration of treatment (British National Formulary, 2019a). Healthcare professionals should be mindful of the following potentially life-threatening presentations for a patient on long-term steroids:

Adrenal suppression

Prolonged use of corticosteroids causes suppression of the adrenal gland in cases where the 'fight or flight' response would usually result in stimulation (see Figure 13.10). This is a condition known as adrenal atrophy and can last for many years after treatment with steroids is stopped. Abrupt withdrawal of prolonged courses of exogenous, systemic glucocorticoid can result in refractory hypotension and even death. Healthcare professionals must be mindful of this phenomena when patients present with intercurrent illness, trauma or post-surgery whereby the natural release of cortisol would normally occur. A short course of increased glucocorticoid therapy would be required in these cases; or if the prolonged treatment course had already been stopped, a temporary reintroduction of corticosteroid treatment must be prescribed.

Infections

This patient group is more susceptible to infection, especially those of an atypical nature. Infections such as septicemia and tuberculosis may have reached a very advanced stage before any clinical change is recognised.

Chickenpox

Patients that have not suffered from chickenpox in the past are more susceptible to contracting severe varicella zoster virus infection, which can quickly lead to multi-organ involvement and eventually failure. In those patients who are non-immune to the virus and become exposed to it, immunisation with varicella–zoster immunoglobulin should be initiated when receiving long-term steroid treatment.

Measles

Patients taking corticosteroids in whom measles exposure is likely should be advised to seek immediate medical advice. Prophylaxis with intramuscular normal immunoglobulin may be needed.

Psychiatric reactions

Patients should be advised to seek medical advice if psychiatric symptoms (especially depression and suicidal thoughts) occur and they should also be alert to the rare possibility of such reactions during withdrawal of corticosteroid treatment. Systemic corticosteroids should be prescribed with care in those predisposed to psychiatric reactions.

Source: British National Formulary (2019i).

action upon the release of inflammatory mediators from mast cells, and the reduction of eosinophil and neutrophil chemotaxis, is still widely described within the prescribing literature (Electronic Medicines Compendium, 2019m, n). Current asthma treatment guidelines suggest the mast cell stabiliser sodium cromoglicate is of some benefit in adults and children aged between five and 12 years and nedocromil sodium is of benefit in adults and children under five years of age (BTS/SIGN, 2019).

Leukotriene receptor antagonists

Leukotrienes are a type of inflammatory mediator molecule that are released from mast cells, neutrophils and eosinophils as part of the inflammatory cascade. As explored within Table 13.13, leukotrienes are part of a group known as eicosanoids which have a variety of effects on both the airways and surrounding blood vessels. There are two main groups of leukotrienes, the first acts primarily in conditions where inflammation is concerned, mainly with the granular contents released from neutrophils during inflammation such as CF. The second group of leukotrienes are known as cysteinyl-leukotrienes and are implicated in asthma via their highly selective receptor binding sites (CysLT$_1$) within bronchial smooth muscle and airway macrophages. Cysteinyl-leukotrienes are produced by eosinophils and mast cells, and when bound to CysLT$_1$ receptor sites they induce bronchoconstriction, mucus hypersecretion, microvascular leakage, eosinophil chemotaxis and airway remodelling – all key features in the pathophysiological triad of asthma (see Figure 13.7).

Asthma with a high eosinophil count in both blood and sputum samples (eosinophilia) is a subtype of severe asthma, also known as severe eosinophilic asthma, and is well-recognised as potentially benefiting from leukotriene receptor antagonist drug therapy. Leukotriene receptor antagonists (LKRAs) such as montelukast have a high affinity for binding to CysLT$_1$ receptor sites, which results in a combined bronchodilator and anti-inflammatory effect. These agents are used as a preventer therapy only, and should only be considered if first-line preventer therapies such as long-acting beta-2 agonists and ICS have failed. There is a distinct lack of clinical evidence available to suggest that the use of LKRAs is superior to high-dose ICS (Chauhan et al., 2017). Current guidelines suggest the leukotriene receptor antagonist montelukast be considered if asthma control remains suboptimal despite these agents, or in the case of children under five who are not able to tolerate inhaled corticosteroid treatment (BTS/SIGN, 2019).

Mucolytics

As explored within various sections of this chapter, a common pathological consequence of multiple respiratory disorders is mucous hypersecretion due to goblet cell hyperplasia and hypertrophy. Mucolytics such as carbocisteine and acetylcysteine affect the proteins (mucins) secreted by the goblet cells, breaking them down and in turn reducing sputum viscosity and increased mucus clearance. Recombinant human DNase (dornase alfa) aids in the enzymatic breakdown of intracellular DNA released by invading neutrophils, which would otherwise increase sputum viscosity.

A recent Cochrane review identified that the use of carbocisteine and acetylcysteine is useful for reducing flare-ups, days of disability and hospital admissions in people with COPD or chronic bronchitis (Poole et al., 2019). Current guidelines concerning the management of non-cystic fibrosis related bronchiectasis suggest that there is little evidence to support routine use of either carbocisteine, acetylcysteine or dornase alfa mucolytic agents, but in those patients with difficulty in sputum expectoration a trial of therapy may be considered (British Thoracic Society, 2019). Current guidance for the management of CF, however, suggests that dornase alfa should be the first-line mucolytic for CF patients who have clinical evidence of lung disease (NICE, 2017a).

The following Table 3.14 details some key prescribing data for the therapies mentioned within the mucolytic section of this chapter. It has been composed using the most up-to-date resources at the time of publishing. However, it should only serve as a guide and the latest versions of the British National Formulary and relevant guidelines should be utilised for prescribing in practice within the UK.

Table 13.13   Immune modulator agents and their related pharmacology.

Medication name	Sodium Cromoglicate	Nedocromil sodium	Montelukast
Mode of action	Prevents mast cell degranulation	Prevents mast cell degranulation	CysLT$_1$ receptor antagonist
Route of administration	Inhalation or aerosol	Inhalation or aerosol	
Indications	**ADULTS**		
	Prophylaxis of asthma		
	CHILDREN		
	Prophylaxis of asthma		
Contraindications	• Previous anaphylactic reaction	• Previous anaphylactic reaction	• Previous anaphylactic reaction
Cautions	• Withdrawal should be done gradually over a period of one week – symptoms of asthma may recur • Discontinue if eosinophilic pneumonia occurs • Can be taken as normal during pregnancy	• Withdrawal should be done gradually over a period of one week – symptoms of asthma may recur • Can be taken as normal during pregnancy • Can be taken as normal when breast-feeding	• Manufacturer advises avoidance in pregnancy and when breast-feeding. However, it may be taken as normal in women who have shown a significant improvement in asthma not achievable with other drugs before becoming pregnant
Side effects	• Paradoxical bronchospasm • Cough • Headache • Eosinophilic pneumonia • Rhinitis • Throat irritation	• Paradoxical bronchospasm • Taste alterations • Cough • Gastrointestinal discomfort • Headache • Nausea • Vomiting • Pharyngitis • Throat irritation	Most commonly: • Diarrhoea • Fever • Gastrointestinal discomfort • Headache • Nausea • Skin reactions • Upper respiratory tract infection • Vomiting
Interactions	No interactions with other drugs have been reported since the drug was released on to the market	No interactions with other drugs have been reported since the drug was released on to the market	• Reduces plasma concentration of Phenytoin, phenobarbital and rifampicin

Absorption	• ~10% of inhaled dose is absorbed from the respiratory tract • The remainder is either exhaled or deposited in the oropharynx or swallowed and eliminated via the alimentary tract • ~1% of the dose is absorbed from the gastrointestinal tract • Rate of absorption from the respiratory tract is slower than the elimination rate ($t_{\frac{1}{2}}$ of 1.5–2 h)	• ~10% of inhaled dose is absorbed from the respiratory tract. • The remainder is either exhaled or deposited in the oropharynx or swallowed and eliminated via the alimentary tract. • Plasma concentrations of nedocromil sodium reach a maximum within 1 hour post-dosing and decline with a half-life of 1–2 hours	• Rapidly absorbed following oral administration • Oral bioavailability is 64% (for 10 mg tablets)
Distribution	Moderately and reversibly bound to plasma proteins (≈ 65%)	Moderately (80%) and reversibly bound to human plasma proteins	• >99% bound to plasma proteins
Metabolism	Not metabolised in humans	Not metabolised in humans	• Extensively metabolised by cytochrome P450 2C8 enzymes
Elimination	Excreted unchanged in both urine and bile in approximately equal proportions	Excreted unchanged in the urine (approximately 70%) and in faeces (approximately 30%).	• Montelukast and its metabolites are excreted almost exclusively via the bile • Small amounts excreted in faeces and urine

357

Source: British National Formulary (2019m, n, o); British National Formulary for Children (2019m, n, o); Electronic Medicines Compendium (2019m, n, o).

Table 13.14 Mucolytic agents and their related pharmacology.

Medication name	Carbocisteine	Acetylcysteine (NACSYS® effervescent tablets)	Dornase alfa (Pulmozyme® nebuliser solution)
Mode of action	Mucin cross-link breakdown	Mucin cross-link breakdown	Enzymatic breakdown of neutrophil DNA breakdown
Route of administration	Oral	Oral	Inhalation of nebulised solution
Indications		**ADULTS**	
	Reduction of sputum viscosity	Reduction of sputum viscosity	Management of cystic fibrosis patients with a forced vital capacity (FVC) >40% predicted
		CHILDREN	
	Reduction of sputum viscosity in children aged 2–17 years	Not licensed	Management of cystic fibrosis patients with a forced vital capacity (FVC) of greater than 40% of predicted to improve pulmonary function
Contraindications	• Previous anaphylactic reaction • Active peptic ulceration	• Previous anaphylactic reaction	• Previous anaphylactic reaction
Precautions	• History of peptic ulceration (may disrupt the gastric mucosal barrier) • Manufacturer advises avoid usage in first trimester of pregnancy • Unknown whether carbocisteine and/or its metabolites are excreted in human milk. A risk to the newborn or infant cannot be excluded	• History of peptic ulceration • May be taken in pregnancy and during breast-feeding – available data does not indicate a risk to the child	• No evidence of toxicity to embryo or foetus (teratogenicity); manufacturer advises use only if potential benefit outweighs risk

Side effects	• Gastrointestinal haemorrhage • Skin reactions • Stevens–Johnson syndrome • Vomiting	• Diarrhoea • Fever • Gastrointestinal discomfort • Headache • Hypotension • Nausea • Stomatitis • Tinnitus • Vomiting	• Chest pain • Conjunctivitis • Dyspepsia • Dysphonia • Dyspnea • Fever • Increased risk of infection • Skin reactions
Interactions	No known interactions with other medicinal products	• Simultaneous solution of *NACSYS* 600 mg effervescent tablets with other medicinal products is not recommended • Oral antibiotics should be taken two hours before or after *Acetylcysteine* • Should not be administered concomitantly antitussive medicinal product • May enhance the vasodilatory effects of *nitroglycerin* • Activated charcoal can decrease the effect of *acetylcysteine*	Can be effectively and safely used in conjunction with standard cystic fibrosis therapies such as antibiotics, bronchodilators, pancreatic enzymes, vitamins, inhaled and systemic corticosteroids and analgesics
Absorption	Rapidly absorbed from the GI tract Maximum plasma concentration is reached in two hours	Rapidly absorbed after oral administration and distributed throughout the organism	Human studies show low systemic exposure
Distribution	Bioavailability <10% of the administered dose	Highest tissue concentrations are reached in the liver, kidneys and lungs	Concentrations of dornase alfa in sputum rapidly decline following inhalation
Metabolism	Most likely via intraluminal (gut) metabolism with a significant hepatic first-pass effect	Amino acid metabolism	Proteases present in biological fluids
Elimination	Carbocisteine and its metabolites are excreted primarily through the kidneys	Largely converted into inorganic sulphate, which undergoes renal excretion	No data for inhaled usage

Source: British National Formulary (2019p, q, r); British National Formulary for Children (2019p, q, r); Electronic Medicines Compendium (2019p, q, r).

Clinical considerations

Pulmozyme (dornase alfa) should not be mixed with other drugs or solutions in the nebuliser. It should only be nebulised via a jet nebuliser/compressor system, as an ultrasonic nebuliser may inactivate pulmozyme or have unacceptable aerosol delivery characteristics.

The manufacturers' instructions on the use and maintenance of the nebuliser and compressor should be followed. The majority of jet nebulisers require an optimum gas flow rate of 6–8 L/minute and in hospital can be driven by piped air or oxygen. In acute asthma, the nebuliser should be driven by oxygen. Domiciliary oxygen cylinders do not provide an adequate flow rate; therefore, an electrical compressor is required for domiciliary use.

For patients at risk of hypercapnia, such as those with COPD, oxygen can be dangerous and the nebuliser should be driven by air. If oxygen is required, it should be given simultaneously by nasal cannula.

Source: British National Formulary (2019r), British National Formulary for Children (2019r) and Electronic Medicines Compendium (2019r).

Episode of care (Asthma)

Mr. Wójcik

Mr. Wójcik is a 32-year-old male sales representative who works long hours and has a young family. He enjoys cycling long distances with his family on a regular basis. Mr. Wójcik refers to himself as a 'social smoker' whereby he may partake in up to 10 cigarettes a week while socialising with friends. He attends for an appointment at the asthma clinic at his local general practitioner (GP) surgery after a recent asthma attack which interfered with some important work-related travel, and he has attended the clinic on this occasion to ask about how this can be managed better in the future.

His medical notes indicate that he was diagnosed with asthma in childhood and although this is generally well controlled, he experiences one to two exacerbations a year which require oral steroids. These exacerbations are usually triggered by a viral upper-respiratory tract infection during the winter months lasting up to seven days, but have not required admission to hospital, nor has Mr. Wójcik required any home oxygen or home nebuliser therapy at any point. He is not aware of his usual PEFR readings as he does not monitor this himself, but his medical records state that his PEFR during exacerbations when monitored at the surgery have been around 60% predicted for his height and age. During these occasions he has not had any features of acute severe or life-threatening asthma. On previous examination around 18 months ago, Mr. Wójcik's PEFR had been shown to be >80% predicted for his age and height. He states he is often unable to attend asthma clinic due to his work, but that between exacerbations he reports no daytime symptoms, or nighttime awakenings due to his asthma and no limitations on his activity levels.

Mr. Wójcik's regular prescription includes Fluticasone inhaler 200 micrograms twice daily and Salbutamol inhaler as required. On review of his medications in the asthma clinic it became apparent that Mr. Wójcik did not take his Fluticasone inhaler unless he felt 'unwell'. He reports no side effects from his asthma treatment. Mr. Wójcik does not possess an asthma self-management plan or a PEFR diary.

This case presents many opportunities for improving asthma management, and in turn preventing potential morbidity and mortality. As a busy professional with a young family, Mr. Wójcik appears to have suboptimal control of his disease process which has resulted in multiple exacerbations and a recent 'attack'. This recent unfortunate event which triggered the consultation offers a rare opportunity to engage with him and discuss how he can improve his asthma management. There is an extensive evidence base of asthma self-management in the first instance, for effectively reducing the morbidity and mortality rates from this disease process. Both international and national guidelines emphasise the importance of supporting self-management (BTS/SIGN, 2019; GINA, 2019). The recent *Practical Systematic Review of Self-Management Support*

(PRISMS) meta-review and *Reducing Care Utilisation through Self-management Interventions (RECURSIVE)* health economic review (Pinnock et al., 2017) analysed evidence from 270 randomised-controlled trials and confirmed that supported self-management for asthma:

1. reduces unscheduled care;
2. improves asthma control;
3. can be delivered effectively for diverse demographic and cultural groups;
4. is applicable in a broad range of clinical settings;
5. does not significantly increase total healthcare costs.

There are also other key themes in Mr. Wójcik's asthma management that can be addressed here, such as monitoring, non-pharmacological management and pharmacological management. Each of these key themes, including the aforementioned supported self-management, will be addressed according to the most recent BTS/SIGN (2019) and NICE (2017b) guidelines below. NICE, BTS and SIGN have recently formed an alliance to produce a joint guideline on chronic asthma.

Supported self-management
- Mr. Wójcik should be offered self-management education, including a written **personalised** asthma action plan (PAAP). Free PAAP resources are available via www.asthma.org.uk/advice/manage-your-asthma/action-plan and encourage the asthma sufferer to be aware of their regular treatment, how to monitor and recognise that control is deteriorating, and the action they should take including their personal best PEFR and PEFR during exacerbations.
- Mr. Wójcik should be supported by regular professional review. However, his busy lifestyle may require more flexible arrangements for follow-up via the utilisation of different modes of consultation such as community outreach clinics, telephone or email.

Monitoring
Alongside the use of a PAAP, Mr. Wójcik should be supported in reinforcing the best techniques for monitoring PEFR and encouraged to consider keeping a diary of his regular PEFR readings at both baseline and during exacerbations. The use of a PEFR diary such as those which can be found via the Asthma UK charity may be useful: www.asthma.org.uk/advice/manage-your-asthma/peak-flow.

Non-pharmacological management
- Mr. Wójcik should be supported in identifying and avoiding any triggers which may exacerbate his asthma:
  - Smoking: he should be advised regarding the dangers of smoking and second-hand tobacco smoke exposure. Smoking cessation advice should be offered at every opportunity when in contact with a healthcare professional.
  - Immunisations: Mr. Wójcik's exacerbations tend to occur around the winter months, when there is a potential increased risk of suffering from serious complications of influenza infection. There is also the potential for asthma patients to develop serious complications from pneumococcal infection. The Centre for Disease Control and Prevention (2019) recommend that asthma patients should be offered vaccination against both influenzas and pneumococcus.

Pharmacological management
- Before initiating any new pharmacological treatment with Mr. Wójcik, practitioners should check adherence with existing therapies, check inhaler technique and eliminate trigger factors.
- Asthma management should always follow a step-wise process (see Figure 13.9 on page x).

Conclusion

As a student healthcare practitioner, you will undoubtedly be involved in the care of a number of patients with one or multiple types of respiratory disorder. These disorders can be very complex and have the potential to have detrimental effects on a patient's activities of daily living. The incidence of respiratory disorders continues to rise, but this may in part be due to improvements in diagnostic techniques. As such, it is crucial that the healthcare professionals involved in supporting this patient group have a sound understanding of the pathophysiological, pharmacological and evidence base that underpins the promotion of safe and effective care.

References

Asthma UK (2018). *Stop asthma attacks. Cure asthma. Asthma UK Annual Report.* www.asthma.org.uk/about/annual-report-accounts (accessed September 2019).

Bastin, A.J., Starling, L., Ahmed, R., et al. (2010). *High prevalence of undiagnosed and severe chronic obstructive pulmonary disease at first hospital admission with acute exacerbation.* https://doi.org/10.1177/1479972310364587 (accessed September 2019).

British Compressed Gas Association (2018). *Gas cylinder identification label and colour code requirements. Technical information sheet 6.* www.bcga.co.uk/assets/BCGA%20TIS%206%20-%20Rev%203%20-%20For%20Publication.pdf (accessed September 2019).

British Lung Foundation (2016). *The battle for breath – the impact of lung disease in the UK.* https://cdn.shopify.com/s/files/1/0221/4446/files/The_Battle_for_Breath_report_48b7e0ee-dc5b-43a0-a25c-2593bf9516f4.pdf?7045701451358472254&_ga=2.36864416.1645006389.1567499245-684242941.1567499245 (accessed September 2019).

British Lung Foundation (2017). *Out in the cold. Lung disease the hidden diver of NHS winter pressure.* https://cdn.shopify.com/s/files/1/0221/4446/files/Out_in_the_cold_Dec_2017.pdf?15282568839826487629&_ga=2.235455873.1645006389.1567499245-684242941.1567499245 (accessed September 2019).

British National Formulary (2019). *Oxygen.* https://bnf.nice.org.uk/treatment-summary/oxygen.html (accessed September 2019).

British National Formulary (2019a). *Salbutamol.* https://bnf.nice.org.uk/drug/salbutamol.html (accessed September 2019).

British National Formulary (2019b). *Terbutaline sulfate* https://bnf.nice.org.uk/drug/terbutaline-sulfate.html (accessed September 2019).

British National Formulary (2019c). *Salmeterol.* https://bnf.nice.org.uk/drug/salmeterol.html (accessed September 2019).

British National Formulary (2019d). *Formoterol fumarate.* https://bnf.nice.org.uk/drug/formoterol-fumarate.html#indicationsAndDoses (accessed September 2019).

British National Formulary (2019e). *Ipratropium bromide.* https://bnf.nice.org.uk/drug/ipratropium-bromide.html (accessed September 2019).

British National Formulary (2019f). *Tiotropium.* https://bnf.nice.org.uk/drug/tiotropium.html (accessed September 2019).

British National Formulary (2019g). *Theophylline.* https://bnf.nice.org.uk/drug/theophylline.html (accessed September 2019).

British National Formulary (2019h). *Aminophylline.* https://bnf.nice.org.uk/drug/aminophylline.html (accessed September 2019).

British National Formulary (2019i). *Prednisolone.* https://bnf.nice.org.uk/drug/prednisolone.html (accessed September 2019).

British National Formulary (2019j). *Beclomethasone.* https://bnf.nice.org.uk/drug/beclometasone-dipropionate.html#indicationsAndDoses (accessed September 2019).

British National Formulary (2019k). *Budesonide.* https://bnf.nice.org.uk/drug/budesonide.html (accessed September 2019).

British National Formulary (2019l). *Fluticasone.* https://bnf.nice.org.uk/drug/fluticasone.html#indicationsAndDoses (accessed September 2019).

British National Formulary (2019m). *Sodium cromoglicate.* https://bnf.nice.org.uk/drug/sodium-cromoglicate.html (accessed September 2019).

British National Formulary (2019n). *Nedocromil sodium.* https://bnf.nice.org.uk/drug/nedocromil-sodium.html (accessed September 2019).

British National Formulary (2019o). *Montelukast*. https://bnf.nice.org.uk/drug/montelukast.html (accessed September 2019).

British National Formulary (2019p). *Carbocisteine*. https://bnf.nice.org.uk/drug/carbocisteine.html (accessed September 2019).

British National Formulary (2019q). *Acetylcysteine*. https://bnf.nice.org.uk/drug/acetylcysteine.html (accessed September 2019).

British National Formulary (2019r). *Dornase alfa*. https://bnf.nice.org.uk/drug/dornase-alfa.html (accessed September 2019).

British National Formulary for Children (2019a). *Salbutamol*. https://bnfc.nice.org.uk/drug/salbutamol.html (accessed September 2019).

British National Formulary for Children (2019b). *Terbutaline sulphate*. https://bnfc.nice.org.uk/drug/terbutaline-sulfate.html (accessed September 2019).

British National Formulary for Children (2019c). *Salmeterol*. https://bnfc.nice.org.uk/drug/salmeterol.html (accessed September 2019).

British National Formulary for Children (2019d). *Formoterol*. https://bnfc.nice.org.uk/drug/formoterol-fumarate.html (accessed September 2019).

British National Formulary for Children (2019e). *Ipratropium bromide*. https://bnfc.nice.org.uk/drug/ipratropium-bromide.html (accessed September 2019).

British National Formulary for Children (2019f). *Tiotropium*. https://bnfc.nice.org.uk/drug/tiotropium.html (accessed September 2019).

British National Formulary for Children (2019g). *Theophylline*. https://bnfc.nice.org.uk/drug/theophylline.html (accessed September 2019).

British National Formulary for Children (2019h). *Aminophylline*. https://bnfc.nice.org.uk/drug/aminophylline.html (accessed September 2019).

British National Formulary for Children (2019i). *Prednisolone*. https://bnfc.nice.org.uk/drug/prednisolone.html (accessed September 2019).

British National Formulary for Children (2019j). *Beclomethasone*. https://bnfc.nice.org.uk/drug/beclometasone-dipropionate.html#indicationsAndDoses (accessed September 2019).

British National Formulary for Children (2019k). *Budesonide*. https://bnfc.nice.org.uk/drug/budesonide.html (accessed September 2019).

British National Formulary for Children (2019l). *Fluticasone*. https://bnfc.nice.org.uk/drug/fluticasone.html#indicationsAndDoses (accessed September 2019).

British National Formulary for Children (2019m). *Sodium cromoglicate*. https://bnfc.nice.org.uk/drug/sodium-cromoglicate.html (accessed September 2019).

British National Formulary for Children (2019n). *Nedocromil sodium*. https://bnfc.nice.org.uk/drug/nedocromil-sodium.html (accessed September 2019).

British National Formulary for Children (2019o). *Montelukast*. https://bnfc.nice.org.uk/drug/montelukast.html (accessed September 2019).

British National Formulary for Children (2019p). *Carbocisteine*. https://bnfc.nice.org.uk/drug/carbocisteine.html (accessed September 2019).

British National Formulary for Children (2019q). *Acetylcysteine*. https://bnfc.nice.org.uk/drug/acetylcysteine.html (accessed September 2019).

British National Formulary for Children (2019r). *Dornase alfa*. https://bnfc.nice.org.uk/drug/dornase-alfa.html (accessed September 2019).

BTS/SIGN: British Thoracic Society & Scottish Intercollegiate Guidelines Network (2019). *British guideline on the management of asthma: A national clinical guideline*. https://www.brit-thoracic.org.uk/quality-improvement/guidelines/asthma (accessed September 2019).

British Lung Foundation (2019). *Chronic obstructive pulmonary disease (COPD) statistics*. https://statistics.blf.org.uk/copd (accessed September 2019).

Canning, B.J., Woo, A., and Mazzone, S.B. (2012). Neuronal modulation of airway and vascular tone and their influence on nonspecific airways responsiveness in Asthma. *Journal of Allergy*. https://doi.org/10.1155/2012/108149.

Centre for Disease Control and Prevention (2019). *Flu and people with asthma*. Online. https://www.cdc.gov/flu/highrisk/asthma.htm (accessed September 2019).

Chauhan, B.F., Jeyaraman, M.N., Mann, S. et al. (2017). Addition of anti-leukotriene agents to inhaled corticosteroids for adults and adolescents with persistent asthma. *Cochrane Database of Systematic Reviews* (3): CD010347. https://doi.org/10.1002/14651858.CD010347.pub2.

Chu, D.K., Kim, L.H.N., Young, P.J. et al. (2018). Mortality and morbidity in acutely ill adults treated with liberal versus conservative oxygen therapy (IOTA): a systematic review and meta-analysis. *Lancet* **391**: 1693–1705.

Cole, P.J. (1986). Inflammation: a two-edged sword – the model of bronchiectasis. *European Journal of Respiratory Disease* **147**: 6–15.

Cystic Fibrosis Trust (2019). *UK Cystic Fibrosis Registry Annual Data Report 2018*. https://www.cysticfibrosis.org.uk/~/media/documents/the-work-we-do/uk-cf-registry/2018-registry-annual-data-report.ashx?la=en (accessed September 2019).

Dougherty, L. and Lister, S. (2015). *The Royal Marsden Hospital Manual of Clinical Nursing Procedures*, 9e. West Sussex: Wiley.

Electronic Medicines Compendium (2019a). *Salbutamol*. www.medicines.org.uk/emc/product/6339/smpc (accessed September 2019).

Electronic Medicines Compendium (2019b). *Terbutaline sulfate*. www.medicines.org.uk/emc/product/869/smpc (accessed September 2019).

Electronic Medicines Compendium (2019c). *Salmeterol*. www.medicines.org.uk/emc/product/7228/smpc (accessed September 2019).

Electronic Medicines Compendium (2019d). *Formoterol fumarate*. www.medicines.org.uk/emc/product/312/smpc (accessed September 2019).

Electronic Medicines Compendium (2019e). *Ipratropium bromide*. www.medicines.org.uk/emc/product/3213/smpc (accessed September 2019).

Electronic Medicines Compendium (2019f). *Tiotropium*. www.medicines.org.uk/emc/product/1693/smpc (accessed September 2019).

Electronic Medicines Compendium (2019g). *Theophylline*. www.medicines.org.uk/emc/product/7719/smpc (accessed September 2019).

Electronic Medicines Compendium (2019h). *Aminophylline*. www.medicines.org.uk/emc/product/6560/smpc (accessed September 2019).

Electronic Medicines Compendium (2019i). *Prednisolone*. www.medicines.org.uk/emc/product/1742/smpc (accessed September 2019).

Electronic Medicines Compendium (2019j). *Beclometasone*. www.medicines.org.uk/emc/product/6975/smpc (accessed September 2019).

Electronic Medicines Compendium (2019k). *Budesonide*. www.medicines.org.uk/emc/product/9723/smpc (accessed September 2019).

Electronic Medicines Compendium (2019l). *Fluticasone*. www.medicines.org.uk/emc/product/7601/smpc (accessed September 2019).

Electronic Medicines Compendium (2019m). *Sodium cromoglicate*. www.medicines.org.uk/emc/product/6320/smpc (accessed September 2019).

Electronic Medicines Compendium (2019n). *Nedocromil sodium*. www.medicines.org.uk/emc/product/163/smpc (accessed September 2019).

Electronic Medicines Compendium (2019o). *Montelukast*. www.medicines.org.uk/emc/product/1243/smpc (accessed September 2019).

Electronic Medicines Compendium (2019p). *Carbocisteine*. www.medicines.org.uk/emc/product/6973/smpc (accessed September 2019).

Electronic Medicines Compendium (2019q). *Acetylcysteine*. www.medicines.org.uk/emc/product/2488/smpc (accessed September 2019).

Electronic Medicines Compendium (2019r). *Dornase alfa*. www.medicines.org.uk/emc/product/1112 (accessed September 2019).

Erjefält, J.S. (2014). *Mast cells in human airways: the culprit?*. European Respiratory Review **23**: 299–307. doi: 10.1183/09059180.00005014.

GINA: Global Initiative for Asthma (2019). *2019 GINA Report, Global Strategy for Asthma Management and Prevention*. https://ginasthma.org/wp-content/uploads/2019/06/GINA-2019-main-report-June-2019-wms.pdf (accessed September 2019).

Graeme-Smith, D.G. and Aronson, J.K. (2002). *Oxford Textbook of Clinical Pharmacology and Drug Therapy*, 3e. Oxford: Oxford University Press.

Hardinge, M., Annandale, J., Bourne, S., et al. (2015). *British Thoracic Society guidelines for home oxygen use in adults*. https://thorax.bmj.com/content/thoraxjnl/70/Suppl_1/i1.full.pdf (accessed September 2019).

Hiley, E., Rickards, E., and Kelly, C.A. (2019). Ensuring the safe use of emergency oxygen in acutely ill patients. *Nursing Times* **115**: 18–21.

Hill, A.T., Sullivan, A.L., Chalmers, J.D., et al. (2019). *British Thoracic Society guideline for bronchiectasis in adults*. https://thorax.bmj.com/content/74/Suppl_1/1 (accessed September 2019).

Hurst, J.R., Elborn, S. and De Soyza, A. on behalf of the BRONCH-UK Consortium. (2015). COPD-bronchiectasis overlap syndrome. *European Respiratory Journal* **45**: 310–313. doi: 10.1183/09031936.00170014.

Ibrahim, I. and Choong See, K. (2018). *BMJ Best Practice: Asthma in adults*. https://bestpractice.bmj.com/topics/en-gb/44 (accessed September 2019).

Maselli, D.J., Amalakuhan, B., Keyt, H. and Diaz, A.A. (2017). Suspecting non-cystic fibrosis bronchiectasis: What the busy primary care clinician needs to know. *International Journal of Clinical Practice* **71** (2): e12924.

Miller, M.R., Hankinson, J., Brusasco, V. et al. (2005). Standardisation of spirometry. *European Respiratory Journal* **26**: 319–338.

National Health Service (2018). *Peak flow test.* https://www.nhs.uk/conditions/peak-flow-test (accessed September 2019).

National Institute for Clinical Excellence (2017a). *Cystic fibrosis: diagnosis and management. NICE guideline [NG78].* https://www.nice.org.uk/guidance/ng78 (accessed September 2019).

National Institute for Health and Care Excellence (2017b). *Asthma: diagnosis, monitoring and chronic asthma.* https://www.nice.org.uk/guidance/ng80/chapter/Recommendations#principles-of-pharmacological-treatment (accessed September 2019).

National Institute of Clinical Excellence (2018). *Chronic obstructive pulmonary disease in over 16s: diagnosis and management.* NICE Guideline [NG115]. https://www.nice.org.uk/guidance/ng115 (accessed July 2020).

National Institute of Clinical Excellence (2019a). *Asthma, acute. Levels of severity.* https://bnf.nice.org.uk/treatment-summary/asthma-acute.html (accessed September 2019).

National Institute for Clinical Excellence (2019b). *Chronic obstructive pulmonary disease in over 16s: diagnosis and management.* https://www.nice.org.uk/guidance/ng115 (accessed September 2019).

Neal, M.J. (2015). *Medical Pharmacology at a Glance,* 8e. New York: Wiley.

Nelson, H.S., Weiss, S.T., Bleecker, E.R. et al. (2006). The salmeterol multicenter asthma research trial: a comparison of usual pharmacotherapy for asthma or usual pharmacotherapy plus salmeterol. *Chest* **129** (1): 15–26.

NHS Improvement (2016). *Patient safety alert: Reducing the risk of oxygen tubing being connected to air flowmeters.* https://improvement.nhs.uk/documents/408/Patient_Safety_Alert_-_Reducing_the_risk_of_oxygen_tubing_being_connected_to_a_bDUb2KY.pdf (accessed September 2019).

NHS Improvement (2018a). *Patient safety alert: Risk of death and severe harm from failure to obtain and continue flow from oxygen cylinders.* https://improvement.nhs.uk/documents/2206/Patient_Safety_Alert_-_Failure_to_open_oxygen_cylinders.pdf (accessed September 2019).

NHS Improvement (2018b). *Never events list 2018.* https://improvement.nhs.uk/documents/2266/Never_Events_list_2018_FINAL_v5.pdf (accessed September 2019).

NHS: The National Health Service (2019). *The NHS Long Term Plan.* https://www.longtermplan.nhs.uk/wp-content/uploads/2019/08/nhs-long-term-plan-version-1.2.pdf (accessed September 2019).

O'Donnell, A.E. (2018). *BMJ best practice: bronchiectasis.* https://bestpractice.bmj.com/topics/en-gb/1007 (accessed September 2019).

O'Driscoll, B.R., Howard, L.S., Earis, J. et al. (2017). British Thoracic Society guideline for oxygen use in adults in healthcare and emergency settings. *Thorax* **72** (Supplement 1): 1–90.

Office for National Statistics (2018). *Deaths from asthma, respiratory disease, chronic obstructive pulmonary disease and flu, England and Wales, 2001 to 2017 occurrences.* www.ons.gov.uk/peoplepopulationandcommunity/birthsdeathsandmarriages/deaths/adhocs/009014deathsfromasthmarespiratorydiseasechronicobstructivepulmonarydiseaseandfluenglandandwales2001to2017occurrences (accessed September 2019).

Pinnock, H., Parke, H.L., Panagioti, M., et al. (2017). Systematic meta-review of supported self-management for asthma: a healthcare perspective. *BioMed Central Medicine* **15** (1): 64. doi: 10.1186/s12916-017-0823-7.

Poole, P., Sathananthan, K., and Fortescue, R. (2019). Mucolytic agents versus placebo for chronic bronchitis or chronic obstructive pulmonary disease. *Cochrane Database of Systematic Review* (7): CD001287. https://doi.org/10.1002/14651858.pub6.

Preston, W. and Kelly, C. (2016). *Respiratory Nursing at a Glance.* West Sussex: Wiley.

Public Health England (2015). *Respiratory disease: applying 'All Our Health'.* https://www.gov.uk/government/publications/respiratory-disease-applying-all-our-health/respiratory-disease-applying-all-our-health (accessed September 2019).

Qunit, J.K., Millett, R.C., Joshi, M., et al. (2016). Changes in the incidence, prevalence and mortality of bronchiectasis in the UK from 2004 to 2013: a population-based cohort study. *European Respiratory Journal* **47**: 186–193. doi: 10.1183/13993003.01033-2015.

Ritter, J.M., Flower, R., Henderson, G. et al. (2012). *Rang and Dale's Pharmacology,* 9e. Oxford: Elsevier Ltd.

Siemieniuk, R.A.C., Chu, D.K., Kim, L.H., et al. (2018). *Oxygen therapy for acutely ill medical patients: a clinical practice guideline.* https://www.bmj.com/content/363/bmj.k4169 (accessed September 2019).

Snell, N., Strachan, D., Hubbard, R., et al. (2016). Burden of lung disease in the UK; findings from the British Lung Foundation's 'respiratory health of the nation' project. *European Respiratory Journal* **48**: PA4913. doi: 10.1183/13993003.congress-2016.PA4913.

Soar, J., Deakin, C., Lockey, A. et al. (2015). *Resuscitation Guidelines 2015 Adult Life Support*. London: Resuscitation Council UK.

World Health Organisation (2011). *Pulse Oximetry Training Manual*. https://www.who.int/patientsafety/safesurgery/pulse_oximetry/who_ps_pulse_oxymetry_training_manual_en.pdf?ua=1 (accessed September 2019).

World Health Organisation (2016). *Oxygen therapy for children*. https://apps.who.int/iris/bitstream/handle/10665/204584/9789241549554_eng.pdf;jsessionid=20408069BC3191A6FC42826A2CEAA000?sequence=1 (accessed September 2019).

Further reading

British Thoracic Society (BTS) Guidelines
https://www.brit-thoracic.org.uk/quality-improvement/guidelines
BTS has been at the forefront of guideline production in respiratory medicine for over 30 years. Their guideline production process is accredited by NICE (awarded 2011, renewed 2017).

National Institute of Clinical Excellence (NICE) Guidelines
www.nice.org.uk
NICE provides national guidance and advice to improve health and social care. They provide a number of guidelines concerning all aspects of healthcare delivery. Their aim is to improve health and social care through evidence-based guidance.

Multiple choice questions

1. Which of the following is <u>NOT</u> a characteristic of asthma?
   (a) Decreased airway smooth muscle relaxation
   (b) Increased airway resistance
   (c) Infiltration of immune-active substances into the airways
   (d) Increased mucus production

2. The U-shaped rings that form the framework of the trachea and help to keep it open are composed of:
   (a) Skeletal muscle
   (b) Bone
   (c) Cartilage
   (d) Fibro-elastic tissue

3. Which of the following is <u>NOT</u> part of the conducting zone within the respiratory system?
   (a) Trachea
   (b) Alveoli
   (c) Bronchus
   (d) Tertiary bronchus

4. Naturally occurring (endogenous) glucocorticoids:
   (a) Control salt and water homeostasis (osmoregulation)
   (b) Are released from medulla of the adrenal gland in response to stressor
   (c) Are released from the cortex of the adrenal glands in response to stressor
   (d) Are part of a positive feedback loop that involves the hypothalamus, pituitary gland and the adrenal glands

5. Montelukast mode of action is upon which of the following?
   (a) Cysteinyl-leukotrienereceptor binding sites ($CysLT_1$)
   (b) β_1 receptor binding sites
   (c) Mucin cross-links
   (d) Cytoplasmic Glucocorticoid Receptors

6. Sodium cromoglicate belongs to which class of respiratory drugs?
   (a) Long-acting β_2 agonists (LABA)
   (b) Xanthines
   (c) Mast cell stabilisers
   (d) Leukotriene receptor antagonists
7. Which of the following is NOT part of the NICE diagnostic criteria for COPD?
   (a) Typical symptoms such as chronic cough
   (b) Typical symptoms such as exertional breathlessness
   (c) Presence of a risk factor, e.g. history of smoking
   (d) Age < 35 years
8. Which of the following is a term used for low blood oxygen content?
   (a) Hyperoxia
   (b) Hypoxia
   (c) Hypercarbia
   (d) Hypoxemia
9. Pulse oximetry gives an indication of which of the following?
   (a) Respiratory ventilation in terms of respiratory rate, tidal volume and arterial carbon dioxide
   (b) The percentage of haemoglobin saturated within the blood
   (c) The amount of oxygen dissolved within the arterial content of the blood
   (d) Carbon monoxide poisoning

10. Type II respiratory failure is demonstrated on an arterial blood gas as:
    (a) Low arterial blood content with high arterial carbon dioxide blood content
    (b) High arterial blood content with low arterial carbon dioxide content
    (c) High arterial blood content with high arterial carbon dioxide content
    (d) Low arterial blood content with low arterial carbon dioxide content
11. Select the correct oxygen device with the appropriate oxygen saturation target:
    (a) Nasal cannulae 2–4 L, oxygen saturation target 98–100%
    (b) Simple facemask 5–10 L, oxygen saturation target 88–92%
    (c) Non-rebreathe mask 15 L, oxygen saturation target 85–87%
    (d) Venturi mask 24–28%, oxygen saturation target 88–92%
12. Which of the following does NOT require oxygen therapy?
    (a) A patient with sepsis and saturations of 89%
    (b) A patient with COPD and saturations of 82%
    (c) A patient with an acute stroke and saturations of 93%
    (d) A neonate within the first few hours of life with saturations of 96%
13. Theophylline belongs to the xanthine class of drugs and causes bronchodilation by the following mechanism:
    (a) β_2-adrenoceptor stimulation
    (b) M_3 receptor stimulation
    (c) Inhibits phosphodiesterase
    (d) Leukotriene receptor stimulation
14. Bronchodilators act upon specific receptors resulting in the following effects:
    (a) β_1-adrenoceptors causing bronchoconstriction and M_3 receptors causing bronchodilatation
    (b) β_2-adrenoceptors causing bronchoconstriction and M_2 receptors causing bronchodilatation
    (c) β_2-adrenoceptors causing bronchodilation and M_3 receptors causing bronchodilatation
    (d) β_1-adrenoceptors causing bronchodilation and M_2 receptors causing bronchodilatation

15. With regards to inhaled therapy via an MDI or DPI, which of the following techniques are correct?
    (a) MDI quick and deep, DPI slow and steady
    (b) MDI slow and deep, DPI quick and steady
    (c) MDI slow and steady, DPI quick and deep
    (d) MDI quick and steady, DPI slow and deep

Find out more

The following are a list of conditions that are associated with people who have an exacerbation of their asthma. Take some time to write notes about each of the conditions. Think about the medications that may be used in order to treat these conditions and be specific about the pharmacokinetics and pharmacodynamics. Remember to include aspects of patient care. If you are making notes about people you have offered care and support to, you must ensure that you have adhered to the rules of confidentiality.

The condition	Your notes
Bronchospasm	
Lower-respiratory tract infection (LRTI)	
Type-1 respiratory failure (T1RF)	
Type-2 respiratory failure (T2RF)	
Eosinophilia	

Chapter 14

Medications and the gastrointestinal system

David Waters and Ian Naldrett

Aim

The aim of this chapter is to provide the reader with an introduction to some of the common gastrointestinal conditions and the pharmacological interventions used in their management.

Learning outcomes

After reading this chapter, the reader will:

1. Demonstrate an understanding of common gastrointestinal diseases and disorders, including their causes and clinical presentation
2. Be able to relate the signs and symptoms of common gastrointestinal conditions to their underlying pathophysiology
3. Understand pharmacological treatment options for common gastrointestinal diseases and disorders
4. Recognise the wider care considerations associated with the administration of medications associated with the gastrointestinal tract

Test your knowledge

1. Describe the components and main functions of the gastrointestinal tract.
2. Write down the common gastrointestinal disorders that you have encountered in clinical practice.
3. What are the common routes for the administration of gastrointestinal medications?
4. Identify common causes for constipation and potential interventions for this condition.

Fundamentals of Pharmacology: For Nursing and Healthcare Students, First Edition. Edited by Ian Peate and Barry Hill.
© 2021 John Wiley & Sons Ltd. Published 2021 by John Wiley & Sons Ltd.

Introduction

Normal physiological function of the body is reliant on the consumption, absorption and metabolism of food; the gastrointestinal tract plays an essential role in all of these processes. There are numerous disorders that can influence the normal functions of the gastrointestinal tract; these can include peptic ulcer disease, dyspepsia, disorders associated with the motility of faeces, such as constipation or diarrhoea, and also conditions such as inflammatory bowel disease (IBD). A significant proportion of the United Kingdom general population will experience some gastrointestinal disorder or disturbance at some point, with medications used to treat gastrointestinal disorders comprising of around 8% of all prescriptions in the United Kingdom (Ritter et al., 2020).

This chapter will focus on some of the most common gastrointestinal disorders, specifically peptic ulcer disease, nausea and vomiting, constipation, diarrhoea and IBD. Each section within the chapter will feature an overview of the gastrointestinal disorder and the common medications that are utilised in its management. Additionally, further discussion will be directed toward some of the wider medication administration considerations associated with gastrointestinal nursing care.

Gastroesophageal reflux disease

Gastroesophageal reflux disease (GORD) is a relatively common condition that occurs when there is an abnormal upward movement of gastric contents from the stomach into the oesophagus, with potential development of inflammation of the oesophageal mucosa. This situation occurs when there is a transient relaxation of the oesophageal sphincter, which can be due to gastric distension after a large meal or delayed gastric emptying due to consumption of fatty food or alcohol (Gladson, 2011). GORD is often associated with symptoms of dyspepsia, which can include upper abdominal pain and discomfort, sensations of 'heart burn' and gastric reflux, nausea or vomiting and are typically present for periods of four weeks or more (National Institute for Health and Care Excellence [NICE], 2014). Initial management of dyspepsia symptoms can often be managed by the patient themselves, who may consult a community pharmacist and purchase over-the-counter medications, such as antacids. If symptoms persist, further input from a general practitioner or specialist is recommended.

Clinical considerations

Initial non-pharmacological management of dyspepsia

Prior to commencing medications for GORD or dyspepsia symptoms, patients should be offered lifestyle modification support, which might include advice concerning healthy eating, smoking cessation and losing weight (NICE, 2014). In addition, patients should attempt to avoid known stimulants for their dyspepsia symptoms, which might include avoiding alcohol, chocolate, coffee, smoking or general fatty foods. Additional non-pharmacological interventions for dyspepsia might include sleeping with several pillows to facilitate a raised head position and also to ensure that an evening meal is eaten several hours before retiring to bed (NICE, 2014).

Common medications utilised to treat symptoms of dyspepsia include the use of H_2 receptor antagonists and proton pump inhibitors (PPIs).

H_2 receptor antagonists refer to a group of medications that directly inhibit histamine and gastrin-simulated acid secretion. Commonly used examples of H_2 receptor antagonists include ranitidine, cimetidine, famotidine and nizatidine. They have been found to reduce both basal and food stimulated acid secretion by 90% or more (Ritter et al., 2020) and to also promote the healing of peptic ulcers. However, relapses of peptic ulcer disease have been noted when H_2 receptor antagonists have been discontinued or in the instance of poor user compliance. Their use has also been shown to promote healing in cases of NSAID-related ulcers (Joint Formulary Committee, 2019). The use of this drug group is recommended for patients presenting with functional dyspepsia and for those with un-investigated dyspepsia in the absence of 'warning signs', i.e. upper gastrointestinal bleeding, sudden weight loss, dysphagia or vomiting, which might be suggestive of some sinister pathology (NICE, 2014). H$_2$ receptor antagonists are typically given orally and are generally well absorbed; however, some medications within this group can also be administered as intramuscular or intravenous preparations (Joint Formulary Committee, 2019). The dosage prescribed can vary according to condition and indication for its use. Currently, low-dose preparations of several H$_2$ receptor antagonists can be purchased over-the-counter from pharmacies for short-term use without a prescription (Ritter et al., 2020). Unwanted or adverse effects associated with this group of medications are rare; however, the following have been reported: constipation, diarrhoea, fatigue, dizziness, headache, muscle pains, transient skin rashes, confusion in the elderly and gynecomastia (Joint Formulary Committee, 2019).

PPIs are further medications that inhibit the secretion of gastric acid. Their mechanism of action relies on the blocking of the hydrogen–potassium adenosine triphosphate enzyme system (sometimes referred to as the proton pump) of the acid-producing gastric parietal cell. Common PPIs include omeprazole, esomeprazole, lansoprazole, pantoprazole and rabeprazole sodium. PPIs are utilised across a number of situations, this includes the short-term treatment of peptic ulcers, the eradication of *Helicobacter pylori* in combination with antibiotics, and the general treatment of dyspepsia and GORD and also for the prevention and treatment of non-steroidal anti-inflammatory drug (NSAID)-associated peptic ulcers. Furthermore, high-dose intravenous PPI medication is also commonly utilised following endoscopic interventions for acute and severe bleeding peptic ulcers. PPIs are commonly administered as oral preparations; however, intravenous options are recommended for certain situations. Unwanted side effects of this medication group are uncommon, however they can include: abdominal pain, constipation, vomiting, headache and insomnia.

371

Clinical considerations

Specific adverse reactions to PPIs
The acid suppression action of PPIs is associated with an increased risk of *Clostridium difficile* diarrhoea, especially in vulnerable patient groups, such as the elderly, those who are immuno-suppressed or those patients who are receiving antibiotic therapy (Ritter et al., 2020). Particular attention should be directed toward to these 'at risk' groups, with any new diarrhoea symptoms being proactively investigated and monitored.

Peptic ulcer disease

Peptic ulcers refer to the development of an ulcer in the lower part of the oesophagus, stomach or duodenum (McErlean, 2017). Peptic ulcers can develop when there is an imbalance between mucosal damaging processes (such as the secretion of stomach acids) and the mucosal protective mechanisms (secretion of bicarbonate and mucus). Excessive gastric acid production, in addition to inadequate mucus, can result in the digestive tract being vulnerable to mucosal erosion and development of peptic ulceration (Nair and Peate, 2015) (see Figure 14.1).

A common cause of peptic ulcers is the bacterium *H. pylori*. *H. pylori* infection has been shown to be a causative factor in the development of gastric and duodenal ulcers, in addition to being a risk factor for gastric cancer. *H. pylori* is a spiral shaped, Gram-negative rod bacterium that can be found deep in the gastric mucosal layer. Around 40% of the United Kingdom population are colonised with *H. pylori* in their stomachs; however, of these only around 15% develop gastric or duodenal ulcers. *H. pylori* infection is noted in around 95% of duodenal ulcers and 70% of gastric ulcers (Neal, 2016).

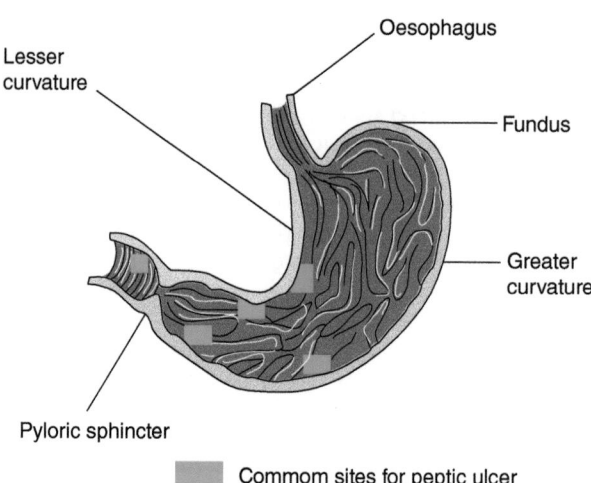

Figure 14.1 Common sites for peptic ulcer. Source: Peate (2018) (3rd Ed) Fundamentals of Applied Pathophysiology Ch 11 Fig 11.16 pp 331.

Clinical considerations

Testing for *H. pylori*

It is recommended practice to test for *H. pylori* in patients that present with symptoms associated with GORD or dyspepsia (NICE, 2014). There are several ways to test for *H. pylori* colonisation, these include:

A blood sample which is sent for serology analysis and aims to detect antibodies specific to the bacterium.

A carbon-13 urea breath test. This involves the oral administration of urea which is made from an isotope of carbon. If *H. pylori* is present in the stomach, the urea is broken up and turned into carbon dioxide. Samples of exhaled breath are collected and the isotopic carbon in the exhaled carbon dioxide is measured.

A stool sample can be gathered and screened for *H. pylori* antibodies.

Alternatively, a biopsy can be taken from the gastric tract during an endoscopy procedure, which can be analysed for the presence of the bacterium.

Following a positive *H. pylori* test result, eradication can be achieved with a one-week course of triple therapy, which includes a PPI (such as esomeprazole, lansoprazole, omeprazole, pantoprazole or rabeprazole) in combination with amoxicillin and either clarithromycin or metronidazole, or for those with a penicillin allergy, clarithromycin and metronidazole (NICE, 2014).

Clinical considerations

Compliance with eradication therapy

A successful eradication of *H. pylori* is achieved in around 90% of patients who undergo triple therapy (Galbraith et al., 2007). To promote an effective eradication process, it is essential that the patient fully adheres to the prescribed regimen. They should be encouraged to take the full week's course of medications and seek advice from their prescribing clinician if they experience any adverse reactions.

Further potential causes for peptic ulcer disease include the use of NSAIDs, which include medications such as aspirin, naproxen and ibuprofen. NSAIDs inhibit prostaglandins, which would normally have a protective effect on the mucosal lining within the gastric tract. Other risk factors for the development of peptic ulcer disease are smoking and alcohol; however, the exact causative mechanism here is unknown. Pharmacological treatment of peptic ulcer disease that is not associated with *H. pylori* does not require an antibiotic, instead the use of an H₂-receptor antagonist (such as ranitidine) usually is effective in promoting ulcer healing.

Episode of care: Peptic ulcer disease

Mohammed Saied is a 32-year-old male, who is employed as a senior manager within an accountancy company. He tends to work long hours, smokes 10 cigarettes a day and eats a diet which often consists of take-away food. Mohammed has recently started experiencing dyspepsia type symptoms, which have included severe 'heart burn' sensations and abdominal discomfort. Initially he managed these symptoms with an antacid preparation which he purchased from his local pharmacy; however, this only brought temporary relief. On recommendation of the pharmacist, Mohammed sought a consultation with his general practitioner, who proposed a potential diagnosis of GORD. To investigate the potential cause of Mohammed's dyspepsia, the GP took a blood sample to detect *H. pylori* antibodies, he also commenced a short course of the PPI medication omeprazole. The *H. pylori* antibody blood test later produced a positive test, so in response the GP later prescribed a week's course of amoxicillin and clarithromycin antibiotics, in addition to continuing the omeprazole. Mohammed was reviewed by his GP following his *H. pylori* eradication therapy and reported a significant improvement in his dyspepsia symptoms, with minimal abdominal discomfort or 'heart burn.' To ensure that his dyspepsia remained controlled, the GP continued the prescription for omeprazole and requested a follow-up appointment in three months.

373

Nausea and vomiting

Nausea and vomiting are known to have many causes, these include medications (i.e. opioids, anaesthetics and chemotherapy agents), migraines, pregnancy and provocative movement (i.e. sea sickness). Consequently, most patients will experience nausea and/or vomiting during their disease journey, either a direct result of pathophysiology, or due to the treatments they are receiving.

Vomiting is considered a defensive response, which is associated with the forceful expulsion of gastric contents through the mouth (Peate, 2013).

Clinical considerations

Anti-emetic prescriptions

Anti-emetic medications should only be prescribed when the cause of the vomiting is known, as administration may mask symptoms and delay diagnosis (Joint Formulary Committee, 2019). In some situations, anti-emetics can be unnecessary and potentially harmful to the patient, especially in cases where the cause of the vomiting/nausea can easily be corrected, i.e. in cases of diabetic ketoacidosis.

There are numerous medications which can be utilised to manage nausea. It is vital, however, that the appropriate anti-emetic is chosen and matched to the aetiology of the nausea or vomiting.

H$_1$ receptor antagonists or antihistamines are the most commonly used anti-emetics, which are effective in treating nausea and vomiting due to a variety of causes, such as motion sickness, because of opioid use or morning sickness associated with pregnancy. Examples of H$_1$ receptor antagonists or antihistamines include cyclizine, cinnarizine and promethazine.

A further group of anti-emetic medications are the 5-HT$_3$ receptor antagonists, which act by blocking serotonin receptors located in the central nervous system and gastrointestinal tract. Their use is often indicated in nausea and vomiting encountered post-operatively and for patients following radiotherapy or chemotherapy (Ritter et al., 2020). Examples include the medications ondansetron, granisetron and palonosetron. 5-HT$_3$ medications can be given orally; however, in the context of nausea and vomiting, intravenous or intramuscular administration may be preferable. Common side effects associated with this medication group include constipation, headache and diarrhoea.

D$_2$ or dopamine receptor antagonists include antipsychotic phenothiazine medications, such as chlorpromazine, perphenazine, prochlorperazine and trifluoperazine. These medications are also effective anti-emetics and are commonly used for the management of nausea and vomiting associated with cancer, due to chemotherapy, opioids or anaesthetic agents. They can be administered orally, but also by intravenous or intramuscular injection, or by suppository. A further D$_2$ receptor antagonist closely related to the phenothiazine group of medications is metoclopramide. In addition to its anti-emetic effect, metoclopramide also increases gastrointestinal tract motility.

374

Gut motility and defaecation

The large intestine is made up of five key sections:

- the ascending colon
- the transverse colon
- the descending colon
- the sigmoid colon
- the rectum
- the anus.

See Figure 14.2.

The large intestine's constituent parts all have a role in either the formation of stool or the holding/storage of stool before defaecation. Within the large intestine itself, three to four days' worth of meals will be present. The ascending colon receives faeces from the cecum where 90% of the absorption of nutrients will have already happened. The transverse colon plays a large role in processing the faeces and the descending colon acts a holding area for faeces for up to 24 hours. The sigmoid colon and rectum also act as reservoirs for stool before defaecation.

Constipation

Constipation is defined as passing fewer than three stools per week and/or straining, hard stools or a sense of incomplete evacuation ≥25% of the time (NHS, 2019).

Symptoms that can be associated with constipation include:

- Abdominal discomfort, pain and bloating.
- Lethargy and malaise.
- 'Spurious diarrhoea' in frail faecally impacted patients.

(NICE 2019)

The prevalence of constipation is thought to affect around 20% of UK adults (Bladder and Bowel UK, 2019). It is important to remember that constipation is a symptom rather than an illness in its own right. Constipation can have a different definition between patients, as patients recognise their own bowel habit and major changes to that. There is a great variation

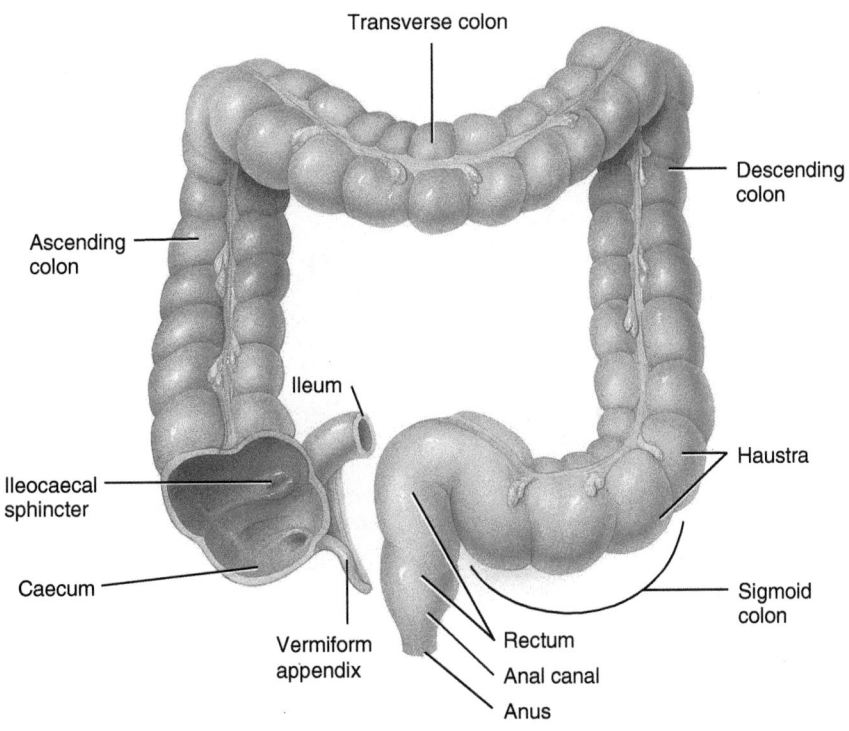

Figure 14.2 The large intestine. Source: Fundamentals of Anatomy and Physiology: For Nursing and Healthcare Students. Peate and Nair (2017) (2nd ed), Chapter 9 figure 9.15, page 279.

in the normal range of bowel movements in adults ranging from three to 12 per week. Therefore, changes to normal bowel habit should be noted alongside the objective definition of constipation when treating patients.

The assessment of constipation should include

- What the person means by 'constipation' and their normal pattern of defaecation.
- The person's perception of a normal bowel habit may influence the diagnosis of constipation.
- The duration of constipation and the frequency and consistency of stools, such as hard/small (pebble-like) or large stools (for example, do they block the toilet); any nocturnal symptoms.
- Consider the use of the Bristol Stool Chart to provide an objective record of the person's stool form.
- Associated symptoms such as rectal discomfort, excessive straining, feeling of incomplete evacuation or rectal bleeding; abdominal pain or distension.
- Note: pelvic floor dyssynergia may be suggested by straining and a feeling of incomplete evacuation.
- Associated fever, nausea, vomiting, loss of appetite and/or weight.
- Associated urinary symptoms, urinary incontinence or retention, dyspareunia.
- Any family history of colorectal cancer or IBD.
- How symptoms affect the person and impact on quality of life and daily functioning.
- Any self-help measures or drug treatments tried, including over-the-counter medication and symptom response.

Source: NICE 2019.

Commonly prescribed medications taken for other indications can also cause constipation, these include opiate analgesics (such as morphine and codeine), anticholinergic drugs (such as antidepressants and anxiolytics) and other drug classes (such as ferrous sulphate). These should be reviewed by the nursing and medical team when treating patients suffering from constipation.

Medications used in constipation

Medications used to relieve constipation can be put in to the following classes:

- bulk laxatives
- emollients/faecal softeners
- stimulant laxatives
- osmotic laxatives
- saline laxatives
- peripheral opioid antagonists.

The choice of medication should both be based on the best available evidence of efficacy, the suspected mechanism of constipation and patient choice and lifestyle assessment.

Bulk laxatives

Bulk laxatives work by increasing the bulk of the stool through absorbing water into a viscous solution or gel. The result being that increased bulk can stimulate peristalsis and the water that has been absorbed softens the stool. Equally bulk laxatives increase the bacterial growth and weight of the stool, further stimulating the intestinal wall to cause peristalsis. These laxatives can take up to 72 hours to work in action and can be combined with other laxative classes. This class can be useful when fibre intake cannot be increased further. Bulk laxatives are given orally in either tablet form or powder for oral solution.
Medications in this class include:

- ispaghula husk, oral solution – Fybogel®
- methylcellulose, oral tablet – Celevac®
- sterculia, oral solution – Normacol®.

Emollients and faecal softeners

This class of drugs works by reducing the surface tension of the faecal mass allowing it to be penetrated by aqueous intestinal fluids, they also reduce the re-absorption of fluid and electrolytes by the intestinal wall. Different examples of this class of drug can be given by multiple routes, such as docusate sodium that can be given orally or per rectum in the form of a suppository. Other rectal preparations include enemas containing arachis oil that lubricate and soften the stool; however, this should not be administered to those with nut allergies as this originates from ground nut oil.
Medications in this class include:

- docusate sodium – oral capsule, liquid or rectal suppository
- arachis oil – enema
- liquid paraffin – oral liquid
- stimulant laxatives.

These drugs work in different ways depending on their subtype to stimulate peristalsis of the intestine. They have a direct action on the mucosa or the nerve plexus. A considerable drawback of these medications is that they cause abdominal cramping and are not recommended in abdominal obstruction. Bisacodyl can be given orally or rectally as a suppository, orally acting within 10–12 hours, rectally acting in less than 60 minutes.
Senna is an anthraquinone that contains sennosides which are activated by bacteria in the intestine that then irritate the mucosal lining to produce peristalsis. Senna itself comes from a

plant extract; overuse of senna can cause drug dependence, damaging the intestine's haustral folds, making the intestine less able to move stool through peristalsis.

Co-danthramer is a combination of Dantron (a stimulant laxative) and Poloxamer 188 (stool softener) and is primarily used in palliative care to alleviate constipation related to opioid use; it is not recommended for other types of constipation due to concerns regarding its potential carcinogenic properties.

Medications in this class include:

- Bisacodyl – oral capsule or rectal suppository
- senna – oral solution/tablet – Sennakot®
- co-danthramer – oral capsule
- osmotic laxatives.

These medications are mainly non-absorbable solutions. They work by increasing the amount of water in the intestine.

Lactulose is an osmotic laxative of note, a disaccharide sugar of fructose and galactose it produces an osmotic effect and a low faecal pH; it discourages the proliferation of ammonia-producing bacteria and therefore is useful in the treatment of hepatic encephalopathy. Lactulose is metabolised in the intestinal lumen by enteric bacteria as it is not able to broken down by human enzymes, it is broken down in to short chain fatty acids including lactic acid and acetic acid. Its metabolites also increase peristalsis and have further osmotic effect until they leave the body in the faeces.

Sorbitol, a sugar alcohol and a sweetener used in some diet foods, is also an osmotic laxative that can be used to treat constipation and can also cause diarrhoea in excessive consumption.

Medications in this class include:

- lactulose – oral solution
- macrogol 3350 in combination with other electrolyte solutions – oral powder Movicol® Moviprep®
- phosphate – oral solution and enema Fleet®.

Saline laxatives

Saline laxatives attract and retain water in the intestine. They are made up of magnesium in different preparations. Excessive ingestions of orally supplemented magnesium to correct electrolyte imbalance can cause diarrhoea through the same action. Magnesium-based saline laxatives also stimulate the release of cholecystokinin, which increases intestinal motility and fluid secretion.

Medications in this class include:

- magnesium hydroxide
- magnesium sulphate
- sodium phosphate.

Peripheral opioid antagonists

Peripheral opioid antagonists reduce the constipating effects of opioid analgesics while not interfering with the central analgesic action of the opioid medication being given. They are only indicated for constipation which is linked to the use of opioid analgesia after other laxatives have proven ineffective; these medications are considerably more expensive than other laxative classes.

Medications in this class include:

- naloxegal.

Non-pharmacological treatment of constipation

While many medications exist, non-pharmacological options can be used to manage constipation symptoms and help to stop them from re-occurring. Adequate fluid intake is crucial in preventing constipation and in aiding laxative medications to work: 1600 to 2000 mL per day of oral fluids is recommended (BDA, 2017) in aiding gastrointestinal transit. This aids transit of faeces through the small and large intestine; diuretic fluids such as coffee or cola that contain caffeine are less effective at keeping fluid within the colon intestine itself. Adequate fibre intake is also important in maintaining effective gastrointestinal transit. An adult should have an intake of 30 g of dietary fibre per day, slowly increased to this to reduce flatulence and bloating (NICE, 2019), which is best obtained from high fibre and whole grain foods such as fruits, grains that contain bran and vegetables.

The neglect of the call to stool

The cause of constipation may originate from social reasons or may be due to illness or surgery. The result is that large intestine becomes used to being distended by faeces and loses the ability to contract. In short-term constipation, pharmacological treatment orally will usually be sufficient in returning bowel habit; however, in chronic constipation the aim of treatment and health promotion is to re-educate the intestine by increasing the bulk of the faeces by consuming a high fibre diet or by giving prescribed bulk forming laxatives. Equally, ensuring that patients understand that when they have the urge to pass stool not to ignore it, as this can cause functional constipation (Bladder and Bowel UK, 2019).

Episode of care: Constipation

Mr. John Whittingham is a 55-year-old mobile salesman for a telecommunications company. John has been working in the field for the past ten years and recently due to changes in his company his workload and geographical area has increased. He has attended his local walk-in centre due to feeling bloated and a noticeable reduction in bowel activity, he was unable to obtain a GP appointment at his registered surgery.

On subjective assessment by the advanced clinical practitioner (ACP) in the walk-in centre. John reports that he has noticed a change in his bowel habit over the past six months. He used to go 'regularly', which he identified as five to seven bowel movements a week, which has now reduced to three times on average per week with difficulty. He reports that the stool is now hard and difficult to pass at times. He reports driving long distances often without access to toilet facilities and says 'sometimes I have to hold it in whilst driving till my next destination'. He reports that due to his larger area of work his diet has deteriorated and he is eating more 'convenience food' and his weight has increased.

John's past medical history includes: gastritis, gout and hypertension. John does not take any regular medication. On physical examination, the ACP finds no physical abnormality apart from the formation of haemorrhoids which John says has got progressively worse with excessive straining. There are no red flags present such as bleeding or abdominal masses. There is no family history of bowel cancer; however, screening advice was given that he would enter the NHS bowel screening program at 55.

The ACP asks if John has been self-managing his symptoms at all by taking over-the-counter medications or performing any lifestyle changes. John reports he has not currently and this is his first contact with health services since his bowel habit has changed.

The ACP diagnoses John with chronic constipation as these symptoms have been ongoing for more than three months. Therefore the ACP gives the following advice: that constipation itself is a condition that can be influenced by lifestyle changes, such as having a high fibre diet that is rich in fruit vegetables and legumes, and suggesting John pre-makes meals such as breakfast with oat based recipes to fit around his working life; that he should make regular and scheduled toilet breaks and avoid ignoring it when he feels the need to pass stool and to avoid straining; ensure that he has sufficient fluid intake of at least 1500 mL of water per day and increase his amount of physical exercise. Also, that if symptoms change or do not resolve, he must report back to his general practice or local health services.

The ACP advises following this lifestyle advice before taking over-the-counter medications for constipation, or returning for further investigation and prescription of medication.

Skills in practice: How to administer a phosphate enema

Preparation and equipment

The nurse should have an understanding of the anatomy of the rectum prior to administering. All equipment required should be available and to hand including:

- prescription
- the prescribed enema (checking the expiration date)
- a jug of lukewarm water
- tissues
- lubricating gel
- bed cover/incontinence sheet
- there should be a good source of light
- personal protective equipment.

Procedure

- Confirm the patient's identity against their medicine administration record, explain to the patient the procedure and gain consent.
- Assess the patient's need for assistance to assume the correct position.
- Ask the patient to empty their bladder before administration if necessary.
- Assist patient to remove clothing from waist down, ensuring they are not unduly exposed and maintaining warmth and dignity.
- Assist patient to adopt the left lateral position with knees up drawn to chest (check patient has no musculoskeletal disorder that contraindicates this position).
- Warm the enema in the jug of water (following manufacturer's instructions).
- Wash hands and don personal protective equipment, place incontinence sheet under patient.
- Continually explain what you are doing, remembering the patient is facing away from you and cannot see what you are doing, pay particular attention if the patient has a sensory deficit such as hearing disorders.
- Gently part the buttocks, inspecting the perineal area for abnormality.
- Remove the protective cap, placing lubricating gel on the end of the enema nozzle.
- Expel excess air from the enema.
- Gently introduce the enema nozzle into the anus and rectum, usually around 5 cm.
- Deploy the contents of the enema slowly continually informing the patient of what you are doing.
- Stop if the patient experiences pain or bleeding and seek further advice at this time from a senior clinician.
- Slowly remove the nozzle.
- Ensure the patient is clean; if they are able to clean themselves, ensure they have appropriate tissue and assist them in disposing of this.
- Cover the patient ensuring dignity, asking the patient to retain the enema for 10–15 minutes before using the commode or toilet.
- Dispose of equipment safely, adhering to local polices and guidelines.
- Ensure the patient has access to a call bell or way of alerting you if they need assistance.
- Document administration of the enema and the result of administration, utilising the Bristol stool chart to document any bowel movement.

Source: Adapted from Peate (2015).

Diarrhoea

Diarrhoea is an unpleasant condition where stools are loose, without solids, and watery; it can have many causes and can be a symptom of other conditions. Most people get diarrhoea at some point in their lives and most of the time it can be self-managed without medications (NICE, 2019). However it can have profound consequences for morbidity and mortality in at risk groups such as the elderly and the very young (Crombie et al., 2013).

It can be classified into acute diarrhoea – of which the duration of symptoms are less than four weeks – and chronic diarrhoea – of which the symptoms have a duration of over four weeks (NICE, 2018).

The condition can be placed in a subgroup, relating to the cause of the diarrhoea.

Osmotic diarrhoea	Secretory diarrhoea	Inflammatory diarrhoea
Osmotic diarrhoea is caused when too much water is drawn into intestine by osmosis, when a non-absorbable substance such as an osmotic laxative has been ingested. This could also be related to malabsorption such as in coeliac disease and pancreatic insufficiency	Secretory diarrhoea occurs when there are increased secretions from the intestinal tract, including electrolytes. There can also be decreased absorption. This is caused by abnormal mediators such as bacterial enterotoxins, bile salts (after ileal resection) and some laxative medications	This is caused by damage to the intestinal mucosal cells leading to a loss of fluid, blood and defective absorption of fluid and electrolytes. Common causes include infective conditions such as dysentery due to shigella and inflammatory conditions such as ulcerative colitis, Crohn's disease and coeliac disease

Source: Adapted from Crombie et al. (2013).

The Bristol stool chart can be used to classify stool form and help in the assessment and treatment of diarrhoea (see Figure 14.3).

Type	Description
1	Separate hard lumps, similar to nuts and difficult to pass
2	Sausage-shaped, but lumpy
3	Like a sausage but with cracks on its surface
4	Like a sausage or snake, smooth and soft
5	Soft blobs with clear cut edges (easy to pass)
6	Fluffy pieces with ragged edges, a mushy stool
7	Watery, no solid pieces, entirely liquid

NICE have developed assessment questions to assist in the assessment of acute diarrhoea.

Type	Description
1	Separate hard lumps, similar to nuts and difficult to pass
2	Sausage-shaped, but lumpy
3	Like a sausage but with cracks on its surface
4	Like a sausage or snake, smooth and soft
5	Soft blobs with clear cut edges (easy to pass)
6	Fluffy pieces with ragged edges, a mushy stool
7	Watery, no solid pieces, entirely liquid

Figure 14.3   The Bristol stool chart.

Determine the onset, duration, frequency and severity of symptoms

Enquire about the presence of red flag symptoms:
   Blood in the stool.
   Recent hospital treatment or antibiotic treatment. For more information, see the CKS topic on diarrhoea – antibiotic associated.
   Weight loss.
   Evidence of dehydration.
   Nocturnal symptoms – organic cause more likely.

Attempt to ascertain the underlying cause. Assess for:
   Quantity and character of stools (watery, fatty, containing blood or mucus).
   Features suggesting infection, such as fever and vomiting.
   Recent contact with a person with diarrhoea.
   Exposure to possible sources of enteric infection (for example, having eaten meals out, or recent farm or petting zoo visits).
   Travel abroad – increases the likelihood of infection. Ask about potential exposures such as raw milk or untreated water.
   Being in a higher risk group, such as food handlers, nursing home residents and recently hospitalised people.
   Any new drugs, especially antibiotics or laxatives.
   Stress or anxiety.
   Abdominal pain, which is often present in IBD, irritable bowel syndrome and ischemic colitis.
   History of recent radiation treatment to the pelvis.
   Factors increasing the risk of immunosuppression (for example, human immunodeficiency virus infection, long-term steroid use or chemotherapy).
   Any surgery or medical conditions (for example, endocrine disease) accounting for the diarrhoea.
   Diet and use of alcohol or substances such as sorbitol.
   Assess for complications of diarrhoea, such as dehydration.
   Features indicating dehydration include increased pulse rate, reduced skin turgor, dryness of mucus membranes, delayed capillary refill time, decreased urine output, hypotension (check for postural changes) and altered mental status. For more detail, see Clinical Features of dehydration.
   Also consider underlying conditions that may increase the risk of complications.
   If trained to do so and it is safe to proceed, perform an abdominal examination to assess for pain or tenderness, distension, mass, increased or decreased bowel sounds, or liver enlargement.
   Consider a rectal examination to assess for rectal tenderness, stool consistency, and for blood, mucus and possible malignancy (caution patients at risk of autonomic dysreflexia).
   If acute causes have been excluded and the person has features suggestive of an early presentation of a chronic cause, see chronic diarrhoea (more than four weeks).

Source: (NICE 2018)

Drugs used in the treatment of diarrhoea

It is important to note although medications exist for the treatment of diarrhoea, the cause of the diarrhoea should be assessed and infective diarrhoea should be excluded, as antidiarrhoeal medication could impede recovery. Furthermore, it should be noted that most episodes of diarrhoea will settle without treatment.

381

The management of diarrhoea should focus on the assessment and then reversal of fluid and electrolyte depletion, this is particularly important in the frail, elderly population and children.

Oral rehydration salts are widely available and contain a combination of electrolytes and sugars made up with water to replace sodium, potassium and fluids. These should be made as per instructions to ensure that they are of the correct concentration to aid absorption and correction of body fluid composition.

Loperamide

The main antidiarrhoeal drug that is widely used is loperamide; this drug is an opioid receptor agonist that acts on the myenteric plexus of the intestine. This then slows peristalsis allowing more time for the intestine to absorb water from the contents of the intestine, which leads to less watery and more formed stool. It is taken orally; however, it behaves differently to other opiates in that its efflux by P-glycoprotein in the intestinal wall reduces its passage into the circulation, equally first-pass metabolism by the liver further reduces its distribution. This reduction and efflux by the P-glycoprotein prevents circulating loperamide from effectively crossing the blood–brain barrier and exerting the neurological effects of the other opioid class of drugs.

Caution should be taken with patients taking loperamide in large doses or in an overdose situation, as it can prolong the QTc segment of the ECG, leading to life-threatening arrhythmias including Torsade's de pointes leading to cardiac arrest. However, these effects are only seen in large or overdoses and at recommended doses this does not normally occur. The recreational use of loperamide can have central nervous system affects and dependency can occur.

Loperamide in excessive doses can be a drug of abuse due to its opioid properties, in overdose the effects can be reversed using naloxone; however, it is important to note that the half-life of naloxone (around 1–3 hours) is shorter than that of Loperamide and repeated dosing may need to take place and the patient observed for up to 48 hours after the overdose for CNS depression (MacDonald et al., 2015).

Inflammatory bowel disease

IBD is an umbrella term that includes two main long-term conditions: ulcerative colitis and Crohn's disease. Although IBD mainly includes these two diseases, there are less common diseases also under the umbrella of IBD that include microscopic colitis. Most diagnoses for IBD occur between the ages of 15 and 45 years.

Ulcerative colitis

This is a long-term condition that affects the intestine up to the rectum. The intestine becomes inflamed and small ulcers appear that can bleed and have pus-like exudate. This causes symptoms including diarrhoea with blood and mucus in the stool, weight loss and anaemia.

The cause of ulcerative colitis is unknown; it affects about one in every 420 people in the UK (Crohns and Colitis UK, 2019). The management of ulcerative colitis depends on the extent of the disease and can include medications, surgery and diet/lifestyle changes.

Crohn's disease

Crohn's disease is a long-term condition that can affect any part of the gastrointestinal (GI) tract from mouth to anus. It affects up to one people in every 650 people in the UK population (Crohn's and Colitis UK, 2019). Symptoms can include abdominal pain, increased frequency of bowel movements (up to 20 a day) and diarrhoea, which can be watery or porridge like in consistency depending on where the majority of the disease sits in the GI tract.

The cause of Crohn's disease is unknown but is thought to be multifactorial including environmental factors and genetic predisposition.

Main medications used in IBD include the following.

Glucocorticoid

The glucocorticoid class of medication can be used to manage inflammation both in ulcerative colitis or Crohn's disease. These can be administered orally or intravenously in severe cases. These medications when used long term can have profound side effects including weight gain and steroid-induced diabetes (prolonged hyperglycaemia). Their use is recommended in acute severe ulcerative colitis by NICE (2019) and for the management of Crohn's disease in inducing remission.

Aminosalicylates

Aminosalicylates are drugs with anti-inflammatory properties that are similar in structure to aspirin. They are used in the control of inflammation once the patient is in remission and are effective in ulcerative colitis and colonic Crohn's disease. They can have side effects including serious blood disorders where the white blood cell count is reduced.

Drugs in this class include:

- sulfasalazine
- mesalazine.

Immunosuppression

Immunosuppressants reduce the action of the immune system, which with IBD causes the inflammation. These drugs inhibit either the production of immune cells or proinflammatory proteins that cause inflammation. There are risks of being immunocompromised that leave the patient more susceptible to infection, but this is often outweighed by the benefits in severe disease. They are often used in conjunction with steroid medication and can reduce the dose of steroids the patient needs to manage the disease, thus reducing the side effects of taking high dose steroids.

Drugs in this class include:

- azathioprine
- methotrexate.

Infliximab and adalimumab

These drugs are known as mono-clonal antibodies, they inhibit the powerful proinflammatory protein Tissue Necrosing Factor Alpha or TNF-α, which is a proinflammatory cytokine that signals the release of further inflammatory cascade. These drugs are administered intravenously. Usually the patient is admitted to a day unit where the patient can be monitored while administration is taking place as they are at risk of severe immunological reactions; resuscitation facilities should be available in areas that administer these drugs intravenously (Joint Formulary Committee, 2019). These drugs are used in severe disease non-responsive to other medications.

Clinical considerations

With immunosuppressant medication and aminosalicylates, there is a risk of suppressed white blood cell and platelet counts leading to infection, bleeding and bruising. If patients experience these symptoms, they should seek medical help immediately.

Conclusion

This chapter has provided an overview of medication used in the treatment of common gastrointestinal disorders. A short overview of each disorder has been provided, followed by the evidence that supports the use of specific drugs, their actions, adverse effects and the administration considerations. The wider issues associated with medication administration in gastrointestinal care, including patient education, referral onto specialist services and other treatment options has been explored.

References

Bladder and Bowel UK (2019). *Constipation in adults*. www.bbuk.org.uk (accessed 16 October 2019).

British Dietetic Association (BDA) (2017). *Food fact sheet: fluids*. www.bda.uk.com/foodfacts/fluid.pdf (accessed 9 November 2019).

Joint Formulary Committee (2019). *British National Formulary*, 78e. BMJ Group and Pharmaceutical Press: London.

Crohns and Colitis UK (2019). *How common is Crohns disease*. www.crohnsandcolitis.org.uk/about-crohns-and-colitis/publications/crohns-disease (accessed 9 November 2019).

Crombie, H., Gallagher, R. and Hall, V. (2013). Assessment and management of diarrhoea. *Nursing Times* **109** (30): 22–24.

Galbraith, A., Bullock, S., Manias, E. et al. (2007). *Fundamentals of Pharmacology. An Applied Approach for Nursing and Health*, 2e. Pearson Education Ltd: Harlow.

Gladson, B. (2011). *Pharmacology for Rehabilitation Professionals*, 2e. Elsevier Saunders: St Louis, USA.

MacDonald, R., Heiner, J., Villarreal, J. and Strote, J. (2015). *Loperamide dependence and abuse*. BMJ Case Reports: pp. bcr2015209705-bcr2015209705.

McErlean, L. (2017). The gastrointestinal system and associated disorders. In: *Fundamentals of Applied Pathophysiology. An Essential Guide for Nursing and Healthcare Students*, 3e (eds. M. Nair and I. Peate), 306–337. Oxford: Wiley Blackwell.

Nair, M. and Peate, I. (2015). *Pathophysiology for Nurses at a Glance*. Oxford: Wiley Blackwell.

National Health Service (NHS) (2019). *Constipation*. https://www.nhs.uk/conditions/constipation (accessed 16 October 2019).

National Institute for Health and Care Excellence (NICE) (2014). *Gastro-oesophageal reflux disease and dyspepsia in adults: investigation and management. Clinical guideline [CG184]*. www.nice.org.uk/guidance/cg184 (accessed 16 October 2019).

National Institute for Health and Care Excellence (NICE) (2018). *Scenario: Acute diarrhoea (less than 4 weeks)*. https://cks.nice.org.uk/diarrhoea-adults-assessment#!scenario (accessed 16 October 2019).

National Institute for Health and Care Excellence (NICE) (2019). *Scenario: Constipation in adults*. https://cks.nice.org.uk/constipation#!scenario (accessed 16 October 2019).

Neal, M.J. (2016). *Medical Pharmacology at a Glance*, 8e. Wiley Blackwell: Oxford.

Peate, I. (2013). Fluid and electrolyte balance and associated disorders. In: *Fundamentals of Applied Pathophysiology. An Essential Guide for Nursing and Healthcare Students*, 2e (eds. M. Nair and I. Peate), 500–525. Oxford: Wiley Blackwell.

Peate, I. (2015). How to administer an enema. *Nursing Standard* **30** (14): 34–36.

Ritter, J.M., Flower, R., Henderson, G. et al. (2020). *Rang and Dale's Pharmacology*, 9e. Elsevier: Edinburgh.

Tortora, G., Gerard, J. and Derrickson, B. (2017). *Principles of Anatomy and Physiology*, 15e. Wiley: Chichester.

Further reading

If you would like to explore any specific areas of gastrointestinal care and medications used within this specialism in more depth, you may want to consult some of the following resources and organisations:

The National Institute for Health and Care Excellence
The Scottish Inter Collegiate Guidelines Network
British Society of Gastroenterology
British Pharmacological Society.

Multiple choice questions

1. Dyspepsia refers to symptoms of
   (a) Constipation
   (b) Upper abdominal pain and discomfort, sensations of 'heart burn', nausea and vomiting
   (c) Diarrhoea
   (d) Lower abdominal discomfort and bloating
2. An example of a H_2 receptor antagonist medication is:
   (a) Cimetidine
   (b) Esomeprazole
   (c) Pantoprazole
   (d) Omeprazole
3. The use of PPIs is associated with an increased risk of what condition:
   (a) Atrial fibrillation
   (b) *Clostridium difficile* diarrhoea
   (c) Migraine headaches
   (d) Hair loss
4. How do NSAIDs contribute to the development of peptic ulcers?
   (a) NSAIDs promote acid production by parietal cells
   (b) Due NSAIDs promotion of motility through the GI tract
   (c) NSAIDs increase the risk of *H. pylori* infections, which are associated with the development of peptic ulcers
   (d) NSAIDs inhibit prostaglandins, which normally have a protective effect on the mucosal lining of the GI tract
5. A course of *H. pylori* eradication therapy will commonly consist of
   (a) A H_2 receptor antagonist, a PPI and an antibiotic
   (b) A PPI and one antibiotic
   (c) A PPI and two antibiotics
   (d) Two antibiotics only
6. A course of *H. pylori* eradication therapy is recommended to be for how long
   (a) One month
   (b) One week
   (c) Two weeks
   (d) Six months
7. An example of a H_1 receptor antagonist antiemetic is:
   (a) Chlorpromazine
   (b) Ondanestron
   (c) Metaclopramide
   (d) Cyclizine
8. Which anti-emetic also increases gastrointestinal tract motility?
   (a) Metoclopramide
   (b) Prochlorperazine
   (c) Granisetron
   (d) Cyclizine
9. Chronic constipation is classified as an episode of symptoms lasting over:
   (a) Two weeks
   (b) Three weeks
   (c) One month
   (d) Three months

10. Shigella is an organism that's is associated with the causation of which subtype of diarrhoea?
    (a) Osmotic diarrhoea
    (b) Secretory diarrhoea
    (c) Inflammatory diarrhoea
    (d) Its associated with constipation not diarrhoea

11. Loperamide is an antidiarrhoeal drug that is associated with the following complications when taken in extreme doses:
    (a) Urticarial rash
    (b) Long QT syndrome leading to risk of cardiac arrhythmia
    (c) Hair loss
    (d) Postural hypotension

12. The immunosuppressant medication infliximab binds to which cytokine preventing it from binding to its receptor in cells?
    (a) TNF-α
    (b) Bradykinin
    (c) TGF-β1
    (d) Interleukin-1

13. Senna is a plant extract that is used as a laxative medication, what statement best describes its action within the body?
    (a) Bulk forming laxative; senna adds bulk to the stool to distend the intestinal wall
    (b) Stimulant laxative; the metabolites of senna irritate the intestinal wall increasing peristalsis
    (c) Osmotic laxative; senna causes the movement of water into the bowel
    (d) Peripheral opioid antagonist, senna binds to peripheral opioid receptors in the intestine to reduce the constipating effects of opioid medications

14. Lactulose is an osmotic laxative used to treat constipation; it can also be used for another indication, choose the correct answer below:
    (a) Lactulose is a sugar, therefore it is indicated in hypoglycaemia
    (b) Lactulose also has antibiotic properties
    (c) Lactulose has antihypertensive properties when used with senna
    (d) Lactulose metabolites reduce ammonia absorption; therefore, it can be used to treat hepatic encephalopathy

15. Constipation is a common complaint that's treatment includes holistic assessment and can be modified by lifestyle choices. What health promotion advice is relevant for advising an adult how to avoid constipation?
    (a) Adequate oral fluid intake (1600–2000 mL/day)
    (b) A diet rich in fruit, vegetables and other sources of dietary fibre
    (c) Always answering the body's call to pass stool, avoiding stool holding
    (d) All of the above

Find out more

The following are a list of conditions that are associated with people who have GI tract disorders. Take some time and write notes about each of the conditions. Think about the medications that may be used in order to treat these conditions and be specific about the pharmacokinetics and pharmacodynamics. Remember to include aspects of patient care. If you are making notes about people you have offered care and support to, you must ensure that you have adhered to the rules of confidentiality.

The Condition	Your Notes
Coeliac disease	
Microscopic colitis	
Toxic mega colon	
Barrett's oesophagus	
Diverticulitis	

Chapter 15

Medications used in cancer
Elaine Walls and Leah Rosengarten

Aims

The aim of this chapter is to help the reader understand the pharmacology and pharmaceutical treatment options commonly used in cancer care.

Learning outcomes

After reading this chapter, the reader will:

1. Understand how cancer occurs in relation to the cell cycle
2. Discuss the use of chemotherapies in the treatment of cancer
3. Appreciate the role of immunotherapies in the management of cancer
4. Recognise how corticosteroids are used in cancer care

Test your knowledge

1. What is the difference between normal cells and cancer cells?
2. What medicines are used in the treatment of cancer?
3. What considerations are relevant when prescribing and administering chemotherapy?
4. How is the immune system used in the treatment of cancer?
5. Why use corticosteroids in cancer care?

Fundamentals of Pharmacology: For Nursing and Healthcare Students, First Edition. Edited by Ian Peate and Barry Hill.
© 2021 John Wiley & Sons Ltd. Published 2021 by John Wiley & Sons Ltd.

Introduction

Over recent years, the NHS has seen a year on year increase in the number of cancer diagnoses but a year on year decrease in the number of people dying from cancer (Office for National Statistics (ONS), 2019). Consistently statistics have shown that more males in England are diagnosed with cancer than females and just over half (52.6%) of all cancers diagnoses in 2017 were either breast, prostate, lung or colorectal cancer (ONS, 2019).

The goal of cancer treatment in the UK is to cure patients of their cancer through eradication of all cancer cells in their body (Cancer Research UK, 2017). In situations where this is not possible, treatments can be focused on prolonging life or improving the patient's quality of life through symptom management. Treatment options for cancer are not limited to drugs and may include surgery, radiotherapy, bone marrow or stem cell transplants and gene therapies, among others. This chapter will consider the different drugs used in the treatment of cancer.

First, it is important that we develop a baseline understanding of what cancer is and the process of the normal cell cycle before we can appreciate the roles and mechanisms of drugs used in cancer.

Cancer

Cancer is a condition which occurs when cells in a certain part of the body grow and divide uncontrollably. When these cells grow abnormally, they can form a lump, which is called a tumour. Not all tumours are cancerous; tumours can be benign (not cancerous) or malignant (cancerous). The difference between these is that benign tumours will not spread to other areas of the body, but malignant tumours can spread to other tissues and organs.

Tumours that are benign will still continue to grow but typically only cause problems if they place pressure on nearby organs when they grow. Malignant or cancerous tumours in one part of the body can cast off cells which travel around the body and invade other organs. When these cells invade other organs, they may start to grow and form a second tumour, which is called a metastasis. In blood cancer, cancerous cells behave in the same way as other cancer cells and build up in the blood or bone marrow but do not form tumours.

There are certain 'hallmarks' which are said to distinguish cancer cells from normal cells; these are displayed in Figure 15.1 (Hanahan and Weinberg, 2011). Though it has been argued

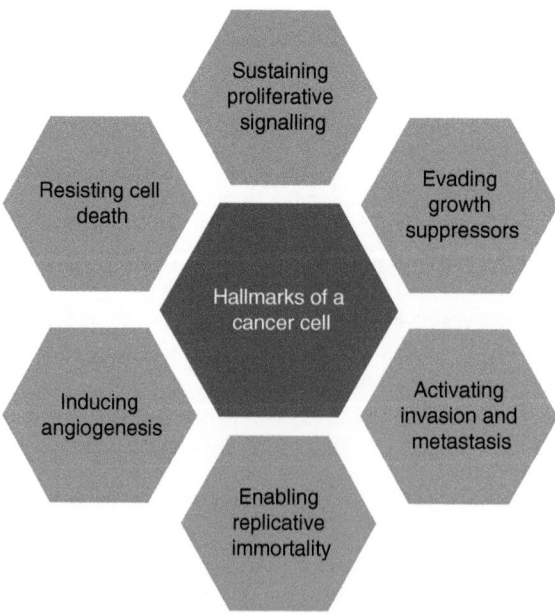

Figure 15.1   Hallmarks of a cancer cell. Source: Hanahan and Weinberg (2011).

390

that not all cancers can be defined by the same six biological capabilities, appreciation of these common traits can lead to a greater understanding of the difference between cancer cells and normal cells and enhance the quality of care provided.

Sustaining proliferative signalling describes how a cancer cell ignores signalling to control growth. Where a normal cell's growth is carefully controlled through the production of growth promoting signals, a cancer cell becomes self-sufficient in providing its own growth signals and does not require signalling from external cells to continue to grow. In addition to this, cancer cells also become resistant to antigrowth signals, which is the second hallmark: evading growth suppressors.

Activating tissue invasion and metastasis refers to the cancer cell's ability to invade and spread to surrounding tissues and organs rather than remaining in set boundaries, as normal cells do. Additionally, cancer cells do not have a limit to how many times they can multiply and grow as a normal cell does; this is termed enabling replicative immortality.

The hallmark inducing angiogenesis identifies that the cancer cell can draw blood cells in to a tumour in order to feed it and ensure it can continue to grow, where a normal cell will attract blood vessels only when they need to grow and feed. Lastly, the resisting cell death hallmark recognises that the cancer cell has an ability to ignore signals to die. While a normal cell has a program of self-destruction, called apoptosis, which is activated in occasions such as when DNA is damaged, a cancer cell can evade this process.

In short, a normal cell will: multiply and divide only when signalled to do so; stop multiplying and dividing when signalled to do so; perform one function that they were designed to perform; reproduce only a set number of times; attract blood vessels only when they need to grow; and self-destruct when necessary. A cancer cell will: multiply and divide uncontrollably; ignore signals to stop growing; invade other tissues and organs; continue to multiply and divide indefinitely; attract blood vessels to nourish itself constantly; and resist cell death.

391

Cell cycle

The purpose of the cell cycle is for cells to reproduce themselves, to replace dead or injured cells and add new ones for tissue growth. The cell cycle is an ordered series of events which consists of two main periods: interphase, when the cell is not dividing and the mitotic (M) phase when the cell is dividing. Figure 15.2 below shows the cell cycle.

The interphase is a period of rapid growth during which the cell replicates its deoxyribonucleic acid (DNA). There are three phases within this period: G_1, S and G_2. The G phases are gaps or interruptions in DNA replication and the S phase involves the replication of DNA.

The G_1 phase is the gap between the mitotic stage and the S phase, during which the cell is preparing for DNA synthesis through genes directing the synthesis of ribonucleic acid (RNA) and proteins. This stage may last from 8 to 10 hours, though some cells remain in this phase for a longer time and are considered to be in the G_0 or resting phase. The S phase is between G_1 and G_2 and lasts approximately eight hours, during which time all 46 chromosomes containing genetic DNA are copied, so both new cells that are formed will have matching DNA. Once a cell enters this phase, it is committed to going through cell division. The G_2 phase is the gap between the S phase and mitosis, this phase may last for four to six hours, during which time cell growth continues and enzymes and other proteins are synthesised in preparation for cell division.

The M phase or mitosis is characterised by chromosomes passing through phases of change (cytokinesis) to form two genetically identical cells. Mitosis may be broken down into four distinct phases; prophase where chromosomes form identical pairs, called chromotids; metaphase where spindle fibres attach to chromosomes and chromatids begin to separate; anaphase where two sets of new single-stranded chromosomes move to opposite ends of the cell; and telophase where a nuclear membrane forms around each set of chromosomes dividing the cell in two.

Understanding the process of the cell cycle is important as certain drugs used in the treatment of cancer impact on specific points in the cell cycle. These drugs interrupt the process of

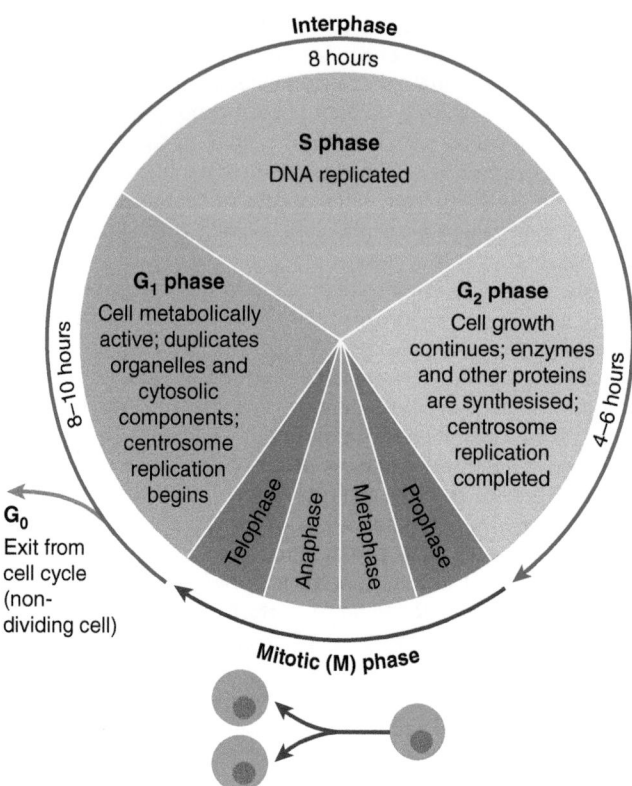

Figure 15.2   The cell cycle. Source: The cell cycle page 290 in Peate and Wild Nursing Practice Knowledge and Care 2nd Ed.

the cell cycle in order to prevent the cancer from growing further or to kill the cancer cell completely.

Chemotherapies

Chemotherapy is the name given to the group of drugs which are cytotoxic, meaning that they are toxic to cells. Chemotherapy has been used in the treatment of cancer since the 1940s and today there are more than 100 different types of chemotherapy used in the UK. Chemotherapy destroys cancer cells by interrupting the cell cycle and preventing the cells from multiplying further, though chemotherapy cannot distinguish between normal and abnormal cells so healthy cells can also be affected. The point at which a chemotherapy will interrupt the cell cycle differs depending on the type of chemotherapy.

Preparations of chemotherapy

Chemotherapy is most commonly given intravenously as either a bolus or infusion but can also be administered through the following routes:

- Orally – swallowed in pill, tablet, capsule or liquid form.
- Subcutaneous – into the space between the skin and the muscle.
- Intramuscular – into the muscle.
- Intrathecal – into the spinal fluid.

Clinical considerations

Types of chemotherapy are broken down into groups according to: their chemical structure, how they work and their relationships to other drugs. Some chemotherapies may belong to more than one group as they work in more than one way. Different chemotherapy agents are often given in combination with each other, to interrupt different points within the cell cycle.

Tables 15.1–15.4 display the commonly used chemotherapy agent for each group.

- Intraperitoneal – into the abdominal cavity.
- Intravesicular – into the bladder.
- Intrapleural – into the space between the lung and the lining of the lung.
- Intra-arterial – into the artery that is supplying blood to the tumour.
- Topical – onto the skin.

Types of chemotherapy

The British National Formulary (BNF) (Joint Formulary Committee, 2019) identifies four classes of chemotherapy;

1. alkylating drugs
2. antimetabolites
3. anthracyclines and other antibiotics
4. vinca alkaloids.

Alkylating drugs

Alkylating drugs or alkylating agents were the first chemotherapy drugs to be used to treat chemotherapy. The use of alkylating drugs to treat cancer was first discovered in the First World War, when sulphur mustards (mustard gas) were used as chemical weapons. As such, alkylating drugs are some of the most studied drugs used to treat cancer and still remain one of the most commonly used group of drugs for this purpose (Almeida et al., 2005).

Table 15.1 Commonly used alkylating drugs.

Drug	Licensed for treatment of
Cyclophosphamide *oral or intravenous*	A wide range of malignancies including leukaemia, lymphomas and solid tumours
Ifosfamide (related to cyclophosphamide) *Intravenous*	Malignant disease
Melphalan *Intravenous*	Multiple myeloma, polycythemia vera, childhood neuroblastoma, advanced ovarian adenocarcinoma and advanced breast cancer
Lomustine *Oral*	Hodgkin's disease resistant to conventional therapy, malignant melanoma and certain solid tumours
Carmustine *Intravenous*	Multiple myeloma, non-Hodgkin's lymphoma and brain tumours
Estramustine phosphate *Oral*	Prostate cancer

Source: Joint Formulary Committee (2019).

Alkylating drugs are generally considered non-cell specific as their activity is not restricted to one specific point in the cell cycle (Pires et al., 2018). These drugs work through transferring alkyl carbon groups onto a wide range of biological molecules, preventing the proteins in the DNA from joining together as they should and eventually breaking the strands of DNA, stopping the cell from continuing to multiply and killing the cell (Fu et al., 2012).

As every aspect of the cell cycle is concerned with the replication of DNA, alkylating drugs can impact on every point in the cell cycle; but their biggest impact is thought to be within the S phase of the cell cycle where all 46 chromosomes are copied (Bignold, 2006). Table 15.1 identifies some of the commonly used alkylating drugs in cancer care.

Antimetabolites

Antimetabolites structurally resemble normal biological molecules within a cell and work through interfering with the processes that require the use of that normal biological molecule (Gmeiner, 2002). As antimetabolites structurally resemble essential molecules, enzymes will mistake antimetabolites for other essential molecules and combine with them; this results in the exclusion of essential molecules from their normal role and creates a deficiency of that molecule (Woolley, 1959).

Antimetabolites attack cells at specific parts of the cell cycle, but the point at which this occurs in the cycle depends on which substance the antimetabolite interferes with. These drugs tend to be further classified according to which substance they inhibit, which can include: dihydrofolate reductase, tetrahydrofolate, purines and pyrimidines (Gmeiner, 2002). Table 15.2, identifies some of the commonly used antimetabolites in cancer care.

Anthracyclines and other antibiotics

Anthracyclines have been widely used in cancer treatment for over 50 years and are derived from antibiotics.

Table 15.2   Commonly used antimetabolites.

Drug	Licensed for use in
Methotrexate *Intramuscular, subcutaneous, intravenous, oral and intrathecal*	Neoplastic diseases
6-mercaptopurine *Oral*	Acute leukaemia's and chronic myeloid leukaemia
6-tioguanine *Oral*	Acute leukaemia and chronic myeloid leukaemia
Fludarabine phosphate *Oral or intravenous*	Advanced B-cell chronic lymphocytic leukaemia (CLL)
Pentostatin *Intravenous*	Hairy cell leukaemia
Cladribine *Subcutaneous, intravenous or oral*	Hairy cell leukaemia and chronic lymphocytic leukaemia
5-fluorouracil *Intravenous or intra-arterial*	Some solid tumours including gastrointestinal tract cancers and breast cancer and in combination with folinic acid in advanced colorectal cancer
Cytarabine *Intravenous or subcutaneous*	Acute myeloid leukaemia
Gemcitabine *Intravenous*	Locally advanced or metastatic non-small cell lung cancer, locally advanced or metastatic pancreatic cancer and advanced or metastatic bladder cancer

Source: Joint Formulary Committee (2019).

Table 15.3   Commonly used anthracyclines and other antibiotics.

Drug	Licensed for treatment of
Daunorubicin *Intravenous*	Acute myelogenous leukaemia and acute lymphocytic leukaemia
Doxorubicin hydrochloride *Intravenous or intravesical*	Acute leukaemia, Hodgkin's and non-Hodgkin's lymphomas, paediatric malignancies and some solid tumours including breast cancer
Epirubicin hydrochloride *Intravenous or Intravesical*	Breast cancer
Idarubicin hydrochloride *Oral or intravenous*	Haematological malignancies
Mitoxantrone *Intravenous*	Metastatic breast cancer, non-Hodgkin's lymphoma, adult acute non-lymphocytic leukaemia and non-resectable primary hepatocellular carcinoma
Pixantrone *Intravenous*	Refractory or multiply relapsed aggressive non-Hodgkin's B-Cell lymphomas
Bleomycin *Intramuscular, intravenous or intra-arterial*	Metastatic germ cell cancer and non-Hodgkin's lymphoma
Dactinomycin *Intravenous*	Paediatric cancers
Mitomycin *Intravenous or intravesical*	Gastrointestinal and breast cancers and by bladder instillation for superficial bladder tumours

Source: Joint Formulary Committee (2019).

Though anthracyclines can induce many intracellular effects, their main mechanism of action is inhibition of topoisomerase II (Neilsen et al., 1996). Topoisomerase II is an enzyme which generates breaks in strands of DNA in order to regulate DNA processes (McClendon and Osheroff, 2007). Anthracyclines inhibit topoisomerase II through intercalating (inserting molecules) between base pairs of adjacent DNA, damaging the DNA and ultimately inducing apoptosis (Hortobágyi, 1997). Table 15.3 identifies some of the commonly used anthracyclines and other antibiotics in cancer care.

Vinca alkaloids

Vinca alkaloids are derived from certain types of plant and work through the inhibition of tubulin into microtubules (Zhou and Rahmani, 1992). Microtubules are needed to provide structure and shape to cells and when vinca alkaloids bind to tubulin, they prevent the tubulin from then being able to bind to microtubules (Moudi et al., 2013). This process ultimately blocks the ability of the cell to divide and causes apotosis (Moudi et al., 2013). Table 15.4, identifies some of the commonly used vinca alkaloids in cancer care.

Side effects of chemotherapy

It has been noted that the effects of chemotherapy are not limited to only cancer cells but also impact on healthy cells. As chemotherapy affects the fastest dividing cells in the human body most, side effects of chemotherapy are more likely to occur in areas of the body where cells are fast dividing. Though individual chemotherapies will have differing side effects, common side effects are below:

- nausea and vomiting
- alopecia

Table 15.4   Commonly used vinca alkaloids.

Drug	Licensed for use in
Vinblastine sulphate *Intravenous*	Variety of cancers including leukaemias, lymphomas and some solid tumours (e.g. breast and lung cancer)
Vincristine sulphate *Intravenous*	Variety of cancers including leukaemias, lymphomas and some solid tumours (e.g. breast and lung cancer)
Vindesine sulphate *Intravenous*	Variety of cancers including leukaemias, lymphomas and some solid tumours (e.g. breast and lung cancer)
Vinorelbine *Oral or intravenous*	Advanced breast cancer and advanced non-small cell lung cancer

Source: Joint Formulary Committee (2019).

- bone marrow suppression leading to:
  - anaemia (low red blood cell count)
  - thrombocytopenia (low platelets)
  - leukopenia (low white blood cell count)
- mucositis
- skin changes.

As chemotherapy is usually given in cycles or set regimens, patients are clinically assessed before commencing every regimen to ensure that side effects are manageable. These assessments change depending on the point in treatment but frequently include blood tests and a full clinical exam. Healthcare professionals need to assess the patient to ensure that the impact of the patient's experienced side effects do not outweigh the benefit of the chemotherapy. Some side effects, such as nausea and vomiting, can be managed but others, such as mucositis, require the patient to be given time to recover before commencing more chemotherapy.

Clinical considerations

According to the Control of Substances Hazardous to Health Regulations 2002 (COSHH), cytotoxic drugs are hazardous substances (see the Health and Safety Executive (HSE, 2019) website). Due to this, staff administering these drugs should: control their exposure to the substance, wear personal protective equipment (PPE), monitor exposure in the workplace, use occupational health services to help identify risks if necessary, deal with spillages and contamination appropriately, dispose of waste correctly and report incidents as necessary according and in line with local policy and procedure (HSE, 2019).

Prescription and administration of chemotherapy

The National Chemotherapy Advisory Group (NCAG, 2009) give recommendations on the prescription of chemotherapy. They advise that the decision to initiate a program of chemotherapy should be made by a consultant and that all patients must have a treatment plan in place for each cycle of chemotherapy they are given. NCAG (2009) direct that chemotherapy should only be prescribed by appropriately trained staff, according to predefined protocols and should be on preprinted forms. Practice areas should keep an annually updated list of all staff who can prescribe chemotherapy and an oncology pharmacist should check all chemotherapy prescriptions. Exceptions may be made to the above in emergencies and extraordinary circumstances.

Table 15.5 Properties of cyclophosphamide.

Use	Can be used in the treatment of a wide range of malignancies, including some leukaemias, lymphomas and solid tumours (Joint Formulary Committee, 2019)
Dose	Must be individualised. The dose, duration of treatment and treatment intervals are adjusted according to the therapeutic indication of the patients scheme of chemotherapy (Electronic Medicines Compendium [EMC], 2017)
Administration	Can be given orally or intravenously (IV) as a bolus or an infusion
Pharmacodynamics	An alkylating agent which affects the cell at the S or G2 phase of the cell cycle. It is not known whether cyclophosphamide works *only* through the alkylation of DNA, but this is the drugs main known method of action (EMC, 2017)
Pharmacokinetics	Cyclophosphamide is inactive at administration but activated in the liver Absorption – quickly and almost completely absorbed parenterally and well absorbed orally Distribution – distributed widely around the body and can cross the blood–brain barrier, the placental barrier, and is found in ascites. The parent compound binds poorly to plasma protein but the active metabolites are significantly protein bound Metabolism – Activated in the liver. 2–4 hours after administration, the plasma concentrations of the active metabolites are maximal, after which plasma concentrations rapidly decrease Excretion – The plasma half-life is about 4–8 hours in adults and children. Cyclophosphamide and its metabolites are primarily excreted by the kidneys (EMC, 2016, 2017)
Side effects (common or very common)	Bone marrow suppression and problems associated low blood counts, alopecia, physical weakness or lack of energy, cystitis, haemolytic uremic syndrome, hepatic disorders, mucosal abnormalities, sperm abnormalities and progressive multifocal leukoencephalopathy (PML) (Joint Formulary Committee, 2019)

397

Episode of care

Jasmine

Jasmine was 16 years old when she presented to hospital with a seizure. On admission to hospital Jasmine also identified a month history of dizziness and vomiting. After initial testing, Jasmine was diagnosed with an ependymoma (a type of brain tumour); Jasmine is now 20 years old and has recently relapsed with her ependymoma.

Jasmine has a moderate learning disability and lives in assisted living where she is visited regularly by her parents and older sister.

Jasmine is being treated with a combination of oral chemotherapies at home. Jasmine was prescribed 50 mg/m² of etoposide orally every day for a period of three weeks. She is now due to start taking 2.5 mg/kg of cyclophosphamide orally every day.

Jasmine was given the correct number of tablets of etoposide to last for three weeks, but on return to clinic to collect her cyclophosphamide tablets, Jasmine still has half of her tablets left in the bottle.

Jasmine was previously assessed as having capacity to manage her own medications, but she now seems confused by which medications she should take and when. Jasmine isn't able to remember which days she has taken her medications and which days she may have forgotten.

Before Jasmine can be discharged home, healthcare professionals need to reassess Jasmine's capacity to manage her own medications at home and develop a plan to ensure that she is compliant with her treatment regimen.

Drug resistance

It is possible for cancer cells to be or become resistant to chemotherapy treatment. Occasions when cancer does not respond to chemotherapy treatment may be termed 'refractory.' Some cancer cells may initially respond to chemotherapy, but later develop the ability to prevent chemotherapy drugs from entering the cell, or limit the amount of drug that enters the cell to stop or minimise the amount of damage the drug can do.

Cyclophosphamide

Using the above categories, cyclophosphamide can be used as an example to gain a deeper insight into the use of a chemotherapy as an anticancer drug. Table 15.5 explains the properties of cyclophosphamide.

Immunotherapies in treating cancer

The immune system

In immunotherapy, it is essential to understand the role of the immune system and how this line of therapy may influence cancer management plans.

The immune system plays a significant role in the development and progression of cancers (Coosemans et al., 2019; Hanahan and Weinberg, 2011). Natural antibodies within the immune system are proteins that fight infection when the body recognises something harmful, such as viruses and bacteria. In response to these harmful cells, signals are sent by the immune system to interrupt growth and kill the invading cell (Figure 15.3).

While some of the body's own malformed cells will be destroyed by the immune system responses, many cancers are able to avoid this process as they act as part of the body's own structure rather than an invading cell. This allows the cancer cell to avoid attack and escape immune system pathways that are in place to block and reduce harm.

Though the immune system sometimes fails to destroy cancer cells initially, it can still be useful in the management and treatment of cancer. Immunotherapy uses substances that are naturally made by the body or made synthetically in a laboratory, to improve or restore the immune system in order to elicit or amplify an immune response.

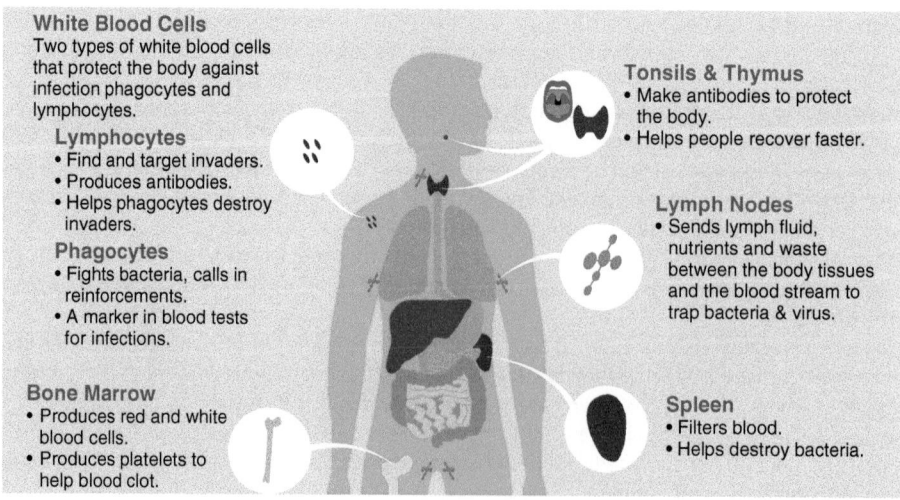

Figure 15.3   The immune system.

Immunotherapy

Immunotherapy is a relatively new form of cancer therapy. Although first recognised by Dr. William Coley in the 1800s, it was initially approved as part of cancer treatment in 1990. This was in the form of a cancer-based vaccine for tuberculosis (Cancer Research Institute, 2019) and since then advances in research and use of immunotherapy in cancer care has increased exponentially.

Immunotherapy is a form of treatment that can act to support the immune system in recognising specific cancer cells and either destroying them or stopping or slowing growth within the cancer cell (Schreiber and Smyth, 2011).

Immunotherapy can act to block the pathways that cancer cells often use to avoid immune responses and encourage the immune system to form memory cells against specific types of cancer. In certain cancers, it is thought that immunotherapy relaunches the immune system, allowing it to re-form and therefore producing cancer specific antibodies that will be retained in the immune memory and attack any returning cancer cells. Currently immunotherapy has been formulated to be suitable only for certain cancers due to cell composure within these cancer cells. Cancer immunotherapy is an artificial interaction with the immune system in an attempt to fight cancer.

The use of immunotherapy

Immunotherapy may be used independently or as part of a treatment regimen (with chemotherapy and or surgery), both in active and supportive pathways (see below). Using the body's own immune responses allows immunotherapy to respond to cancer only cells, preventing their growth and sparing healthy cells from this invasion, therefore reducing the severe side effects as commonly seen in chemotherapy.

- Active immunotherapy primes the immune system to recognise cancer cells as foreign, encouraging the production of antibodies or cytotoxic T cells to fight cancer, which aims to stop growth within the cancer cell (Yao et al., 2018).
- Supportive immunotherapy is non-specific strengthening of the innate immune system and acts as a secondary treatment line in slowing cancer growth (Vansteenkiste, 2012).

Immunotherapy is considered in addition to chemotherapy and radiotherapy for more resistant cancers as part of an aggressive treatment plan, and the effects of such treatment regimens remain under scrutiny (Coosemans et al., 2019).

Immunotherapy is used in a variety of treatment methods, including:

- targeted antibodies
- checkpoint inhibitors
- bone marrow/stem cell transplant
- adoptive cell transfer
- cytokines.

The role of each of the above are now discussed.

Targeted antibodies

Advances in technology have allowed for the identification of proteins that are uniquely expressed within tumour cells. There are several types of targeted antibodies, each acting on different proteins. Monoclonal antibodies are manufactured antibodies that act by targeting specific proteins so the immune system can destroy these abnormal proteins. The purpose being to return cellular growth, differentiation and proliferation back to its healthy state. Monoclonal antibodies are made up of one protein type and bind to this particular epitope within the cell (Figure 15.4). Some monoclonal antibodies work by stimulating the immune system to respond and attack the cancer, rather than allowing natural immune regulation to

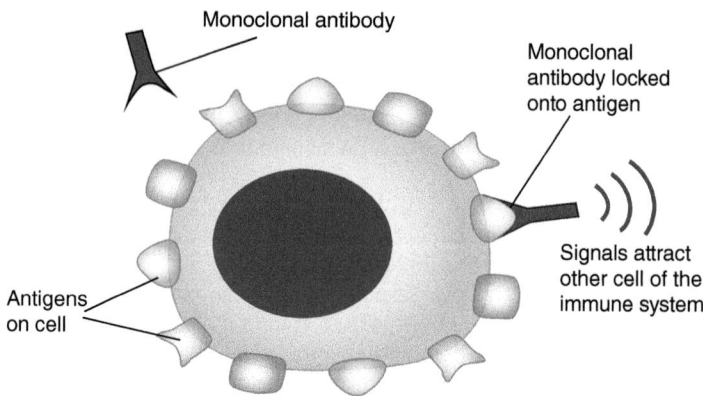

Figure 15.4 Mononuclear antibodies.

see cancer proteins as part of the self and preventing continued antigen assault. Monoclonal antibodies target cancer cells by driving the immune system to release its brakes and remain active in the fight against harmful antigens (National Centre for Biotechnology Information, NCBI, 2019). Table 15.6, identifies some of the commonly used monoclonal antibodies in cancer care.

Checkpoint inhibitors

Check point inhibitors can also be considered a form of monoclonal antibody. There are pathways in the immune system which are crucial in preventing cancer from being able to avoid immune responses and continue to grow. These pathways would normally contain a checkpoint to recognise and block invading organisms (such as cancer) and to allow immune responses to identify and destroy harmful cells.

Some cancers are able to fool the immune system and move through these pathways or checkpoints (PD-1/DD-L1, CTLA-4), which is where checkpoint inhibitor drugs may be useful. Checkpoint inhibitors are antibodies that act by stimulating the immune system to block these checkpoints, enticing immune recognition and response to occur, aiming to stop or slow growth of cancer cells (Johnson et al., 2019).

Figure 15.5 shows the action that occurs when checkpoint inhibitors such as Anti PD1 occur within the cell. Table 15.7 identifies some of the commonly used checkpoint inhibitors in cancer care.

See Table 15.8 for examples of checkpoint inhibitors.

Table 15.6 Examples of monoclonal antibodies.

Drug and route	Indication	Pharmacodynamics
Trasruzumab (Herceptin) *Intravenous infusion*	Breast cancers that over-express HER2	Attach to HER2 cells to block growth signals
Rituximab *Intravenous infusion*	Chronic lymphocytic leukaemia (CLL) Non-Hodgkin's lymphoma	Target CD20 on B cells' immune responses then attach and kill CD20 (young cells in the bone marrow do not have CD20)

Source: Joint Formulary Committee (2019).

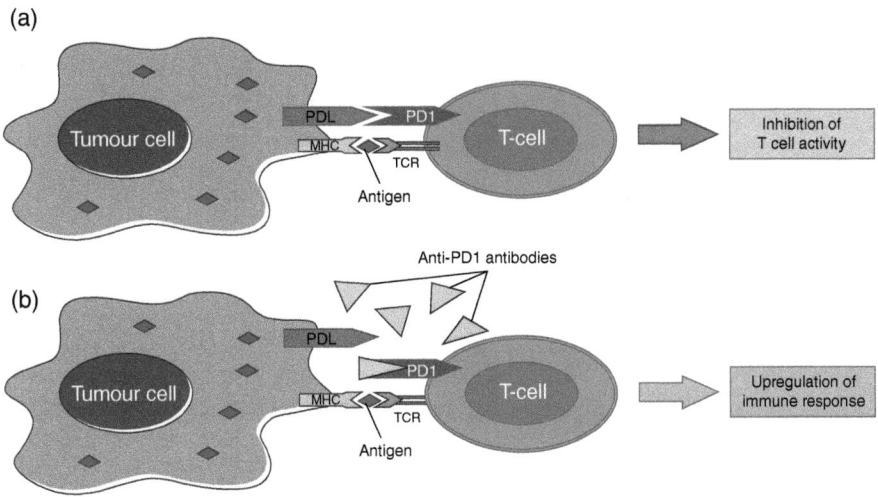

Figure 15.5   Cell activity with checkpoint inhibitor.

Table 15.7   Demonstrates properties of Rituximab as a monoclonal antibody.

Use	Cancers such as: follicular lymphoma, B cell non-Hodgkins lymphoma, chronic lymphocytic leukaemia (CLL)
Dose	Adults 375 mg/m² body surface Child dose is strictly guided by individual protocols, weight of child and clinical presentation
Administration	Always given as IV or Subcutaneous infusion Patients must have close monitoring by a healthcare professional and be in an environment where full resuscitation facilities are available Pre-medication of antipyretic and antihistamine is required alongside pre-hydration
Pharmacodynamics	Rituximab is a monoclonal antibody that binds to transmembrane antigen CD20 on B cells. CD20 is present on normal and malignant B cells, but not on stem cells
Pharmacokinetics	Absorption – circulating B cells are depleted by Rituximab within 3 weeks, effects can last up to 6 months Distribution-binding to B cells is seen on lymphoid cells in thymus, spleen, peripheral blood and lymph nodes Excretion – half-life varies depending on disease, with an average of 22 days. This is increased in patients with large tumour mass, in CLL can be up to 32 days. Serum concentrate after 4 doses can be detected after 3–6 months
Common or very common side effects (a selection only listed)	Decreased appetite Bone marrow disorders Anxiety Myocardial infarction Conjunctivitis Insomnia Ear pain Dizziness Migraine Sepsis Multi-organ failure

Source: Joint Formulary Committee (2019), EMC (2019), Drugs.com (2019).

Table 15.8 Other checkpoint inhibitors.

Drug and route	Indication	Pharmacodynamics
Ipilimumab *Intravenous infusion*	Melanoma	Stimulates T cell activation to destroy cancer cell
Avelumab *Intravenous infusion*	Merkel cell carcinoma	Binds to PD1 (programmed death) receptor–at checkpoint to stimulate immune response

Source: Joint Formulary Committee (2019); Kirkwood et al. (2001).

Bone marrow and stem cell transplant

Bone marrow transplants (BMT), also referred to as stem cell transplants, are used to replace diseased bone marrow with new healthy cells. This is a form of immunotherapy, as the transplanted marrow elicits the immune system to re-evaluate and re-launch, making it more able to respond to harmful cells following significant attack from diseases such as cancer. BMT is also used to replace cells within the immune system which have been permanently destroyed by cancer treatments (such as chemotherapy).

Bone marrow or stem cells can be donated from a matched donor or autologous, meaning they have been harvested, cleaned, and stored and are later given back to the same person (Figure 15.6).

BMT and stem cell transplantation are used in conjunction with robust pharmaceutical regimens. Treatment to destroy the damaged immune system occurs pre BMT, alongside post-BMT therapies which support the new cells to be established and minimise risk of rejection from the body's original immune system. Table 15.9, identifies the indication for stem cell transplant or bone marrow transplant in cancer care.

Adoptive cell transfer (ACT)

Adoptive cell transfer is the autologous use of genetically modified T cells to help activate T cell activity, by stimulating T cells to recognise and target specific proteins on cancer cells. Before ACT can occur, depletion of lymphocytes is required to support the immune system's ability to accept replaced T cells (Rosenberg et al., 2008). This is achieved through chemotherapy agents which destroy lymphocytes.

T cells without tumour activity are harvested via blood from the cancer patient (autologous); the T cell is separated from other components within the blood then genetically modified *in vitro* and allowed to multiply. A larger collection of stronger T cells now with tumour

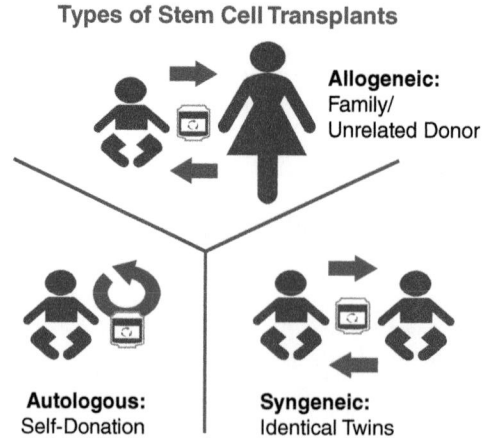

Types of Stem Cell Transplants

Allogeneic:
Family/
Unrelated Donor

Autologous:
Self-Donation

Syngeneic:
Identical Twins

Figure 15.6 Types of bone marrow transplant.

Table 15.9   Indications for use of transplant.

Route	Indication
Bone marrow/stem cells *Intravenous infusion*	leukaemia Lymphoma Multiple myeloma

Table 15.10   Examples of adoptive cell transfer drugs.

Form of ACT	Indication
Tisagenlecleucal	Acute lymphoblastic leukaemia in patients up to aged 25 years only
Axicabtagene	T cell lymphomas for patients who have failed conventional treatment twice

Source: National Institute for Health and Care Excellence, NICE (2018a, b).

Table 15.11   Examples of cytokines.

Drug and Route	Indication	Pharmacodynamics
Interferon alpha *Subcutaneous injection or intravenous injection*	Hairy cell leukaemia Non-Hodgkin's lymphoma Myeloma Liver or lymph metastasis of carcinoid tumour	Boosts immune systems response and reduce growth of cancer by interfering with action of proteins that affect growth
Interleukin 2/proleukin *Subcutaneous injection or intravenous infusion*	Metastatic renal cancer	Aims to produce tumour shrinkage by inhibiting cell growth

Source: Joint Formulary Committee (2019).

activity is infused back into the cancer patient. These engineered T cells have an enhanced ability to attack the proteins on the cancer cell (Restifo et al., 2012).

Table 15.10 identifies some of the commonly used ACT drugs in cancer care.

Cytokines

Cytokines are memory bound proteins that act as a mediator of intercellular activity. Cytokines are responsible for signalling between cells and maintaining the balance of the immune system. Cytokines act as messenger cells communicating and coordinating responses to targeted antigens within the immune system (Lee and Margoln, 2011).

Engineered cytokine drugs stimulate the immune system to encourage T cell activity, they are able to interfere with the cancer cell by enticing it to produce chemicals that are easily recognised as harmful within the immune system, stimulating T cell attack. Cytokines also interfere with the way the cancer cell multiplies, attempting to reduce growth (Castro et al., 2018). Table 15.11 identifies some of the commonly used cytokines in cancer care.

Side effects of immunotherapy

The side effects associated with immunotherapies vary between person to person and differ with each therapeutic agent. Table 15.12 details possible side effects from immunotherapy. The majority of side effects from immunotherapy are mild, due to the composition of immunotherapies in targeting cancer cells, thereby protecting healthy cells within the body. However, there are recorded incidences of severe and life threatening effects from some

Table 15.12 Side effects of immunotherapy.

Mild side effects	Severe side effects
Minor inflammation	Auto-immune response
Flu-like symptoms	Skin breakdown
Nausea	Mucositis
Headaches	Blood pressure irregularity
Body aches	Vomiting
Fatigue	Colitis
Itching (rash on less than10% of body)	Paralysis
	Myocarditis
	Neurological disorders

Source: Haanen et al. (2017), Kirkwood et al. (2001), Joint National Formulary (2019).

patients. As immunotherapies stimulate the immune system, certain reactions should be expected (Kirkwood et al., 2001; Joint Formulary Committee, 2019).

Immunotherapies (in particular checkpoint inhibitors) take the brakes off the regulation of the immune system; it is therefore crucial when administering immunotherapy that close monitoring of the patient occurs. This monitoring is needed because releasing the immune system control may entice attack from the immune system onto healthy functioning parts of the body. This could cause unpredictable, life-threatening side effects if early identification and treatment did not occur (Potter et al., 2014). Monitoring of the patient by healthcare professionals should seek to recognise any allergic responses or flu-like symptoms which may occur during or shortly after treatment.

Clinical considerations

Immunotherapy treatments are increasingly becoming a popular choice in cancer care. They have expended treatment possibilities and are associated with less toxicity than traditional approaches. Guidelines for their use are differentiated by diagnosis, age and prognosis of each patient. Not all cancers and patients are responsive to immunotherapy. The risks and benefits of treatment as always is the priority in any consideration for immunotherapy (Haanen et al., 2017).

Episode of care

Oluchi
Oluchi was 45 years old when she presented to her GP with a lump in her breast. Oluchi was the mother of three girls and lived in the city centre with her husband and children. After initial testing, Oluchi was diagnosed with breast cancer. Further testing showed that Oluchi's cancer staging was 2a and was HER2 positive.

Oluchi was initially given Trasruzumab (targeted antibody) to reduce the size of her tumour, before she had surgery to remove the tumour completely.

Throughout her treatment, Oluchi's experienced various side effects, including:

- hot flushes and sweating
- disinterest in sex
- vaginal dryness

- nausea and vomiting
- pain in her joints
- mood changes
- fatigue.

Oluchi will continue to receive oral Trasruzumab at 6 mg/kg for at least two years after her surgery and will continue to see her specialist team in the long-term follow-up clinic.

Healthcare professionals will need to offer ongoing psychological and physical support for Oluchi, monitoring her for side effects of treatment and to ensure that her cancer does not recur.

Corticosteroid use in cancer

Steroids

Steroids are hormones that are naturally produced within the body, these are produced in small amounts during physiological or emotional stress. Stress sends signals to the brain for the pituitary gland to release the adrenocorticotropic hormone (ACTH). ACTH acts by instructing the adrenal glands (located above the kidney) to release cortisol, the body's natural steroid. Cortisol once released is picked up by cell receptors to respond to specific stress issues around the body (Ly and Wen, 2017).

Cortisol has several functions, it can help reduce inflammation, help control blood glucose, regulate the metabolism, control salt and water balance, maintain blood pressure and assist memory function. Cortisol receptors are present in a majority of body cells, each using the cortisol in a different way.

Although there is currently limited knowledge on the pharmacodynamics of steroids, it is reported that corticosteroids act in the body by altering transcription and protein synthesis within cellular activity (Wooldridge et al., 2001), thereby inhibiting the release of specific inflammatory mediators such as arachidonic acid.

Corticosteroids are manmade replicas of natural cortisol hormones (steroids). Corticosteroids are used as a means of supplying the body with an increased source of steroid, in order to encourage and produce the same effects within cells of the body that cortisol stimulates (Twycross, 1994). Corticosteroids act through genomic and non-genomic mechanisms. Genomic effects occur through gene translation or transcription. These include anti-inflammatory and immune suppression by excretion of anti-inflammatory cytokines and metabolic effects through suppression of the hypothalamic–pituitary–adrenal axis (Czock et al., 2005). Non-genomic effects occur through interaction with specific receptors such as glucocorticoids within cell membranes (Yu et al., 1981; Ly and Wen, 2017).

Using corticosteroids to treat cancer

Corticosteroids act in a variety of ways; in cancer they are used for two principal functions: providing important components for modifying the fluid membrane and signalling molecules within the cell. These functions aim to reproduce responses within the immune system that are initiated by steroid activity, such as:

- reduce inflammation;
- suppress immunity;
- reduce allergic reactions;
- stimulate appetite (metabolic effects);
- control the balance of water and salt;
- regulate blood pressure;
- control mood and behaviour (Walsh et al., 2000; Zhou and Cidlowski, 2005).

Table 15.13   Examples of corticosteroid use in cancer.

Therapeutic plan	Desired effect
In conjunction with chemotherapy	Inhibit inflammatory responses, reduce allergic reactions, help reduce sickness, increase appetite Maintain blood pressure Control balance of water and salt
Pre and post surgery	Reduce inflammatory responses
Post bone marrow transplant	Suppress immune system and reduce risk of rejection
Autonomously (advanced cancer)	Reduce inflammatory responses as part of symptom relief Increase appetite

The use of corticosteroids in cancer is part of well-established treatment protocols. The type and stage of cancer often determines how corticosteroids will be used within pharmaceutical therapy plans (Table 15.13). Corticosteroids are used in cancer to achieve a variety of effects, such as to reduce inflammation, suppress immune responses, treat the cancer (by attacking the cell), help alleviate sickness and improve appetite. Type and stage of cancer often indicates corticosteroid use within treatment or management plans. Corticosteroids can be prescribed from diagnosis, throughout therapy or in palliative care (Ryken et al., 2010; Cancer Network, 2019). Anti-inflammatory and immune suppression are the main functions that signal use of corticosteroids in cancer patients. Reducing the inflammation around tumours can help decrease the pressure on nerve endings, brain, spine or bone which are caused by the tumour. The corticosteroids' ability to suppress the immune system by altering normal immune responses, although making the patient more susceptible to infection, allows the immune system to be re-programmed and other therapeutic agents to fight cancer cells. It is also thought that corticosteroids can induce programmed death within certain cells and help fight cancer (Joint Formulary Committee, 2019).

In cancer treatment there are four main corticosteroids in use. These are prednisolone, methylprednisolone, dexamethasone and hydrocortisone as identified in Table 15.14.

Corticosteroids can be administered through oral, topical, intravenous and eye drops. Oral tablets or liquids and intravenous methods are the most common routes in cancer care. Each corticosteroid has its own half-life and intermediate acting properties, defining differential indications for use (NICE, 2017).

Table 15.14   Examples of corticosteroid.

Route	Example of corticosteroid	Indication
Oral	• Prednisolone • Methylprednisolone • Dexamethasone	• Acute lymphoblastic leukaemia • Chronic lymphocytic leukaemia • Hodgkin's lymphoma • Non-Hodgkin's lymphoma • Mycosis lymphoma • Aplastic anaemia
Intravenous	• Hydrocortisone • Methylprednisolone • Dexamethasone	• Brain tumours • Spine tumours • Cerebral oedema caused by tumours
Topical	• Dexamethasone • Hydrocortisone	• Basal and squamous cell skin cancers
Eye drops	• Dexamethasone	• Prevent eye inflammation in leukaemia and lymphoma patients

Table 15.15   Dexamethasone.

Use	Dexamethasone is a corticosteroid that can be used for its anti-inflammatory, immune suppression and membrane stabilising properties within most cancers. It is also often used for the reduction of nausea and vomiting in patients undergoing chemotherapy (EMC, 2019)
Dose	Adult doses range from 0.5–10 mg daily, depending on severity of disease. When used to treat nausea and vomiting, doses can range from 8–16 mg/day (Joint Formulary Committee, 2019) Children's doses are calculated dependent on reason for use, stage of cancer, alongside the child's weight. Each individual child must be prescribed a dose accordingly while considering how they will manage the treatment
Administration	Can be given as IV infusion, or oral in tablets and liquid form. Oral treatment should be taken as one dose each morning with or after food. Patients on high doses may be required to have doses more than once day (EMC, 2019; Joint Formulary Committee, 2019)
Pharmacodynamics	Dexamethasone activates the transcription of corticosteroid sensitive genes. Effects of anti-inflammatory, immune suppression and cell anti-proliferation are caused by a decrease in the formation, release and activity of inflammatory mediators, inhibiting the specific function and migration of inflammatory cells
Pharmacokinetics	Absorption – oral dexamethasone is rapidly absorbed in the stomach and small intestine. Creating a bioavailability of 80–90% Distribution – it binds to plasma albumin, high doses give the largest portion of drug that circulates within the blood Metabolism – partly metabolised by the kidneys. Half-life is up to 36 hours Excretion – metabolites are excreted as gluconates or sulphates and excreted by the kidneys (EMC, 2019)
Common or very common side effects	Adrenal suppression Anxiety Appetite increased Abnormal behaviour Cataract Cushing's syndrome Electrolyte imbalance Fluid retention Headache Increased risk of infection Osteoporosis (Joint Formulary Committee, 2019)

407

Dexamethasone is one of the strongest corticosteroids. Dexamethasone holds 7.5 times greater effect opposed to prednisolone and hydrocortisone. The use of dexamethasone in cancer is a popular choice during initial treatment protocols. Long term use is mainly restricted to palliative care (EMC, 2019). Table 15.15 outlines the properties of oral dexamethasone.

Side effects of Corticosteroids

Corticosteroid use has several mild and severe associated side effects. It is well known that Corticosteroids can mask the symptoms of infection and reduce immunity; therefore, stringent procedures should be in place to ensure safe use in cancer patients. Short-term use with low doses of Corticosteroid have less complicated and more often immediate, short-term side effects. Long-term use with a high dose of Corticosteroids, as is common in cancer patients, can present severe side effects that may take a prolonged time to resolve once treatment has ceased.

Table 15.16   Side effects of Corticosteroids.

Side effects in short-term use (often lower dose)	Side effects in long-term and high-dose use
Insomnia	Weight gain
Gastrointestinal ulcers	Thinning of skin
Oral and vaginal candida	Cushingoid appearance
Anxiety	Osteoporosis *This may be permanent*
Glucose intolerance	Proximal myopathy
	Infection
	Impaired wound healing
	Gastrointestinal bleed
	Cardiac arrhythmias *This may be permanent*
	Cataracts *This may be permanent*
	Acne
	Increased risk of bone fracture
	Depression, suicidal thoughts
	Growth deceleration in children

Source: Yasir and Sonthalia (2019), Schäcke et al. (2002).

Clinical considerations

High dose and long-term use of corticosteroids requires healthcare practitioners to be alert to not only common side effects but also to the more uncommon and rare effects on an individual's physical and mental health that can be attributed to this form of treatment. The elderly population are at increased risk of osteoporosis and children are more susceptible to retarded growth. Pre-term infants may suffer extra complications such as cognitive impairment (EMC, 2019).

Certain side effects may cause adverse reactions and irreversible damage (Yasir and Sonthalia, 2019). Table 15.16 details some of the more common side effects of long- and short-term use of Corticosteroids; this list is not exhaustive. When administering Corticosteroids, factors such as dose, duration and route alongside each patient's condition and health status need consideration for potential risk of side effects and adverse reactions.

Clinical considerations

NICE (2017) stipulate that consideration for the use of Corticosteroids should consider the age of the person (children and elderly being more susceptible to adverse side effects), and certain conditions, (diabetes mellitus, hypertension and hepatic impairment require caution and close monitoring) in conjunction with the indication for use to ensure patient safety.

Conclusion

Treatment of cancer can occur using a number of different pharmaceutical options. Understanding of the difference between cancer cells and normal cells allows for greater appreciation of the pharmacodynamics of each of these treatment options. When caring for

Episode of care

Alex

Alex was 3 years old when he presented to hospital with a month history of flu-like symptoms and a recent development of a purpuric rash. After initial testing, Alex was diagnosed with acute lymphoblastic leukaemia (ALL).

Alex lives at home on a farm with his mother, father and one sister, aged 2 years. The family are struggling with income due to recent floods.

Alex was treated according to the UKALL 2011 trial guidelines which combines the use of corticosteroids and chemotherapy. As Alex's cancer was low risk, he was assigned to regimen A of the trial.

Alex was initially given a four-week period of bi-daily, high-dose oral dexamethasone, along-side intravenous vincristine (weekly). Following this initial induction period (six weeks), Alex was given a combination of intravenous and oral chemotherapy and oral corticosteroids over a period of three years to cure his leukaemia.

Throughout his treatment, Alex experience various side effects including:

* initial weight gain
* nausea and vomiting
* alopecia
* mucositis
* weight loss (later in treatment)
* decelerated growth.

Prior to discharge, a nurse will need to ensure that Alex's family are educated and competent in recognising the side effects of treatment and when to seek medical help.

Alex will continue to be followed up after his treatment by his specialist team in long-term follow-up. Healthcare professionals will need to offer ongoing psychological and physical support for Alex, monitoring him for side effects of treatment and ensuring that his cancer does not recur.

patients with cancer, it is important that the nurse understands how each treatment regimen works and the side effects of these. The nurse also needs to be able to provide those receiving cancer treatment and, if appropriate, their families, with high-quality safe and effective care in a compassionate manner. A holistic approach is advocated with the patient at the centre of all that is done.

Different cancers have different properties and result in different abnormalities during the growth and multiplication of the cell. Not all treatments will be appropriate for all cancers; instead, treatment must be tailored to the individual patient's cancer. While one patient may have a single approach to treatment, other patients will require a combination of many different forms of treatment. Cancer care must be managed to ensure that the benefit of treatment outweighs the risk from adverse reactions or side effects.

This chapter has outlined some of the main pharmaceutical treatment options currently used for cancer in the UK. Advances in cancer research are continually developing and improving the care that can be offered to patients with cancer.

Glossary

Alopecia	The partial or complete loss of hair from areas of the body where it normally grows.
Antibodies	A blood protein produced in response to and counteracting a specific antigen. Antibodies combine chemically with substances which the

	body recognises as alien, such as bacteria, viruses and foreign substances in the blood.
Antigen	A toxin or other foreign substance which induces an immune response in the body, especially the production of antibodies.
Auto-immune	Relating to disease caused by antibodies or lymphocytes produced against substances naturally present in the body, producing the body's own auto-immune response.
Differentiation	The process by which cells, tissue and organs acquire specialised features, especially during embryonic development.
Epitope	The part of an antigen molecule to which an antibody attaches itself.
Molecule	A group of atoms bonded together, representing the smallest fundamental unit of a chemical compound that can take part in a chemical reaction.
Mucositis	Inflammation of a mucus membrane, especially that caused by cytotoxic therapy (radiation or chemotherapy).
Organism	An individual animal, plant or single-celled life form.
Proliferation	Rapid reproduction of a cell, part or organism.
Protein	Proteins are large molecules, composed of one or more chains of amino acids in a specific order, and are required for the structure, function and regulation of the body's cells, tissues and organs.
T cell	A lymphocyte of a type produced or processed by the thymus gland and actively participating in the immune response.
Toxic	Relating to or caused by poison.

References

Almeida, V.L., Leitão, A., Reina, L.C.B.., Montanari, CA., Donnici, CL. and Lopes MTP. (2005). Cancer and nonspecific cycle-cell and nonspecific cycle-cell antineoplastic agents interacting with DNA: an introduction. *New Chemistry* **28** (1): 118–129.

Bignold, L.P. (2006). Alkylating agents and DNA polymerases. *Anticancer Research* **26**: 327–1336.

Cancer Network (2019). *Corticosteroids*. www.cancernetwork.com/view/corticosteriods-advanced-cancer (accessed August 2019).

Cancer Research Institute (2019). *Homepage*. https:www.cancerresearchuk.org (accessed August 2019).

Cancer Research UK (2017). *Treatment*. https://www.cancerresearchuk.org/about-cancer/cancer-in-general/treatment (accessed August 2019).

Castro, F., Cardoso, A., Goncalves, R. et al. (2018). Interferon gamma at the crossroads of tumour surveillance or evasion. *Frontiers in Immunology*. https://doi.org/10.3389/fimmu.2018.00847.

Coosemans, A., Vankerckhoven, A., Baert, T. et al. (2019). Combining conventional therapy with immunotherapy: a risky business? *European Journal of Cancer* **113**: 41–44.

Czock, D., Keller, F., Rasche, F. et al. (2005). Pharmacokinetics and pharmacodynamics of systemically administered glucocorticoids. *Clinical Pharmokinetics* **44**: 61–98. https://doi.org/10.2165/00003088-2 00544010-00003.

Electronic Medicines Compendium (EMC) (2016). *Cyclophosphamide tablets 50mg*. www.medicines.org. uk/emc/product/1813/smpc (accessed August 2019).

Electronic Medicines Compendium (EMC) (2017). *Cyclophosphamide 1000mg powder for solution for injection or infusion*. www.medicines.org.uk/emc/product/3525/smpc (accessed August 2019).

Electronic Medicines Compendium (EMC) (2019). *MabThera 100 mg concentrate for solution for infusion*. https://www.medicines.org.uk/emc/product/3801/smpc (accessed August 2019).

Fu, D., Calvo, J.A., and Samson, L.D. (2012). Genomic instability in cancer balancing repair and tolerance of DNA damage caused by alkylating agents. *Nature Reviews Cancer* **12** (2): 104–120.

Gmeiner, W.H. (2002). Antimetabolite incorporations into DNA: structural and thermodynamic basis for anticancer activity. *Biopolymers* **65**: 180–189.

Haanen, J.B.A.G, Carbonnel, C., Robert, C., et al. (2017). Management of toxicities from Immunotherapy: ESMO Clinical Practice Guidelines for diagnosis, treatment and follow-up. *Annals of Oncology* **28** (suppl_4): iv119–iv142. doi: 10.1093/annonc/mdx225.

Hanahan D and Weinberg RA. (2011). 'The hallmarks of cancer: the next generation' doi:10.1016/j.cell.2011.02.013

Health and Safety Executive (HSE) (2019). *Safe handling of cytotoxic drugs in the workplace*. www.hse.gov. uk/healthservices/safe-use-cytotoxic-drugs.htm (accessed July 2019).

Hortobágyi, G.N. (1997). Anthracyclines in the treatment of cancer. *Drugs* **54** (Supplement 4): 1–7.

Drugs.com (2019). *Rituximab*. https://drugs.com/monograph/rituximab.html (accessed August 2019).

Johnson, B., Manoucher, A., Haugh, A. et al. (2019). Neurological toxicity associated with immune checkpoint inhibitors: a pharmacoconveince study. *Journal for Immunotherapy of cancer* **7** (134). https://doi. org/10.1186/s40425-019-0617-x.

Joint Formulary Committee (2019). *Cytotoxic drugs*. https://bnf.nice.org.uk/treatment-summary/cytotoxic-drugs.html (accessed July 2020).

Kirkwood, J., Lotze, M., and Yasko, J. (2001). *Current Cancer Therapeutics*, 4e. Philadelphia: Port City Press.

Lee, S. and Margoln, K. (2011). Cytokines in cancer immunotherapy. *Journal of Cancer* **3** (4): 3856–3893. https://doi.org/10.33901/cancers3043856.

Ly, I.K. and Wen, P. (2017). Clinical relevance of steroid use in Neuro-Oncology. *Current Neurology and Neuroscience Reports* **17** (1): 5. doi: 10.1007/s11910-017-0713-6.

McClendon, A.K. and Osheroff, N. (2007). DNA topoisomerase II, genotoxicity, and cancer. *Mutation Research* **623** (1–2): 83–97.

Moudi, M., Rusea, G., Yien, C.Y.S., and Nazre, M. (2013). Vinca Alkaloids. *International Journal of Preventative Medicine* **4** (11): 1231–1235.

National Chemotherapy Advisory Group (NCAG) (2009). *Chemotherapy services in england: ensuring quality and safety*. http://webarchive.nationalarchives.gov.uk/20130107105354/http://www.dh.gov.uk/prod_consum_dh/groups/dh_digitalassets/documents/digitalasset/dh_104501.pdf (accessed July 2020).

NCBI (2019). *Homepage*. www.ncbi.nlm.nih.gov (accessed August 2020).

Neilsen, D., Maare, C., and Skovsgaard, T. (1996). Cellular resistance to anthracyclines. *General Pharmarcology: The Vascular System* **27** (2): 251–255.

NICE (2017). *Glucocorticoid*. bnf.nice.orh.uk/treatment-summary/glucocorticoid (accessed August 2020).

NICE. (2018a). *Guidance*. Nice.org.uk/guidanceta576 (accessed August 2020).

NICE (2018b). *Guidance. Nice.org.uk/guidanceta559* (accessed August 2020).

Office for National Statistics (ONS) (2019). *Cancer registration statistics, England: 2017*. www.ons.gov.uk/peoplepopulationandcommunity/healthandsocialcare/conditionsanddiseases/bulletins/cancerregistrationstatisticsengland/2017 (accessed July 2019).

Pires, J., Kreutz, O.C., Sayuri Suyenaga, E., and Perassolo, M.S. (2018). Pharmacological profile and structure-activity relationship of alykylating agents used in cancer treatment. *International Journal of Research in Pharmacy and Chemistry* **8** (1): 6–17.

Potter, E.A., White, A.L., Dou, L. et al. (2014). Fc gamma receptor dependency of agonistic CD40 antibody in lymphoma therapy can be overcome through antibody multimerization. *Journal Of Immunology* **193** (4): 1828–1835.

Restifo, N., Dudley, M., and Rosenberg, S. (2012). Adoptive immunotherapy for cancer: harnessing the T cell response. *Nature Reviews Immunology* **12**: 269–281.

Rosenberg, S., Restifo, N., Yang, J. et al. (2008). Adoptive cell transfer: a clinical path to effective cancer immunotherapy. *Nature Reviews Cancer* **8**: 299–308.

Ryken TC, McDermott M, Robinson P, Ammirati M, Andrews D, Asher A, Burri S. (2010).'The role of steroids in management of brain metastases: A systemic review*. doi:10.1007/s11060-009-0057-4

Schäcke, H., Dacke, W., and Asadullah, K. (2002). Mechanisms involved in the side effects of glucocorticoids. *Pharmacology* **961**: 23–43.

Schreiber, R.D. and Smyth, M.J. (2011). Cancer immunoediting: integrating immunity's role in cancer suppression and promotion. *Science* **331** (6024): 1565–1570. doi: 10.1126/science.1203486.

Twycross, R. (1994). Risks and benefits of corticosteroids in advanced cancer. *National Library of Medicine* **11** (3): 163–168.

Vansteenkiste J. (2012). *Immunotherapy*. Lung Cancer doi:10.1016/j.lungcan.2012.05.029 (accessed August 2019).

Walsh, D., Doona, M., Molnar, M., and Lipnickey, V. (2000). Symptom control in advanced cancer: important drugs and routes of administration. *Oncology* **27** (1): 69–83.

Wooldridge, J., Anderson, M., and Parry, M. (2001). Corticosteroids in advanced cancer. *Cancer Network* **15** (2): 225–234.

Woolley, D. (1959). Antimetabolites. *Science* **129**: 3349.

Yao, H., Wang, H. Fang, J.Y. et al. (2018). *Cancer cell intrinsic PD-1 and implications in combinatorial immunotherapy*. Frontiers in Immunology 9. doi:10.3389/fimmu.2018.01774.

Yasir, M., Goyal, A.; Bansal, P. and Sonthalia, S. (2019). Corticosteroid Adverse Effects. *StatPearls*. https://www.ncbi.nlm.nih.gov/books/NBK531462/#:~:text=Glucocorticoids%20increase%20the%20risk%20of,ulcer%20formation%2C%20and%20GI%20bleeding (accessed October 2020).

411

Yu, Z.Y., Wrange, O., Boëthius, J. et al. (1981). A study of glucocorticoid receptors in intracranial tumours. *Journal of Neurosurgery* **55** (5): 757–760. doi: 10.3171/jns.1981.55.5.0757.

Zhou, J. and Cidlowski, J.A. (2005). The human glucocorticoid receptor: one gene, multiple proteins and diverse responses. *Steroids* **70** (5–7): 407–417. doi: 10.1016/j.steroids.2005.02.006.

Zhou, X.J. and Rahmani, R. (1992). Preclinical and clinical pharmacology of Vinca alkaloids. *Drugs* **44** (Supplement 4): 1–16.

Further reading

National Cancer Peer Review – National Cancer Action Team

The NCAT have written a Manual for Cancer Services which supports the National Cancer Peer Review quality assurance program for cancer services to enable quality improvement in terms of both clinical and patient outcomes.

NICE guidelines

The National Institute for Health and Care Excellence (NICE) writes evidence-based recommendations for healthcare in England. They provide a number of guidelines for the care and services suitable for most patients with certain types of cancer.

SIGN Guidelines

The Scottish Intercollegiate Guidelines Network (SIGN) develops and disseminates clinical guidelines for evidence-based healthcare practice in Scotland. They have developed a range of guidelines for use in cancer care.

Royal Pharmaceutical Society

The RPS provides pharmaceutical guidance for all healthcare practitioners in the UK. Information is available on current treatments for cancer.

Multiple choice questions

1. Over recent years, the UK has seen:
   - (a) A decrease in the number of females diagnosed with cancer
   - (b) An increase in the number of people dying from cancer
   - (c) A decrease in the number of people dying from cancer
   - (d) No change in the number of people diagnosed with cancer
2. Which of these is a 'hallmark of a cancer cell'?
   - (a) Inducing angiogenesis
   - (b) Apoptosis
   - (c) Activating growth suppressors
   - (d) Limited multiplication
3. At what stage in the cell cycle does the cell completely divide?
   - (a) M
   - (b) G1
   - (c) G2
   - (d) S
4. What does cytotoxic mean?
   - (a) Nourishes the cell
   - (b) Stops the cell receiving messages
   - (c) Stimulates the cell to grow
   - (d) Poisonous to cells
5. Which of these is not a route that chemotherapy can be administered?
   - (a) Oral
   - (b) Intravenous
   - (c) Intrafollicular
   - (d) Intrathecal

6. How does an antimetabolite work?
   (a) Inhibits topoisomerase II
   (b) Creates a deficiency of essential molecules
   (c) Transfers alkyl carbon molecules
   (d) Binds to tubulin
7. What are vinca alkaloids derived from?
   (a) Plants
   (b) Hormones
   (c) Horse urine
   (d) Synthetic compounds
8. Which of these is a common side effect of chemotherapy?
   (a) Changes to eye colour
   (b) Death
   (c) Hair loss
   (d) Perforated ear drum
9. What are the two main functions of the immune system?
   (a) Increase bone strength and fight infection
   (b) Fight infection and reduce inflammation
   (c) Stimulate growth and reduce inflammation
   (d) Control hair growth and support vision

10. Which one of the following is not part of the immune system?
    (a) White blood cells
    (b) Spleen
    (c) Lymph nodes
    (d) Liver
11. How does immunotherapy work?
    (a) Targets proteins on cancer only cells
    (b) Suppresses the immune system
    (c) Attracts cancer cells
    (d) Opens checkpoints in cancer cells
12. What is the role of supportive immunotherapy?
    (a) To prime the immune system
    (b) To stop growth within the cancer cell
    (c) To reduce growth in the cancer cell
    (d) To reduce inflammation
13. Who is the donor for an autologous bone marrow transplant?
    (a) Identical twin
    (b) Unrelated
    (c) Family
    (d) Self
14. Where are steroids naturally produced in the body?
    (a) The adrenal glands
    (b) Lymphocytes
    (c) The bone marrow
    (d) Testes
15. Why are corticosteroids used in the treatment of cancer?
    (a) To regulate heart and kidney function
    (b) To increase immunity and inflammatory responses
    (c) To reduce inflammation and allergic reactions
    (d) To support bone strength and growth

Find out more

The following is a list of some of the cancers that are included in this chapter. Take some time and write notes about the treatment of each of the cancers and be specific about the pharmacodynamics and possible side effects of the medicines that would be used to treat this.

Acute lymphoblastic leukaemia (ALL)	Your Notes
Myeloma	
Hodgkin's lymphoma	
Breast cancer	
Melanoma	

Chapter 16

Medications and the nervous system

Julie Derbyshire

Aim

The aim of this chapter is to provide the reader with an introduction to the pharmacology linked to common neurological disorders.

Learning outcomes

After reading this chapter, the reader will be able to:

1. Discuss the complexity of neurology and the importance of medication in the treatment of some key neurological disorders
2. Explain the main medications, including their use, side effects and contraindications, used in the management of strokes, epilepsy, Parkinson's disease and multiple sclerosis
3. Appreciate the importance of patient education and medication concordance in managing their neurological disorder effectively
4. Acknowledge other treatment options to support medication in the management of key neurological disorders

Test your knowledge

1. Can you identify the first line anti-epileptic drugs used to treat focal seizures?
2. What anti-epileptic drugs are recommended in the management of an acute seizure?
3. Why is it important for those with Parkinson's disease to have their medication on time?
4. How does levodopa work in the treatment of Parkinson's disease?
5. What is the aim of intravenous thrombolytic therapy in the treatment of acute ischaemic stroke?

Fundamentals of Pharmacology: For Nursing and Healthcare Students, First Edition. Edited by Ian Peate and Barry Hill.
© 2021 John Wiley & Sons Ltd. Published 2021 by John Wiley & Sons Ltd.

Introduction

Neurological disorders affect the peripheral and central nervous system – which includes the brain, spinal cord and the nerves that connect them – and it is this system that controls and coordinates many of the body's actions. Neurology is the medical science that deals with the nervous system and disorders that affect it, including investigations, diagnosis and treatment. Although some mental health conditions are categorised as neurological disorders and can affect the nervous system, they are classified differently and managed by psychiatrists, so will not be included in this chapter. There are over 600 neurological disorders, and for many of them treatment is often limited due to the complexity and sophistication of the nervous system. However, medication in the treatment of neurological disorders is recognised as an important part of the management plan. Therefore, this chapter will help nurses develop an understanding of pharmacology used in the management of neurological disorders, which is essential to provide care that is safe and effective. As well as an understanding of pharmacology, nurses are also required to work with patients and their families in explaining how to administer the medication, the action(s) of the medications, potential side effects and the contraindications. It is also important that nurses look at the wider issues associated with medication optimisation, including other treatment options, lifestyle issues, and the physical and psychological impact of the neurological disorder on both the patient and their family. This chapter will focus on four of the most common neurological disorders: epilepsy, Parkinson's disease, strokes and multiple sclerosis. Each section will include an overview of the neurological disorder, how medications work to treat the disorder, including consideration of other issues important to managing the disorder effectively.

Epilepsy

Epilepsy is one of the most common chronic neurological condition (WHO, 2017) and is characterised by recurrent and unprovoked seizures originating in the brain, with the dysfunction caused by excessive and abnormal neuronal discharge (Hickey, 2017). Accurate estimates of incidence and prevalence are difficult to achieve, but it is estimated that approximately 600 000 people in the UK have epilepsy (Epilepsy Research UK, 2017). Some causes of epilepsy include neonatal onset (e.g. congenital), previous cerebral trauma or a neurological condition and/or drug toxicity. However, in many cases a cause of the epilepsy is not identified, and this is referred to as unknown or idiopathic. Treatment of epilepsy varies widely and most often depends on the clinical manifestation, particularly diagnosis of seizure type which are most often categorised into two main categories: focal or generalised (see further divisions in Table 16.1).

The mainstay of treatment for epilepsy is directed at the management of seizures through medication (Karch, 2017). The drugs that are used to manage seizures are referred to as anticonvulsants or more commonly anti-epileptic drugs (AEDs). These drugs aim to control epilepsy in one of three ways (Greenstein, 2009):

Table 16.1   Classification of seizures

Focal Seizures	Generalised seizures
• Focal aware seizures without impaired consciousness level • Focal impaired awareness seizures with impaired consciousness level	• Absence seizures • Myoclonic seizures • Clonic seizures • Tonic seizures • Tonic–clonic seizures • Atonic seizures

Source: Modified from Epilepsy Action (2017).

- Enhancing the activity of the inhibitory neurotransmitter gamma-aminobutyric acid (GABA).
- Enhancing the activity of the excitatory brain neurotransmitter glutamate.
- Directly blocking sodium and/or calcium channels in the nerve cell membrane.

Medications prescribed for epilepsy should be individualised according to the seizure and epilepsy type, the person's lifestyle, age, co-morbidities and preferences of the person, their family and/or carers as appropriate (NICE, 2018). Effective management is aimed at the prevention of seizure occurrence, the use of single or combination drug therapy with the least side effects, choice in medication and frequency to optimise compliance and regular monitoring. Hickey (2017) states that 75% of patients with epilepsy can have seizures reduced or controlled effectively by medication. Although there are now a number of drugs used in the treatment of epilepsy, it is best for practitioners to prescribe one drug (monotherapy), at a low dose, with a gradual increase until seizures are controlled or adverse effects develop. If seizures are not controlled with a single drug, another drug might be added until optimum management is achieved (Epilepsy Society, 2018). NICE (2018) categorises AED options into seizure type to guide practitioners who are prescribing medication as part of a person's treatment plan, with approximately 25 AEDs currently licensed for use in the UK (Epilepsy Society, 2018). These are summarised in Table 16.2, but only five AEDs, their mechanism of action, therapeutic use and potential adverse effects will be discussed in more detail.

Carbamazepine

Carbamazepine is one of the older AEDs but is still used widely to treat generalised tonic–clonic and focal seizures, often as monotherapy. It works by blocking sodium channels in the nerve membranes, maintaining the conducting nerve in an inactive state. It is most often given orally; it is absorbed in the gastrointestinal (GI) tract and is metabolised in the liver. It is introduced at a lower dose initially and gradually increased to achieve optimum effect

Table 16.2 AED by seizure type

Seizure type	First-line AED	Adjunct AED
Focal (partial, complex partial, secondary generalised)	Carbamazepine Lamotrigine Levetiracetam Oxcarbazepine Gabapentin Sodium valproate	Levetiracetam Clobazam (and many other AEDs)
Generalised tonic–clonic	Carbamazepine Lamotrigine Oxcarbazepine Sodium valproate	Clobazam Lamotrigine Levetiracetam Sodium valproate Topiramate
Absence	Ethosuximide Lamotrigine Sodium valproate	Ethosuximide Lamotrigine Sodium valproate Benzodiazepines Levetiracetam Topiramate
Myoclonic	Levetiracetam Sodium valproate Topiramate	Levetiracetam Sodium valproate Topiramate Levetiracetam Clonazepam topiramate

Source: NICE (2018).

(Greenstein, 2009). Adverse effects can include drowsiness, rashes, dizziness, dry mouth, fatigue and GI disturbances (Joint Formulary Committee, 2019). Drug interactions can vary and the Joint Formulary Committee (2019) list them as mild, moderate and severe with manufacturer recommendations; however, Greenstein (2009) states that only 5% of patients on carbamazepine need to discontinue treatment due to an interaction or adverse effect.

Sodium valproate

Sodium valproate is another one of the older AEDs licensed to treat all types of seizures, but it is thought to be particularly effective in tonic–clonic, absence and myoclonic seizures (Crouch and Chapelhow, 2008). Sodium valproate works by enhancing the activity of the neurotransmitter GABA, reducing neuronal discharge and hence seizure activity. It can be administered intravenously initially in some cases but is most often taken orally and metabolised in the liver. Sodium valproate is relatively free of side effects but these can include GI disturbances, aggression alopecia, and anaemia with more severe ones including thrombocytopenia and liver failure (Joint Formulary Committee, 2019). Valproate medicines are contraindicated in women and girls of childbearing potential unless the conditions of the Pregnancy Prevention Program are met (NICE, 2018).

Lamotrigine

Lamotrigine inhibits the release in the brain of the excitatory neurotransmitters glutamate and aspartate in order to prevent seizure activity and is most effective in the management of focal and tonic–clonic seizures (Joint Formulary Committee, 2019). It appears to be used more commonly as an alternative to carbamazepine. It is licensed as monotherapy in those with newly diagnosed epilepsy, as it is tolerated well with very few side effects. Lamotrigine is also prescribed when other AEDs have failed or as an adjunct to other AEDs and, in these cases, the initial dose may need to be adjusted (Greenstein, 2009). Adverse effects can include agitation, drowsiness, ataxia, headaches, nausea and rashes. Serious skin reactions can be dangerous, particularly in children, causing a condition called "Stevens Johnson" syndrome resulting in hypersensitivity, and lamotrigine should be withdrawn if this occurs (Joint Formulary Committee, 2019).

Levetiracetam

Levetiracetam is one of the newer AEDs approved for those over 16 years of age as monotherapy or as an adjunct to other AEDs with all individuals over one month of age for the treatment of focal seizures with or without generalised seizures (Joint Formulary Committee, 2019). Although the mechanism of action with levetiracetam is relatively unknown, it is believed that it interferes with neurotransmitter release at the synapse to reduce seizure activity (Lewis, 2014). Some of the adverse effects of levetiracetam include skin rashes nausea, dizziness, drowsiness, headache and loss of appetite. Caution is to be exercised with patients who have a history of depression as it can exacerbate symptoms and those who are pregnant or breast-feeding (Greenstein, 2009). Interestingly, Lewis (2014) discusses a review of levetiracetam in five randomised controlled trials with adults and children who had focal epilepsy and they demonstrated that the frequency of seizure activity was reduced in 50% of the patients.

Gabapentin

Gabapentin is also a newer AED with an unclear mechanism of action, but it appears to work by either mimicking the actions of the inhibitory neurotransmitter GABA or blocking the calcium channels – both which are known to reduce neuronal damage and seizure activity (Greenstein, 2009). It is used for the treatment of focal seizures with or without generalised seizures, both as monotherapy and as an adjunct therapy with other AEDs. It is not used in children under 6 years of age and in those over 6 years of age it is used with caution in higher doses. Some of the adverse effects include drowsiness, fatigue, ataxia, confusion and loss of appetite. Gabapentin has been associated with a rare risk of respiratory depression, so should be used with caution in patients with pre-existing respiratory conditions, CNS disorders and older people. Following concerns about dependence and abuse of gabapentin, it is now a class C drug and, similarly to pregabalin, it is only prescribed for individuals following accurate assessment by a healthcare practitioner (Joint Formulary Committee, 2019).

Clinical considerations

Branded and generic drugs
AEDs should always be prescribed by brand name to ensure consistency of the drug rather than generic substitutions, which could affect the bio-equivalency of the drug and subsequently reduce the therapeutic effect resulting in seizures or enhancing the effect and causing toxicity.

Clinical considerations

Medication concordance
Patient education is essential for those with epilepsy to ensure concordance with medication and prevention of seizure activity. Patients should be advised to take their medication at the same time every day and not to stop taking any of their medication suddenly. They should gain advice from a healthcare professional if they experience unwanted adverse effects from their medication. They should be advised not to take over-the-counter medication and alcohol without consulting with a healthcare professional, as they may interact with current medications. Each seizure should be recorded and any triggers noted. Regular medical follow-up is recommended, including blood tests to monitor the therapeutic effect of their medication.

Status epilepticus

Status epilepticus is a medical emergency that requires immediate treatment as it has a morbidity and mortality rate of about 10%. The causes of status epilepticus are withdrawal or poor concordance to medication, dosage changes, ill health and/or infection. It is mainly associated with generalised tonic–clonic seizures and characterised by prolonged and repeated seizures without recovery lasting 30 minutes or more (Queally and Lailey, 2007). However, the time period for treatment may vary depending on individual usual seizure presentation with most seizures lasting less than five minutes. Therefore, practitioners often initiate treatment before 30 minutes to ensure seizures are controlled promptly. In the hospital setting, the recommended medication is diazepam or lorazepam, which when administered intravenously should control the seizure within 10 minutes (Greenstein, 2009). Alternatively, NICE (2018) discuss the use of diazepam rectally or buccal midazolam, particularly in the pre-hospital phase and community setting where access to medical equipment is more limited. Phenytoin is also recommended by NICE (2018) to be given intravenously, prescribed for seizure relapse in hospital and used with caution due to its action on the heart; thus, cardiac monitoring is required. Other nursing care interventions during status epilepticus should be focused on preserving safety (NMC, 2015), which includes maintenance of patient airway, prevention of injury and displaying a calm and reassuring approach until the patient is fully recovered or transferred to a neurology or a critical care unit.

Adults with epilepsy should have a written epilepsy care plan that includes details about their medication, any preferences and lifestyle issues, which needs to be agreed between the individual with epilepsy and their healthcare team (NICE, 2012). While epilepsy can be a hidden disability, it is a chronic long-term condition which can have a significant impact on the patients' daily life and well-being and therefore ongoing support is required, often by an epilepsy specialist nurse who should conduct the yearly reviews (NICE, 2018). The prognosis of those with epilepsy is variable, but 70–80% of people who develop epilepsy will at some point be free from seizures with effective treatment predominantly from medication (Greenstein, 2009).

Clinical considerations

Epilepsy and driving

People with epilepsy who experience seizures that result in loss of consciousness may put others at risk if they drive a motor vehicle. Not only can a seizure itself cause an accident, but AEDs can have adverse effects that include drowsiness. These patients must inform the DVLA immediately. A patient may be allowed to drive a car when they are seizure free for a year, and this is assessed on an individual basis. In some instances, when someone with epilepsy is seizure free for three to five years, treatment may be stopped.

Episode of care

Amy is a 20-year-old girl who has had recently been diagnosed with temporal lobe epilepsy (with simple focal, complex focal and secondarily generalised seizures). Carbamazepine and lamotrigine are both first-line treatments in focal epilepsy. However, Amy is using a combined hormonal contraceptive pill. This may be affected by enzyme-inducing drugs such as carbamazepine, so lamotrigine is prescribed. If she is to consider pregnancy in the future, she is informed that treatment with high-dose folic acid will be needed to reduce the risk of neural tube defects during pregnancy. The DVLA regulations are discussed with Amy and she is advised that she cannot drive until she has been free of seizures for one year. A written treatment plan is provided, and leaflets are given on different aspects of epilepsy diagnosis, medication management and lifestyle issues which may be affected by epilepsy.

Source: Adapted from NICE (2018).

Parkinson's disease

Parkinson's disease (PD) is a common progressive neurodegenerative disorder that mostly affects people over 60 years of age but can manifest as early as the 40s and 50s with unknown cause. Aging, genetics and environment have been identified as risk factors to development of PD (Ashelford et al., 2016). It is characterised by the gradual and progressive degeneration of the dopamine-producing cells of the substantia nigra located in the basal ganglia of the brain (Donizak and McCabe, 2017). Dopamine is a neurotransmitter that is involved in coordination of motor responses and it is thought that the action of dopamine is opposed by another neurotransmitter called acetylcholine. This is important for the treatment for PD, as many of the therapies against motor loss and progression are aimed at tackling the imbalance between two neurotransmitters (see Figure 16.1). The main symptoms of PD are **tremor,** which occurs at rest and is often described as pill rolling, **rigidity,** where muscle tone is increased and patient complains of stiffness in joints, and **bradykinesia,** which refers to slowness and difficulty in initiating movement (Ashelford et al., 2016). Other signs and symptoms include drooling, slurred speech, difficulty swallowing and a mask-like expression which can occur as more of the dopamine producing cells die. Practitioners often use the terms "on" and "off" periods to describe the different stages of motor fluctuation. The "on" period is the time when PD symptoms are under control and the "off" period is the time when the medication is not working well, causing worsening of PD symptoms (Parkinson's UK, 2019). The imbalance of neurotransmitters can be seen in Figure 16.1.

There is no cure or treatment to stop the degeneration of neurones of PD and therefore drug therapy is the primary treatment to improve quality of life and reduce PD symptoms in most patients. The choice of drug depends on a number of factors, including the patient's

Normal balance between acetylcholine and dopamine

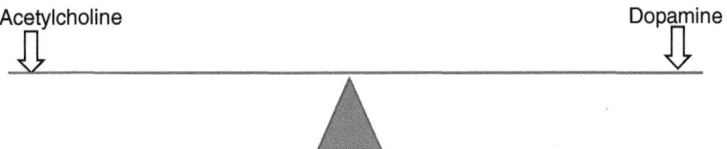

Imbalance showing a lack of dopamine which occurs in PD, and this leads to

increased acetylcholine

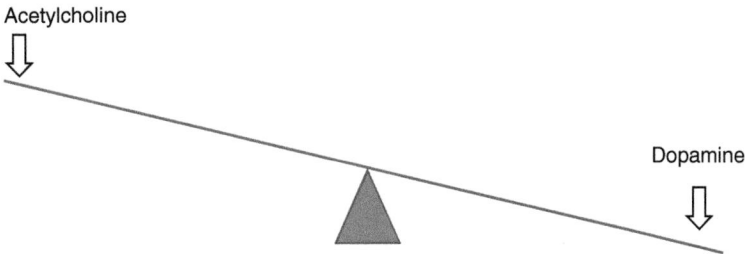

Figure 16.1 The imbalance of neurotransmitters in Parkinson's disease.

co-morbidities, employment status, clinician experience, patient preference and potential adverse effects. The choice should be made following individual assessment and discussion (SIGN, 2010). The main drug categories are outlined in Figure 16.2. Parkinson's UK (2019) state that most PD drug treatments work by doing one or more of the following:

- increasing the amount of dopamine in the brain (dopamine replacements);
- acting as a substitute for dopamine (dopamine agonists) by stimulating the parts of the brain where dopamine works;
- blocking the action of other factors (enzymes) that break down dopamine including drugs, such as Monoamine-oxidase inhibitors (MAOI) B inhibitors, Catechol-O-methyltransferase (COMT) inhibitors and Anti-cholinergics.

Dopamine replacement drugs

The obvious way to increase dopamine in the brain is to administer dopamine; however, alone it cannot cross the blood–brain barrier and enter the brain where it is needed (Ashelford et al., 2016). Instead, it is replaced with a drug called levodopa, which is converted into dopamine in the brain by the enzyme dopa decarboxylase. Levodopa is the main drug used in the management of PD and helps control the motor symptoms of PD. However, levodopa is also converted to dopamine in the rest of the body and causes nausea, vomiting and cardiovascular problems, and therefore is combined with a second drug to prevent these side effects. The most widely used combination drugs to treat PD are Co-careldopa (Sinemet) and Co-beneldopa (madapar) which are often introduced slowly initially and gradually increased to produce the desired effect but without too many adverse effects (SIGN, 2010). These can include nausea and vomiting, postural hypotension, restlessness, involuntary facial movements, increased hand tremor and constipation (Greenstein, 2009). The intervals between taking these medications can be critical in determining the severity of these side effects, and therefore each person is assessed individually for their reaction to the drug.

Dopamine agonists

These group of drugs stimulate dopamine receptors and mimic the effect of dopamine, but are less effective than levodopa at reducing motor symptoms. Therefore, they are only pre-scribed if levodopa is ineffective or the person with PD experiences adverse effects (Ashelford et al., 2016). They can also be used in combination with levodopa and, in these patients, the levodopa dosage is reduced. Dopamine agonists can be divided into ergot-derived (ropinirole, pramipexole and rotigotine) – named after the fungus that they are derived from – and non-ergot derived (bromocriptine, pergolide and cabergoline) and they act on different dopamine receptors in the cells of the basal ganglia. Ergot-derived dopamine agonists should not be given as first-line treatment for PD due to the risk of fibrosis, particularly cardiac fibrosis (NICE, 2017). Apomorphine is another dopamine agonist, which is a powerful drug used to treat "off" times (muscle stiffness, loss of muscle control) in people with advanced Parkinson's disease. It is often given as an intermittent injection or subcutaneous infusion. The adverse effects of all dopamine agonists are very similar and can include nausea, vomiting, postural hypotension, daytime drowsiness or somnolence, hallucinations and confusion. Another reported adverse effect of both types of dopamine agonists are impulse disorders, leading to binge eating, gambling and increased sexual urges (SIGN, 2010; NICE, 2017).

Monoamine-oxidase inhibitors (MAOI)

Monoamine is an enzyme which breaks down the monoamine neurotransmitters, dopamine, serotonin and noradrenaline. MAOI B inhibitors slow the breakdown of dopamine, leading to increased dopamine production and improved motor function (Ashelford et al., 2016). Examples of MAOI B inhibitors include selegiline and rasagaline. Some of the adverse effects include arrhythmias, nausea, abnormal movements, hallucinations, decreased appetite and confusion (Joint Formulary Committee, 2019).

MAOI drugs are also given to people with depression as they also slow the breakdown of serotonin, the neurotransmitter which contributes to the feeling of wellness and influences mood, sleep, appetite and sexuality.

Anticholinergics

Anticholinergics are drugs that block the effects of the excitatory neurotransmitter acetylcho-line at receptor sites in the substantia nigra, helping to restore the dopamine–acetylcholine balance (Karch, 2017). Anticholinergics used to treat PD include benzatropine, trihexyphenidyl and orphenadrine; they are useful in reducing tremor and drooling but are not so effective in reducing rigidity, which is often more challenging for patients with PD (Greenstein, 2009). Anticholinergics are more often prescribed as an adjunct therapy for PD due to their adverse effects, which can include nausea, constipation, dizziness, dry mouth, urinary problems and blurred vision (Joint Formulary Committee, 2019).

Catechol-O-methyltransferase (COMT) inhibitors

COMT inhibitors block the enzyme COMT, which is a naturally occurring enzyme that elimi-nates catecholamines including dopamine (Karch, 2017). Entacapone and tolcapone are the two main COMT inhibitors used either alone in early PD or more commonly as adjunct treat-ments with levodopa for patients who are experiencing end of dose fluctuations in motor functions which often occur with levodopa (Greenstein, 2009). Some of the adverse effects include nausea, vomiting, discoloured urine, dizziness and dry mouth. COMT inhibitors can also cause liver damage and so are contraindicated in those with liver disease (Joint Formulary Committee, 2019).

Amantadine

Amantadine is an antiviral treatment which works by increasing dopamine release by stimulat-ing the release of dopamine from dopaminergic terminals, and it is usually introduced early in

Clinical considerations

PD medication and impulse disorders
"Treatment with dopamine replacement drugs and dopamine agonists are associated with impulse control disorders, including pathological gambling, binge eating and hypersexuality. Patients and their carers should be informed about the risk of impulse control disorders. There is no evidence that ergot- and non-ergot-derived dopamine-receptor agonists differ in their propensity to cause impulse control disorders, so switching between dopamine-receptor agonists to control these side-effects is not recommended. If the patient develops an impulse control disorder, the dopamine-receptor agonist should be withdrawn or the dose reduced until the symptoms resolve" (NICE, 2017).

PD as a single therapy and increased, if necessary, after one week (Greenstein, 2009). However, the Joint Formulary Committee (2019) states that amantadine is usually administered as a combination therapy with other anti-Parkinsonian drugs. Some of the adverse effects include nausea, decreased appetite, skin discolouration, blurred vision, dizziness and dry mouth.

Drugs are an important treatment for those with PD, but many patients choose not to use them as they only relieve symptoms and do not prevent the progression of the disease. About 75% of patients respond to medication and report an improvement in rigidity, a common symptom of PD; however, the efficacy of some PD drugs may reduce with longer term use (Greenstein, 2009). Therefore, NICE (2017) recommend that patients with PD have regular access to clinical monitoring and medicines adjustment to ensure they are receiving the best treatment. They require a point of contact for support and reliable sources of information on PD that should include additional support for their family members and their careers (as appropriate), which in many cases is provided by a Parkinson's disease nurse specialist (NICE, 2017).

Clinical considerations

Deep brain stimulation
Deep brain stimulation (DBS) is a relatively new procedure, introduced in 1997 for people with PD as a treatment to stop tremors. It is also now used for those with advanced PD when other symptoms are not adequately controlled by alternative treatments. This procedure involves inserting electrodes into the parts of the brain affected by PD to control motor symptoms. The electrodes are connected by a wire to a pulse generator, similar to a pacemaker device, that is implanted under the skin in the chest and can be adjusted by the patient to control tremors.

Episode of care

James is a 75-year-old man who has had PD for 12 years. At initial diagnosis he decided not take any medication, but as his symptoms developed he was prescribed selegiline and was better controlled. After five years, his stiffness and tremor returned and Co-beneldopa (Sinemet) was added to his treatment. The dose was gradually increased to four times a day and his symptoms brought under control. James was admitted to his local hospital with a chest infection and did not receive his medication for PD for 24 hours. This had a significant effect on his ability to move; he was slower to get up in the morning and his arms were weak. James and his wife had explained to the nurses the importance of him getting his medication on time, and they had informed him that his medication would be administered during the drug rounds which had set times. The staff did not understand the importance of James receiving his PD drugs while in hospital or the need for timely administration. They did not infer that his physical symptoms were a result of his missed medication. Once he did receive his medication, it was the wrong preparation. The PD nurse specialist was contacted by James's wife and they visited the ward and explained the importance of timely PD medication and the impact on patients if this does not occur. The PD nurse also discussed the importance of ordering the same drug preparation that patients usually take to ensure the duration of action and peak concentration, as administering the wrong drug could result in a deteriorating of PD symptoms – which occurred in James's case. They also discussed the idea of self-medication with the staff for patients with PD, which is recognised as the way forward for patients in hospital and care homes.

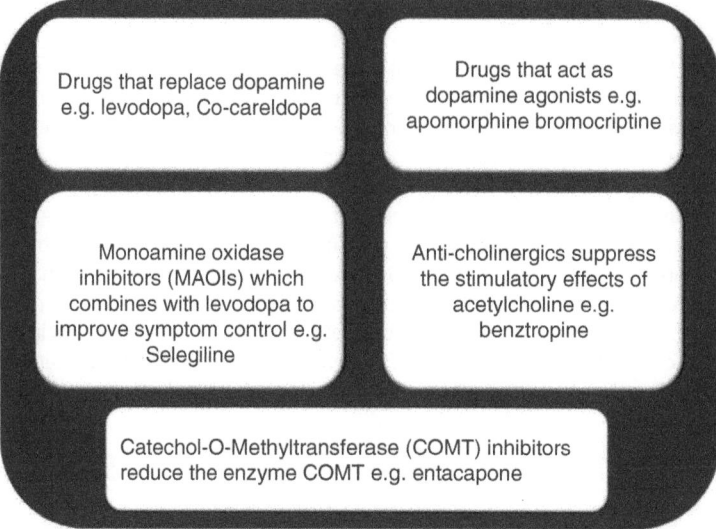

Figure 16.2   Main drugs used in Parkinson's disease.

Clinical considerations

Timing of drugs

In 2006, the Parkinson's Disease Society launched the "Get in on time" campaign to ensure that people with PD in hospitals and care homes receive their medication on time, every time. This was a result of reported incidents where patients were not receiving their prescribed medication at the right time. When those with PD do not receive their medication on time, the balance of chemicals in the body becomes disrupted, which can lead to PD symptoms becoming uncontrolled. This chemical imbalance can render a person unable to move or get out of bed and can take hours, days or weeks to stabilise. Therefore, it is important that healthcare professionals are aware of the importance of timely drug administration.

Strokes

A stroke is defined as a clinical syndrome, of presumed vascular origin, typified by rapidly developing signs of focal or global disturbance of cerebral functions lasting more than 24 hours or leading to death (World Health Organization, 1978). In England and Wales alone, over 80 000 people are hospitalised with acute stroke each year (Intercollegiate Stroke Working Party, 2016).

They are the third most common cause of mortality and are the leading cause of adult disability in the UK. Medical treatment is essential to the management of stroke to reduce neurological deficits, improve functional outcome, reduce the need for ongoing care and prevent the risk of recurrent stroke (Chapman and Bogle, 2014). Over the past 20 years, stroke care had been predominantly directed toward rehabilitation and social care with less attention focused on the emergency care in the "hyper acute" stage of admission (Fitzpatrick, 2013). However, medical and technological advances have transformed stroke care, with access to advanced imaging, the initiation of stroke protocols in the emergency department and the introduction of hyperacute services Royal College of Physicians (RCP) (2016). A stroke is now recognised as a medical emergency, and if outcomes are to be optimised, there should be no time delays in diagnosis and treatment, which was the rationale for the introduction of the FAST tool to educate the public on how to recognise a stroke promptly.

Clinical considerations

FAST
FAST (face, arms, speech and time) is the validated tool that should be used outside of hospital to screen people with a sudden onset of neurological symptoms for a diagnosis of stroke or transient ischaemic attack (TIA). This campaign has increased the awareness of stroke recognition among the public and hence led to quicker access to treatment.

425

There are two main types of stroke: ischaemic and haemorrhagic. An ischaemic stroke accounts for 85% of all strokes and is related to a blockage in an artery from a thrombus, reducing the blood supply to the brain. An ischaemic stroke is most often caused by atheroma in the blood vessel walls developed through aging with additional risk factors such as smoking, obesity, high cholesterol and diabetes. A haemorrhagic stroke accounts for 15% of strokes, resulting in an intracerebral hematoma caused by hypertension or an abnormal blood coagulation, or from a spontaneous rupture of a weakened artery, e.g. an aneurysm causing a subarachnoid haemorrhage. Both types of stroke present with similar neurological signs and symptoms; therefore, anyone with the acute onset of neurological deficits with persisting symptoms and signs (i.e. suspected stroke) should undergo urgent diagnostic assessment (CT scan). This is essential to differentiate between the type of stroke, so effective treatment can be initiated promptly (RCP, 2016; Birns, 2017).

Clinical considerations

Trans-ischaemic attack (TIA)
A TIA is often referred to as a "mini stroke" caused by a temporary disruption in the blood supply to the brain. A TIA presents with similar neurological deficits to an ischaemic stroke, often lasting a few minutes or a few hours but completely subsiding within 24 hours. Aspirin 300 mg is recommended for the initial management of suspected and confirmed TIA, and people should be referred for specialist assessment and secondary prevention (NICE, 2019a) as they are at high risk of a recurrent stroke that may result in more severe outcomes.

Medical treatment is aimed at restoring blood flow and enhancing brain function, with research and clinical guidelines supporting the use of medication as early as possible to reduce damage and improve outcomes, particularly in acute ischaemic stroke (Birns, 2017). In haemorrhagic strokes, treatment is often aimed at reversing any anticoagulants, removing the cause of the haemorrhage (if possible), blood pressure lowering drugs and surgery if clinically indicated

(RCP, 2016). Most of the medications discussed in the clinical guidelines for stroke are aimed at the management of acute ischaemic stroke, and include thrombolytic therapy, anticoagulants and antiplatelet treatments. In addition, cholesterol lowering therapies and antihypertensive medication are used to reduce long-term complications and the risk of recurrent stroke.

Thrombolytic (clot busting) therapy

The aim of acute thrombolytic therapy used in the management of ischaemic stroke is to break up the clot or thrombus to restore perfusion/blood flow, which will reverse the ischemia and reduce the damage to brain tissue (Birns, 2017). Thrombolytic medications are plasminogen activators that boost the action of plasmin, which breaks up the mesh network of fibrin within the clot and allows the accumulated platelets to disperse, restoring normal blood flow (Crouch and Chapelhow, 2008). The recommended plasminogen activator used in the treatment of ischaemic stroke is alteplase, which was approved for use in 1996. However, it has been recently been reviewed by an independent inquiry of the Medicines and Healthcare Products Regulatory Agency (MHRA), which has reaffirmed the benefit of alteplase in the treatment of ischaemic stroke. NICE (2019a) recommend alteplase for treating ischaemic stroke in adults if it is commenced within 4.5 hours of the onset of stroke symptoms, and only when intracerebral haemorrhage has been excluded by appropriate imaging techniques. Alteplase is now administered to one in nine patients with acute ischaemic stroke in the UK (Intercollegiate Stroke Working Party, 2016). Fast-track systems have been developed involving protocol-based rapid response by paramedics, emergency department clinicians and stroke specialist teams to facilitate timely administration (Birns, 2017). These staff should be experienced in the provision of stroke thrombolysis, with a thorough knowledge of the contraindications to treatment and the management of complications (Intercollegiate Stroke Working Party, 2016; NICE, 2019a).

Alteplase is administered intravenously over one hour as it has a short half-life. It is given via a peripheral cannula with the initial 10% of dose administered by intravenous injection and the remainder by intravenous infusion. The dosage is calculated based on weight with a maximum dose of 90 mg (Joint Formulary Committee, 2019). Alteplase is less problematic for patients than other thrombolytic drugs and its action targets the clot better with less risk of an allergic reaction (Crouch and Chapelhow, 2008). The main adverse effect of alteplase is potential bleeding, and therefore it is contraindicated in patients with previous haemorrhagic stroke, GI bleeds, recent surgery, uncontrolled hypertension and coagulation defects.

Combined intravenous thrombolytic therapy and endovascular therapy to remove the clot (thrombectomy) are now being recommended by NICE (2019a) as an effective treatment strategy for large vessel occlusions up to 24 hours from symptom onset.

Antiplatelets

Antiplatelet medications are key to secondary prevention of ischaemic stroke and are used to reduce the platelet "stickiness" associated with clot formation so that aggregation is less likely to occur (Greenstein, 2009). Evidence exists for three different antiplatelet agents used in the management of ischaemic stroke: aspirin, dipyramidamole and clopidogrel, which all have different mechanisms of action (Birns, 2017). Aspirin prevents the formation of a chemical thromboxane, which is released by platelets and makes them stick together; therefore, with no thromboxane platelets are unable to signal to each other to stick together and this prevents clot formation (Ashelford et al., 2016). NICE (2019a) recommends that patients should be offered aspirin 300 mg orally as soon as possible and definitely within 24 hours if they do not have dysphagia, **or** aspirin 300 mg rectally or by enteral tube if they do have dysphagia. A diagnosis of intracerebral haemorrhage must also be excluded by brain imaging before administering aspirin. Aspirin 300 mg daily should be continued for two weeks after the onset of stroke symptoms, prior to long-term oral antithrombotic treatment (NICE, 2019a). Patients who have been prescribed aspirin following an ischaemic stroke reduce their risk of a further stroke by 13% (Birns, 2017). Adverse effects of aspirin are minimal, but can include bleeding and dyspepsia and it is contraindicated in people with peptic ulcers, clotting disorders and children under 16 years of age. Dipyramidole is most often prescribed as an oral medication, prescribed twice a day (200 mg) and used for the secondary prevention of ischaemic stroke not associated with atrial fibrillation and for TIAs used as a single therapy – but works more effectively when combined with aspirin (Greenstein, 2009). Some of its adverse effects include angina, dizziness diarrhea, nausea and skin reactions (Joint Formulary Committee, 2019). Similarly to aspirin, dipyramidole is contraindicated in patients with clotting disorders and also those with dysrhythmias.

Clopidogrel is the third antiplatelet medication used for both TIAs and acute ischaemic stroke in patients with aspirin hypersensitivity or intolerance. Clopidogrel works differently to aspirin, blocking the binding of adenosine triphosphate (ATP), a different chemical released by the platelets to stop platelets sticking together (Ashelford et al., 2016). Some evidence now suggests that clopidogrel should be the first-line antiplatelet medication (not aspirin) used as a single therapy, or alternatively a combination of aspirin and dypyramidole for those who are unable to take clopidogrel (RCP, 2016). Clopidogrel can take three to seven days to reach its full effect, unlike aspirin that works within 15–20 minutes (Ashelford et al., 2016). Some adverse effects of clopidogrel include bleeding, bruising, diarrhea, nausea, vomiting and skin reactions. It is contraindicated if active bleeding occurs and is not recommended for patients with liver or kidney problems, and there may be some interactions with other medications, e.g. non-steroidal anti-inflammatories (Joint Formulary Committee, 2019).

Oral anticoagulants

Vitamin K antagonists are the most common anticoagulants and are used in the primary and secondary prevention of strokes, particularly for those with a history of atrial fibrillation. The best known vitamin antagonist is warfarin, which exerts its anticoagulation effect by interfering with the synthesis of vitamin K-dependent clotting factors, including factors V11, 1X, X and X1 (Greenstein, 2009). Warfarin is given orally, but its onset of action is delayed, and for this reason anticoagulant therapy – such as low molecular weight heparin subcutaneously – is given as this acts immediately. Patients on warfarin need to be monitored regularly for their response to the medication, which is often in the hospital environment for patients with an acute ischaemic stroke. It is monitored through a blood test known as the international normalised ration (INR) which evaluates a patient's prothrombin levels against the normal prothrombin time. The warfarin dose is adjusted to keep the INR between two and three, depending on the clinical situation, with an aim of effective coagulation and low risk of bleeding (Greenstein, 2009). Once the INR level is stable, the low molecular weight heparin is withdrawn. Concordance with vitamin K antagonists like warfarin is challenging as they interact with certain foods and other medication and there is a need for frequent blood tests (INRs). Therefore, patient education is essential to ensure that the patient understands the importance of taking the correct dose at the right time, reporting any adverse effects such as bruising/bleeding, potential interactions with foods, alcohol or other medications, regular INR tests and carrying a warfarin alert card (Stroke Association, 2015).

Newer oral anticoagulants have been introduced as a result of more recent evidence and are classified as non-vitamin K oral antagonists. The advantages of these new drugs are the use of a consistent oral dosage and no need for INR monitoring. These include dabigatran, rivaroxaban and apixaban, which are most commonly used in prophylaxis and treatment of venous thromboembolism (VTE) but can be used in stroke prevention in patients with non-valvular atrial fibrillation with other risk factors, including previous stroke or TIA (Joint Formulary Committee, 2019). Current guidelines advocate that anticoagulants should not be commenced for ischaemic secondary stroke prevention until after 14 days from stroke diagnosis, unless under specialist supervision (Birns, 2017).

Antihypertensives

Antihypertensive treatment in people with acute ischaemic stroke is recommended only if there is a hypertensive emergency with the presence of hypertensive encephalopathy, hypertensive nephropathy, cardiac failure/myocardial infarction, aortic dissection or pre-eclampsia (NICE, 2019a). However, blood pressure control must be lower than 185/110 mmHg if they are being considered for intravenous thrombolysis. Patients with primary intracerebral haemorrhage who present within six hours of onset with a systolic blood pressure greater than 150 mmHg should be treated urgently using a locally agreed protocol for blood pressure lowering to a systolic blood pressure of 140 mmHg for at least seven days. Exceptions include a Glasgow Coma Score of five or less, a large hematoma with expected death, if a structural cause for the hematoma is found, or they undergo immediate surgery to evacuate the hematoma (RCP, 2016).

Statins

The use of immediate statin treatment aims to lower cholesterol, as a high level in the blood – especially in the form of low density lipoproteins (LDL) – is associated with an increased risk of atheroma and potential strokes (Greenstein, 2009). It therefore would seem that drugs to lower the cholesterol concentration would reduce the risk of further strokes. However, NICE (2019a) state that statins are not recommended for people with an acute stroke, unless they are already receiving statins – where they are advised to continue. This is often reviewed later in the stroke rehabilitation process where statins may be prescribed, as they are relatively free of side effects and combined with a reduction of saturated fats in a patient's diet can help to reduce the risk of a further stroke (Stroke Association, 2015).

Other medications used in the management of stroke focus on the common problems experienced by patients following their stroke from the initial diagnosis in the first 24 hours to the weeks and months as they recover (RCP, 2016). They can encounter physical problems such as seizures, pain and limb spasticity and/or psychological problems including depression, which can all impact on the rehabilitation process. However, medication is only one aspect of acute stroke management; other interventions are delivered in specialist stroke units where there is a reliance on nurses and other healthcare professionals to deliver high-quality care to improve recovery and reduce long-term complications (Birns, 2017). In addition, health promotion strategies focusing on lifestyle factors are important for the prevention of further strokes, which is often the remit of nurses within specialist stroke units.

Episode of care

Richard is a 62-year-old who was admitted after a two-hour history of headache, slurred speech, facial drooping and left arm weakness. The paramedics performed the FAST tool and he was transferred to hospital. A CT scan was performed and a diagnosis of an ischaemic stroke was given following exclusion of an intracerebral haemorrhage. He was seen promptly in the emergency department by the stroke specialist nurse and prescribed aspirin 300 mg and was eligible for thrombolysis because of the two hour onset of symptoms. His blood pressure was 150/90 and he received alteplase 90 mg and was admitted to the hyperacute stroke service for ongoing care and rehabilitation, although he was making a good recovery with most symptoms subsided within 48 hours. Richard was given information, advice about risk factors in his lifestyle that may have been linked to his stroke and the need for secondary prevention. He was advised about smoking cessation and the importance of a healthy diet and physical activity to reduce his risk of a recurrent stroke. Consideration was also been given to assessment to identify the extent of carotid stenosis with a view to surgery (carotid endarterectomy) in the future.

Multiple sclerosis

Multiple sclerosis is a chronic, progressive disabling condition usually affecting young adults between 15 and 50 years of age. It is more common in females than males with a 3 : 1 ratio and more prevalent in temperate climates (Murray, 2005; Scolding and Wilkins, 2012). It only affects the myelinated nerves of the central nervous system, where the myelin sheaths that cover the

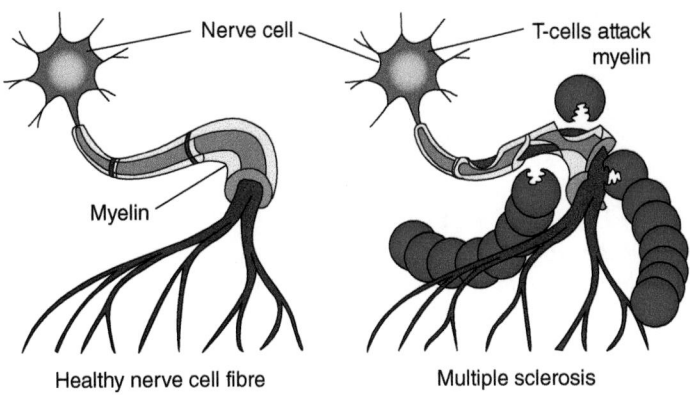

Figure 16.3 Multiple sclerosis.

nerves are damaged. When myelin is damaged or stripped away from the axon of the nerve, the messages become delayed or blocked. It is an unknown process/trigger that alters the response of the immune system and allows this damage to occur. Activated T cells within the immune system regard the myelin sheath as foreign (see Figure 16.3). The immune response leads to inflammation and demyelination, which becomes a self-perpetuating autoimmune process. Some regeneration of myelin occurs, but after repeated relapses the capacity for remyelination decreases, resulting in scar/plaque formation and neurodegeneration. Symptoms experienced by patients depend on what part of the CNS has been affected and the function of the damaged nerve. Some of the symptoms include problems with vision, muscle weakness, loss of sensation and coordination problems (MS Society, 2019). There is no definitive test for MS and diagnosis is based on clinical history, neurological examination and MRI scan (Burgess, 2013).

There are four types of multiple sclerosis, which are categorised as:

- **Relapsing remitting MS** (RRMS) – 85% of people present with RRMS, they have periods of relapses followed by periods of remissions.
- **Secondary progressive MS** (SPMS) – approximately 50% of those with RRMS develop SPMS within 10 years with increasing disability.
- **Primary progressive MS** (PPMS) – 10–15% of people at onset have PPMS, symptoms gradually develop but disability increases from the outset.
- **Benign MS** – 10% of those with MS which is categorised as mild attacks separated by long periods with no symptoms.

There is no cure for MS; however, it is not life threatening and medication can be effective in the treatment of relapses, the reduction in the number of relapses and the management of symptoms. The choice of drug depends on the type of MS, the patient's disability status, severity of disease and individual tolerance, with the overall aim of maintaining maximum functional ability and quality of life (NICE, 2019b).

Corticosteroids

Corticosteroids are the mainstay of treatment for MS relapses and work by reducing inflammation to relieve the symptoms of MS; however, not all relapses need treatment with steroids. NICE (2019b) define a relapse of MS as one where the person develops new symptoms or has worsening of existing symptoms. These symptoms need to last more than 24 hours in the absence of infection or other cause and can include optic neuritis, motor disability and acute ataxia (Pandit and Murthy, 2011). They have been used since the 1960s but are still very effective in the treatment of acute relapses. The main corticosteroid used in the treatment of MS relapses is oral methylprednisolone 500 mg for five days, or prescribed more commonly as an

429

intravenous (IV) infusion 1 g daily for three to five days (Joint Formulary Committee, 2019). Benefits and risks of high dose steroids should be explained to patients and this should be supported with written information in a format that is appropriate for them (NICE, 2019b). Corticosteroids are used to shorten the duration of the relapse but not the progression of the condition, which is more the focus of disease-modifying drugs.

Disease-modifying drugs

Disease-modifying drugs are the recommended treatment for active RRMS and can reduce the number of relapses by targeting the inflammatory process in MS, to prevent further decline and to maintain functional status. First-line generation drugs such as Interferon Beta (betaferon, copaxone, rebif) and Glatiramer Acetate are all given by injection and are the preferred choice for most patients due to their established safety profile and clinician experience with their use (NICE, 2019b). Interferon Beta is also licensed for use in SPMS, reducing the risk of relapses, but does not prevent the development of long-term disability and therefore its use is limited. Glatiramer Acetate (copaxone) is currently the most prescribed single drug for RRMS. These drugs are often well tolerated with the main adverse effect of interferon B drugs being flu-like symptoms (Weiner and Stankiewicz, 2012).

Natalizumab (tysabri) was approved in 2004 for RRMS and is classified as a second-generation disease-modifying drug and is an option for treatment only in rapidly evolving severe RRMS (NICE, 2019b). It is given as an intravenous infusion every four weeks and treatment is discontinued if there is no response after six months. Its use has been limited recently as a result of the increased risk of progressive multi-focal-leukoencephalopathy (PML) caused by the JC virus, and if diagnosed then treatment must be discontinued (Joint Formulary Committee, 2019). Other adverse effects include anxiety, fatigue and sinus congestion (Weiner and Stankiewicz, 2012).

The first oral drug licensed for MS was Fingolimod (gilenya), which was approved at the end of 2010 and can reduce relapses by 50% and slow progression of the disease. It must be initiated by a specialist and is prescribed once daily, but is not recommended for patients at risk of cardiovascular events as its main adverse effect is bradycardia, particularly after the first dose (NICE, 2019b). Therefore, patients who commence on Fingolimod are monitored for six hours after the first dose (Weiner and Stankiewicz, 2012). There are also a number of other disease-modifying drugs used in the management of MS, and researchers continue to look for treatments that can change the underlying cause of the disease by slowing, stopping or repairing damage to the myelin sheath (MS Society, 2019).

Symptom management

Other medications used in the management of MS focus on the chronic symptoms experienced by many patients, such as fatigue, spasticity, depression and visual disturbances that may require pharmacological and non-pharmacological interventions (Weiner and Stankiewicz, 2012). For example, physiotherapy can play an important role in reducing spasticity through active and passive stretching; combined with medication such as baclofen, recommended in the treatment of MS, it may help to improve function and comfort. Sativex is a licensed cannabis-based treatment administered as sublingual spray and used as a second-line treatment for spasticity when other treatments have failed, although it is not recommended by NICE (2019b) who suggest that it is not a cost-effective drug. However, the MS Society (2019) state that one in five people with MS surveyed in 2014 believed that cannabis helped with their symptoms of muscle spasms or stiffness (spasticity) and pain. Regular exercise may have positive effects on mobility and fatigue in patients with MS, which should be supported with psychological therapies such as cognitive behavioural techniques (NICE, 2019b). In addition, drugs such as amantadine are known to help to reduce fatigue in MS (Weiner and Stankiewicz, 2012).

Shared decision-making and a collaborative approach between patients and healthcare professionals is important for adherence to treatment in MS care, as efficacy of medication

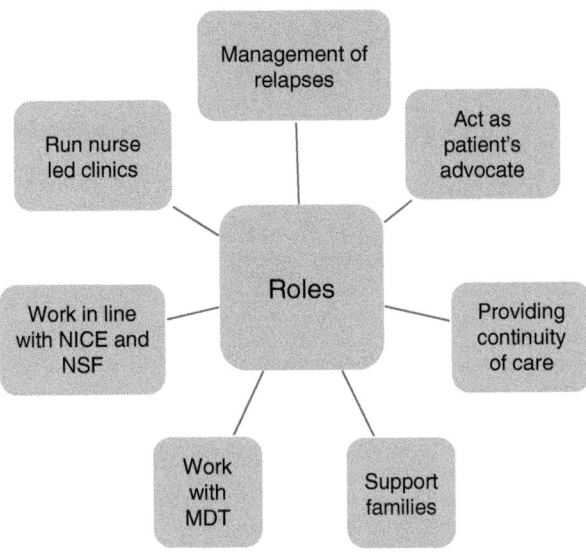

Figure 16.4 Role of the MS specialist nurse.

depends on high levels of concordance. The importance of a coordinated approach to care led by a MS specialist nurse can help the patient and their family better understand their disease, treatment options and adherence to therapy (see Figure 16.4).

Episode of care

Jane Fox is a 42-year-old married lady with two teenage daughters who was diagnosed with RRMS following an initial diagnosis of MS five years ago. At this point she had an MRI scan, which showed two lesions on her spinal cord, and a lumbar puncture identified the presence of oligoclonal bands (both indicators of MS). Jane was admitted to the ward on this occasion with a relapse of her condition, with some weakness of both legs and episodes of urinary incontinence. Jane has had two previous relapses where she received courses of methylprednisolone, with a good recovery, and is currently prescribed Glatiramer Acetate (copaxone). On this admission, Jane is prescribed methylprednisolone intravenously and consideration is being given to the use of a disease-modifying drug, Natalizumab (tysabri), which she will receive once a month as an intravenous infusion. Jane is referred to the physiotherapist and is seen with her family by the MS specialist in relation to support needed on discharge.

Conclusion

This chapter has provided an overview of the medication used in the treatment of four key neurological disorders to help nurses understand the importance of pharmacology and medicines management in the treatment of neurological disorders. A brief overview of each neurological disorder has been given, followed by the evidence to support the use of specific drugs, their actions, adverse effects and the contraindications. The wider issues associated with medication optimisation, including patient education, specialist support, other treatment options and the psychological impact of the neurological disorder on both the patient and their family have also been explored.

References

Ashelford, S., Raynsford, J. and Taylor, V. (2016). *Pathophysiology and Pharmacology for Nursing Students*. London: Sage.

Birns, J. (2017). Anti-thrombotic treatment for ischaemic stroke. *British Journal of Neurosciences Nursing* **13** (supp 5): 526–533.

Burgess, M. (2013). Diagnosing multiple sclerosis: recognising symptoms and diagnostic testing. *British Journal of Neurosciences Nursing* **6** (3) 5: 112–115.

Chapman, B. and Bogle, V. (2014). Adherence to medication and self-management in stroke patients. *British Journal of Nursing* **23** (3): 158–166.

Crouch, S. and Chapelhow, C. (2008). *Medicines Management: A Nursing Perspective*. Harlow: Pearson Education.

Donizak, J. and McCabe, C. (2017). Pharmacological management of patients with Parkinson's disease in the acute hospital setting: a review. *British Journal of Neurosciences Nursing* **13** (5): 220–225.

Epilepsy Action (2017). *Seizure classification*. https://www.epilepsy.org.au/wp-content/uploads/2017/10/ILAE-Seizure-Classifications-2017.pdf (accessed 23 September 2019).

Epilepsy Research UK (2017). *What is epilepsy?* https://epilepsyresearch.org.uk/about-epilepsy/ (accessed 11 August 2020).

Epilepsy Society (2019). *Epilepsy treatment*. https://www.epilepsysociety.org.uk/treatment (accessed 11 August 2020).

Fitzpatrick, M. (2013). Hyper-acute stroke care provision in London: the journey to improvement. *British Journal of Neurosciences Nursing* **9** (3): 120–124.

Greenstein, B. (2009). *Clinical Pharmacology for Nurses*. London: Churchill Livingstone.

Hickey, J.V. (2017). *The Clinical Practice of Neurological and Neurosurgical Nursing*, 7e. Philadelphia: Lippincott.

Intercollegiate Stroke Working Party (2016). *Sentinel Stroke National Audit Programme. Annual results portfolio*. https://www.strokeaudit.org/Documents/National/AcuteOrg/2016/2016-AOANationalReport.aspx (accessed 3 October 2019).

Joint Formulary Committee (2019). *BNF British National Formulary*. bnf.nice.org.uk (accessed August 2020).

Karch, A.M. (2017). *Focus on Nursing Pharmacology*, 7e. New York: Wolters Kluwer.

Lewis, S.A. (2014). Newer drug treatments for focal-onset epilepsy. *British Journal of Neurosciences Nursing* **10** (1): 9–12.

MS Society (2020). *MS symptoms and signs*. https://www.mssociety.org.uk/about-ms/signs-and-symptoms (accessed 11 August 2020).

Murray, T.J. (2005). *Multiple Sclerosis: The History of the Disease*. New York: Demos Publishing.

NICE (2012). *Epilepsies: diagnosis and management (adult case scenarios)* www.nice.org.uk/guidance/cg137/resources (accessed 25 September 2019).

NICE (2017). *Parkinson's disease*. www.nice.org.uk/guidance/ng71 (accessed 30 September 2019).

NICE (2018). *Epilepsies: diagnosis and management*. www.nice.org.uk/guidance/cg137/chapter/Appendix-E-Pharmacological-treatment (accessed 23 September 2019).

NICE (2019a). *Stroke and transient ischaemic attack in over 16s: diagnosis and initial management*. www.nice.org.uk/guidance/ng128 (accessed 3 October 2019).

NICE (2019b). *Multiple sclerosis in adults: management*. www.nice.org.uk/guidance/cg186 (accessed 3 October 2019).

Nursing and Midwifery Council (2015). *The Code Professional Standards of Practice and Behaviour for Nurses and Midwives* https://www.nmc.org.uk/globalassets/sitedocuments/nmc-publications/nmc-code.pdf (accessed 23 September 2019).

Pandit, L. and Murthy, J.K. (2011). Treatment of multiple sclerosis. *Annals of Indian Academy of Neurology* **14**: 65–69.

Parkinson's UK (2019). *Parkinson's drugs*. parkinsons.org.uk/information-and-support/parkinsons-drugs (accessed August 2020).

Queally, C. and Lailey, S. (2012). Care of the person with epilepsy in the hospital environment – getting it right. *British Journal of Neurosciences Nursing* **8** (1): 14–20.

Royal College of Physicians (2016). *National clinical guideline for stroke*. https://www.strokeaudit.org/SupportFiles/Documents/Guidelines/2016-National-Clinical-Guideline-for-Stroke-5t-(1).aspx (accessed 3 October 2019).

Scolding, N. and Wilkins, A. (2012). *Multiple Sclerosis*. Oxford: Oxford University Press.

Scottish Intercollegiate Guidelines Network (SIGN) (2010). *Diagnosis and pharmacological management of Parkinson's disease: A national clinical guideline*. https://www.sign.ac.uk/assets/sign113.pdf (accessed 30 September 2019).

Stroke Association (2015). *Blood thinning medication after stroke*. https://www.stroke.org (accessed 3 October 2019).

Weiner, H.L. and Stankiewicz, J.M. (2012). *Multiple Sclerosis: Diagnosis and Treatment*. London: Wiley Publications.

WHO (1978). *Cerebrovascular Disorders*. Geneva: World Health Organization.

WHO (2017). *Epilepsy*. http://www.who.int/mental_health/neurology/epilepsy/en (accessed 23 September 2019).

Further reading

It should also be remembered that there may be a need to consult other sources of guidance concerning specific areas of practice, such as:

- the National Institute for Health and Care Excellence and Scottish Inter Collegiate Guidelines Network;
- publications by the British National Formulary;
- the Royal College of Nursing;
- specialist associations such as the Stroke Association, Epilepsy UK, Parkinson's UK, and the Multiple Sclerosis Trust;
- the British Pharmacological Society;
- the Nursing and Midwifery Council.

Multiple choice questions

1. Which of the following would the nurse be least likely to include as a type of generalised seizure?
    (a) Petit mal
    (b) Complex
    (c) Tonic–clonic
    (d) Focal

2. Which AED can be prescribed for all types of seizures?
    (a) Topiramate
    (b) Sodium valproate
    (c) Gabapentin
    (d) Carbamazepine

3. What percentage of patients with epilepsy can have it controlled with medication?
    (a) 10%
    (b) 25%
    (c) 50%
    (d) 75%

4. How long is it before patients with epilepsy are allowed to drive once they are seizure free?
    (a) 3 years
    (b) 2 years
    (c) 5 years
    (d) 1 year

5. Many of the drugs used to treat PD act to increase which neurotransmitter?
    (a) Dopamine
    (b) Serotonin
    (c) Acetylcholine
    (d) Glutamate

6. Nausea is a common side effect of PD drugs caused by:
   (a) Stimulation of the gastrointestinal tract
   (b) Increased dopamine in the brain
   (c) Stimulation of the vomiting centre of the brain
   (d) Stimulation of the chemoreceptors in the brain
7. Why is dopamine not given directly as an oral medication?
   (a) It is not a licensed drug
   (b) It is destroyed by gastric enzymes
   (c) It does not cross the blood–brain barrier
   (d) It has to be given as an injectable drug
8. What might be the benefits of medications being self-administered by patient with PD:
   (a) Staff have more time for other duties
   (b) The patient gains more control and will get their medication on time
   (c) There is a reduction in the number of medication errors
   (d) There is less risk of infection
9. What is the recommended time frame for patients to receive thrombolysis following an ischaemic stroke?
   (a) Within 24 hours of diagnosis
   (b) Within 12 hours of onset of symptoms
   (c) Within 4.5 hours of onset of symptoms
   (d) Within 1 hour of diagnosis
10. What is the recommended time period for the patient to receive thrombolysis following the diagnosis of ischaemic/thrombotic stroke?
    (a) Within 24 hours of diagnosis
    (b) Within 12 hours of onset of symptoms
    (c) Within 4.5 hours of onset of symptoms
    (d) Within 1 hour of diagnosis
11. What is the advantage for patients receiving thrombolytic medication?
    (a) They will not require hospitalisation
    (b) It can be given by any healthcare professional
    (c) It will dissolve the clot, aid recovery, and reduce long-term complications
    (d) It does not need to be prescribed
12. What is the recommended drug to be used on admission to hospital for all stroke patients?
    (a) Tinzaparin
    (b) Clopidogrel
    (c) Aspirin
    (d) Alteplase
13. What is the most common type of multiple sclerosis?
    (a) Benign multiple sclerosis
    (b) Relapsing remitting multiple sclerosis
    (c) Secondary progressive multiple sclerosis
    (d) Idiopathic multiple sclerosis

14. What was the first oral disease-modifying drug to be introduced to treat MS?
- **(a)** Methylprednisolone
- **(b)** Baclofen
- **(c)** Glatiramer Acetate
- **(d)** Fingolimod

15. What is the main drug treatment to treat spasticity in MS?
- **(a)** Baclofen
- **(b)** Morphine
- **(c)** Paracetamol
- **(d)** Methylprednisolone

Chapter 17

Medications used in mental health

Laura Stavert

Aim

To develop a fundamental understanding of psychotropic medication used to treat common mental health conditions.

Learning outcomes

After reading this chapter, the reader will be able to:

1. Categorise and evaluate the different groups of medications used in psychosis, affective disorders, anxiety disorders and dementia
2. Have an understanding of the risks associated with identified drug classes
3. Have an understanding of the pharmacokinetics associated with each drug class
4. Have an understanding of the physical health monitoring necessary for identified drug classes and why this is necessary

Antidepressants

Depression is an affective disorder which manifests in many different ways but usually has depressed mood and/or loss of pleasure in most activities central to the presentation (NICE, 2009). The current evidence base recommends that antidepressant medications are used for patients whose depression is moderate–severe as evidence shows they are less effective in mild cases (NICE, 2009). Psychological therapies are also useful when treating depression and should be considered alongside pharmacological treatments.

Selective serotonin reuptake inhibitors (SSRIs)

The current evidence base recommends SSRIs as first-line drug treatment due to their efficacy in treating low mood and their relatively good tolerability and side effect profile

Fundamentals of Pharmacology: For Nursing and Healthcare Students, First Edition. Edited by Ian Peate and Barry Hill.
© 2021 John Wiley & Sons Ltd. Published 2021 by John Wiley & Sons Ltd.

(Cleare et al., 2015; Joint Formulary Committee, 2019; NICE, 2009). Examples include sertraline, citalopram and fluoxetine. SSRIs act directly on the brain to block post-synaptic reuptake of the neurotransmitter **serotonin** and most also have minimal effect on other neurotransmitter systems including noradrenaline and dopamine (Smart et al., 2016). Most SSRIs are taken orally, once daily, and many are available in solid oral dosage forms (tablets and capsules) while some are commercially available in liquid form (e.g. citalopram oral drops). SSRIs are commonly associated with headaches and gastrointestinal (GI) disturbances (particularly nausea) and a number are associated with sexual dysfunction including reduced libido, though this varies within the drug class (Gartlehner et al., 2011). SSRIs are well absorbed from the GI tract following oral administration and are highly protein bound. They are hepatically metabolised, but notably fluoxetine has an active metabolite. Most SSRIs have half-lives of 24–36 hours with the exception of fluoxetine, which is significantly longer (four to five days) (ABPI, 2018a; 2019a, b).

Tricyclic antidepressants

Tricyclic antidepressants (TCA) primarily inhibit the reuptake of serotonin and/or noradrenaline with no demonstrable dopaminergic effects. They are antagonists of $5HT_{2A}$, $5HT_{2C}$, histamine (H1), α_1 and muscarinic receptors, though receptor affinity varies greatly between different drugs (Bazire, 2018; Smart et al., 2016). Examples of TCAs include Amitriptyline, Dosulepin and Clomipramine. TCAs are now less commonly used to treat depression as they are usually less well tolerated compared to the more modern SSRIs (Cleare et al., 2015; Taylor et al., 2014) and this often limits their therapeutic use as patients can find these intolerable. Symptoms may include dry mouth, constipation, difficulty passing urine and blurred vision. One of the most common effects noted with TCAs is drowsiness, and patients can experience a "hangover effect" the day after evening administration. Side effects are normally dose-related and so gradual dose increases are required to achieve a therapeutic effect.

Monoamine oxidase inhibitors (MAOI)

Monoamine oxidase (MAO) is an enzyme present throughout body tissues with particularly high concentrations in the gastrointestinal tract (GIT) and the central nervous system (CNS). There are two subtypes:

- MAO-A which metabolises noradrenaline, serotonin, dopamine and tyramine.
- MAO-B which metabolises tyramine, dopamine and phenylethylamine.

Traditional MAOI antidepressants such as Phenelzine, Tranylcypromine and Isocarboxazid irreversibly inhibit both MAO-A and MAO-B and thereby inhibit reuptake of serotonin and noradrenaline. Common side effects include dizziness, drowsiness, peripheral edema, GI disturbances (nausea, vomiting, dryness of the mouth, constipation), insomnia, blurred vision, tremor and postural hypotension. MAOIs are now rarely used in the treatment of depression, partly due to the dietary restrictions required while taking them as outlined in the Clinical Considerations Box below.

Clinical considerations

Dietary restrictions while taking MAOIs

While taking MAOIs patients must avoid foods rich in tyramine in order to avoid potentially fatal hypertensive crisis. Such foods include mature cheese, salami, pickled herring, meat or yeast extracts like Bovril® and Marmite® or fermented soya bean extract, and some beers, lagers or wines. Also to be avoided are foods containing dopamine (such as broad beans). These must be avoided for the duration of treatment with an MAOI and for two to three weeks after stopping.

Clinical considerations

TCAs are particularly toxic in overdose and are associated with increased potential to cause death (compared to SSRIs and newer antidepressants) (Taylor et al., 2014), often due to cardiac arrhythmias which can occur soon after ingestion (NPIS, 2017). As such, TCAs should be avoided in patients who may be at risk of overdose. Symptoms of overdose can include dilated pupils, coma, hypotension, hypothermia, seizures, respiratory failure and cardiac arrhythmias (Joint Formulary Committee, 2019). Lofepramine has the lowest associated risk of fatality following overdose (Cleare et al., 2015; Taylor et al., 2014). Any patient with a suspected TCA overdose must have emergency intervention (NPIS, 2017).

Moclobemide is an MAOI antidepressant, which unlike the traditional agents produces reversible inhibition and is selective for MAO-A. It is often referred to as a Reversible Inhibitor of Monoamine oxidase A (RIMA). This significantly reduces the potential for tyramine interactions.

The pharmacokinetics of MAOI drugs are poorly understood; they are well absorbed after oral administration and are likely to be highly protein bound (though moclobemide is only about 50% bound). They have very short half-lives (approximately two hours) due to rapid hepatic metabolism (ABPI, 2017a).

A washout period after stopping an MAOI is required as their effects are particularly long acting and concurrent use with other antidepressants can bring about toxic reactions (e.g. serotonin syndrome) which are sometimes fatal (Baxter and Preston, 2019). This is particularly important with concurrent use of serotonergic medicines as this further increases the risk. A period of at least two weeks (three if switching to clomipramine or imipramine) must elapse after stopping an MAOI and starting another antidepressant (Bazire, 2018, Joint Formulary Committee, 2019). The required washout periods when switching to an MAOI from another antidepressant are outlined in Table 17.1 below.

It is somewhat difficult to stop MAOI treatment (for example, if these are not tolerated or are ineffective) as they are often associated with discontinuation symptoms; although this can be minimised with a slow and cautious dose taper over a prolonged period. Discontinuation symptoms can include agitation, irritability, ataxia, movement disorders, insomnia, drowsiness, vivid dreams, cognitive impairment and slowed speech. Less commonly, hallucinations and paranoid delusions can occur. Discontinuation effects may occur within five days of stopping treatment and can persist for a prolonged period (Royal College of Psychiatrists, 2019).

Other antidepressants

Serotonin and noradrenaline reuptake inhibitors (SNRIs)

Examples of drugs in this class include Venlafaxine, Duloxetine and Reboxetine (inhibits noradrenaline reuptake only). The exact mechanism of the antidepressant action of Venlafaxine

Table 17.1   Required washout periods when switching to an MAOI

Previous Antidepressant Class	Washout Period
Switching from another MAOI	At least 14 days after stopping previous MAOI then new MAOI introduced at reduced dose
Switching from a TCA or related drug	At least 7–14 days after stopping (3 weeks if using clomipramine or imipramine)
Switching from an SSRI	At least 7 days after stopping (at least 5 weeks if using fluoxetine due to long half-life of 4–5 days)

Source: Joint Formulary Committee (2019).

is unknown, but is thought to prevent the pre-synaptic reuptake of both serotonin and noradrenaline, although it has a greater effect on serotonin reuptake, especially at lower doses (75–150 mg) (Buckingham, 2019; Smart et al., 2016). At higher doses Venlafaxine also inhibits the reuptake of dopamine (Bazire, 2018). Venlafaxine is well absorbed from the GIT and has a very short half-life of one to two hours. It is hepatically metabolised to active metabolites (ABPI, 2019c).

Duloxetine weakly inhibits dopamine reuptake but demonstrates no histaminic, dopaminergic, cholinergic or adrenergic receptor activity (Smart et al., 2016). Its main side effects are nausea, insomnia, headache, dizziness, dry mouth, somnolence, constipation and anorexia. It is metabolised by CYP1A2 and CYP2D6 and is an inhibitor of CYP2D6 (ABPI, 2019d).

Reboxetine is a selective noradrenaline reuptake inhibitor with no other significant effects at therapeutic dosing (8–12 mg/day). Evidence suggests it is not particularly effective and may have increased incidence of side effects (Cleare et al., 2015), including increased level of arousal/alertness and insomnia, which limits its acceptability to patients (Buckingham, 2019).

SNRIs should be used with caution in patients with established cardiovascular disease as they are known to cause hypertension. Common side effects include dizziness, headache, night sweats, sexual dysfunction, nausea, vomiting and abnormal dreams (ABPI, 2015, 2019b,c). SNRI as a drug class tend to be slightly less well tolerated than SSRI (Cleare et al., 2015).

Mirtazapine

Mirtazapine can be considered to be a noradrenergic and specific serotonergic antidepressant (NASSA). The usual dose range of mirtazapine is 15–45 mg and the minimum effective dose is 30 mg (Taylor et al., 2019). The principal therapeutic action is antagonism at pre-synaptic α_2 receptors which increases activity of both noradrenaline and serotonin systems. It is also an antagonist at $5HT_{2A}$, $5HT_{2C}$ and $5HT_3$ receptors and the lower incidence of serotonergic side effects such as nausea, headache and sexual dysfunction is believed to be related to this (Smart et al., 2016). Mirtazapine is also a histamine (H1) receptor antagonist and this is likely to cause the sedative side effects. At higher doses, the arousing effect from increased noradrenergic activity counteracts the sedative effect from central histamine inhibition (Buckingham, 2019). Consideration must always be given to how this side effect might increase potential risks, particularly falls and especially in older adults. Mirtazapine is also commonly known to increase appetite and cause weight gain; this may be useful if a patient is experiencing reduced appetite and/or weight loss as a biological feature of their depressive illness. Although rare, mirtazapine has been associated with agranulocytosis. If patients taking mirtazapine report sore throat, fever or other symptoms suggestive of infection, a full blood count should be measured to exclude blood dyscrasias (Joint Formulary Committee, 2019). Mirtazapine is completely absorbed and is highly protein bound. It is metabolised by the liver with some active metabolites and has a half-life of 20–40 hours (ABPI, 2014; Bazire, 2018).

Vortioxetine

Vortioxetine has a broad and novel mode of action with serotonin receptor antagonism at $5HT_3$ and to a lesser extent $5HT_{1D/7}$, $5HT_1$ agonism and $5HT_{1B}$ partial agonism as well as serotonin reuptake inhibition (Smart et al., 2016) resulting in antidepressant and anxiolytic effect (Joint Formulary Committee, 2019; Montgomery et al., 2014). NICE recommends that use of vortioxetine be reserved for patients with major depression where there has been lack of response to two antidepressants (NICE, 2015). Common side effects can include dizziness, abnormal dreams, constipation, pruritus, vomiting and diarrhoea. Vortioxetine does not appear to cause hyponatremia like many other antidepressants and may be a useful alternative for patients where this is problematic. At lower doses it does not appear to cause significant weight gain or sexual side effects. (Joint Formulary Committee, 2019). Absorption of vortioxetine from the GIT is slow but complete with high protein binding and has a half-life of 66 hours (ABPI, 2019e).

Agomelatine

Agomelatine is a melatonin receptor agonist (M1 and M2) and selective serotonin-receptor antagonist (5HT$_{2B}$ and 5HT$_{2C}$) (Smart et al., 2016); it has a unique mode of action unlike any other antidepressant currently available as it does not affect the neuronal reuptake of serotonin, noradrenaline or dopamine (Taylor et al., 2014). It is not known to cause hyponatremia and does not have a detrimental impact on blood pressure, weight (Joint Formulary Committee, 2019) or sexual functioning (Cleare et al., 2015). Common side effects include abdominal pain, GI upset (nausea, vomiting, diarrhoea or constipation), anxiety, back pain, dizziness, drowsiness, fatigue, headaches and sleep disorders. Liver injury and hepatotoxicity have been reported with agomelatine, and so close monitoring of liver function is required after 3, 6, 12 and 24 weeks of treatment and when clinically indicated thereafter. Treatment should be stopped if serum transaminases are greater than three times the upper limit of reference range or there are symptoms of liver disorder such as dark urine, light coloured stools, jaundice, unexplained bruising, fatigue, abdominal pain or pruritus (ABPI, 2017a; Joint Formulary Committee, 2019). Agomelatine does not appear to be associated with any discontinuation effects on cessation (Taylor et al., 2019) and so can be stopped abruptly without any dose tapering. Agomelatine is well absorbed and rapidly metabolised following oral administration and has a half-life of only one to two hours (ABPI, 2017b).

441

Considerations with antidepressants

All antidepressant drugs are known to lower the seizure threshold and for this reason they need to be used with a degree of caution in patients with a known seizure disorder such as epilepsy.

Patients treated with an antidepressant should begin to see an associated effect within two weeks of starting it, and if no demonstrable response is noted by three to four weeks, a dose increase or drug change should be considered.

Adverse effects

Suicidal behaviour

The use of antidepressants has been associated with an increased risk of suicidal thoughts and behaviour in adolescents under the age of 25 (National Health Service, 2009) and those with a history of suicidality (Joint Formulary Committee, 2019). Patients should be closely monitored for clinical worsening, suicidality and unusual changes in behaviour when commencing antidepressant treatment, following dose changes and where any risks are identified. Suicidal behaviour may include attempted or completed suicide, preparatory acts for suicide and suicidal ideation (National Health Service, 2009).

Hyponatremia

Hyponatremia is a state where a patient has depleted plasma sodium levels. Sodium levels should usually be between 135 and 145 mmol/L though this can vary between biochemistry laboratories so please check with individual local laboratories. It is an uncommon, but potentially severe side effect which is associated with SSRI and TCA. Severe hyponatremia is usually considered to be plasma level less than 125 mmol/L, however patients may be symptomatic even with sodium levels higher than this. Symptoms associated with hyponatremia can be seen in Table 17.2.

Hyponatremia is likely associated with most antidepressants, though not all drug classes have been investigated. The risk appears to be highest with citalopram and lowest with mirtazapine and agomelatine. There are a number of other factors which can increase the risk of developing hyponatremia outlined in Table 17.3.

Table 17.2 Symptoms associated with hyponatremia

1. Restlessness	2. Irritability
3. Drowsiness	4. Lack of energy
5. Muscle cramps and weakness	6. Nausea and vomiting
7. Confusion	8. Seizures

Source: Modified from Meadows (2019).

Table 17.3 Risk factors for developing antidepressant related hyponatremia

• Female gender	• Heart failure
• Increasing age (likely related to higher rates of comorbidities and concurrent medicines)	• Liver cirrhosis
• Low BMI	• Malignancies
• History of hyponatremia	• Reduced circulating volume
• Syndrome of inappropriate antidiuretic hormone secretion (SIADH)	• Urinary loss

Source: Modified from Taylor et al. (2019).

Serotonin syndrome

Serotonin syndrome is a physiological state where there is an excess of the neurotransmitter serotonin in the bloodstream leading to adverse effects. It is relatively uncommon and is the result of using serotonergic drugs. Symptoms (summarised in Table 17.4) develop after starting, dose increase or overdose with a serotonergic drug and can arise after a few hours or even a number of days.

Symptoms can range from being mild in severity to life-threatening and tend to be more severe in cases of overdose. Treatment of serotonin syndrome requires withdrawal of the causative agent(s) and any supportive therapy which may be required, according to presenting symptoms. The risk of developing serotonin syndrome increases where multiple drugs with serotonergic activity are used concurrently and although this may be appropriate in certain circumstances, patients should be made aware of this risk wherever necessary and advised of the symptoms to be vigilant for.

Antidepressant withdrawal

Antidepressant drugs should be withdrawn gradually to avoid precipitating acute discontinuation reactions unless a serious adverse event has occurred or there are serious risks associated with continuing. Current recommendations advise this should be done over at least a

Table 17.4 Symptoms of serotonin syndrome

Autonomic dysfunction	Neuromuscular hyperactivity	Altered mental state
• Increased heart rate	• Tremor	• Agitation
• Changes in blood pressure	• Hyperreflexia	• Confusion
• Hyperthermia	• Clonus	• Mania
• Shivering	• Rigidity	
• Diarrhoea		
• Sweating		

Source: Modified from Taylor et al. (2019).

four-week period (NICE, 2019). The onset of discontinuation effects can vary depending on the antidepressant used and so some patients may experience a degree of symptoms after only one missed dose, or if they do not take the full prescribed dose. Symptoms can vary in duration, type and severity and it is estimated that up to one-third of patients will experience some degree of discontinuation symptoms (Taylor et al., 2019). Some antidepressant drugs appear to be more likely to precipitate discontinuation symptoms, including paroxetine, venlafaxine, amitriptyline and all MAOIs. Agomelatine and vortioxetine are associated with little or no risk of discontinuation symptoms. There is some evidence to suggest fluoxetine discontinuation is well tolerated on account of its long elimination half-life (Taylor et al., 2019). Antidepressant discontinuation symptoms are outlined in Table 17.5 below.

There is now growing evidence to suggest that discontinuation reactions may be experienced even with a gradual taper in dose over a prolonged period of time. Antidepressant withdrawal can be a contentious subject and in the past available evidence has often differed from the lived experience of patients who have encountered significant difficulties when discontinuing antidepressant treatment. It has previously been disputed that discontinuation reactions continue beyond one to two weeks (Davies et al., 2019); however, more recently, bodies such as the Royal College of Psychiatrists (2019) and NICE (2019) are acknowledging that symptoms may persist for much longer. While advice to plan to withdraw over a minimum of four weeks remains relevant, this should be reviewed in the event of patients reporting difficulties with discontinuation symptoms and smaller dose reductions over a longer period of time should be utilised as appropriate.

To reiterate the points in this section, antidepressants should be reserved for moderate to severe depression due to the risk/benefit ratio of treatment. No one antidepressant drug class has superior efficacy, but SSRIs are normally utilised first-line due to their more favourable side effect profile, compared to TCAs and MAOIs which often carry a significant side effect burden and require dietary restrictions respectively. Rarer adverse effects of antidepressants include hyponatremia (not uncommon with SSRIs and Venlafaxine) and mirtazapine and vortioxetine are good alternatives as they are not known to have this effect. Clinical worsening and suicidal behaviour is associated with the introduction of antidepressant treatment and patients should be closely monitored during the initiation period. Antidepressant discontinuation syndrome is associated with most antidepressants, particularly where treatment has been for six weeks or more, and so doses should usually be tapered over a number of weeks or months and adjusted according to patient response.

443

Antipsychotics

The aim of antipsychotic treatment is to alleviate any distress the patient experiences secondary to psychotic symptoms and to improve social and cognitive functioning. Patients will often require life-long treatment with antipsychotic medication, as discontinuation is associated with a high relapse rate. Antipsychotic drugs are effective for treating positive psychotic symptoms, such as thought disorder, hallucinations and delusions, but are often less successful for managing negative symptoms, such as apathy and social withdrawal.

The majority of antipsychotic drugs block the effects of dopamine at D2 receptors. Antipsychotic response may be seen within the first week of treatment and usually continues

Table 17.5   Antidepressant discontinuation symptoms

- Restlessness
- Problems sleeping
- Unsteadiness
- Sweating
- Abdominal symptoms
- Altered sensations (for example, electric shock sensations in the head)
- Altered feelings (for example, irritability, anxiety or confusion)

to improve over the following weeks. Evidence suggests that there is little difference in efficacy between various antipsychotic drugs and so NICE (2014) recommends that the decision regarding which treatment to utilise is made in partnership with patient and professional, with full consideration of the likely benefits and possible side effects.

First-generation antipsychotics (FGAs) include Haloperidol, Zuclopenthixol, Chlorpromazine and Flupentixol. They work by blocking dopamine D2 receptors in the brain; however, they are not specific for the dopamine pathways in the brain and this gives rise to a number of their unpleasant side effects. Second-generation antipsychotics (SGAs) include Risperidone, Olanzapine, Quetiapine and Clozapine. They produce their antipsychotic effects via a number of chemical pathways giving them a different side effect profile to FGAs (Cheng et al., 2016).

There is no evidence to support any clear advantages of using SGAs over FGAs (Stahl, 2008). FGAs are well known to commonly cause extrapyramidal side effects (EPSE). SGAs have a much lower incidence of EPSE, though this is largely offset by their increased association with metabolic side effects. Drugs from both groups are associated with a number of unpleasant side effects, although this profile varies from drug to drug, and this should be taken into consideration when agreeing on choice of antipsychotic treatment.

Aripiprazole

Unlike other antipsychotic drugs, Aripiprazole works via partial agonism (rather than antagonism) at dopamine D2 receptors (Stahl, 2008). It has a reduced incidence of EPSE and does not cause sedation, weight gain or indeed many of the other metabolic side effects to the same extent as other antipsychotics. Aripiprazole is licensed for treatment of schizophrenia and mania and is available in both oral and parenteral forms. Akathisia and restlessness are very common side effects associated with its use. Aripiprazole is well absorbed after oral dosing with minimal first-pass metabolism. It is highly protein bound (>99%) and extensively hepatically metabolised with an active metabolite. In extensive metabolisers of CYP2D6, the elimination half-life is approximately 75 hours, but in poor metabolisers can be as long as 146 hours (ABPI, 2019f).

Development of side effects is the most common reason for discontinuation of antipsychotic medication and these are summarised in Table 17.6. Assessment of side effects should be part of regular review and use of a structured tool such as the Glasgow Antipsychotic Side Effect Scale (Waddell and Taylor, 2008) can be an effective approach to monitoring this during treatment.

Parenteral formulations

Non-adherence with antipsychotic medication is common, with evidence suggesting up to 50% of patients do not take antipsychotic medication as prescribed (Barnes et al., 2011). Depot and long-acting injectable forms of antipsychotics can be useful in addressing this as non-adherence rates are much lower – reported to be around 25% (Barnes et al., 2011). Use of long-acting parenteral formulations is also associated with a reduced risk of relapse (Taylor et al., 2019). Depots are usually given intramuscularly (IM) into a large muscle using the z-track technique, most commonly into the gluteus muscle or deltoid muscle depending on licensing of each injection and patient preference. Some depots may also be administered in the lateral

Table 17.6 Antipsychotic related side effects

Type of Side Effect	Examples
Metabolic	Weight gain, glucose dysregulation, type 2 diabetes
Extrapyramidal	Akathisia, dystonia, parkinsonism, tardive dyskinesia
Cardiovascular	QTc prolongation, venous thromboembolism (VTE), postural hypotension
Hormonal	Increased prolactin, sexual dysfunction
Other miscellaneous effects	Sedation

thigh muscle. The z-track injection technique is shown in Figure 17.1 below. Before introducing an FGA depot, patients should receive a test dose to assess for any side effects. These formulations are very long lasting and difficult to reverse if given in therapeutic doses. They can be administered anywhere from weekly to every four weeks according to clinical response and patient preference. Test doses are not normally required for SGAs as they are less likely to cause problematic EPSEs. The most commonly used SGA depot injections are Aripiprazole and Paliperidone. They are useful as they are normally administered monthly and are also licensed to be administered in the deltoid muscle, which is often much more acceptable to patients. In addition, paliperidone long acting injection (LAI) is very rapid in its onset (Taylor et al., 2018). For patients whose symptoms are well controlled on monthly paliperidone, there is an even longer acting injection which can be administered every three months and this shows similar tolerability and efficacy as the monthly LAI.

Clozapine

Clozapine, although technically an SGA, is reserved for use in **treatment resistant schizophrenia** (TRS) or where other antipsychotics have not been tolerated. It is often extremely effective where other antipsychotic medication has failed with up to two-thirds of patients with schizophrenia who failed to respond to other antipsychotics demonstrating a response to clozapine (Barnes et al., 2011). Psychosis is considered to be treatment resistant if symptoms have failed to respond to at least two different antipsychotic drugs (one of which should be an SGA) each taken at a suitable dose for six to eight weeks (Joint Formulary Committee, 2019).

445

Clinical considerations

Before determining that an antipsychotic medication is ineffective, it is important to ascertain that patients have been adherent with their prescribed antipsychotic medication (ABPI, 2018c).

Initiation

Clozapine needs to be introduced slowly in order to minimise the risk of adverse effects (notably changes in blood pressure, fever and tachycardia) which are more common and severe when starting and in the first four weeks of this treatment. Initial dose is usually 12.5 mg followed by hourly post-dose monitoring of blood pressure, pulse and temperature (ABPI, 2019g). Frequency of monitoring is usually reduced to twice daily for the next 7–14 days if results are satisfactory and as dose escalation continues. Doses are normally titrated in 12.5–25 mg increments every one to two days; however, this depends on individual patient factors including tolerability.

Treatment breaks and reiteration

Reliable adherence with clozapine is necessary as missed doses can reduce tolerance to the adverse effects of clozapine. A treatment break is considered to be omission of clozapine for more than 48 hours (Taylor et al., 2019). After this time, the risk of initiation effects such as tachycardia increase to a similar point as those naïve to clozapine and, if this occurs, patients need to begin dose titration again from 12.5 mg. An expedited titration may be possible, though this should be done with caution and be guided by results of physical health monitoring and patient tolerability.

Adverse effects
Agranulocytosis and blood dyscrasias

Clozapine is associated with a small but clinically significant risk of neutropenia and potentially fatal agranulocytosis. Patients are required to be registered with a monitoring service

Skills in practice

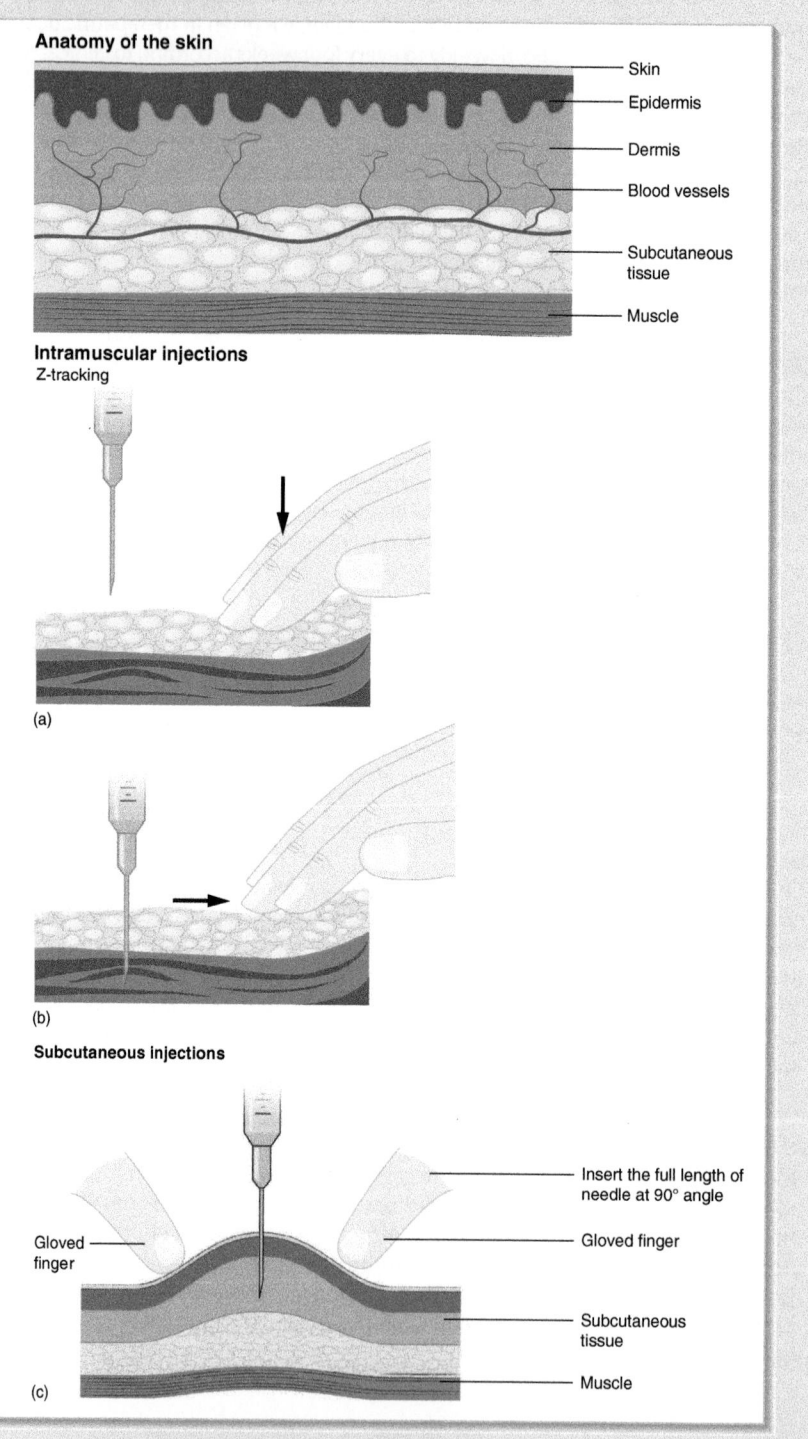

Anatomy of the skin

- Skin
- Epidermis
- Dermis
- Blood vessels
- Subcutaneous tissue
- Muscle

Intramuscular injections
Z-tracking

(a)

(b)

Subcutaneous injections

- Insert the full length of needle at 90° angle
- Gloved finger
- Gloved finger
- Subcutaneous tissue
- Muscle

(c)

Figure 17.1 Z-track injection technique. Source: Midwifery Skills in Practice at a Glance Wiley-Blackwell Lindsay, Bagness and Peate (eds.) (2018) Midwifery Skills Figure 73.1(a) and (b) page 152.

and have regular blood monitoring of leucocytes and differential blood counts. This is initially weekly for 18 weeks as this is when risk of agranulocytosis is highest. Monitoring reduces to fortnightly thereafter, and once treatment has been in place for a year without any abnormal monitoring, this is continued on a monthly basis.

Patients are required to use a specific brand of clozapine and stick to this so that the relevant service can ensure they are appropriately monitored. It should be noted, however, that all brands of clozapine are bioequivalent. The three brands in use in the UK are Denzapine, Clozaril and Zaponex. Check which brand(s) are in use in your area.

Constipation

Constipation is an extremely common side effect associated with clozapine, yet to an extent is normalised and under-reported despite affecting more than one-third of those who take it and its potential to have fatal consequences. The risk is highest within the first few months of treatment, but remains possible throughout. A pre-treatment assessment of bowel function should be documented and any medication causing constipation, such as opioid analgesics, should be stopped wherever possible. Patients must be asked about constipation at every appointment and encouraged to report this as soon as possible in order to prevent serious and potentially fatal consequences such as bowel obstruction, faecal impaction and paralytic ileus (MHRA, 2017).

Sedation

The risk of sedation is known to be highest in the first few months of treatment but can persist for much longer. Doses of up to 900 mg/day are licensed for use and are usually split into two daily doses with a higher dose being given at night to minimise the sedative effect during the day. This is usually dose dependent so, if problematic, dose reduction can be helpful in addressing sedation.

Weight gain

Clozapine is the most likely to cause weight gain of all the antipsychotics currently available in the UK and often to excessive levels (more than 10 lb/4.5 kg) (Taylor et al., 2019). This is usually highly unacceptable to patients and is often cited as a major reason for requesting to discontinue clozapine.

Hypersalivation

Hypersalivation, or sialorrhoea, is commonly associated with clozapine use, occurring in 30–80% of people (Bird et al., 2011). This is thought to be related to dose and is more likely to occur at night-time but can be highly embarrassing for patients, especially when in public. It may also increase the risk of aspiration pneumonia, which can have severe consequences. Where appropriate, dose reduction can be a useful first approach to addressing hypersalivation and should be considered after review by the prescriber. Should dose reduction be ineffective, or not viable, there are a number of treatment options available and the most commonly used approach is hyoscine hydrobromide. Licensed preparations of hyoscine hydrobromide are available in the form of 300 microgram tablets and 1.5 mg/72 hour transdermal patches (Joint Formulary Committee, 2019; Owen, 2017), though use in this indication is unlicensed.

Interactions

The most important interaction with clozapine is the impact of smoking. Smoking causes induction of liver enzymes and increases the clearance of clozapine from the body, resulting in more than 20% higher doses being required compared to non-smokers (Qurashi et al., 2019). This is of significant concern given that patients with a schizophrenia diagnosis are far more likely to be smokers compared to the general population (Lohr and Flynn, 1992).

There are a number of drug interactions listed with clozapine (Baxter and Preston, 2019); however, the most clinically significant are with fluvoxamine, carbamazepine and phenytoin. Fluvoxamine significantly increases clozapine concentrations. Clozapine has also been associated with QT prolongation and fluvoxamine is thought to have the same effect. Concurrent use of fluvoxamine and clozapine should be avoided wherever possible.

Carbamazepine reduces clozapine concentrations and also carries an independent risk of causing blood dyscrasias. The manufacturer of clozapine contraindicates concurrent use with carbamazepine due to this associated increased risk.

High-dose antipsychotic therapy

High-dose antipsychotic therapy (HDAT) is defined as "a total daily dose of a single antipsychotic which exceeds the upper limit stated in the SPC or BNF with respect to the age of the patient and the indication being treated and a total daily dose of two or more antipsychotics which exceeds the SPC or BNF maximum using the percentage method" (RCPsych, 2014a). The use of HDAT has little evidence to demonstrate it is an effective treatment strategy compared to monotherapy (Taylor et al., 2019, p. 17) and so routine use should be avoided. The majority of adverse effects associated with antipsychotic drugs are dose related and HDAT is associated with an increased risk of side effects. Additional physical health monitoring is necessary for patients treated with HDAT and this includes regular ECG and biochemical monitoring.

If HDAT is deemed to be necessary, it should only be used once other treatment options, including clozapine, have been explored. Robust treatment aims should be in place and these should be reviewed regularly.

Physical health monitoring

Patients with serious mental illness (SMI) are known to have a reduced life expectancy and those with schizophrenia have a 20% shorter life expectancy compared to the general population, dying on average 15–20 years earlier (RCPsych, 2014b). A high burden of cardiovascular disease is very much implicated in this, underpinned by an abundance of modifiable risk factors including obesity, dyslipidaemia, diabetes and smoking. As such it is necessary to conduct physical health monitoring for these patients to address and reduce risk factors wherever possible and to help guide the best choice of antipsychotic medication.

NICE guidance for psychosis and schizophrenia outlines the monitoring, which should be conducted before starting antipsychotic medication, and these can be seen in Table 17.7.

Weight should be measured weekly for the first six weeks of treatment and every three months thereafter, as weight gain is commonly associated with a number of antipsychotic drugs.

Blood tests for lipids, prolactin and measure of glucose regulation as well as blood pressure and pulse should be repeated after three months and annually thereafter. A full physical health monitoring screen will also include an assessment of drug therapy in terms of efficacy, tolerability/side effect burden and adherence to medication (NICE, 2014).

To summarise the pertinent points in this section, all antipsychotics appear to have similar efficacy and choice should be made in partnership between professional and patient based

Table 17.7   Antipsychotic pre-treatment monitoring

- Weight and waist circumference
- Fasting blood glucose and HbA_{1c} (glycosylated haemoglobin)
- Prolactin
- Lipid profile
- Assessment of movement disorders
- Assessment of nutritional status, diet and activity level
- ECG (if the patient has a personal history of cardiovascular disease, a physical examination has identified primary risk factors for cardiovascular events or if the person is being admitted as an inpatient)

Source: NICE (2014).

upon comorbid physical health concerns, side effect profile and patient preference. Physical health monitoring should be carried out at specified time points due to the reduced life expectancy of patients with psychosis and the risks associated with using antipsychotic medication, including metabolic diseases such as diabetes. High-dose antipsychotic therapy should be avoided where possible due to increased risks and lack of evidence of efficacy. Clozapine is an effective antipsychotic and should be considered in the event of treatment failure of at least two antipsychotics after a trial or of each at therapeutic dose and for reasonable duration.

Regular blood monitoring is necessary with clozapine due to the small risk of agranulocytosis. There are a number of important side effects associated with clozapine; however, constipation is extremely common, under-reported and can have fatal outcomes. Side effect screening should be carried out routinely as there are a number of unpleasant side effects associated with antipsychotic drugs, including akathisia, dystonia, weight gain, sexual dysfunction, weight gain and hypersalivation; a screening questionnaire such as GASS can be helpful.

Mood stabilisers
Lithium

Lithium is a naturally occurring element licensed for a number of indications, though its exact mode of action is poorly understood. It is principally used to treat affective disorders, including bipolar affective disorder (BPAD) and depression, and especially to prevent their recurrence. It may be less useful in the management of an acute manic episode due to the difficulty in quickly establishing the high doses which are often required.

Unfortunately, it is estimated that approximately 15% of patients with BPAD die of suicide. Treatment with lithium has been shown to reduce the risk of attempted and completed suicide in patients with BPAD by 80% (Taylor et al., 2019).

Unipolar depression

Up to half of patients treated for depression demonstrate an incomplete response to traditional first- and second-line treatment with antidepressants. Lithium is recommended as one of the first-line options for augmenting existing antidepressant therapy and best efficacy is noted when the lithium plasma level is in the range 0.6–1.0 mmol/L (Goodwin et al., 2016).

Lithium is also effective at preventing relapse of depressive illness and was superior to antidepressants in this indication (Taylor et al., 2019).

Formulations

Lithium is taken orally usually once daily at night due to the potential to cause drowsiness. Twice daily administration can be considered where patients experience troublesome side effects, though this may make adherence and therapeutic drug monitoring (TDM) more difficult and is associated with a higher risk of kidney related side effects (Goodwin et al., 2016). Lithium is available in both tablets and liquid, but it is important to note that due to use of different lithium salts the dosage forms are not bioequivalent and cannot be used interchangeably. This means that patients should continue to take the same brand of lithium; if it is necessary to switch from one brand or formulation of lithium to another, then a dose conversion must be carried out. Lithium should always be prescribed by brand and the brands most commonly prescribed in the UK are Priadel and Camcolit. Conversion ratios can be found in the most current edition of the BNF.

Therapeutic drug monitoring (TDM)

Lithium has as a **narrow therapeutic window;** this means that there is only a small difference between doses which are subtherapeutic, therapeutic and toxic. In order to minimise the risk of toxicity, people who take lithium need to have regular monitoring to check the level of lithium in their blood. Blood samples should be collected in a vacutainer with a light green top.

449

The blood level taken is known as a **trough** level, meaning that this reflects the lowest concentration in the blood before the next dose is administered; because of this, blood samples must be taken 12–14 hours after the last dose of lithium in order to have any clinical relevance. Any samples taken outside this window will still provide a lithium level; however, it is not possible to draw any helpful conclusions regarding treatment from them.

Lithium trough levels should normally be between 0.4 and 1.0 mmol/L. The target level will vary greatly for different patients depending on the clinical indication for lithium and their clinical response. In many circumstances it is merely used to ensure prescribed doses do not result in toxicity. There are a number of factors which can affect the level of lithium in the blood, so there can be significant variation in dose ranges for different patients.

Side effects

Adverse reactions include fine tremor, polyuria, weight gain, cognitive impairment, drowsiness, metallic taste, poor coordination and gastrointestinal upset (e.g. nausea). These are often dose dependent and may be alleviated to some extent with dose reduction where this is appropriate. Up to one-fifth of people who take lithium for over 10 years will develop some degree of renal impairment. Lithium is known to cause hypothyroidism, with women more commonly affected than men (Author unknown, 2002). Often, treatment with levothyroxine is required. Hyperparathyroidism is also common with lithium treatment and calcium monitoring is recommended during long-term treatment.

450 Toxicity

Lithium is considered toxic when plasma levels are above 1.0 mmol/L and toxic effects are reliably seen at levels of 1.5 mmol/L and above. Signs of lithium toxicity can include vomiting and diarrhoea, coarse tremor, blurred vision, polyuria, muscle weakness and confusion. Plasma levels above 2.0 mmol/L are associated with increased disorientation and seizures, which may lead to coma and ultimately can be fatal (Goodwin et al., 2016; MHRA, 2018a; Taylor et al., 2019). If lithium toxicity is suspected, patients should have a hospital assessment as an emergency. There is no specific antidote; however, lithium treatment should be discontinued immediately and supportive therapy provided, including correction of electrolyte and fluid balance if indicated. In more serious cases, dialysis may be required to minimise toxic effects (NPIS, 2016).

Lithium blood levels can be greatly affected by fluid balance. This is of particular relevance should people taking lithium become physically unwell resulting in vomiting and/or diarrhoea. In these instances, total body water will reduce, leading lithium levels to increase. As such, any patient taking lithium who reports these symptoms should have a lithium level taken at the earliest opportunity. Any other situations leading to dehydration (e.g. excess sweating, reduced fluid intake) will have the same effect on lithium in the blood. Conversely, if patients dramatically increase their fluid intake, this will likely lead to reduced lithium levels.

The National Patient Safety Association (NPSA) produce a lithium therapy information pack which contains all the important information patients need to be aware of while they are taking lithium (NPSA, 2009). Patients should be given one of these packs prior to starting lithium and at any relevant point throughout their treatment.

Drug interactions

There are certain medicines that must be used with extra caution in those people taking lithium, most notably with drugs which affect how the kidneys handle sodium.

- Angiotensin Converting Enzyme (ACE) inhibitors such as lisinopril, enalapril, ramipril and perindopril. Angiotensin II receptor antagonists (e.g. irbesartan, candesartan and losartan) may be associated with a similar risk.
- Non-steroidal anti-inflammatory drugs (NSAIDs) such as Ibuprofen, Naproxen and Diclofenac.

- Thiazide-type (or related) diuretics such as Bendroflumethiazide, Indapamide and Chlortalidone.

Interactions with NSAIDs are particularly relevant as patients are free to buy these over the counter without prescription in many cases. Advice should be given to avoid all NSAIDs and use other pain relief as appropriate (e.g. paracetamol). Where possible, medicines should either be prescribed or purchased from a pharmacy where a pharmacist can provide advice on what medicines are safe to be used concurrently with lithium.

Physical health monitoring
Baseline monitoring
Lithium can have a number of adverse effects on thyroid, renal and cardiac function and baseline function must be checked before commencing lithium. This would usually include eGFR (estimated glomerular filtration rate) and thyroid and parathyroid function tests (e.g. TSH and calcium) would be expected as a minimum. An ECG is also recommended for those patients who are at increased risk of developing or have existing cardiac disease. Lithium commonly causes weight gain and so baseline measurement of this is helpful for assessing the severity of this side effect. Pregnancy should also be excluded as lithium may have teratogenic effects (Goodwin et al., 2016; NICE, 2018a; Taylor et al., 2019).

Ongoing monitoring
Renal and thyroid monitoring should be checked at least every six months where this is found to be stable. Patients with a degree of impairment or additional concerns (e.g. chronic kidney disease, increasing age) may require more frequent monitoring.

Plasma monitoring of lithium levels should be closely monitored on initiation and once in therapeutic range every three to six months. Plasma monitoring may be helpful following dose changes; however, blood samples should not be taken until at least five days after dose changes to allow the new dose to reach steady state (Goodwin et al., 2016; Taylor et al., 2019). Weight should be monitored due to the propensity for lithium to induce weight gain.

The NPSA lithium pack contains a record book for documenting all results of physical health monitoring and should be taken to every appointment for this purpose.

Discontinuation
Lithium treatment should be gradually reduced as abrupt discontinuation is associated with an increased risk of manic relapse in the first few months following this. Doses should be tapered and withdrawn over four to eight weeks unless there are risks associated with doing so, such as in cases of overdose or toxicity where immediate withdrawal is necessary.

Anticonvulsants
Valproate
Sodium valproate is probably much better known as an anti-epileptic medicine rather than as a mood stabiliser. The way it works to stabilise mood is not well understood but it is thought to modify a number of biochemical pathways. Valproate is recommended for acute mania, acute bipolar depression (in combination with an antidepressant) and for prophylaxis of relapse (NICE, 2018a).

Formulations
In the UK, valproate is available in three different forms; sodium valproate, semi-sodium valproate and valproic acid. Although only semi-sodium valproate is licensed for treating mania (Joint Formulary Committee, 2019), sodium valproate is the form most commonly used in the UK.

Side effects

Valproate may commonly cause weight gain, diarrhoea, drowsiness, hallucinations, headache and hepatic disorders (Joint Formulary Committee, 2019; ABPI, 2018b).

Pharmacokinetics

Sodium valproate is rapidly and completely absorbed from GIT after oral administration, though the rate is delayed by food. There is a low proportion of protein binding and so therapeutic effects may not reflect free drug levels. Valproic acid, however, is highly protein bound. Valproate undergoes extensive hepatic metabolism and in the form of sodium valproate has an elimination half-life of 13–19 hours (ABPI, 2018a; Buckingham, 2019).

Drug interactions

Valproate is an enzyme inhibitor, meaning it slows down some liver enzymes causing certain medicines to be cleared from the body much slower than would be usual with the potential for these to reach toxic levels. These medicines include Clomipramine, warfarin, quetiapine and lamotrigine (Baxter and Preston, 2019).

Teratogenesis

Valproate carries a significant risk of birth defects and developmental disorders in children born to women who take valproate during pregnancy. The current evidence base recommends that its use should be avoided in women under the age of 55 wherever possible for all indications (including epilepsy), but in cases where it is required that a robust pregnancy prevention plan is in place (MHRA, 2018b).

Discontinuation

Abrupt cessation of valproate may give rise to relapse of bipolar disorder, though there is a lack of evidence in this regard, so it is recommended that valproate be reduced over at least a month before stopping (Taylor et al., 2019).

Other anticonvulsant medicines

Carbamazepine

Carbamazepine blocks voltage-gated sodium channels to reduce repetitive neuronal firing and reduces turnover of noradrenaline and dopamine via reduced glutamate release. Carbamazepine is less effective in maintenance treatment than lithium but may sometimes be used as monotherapy if lithium is ineffective and appears to be effective against manic relapse. It is not recommended for use in BPAD in the UK (NICE, 2018a).

GIT absorption of carbamazepine is slow and irregular, but almost complete. It is widely distributed and 70–80% protein bound. Half-life is 36 hours after single dose, though after repeated administration is approximately 12–24 hours (ABPI, 2019i; Buckingham, 2019). There are a number of significant pharmacokinetic interactions that are a particular problem with carbamazepine, as it is a strong inducer of CYP3A4 and will increase clearance of medicines including amitriptyline, clozapine, citalopram, oral contraceptives, tacrolimus, warfarin and theophylline (Baxter and Preston, 2019).

The most common side effects of carbamazepine are double vision, headache, dizziness, drowsiness, nausea and vomiting. Hyponatremia has also been reported with carbamazepine (ABPI, 2019h).

Lamotrigine

Lamotrigine may be an option for treating and preventing relapses of bipolar depression and has similar efficacy to citalopram (Taylor et al., 2019). The effect, however, is modest and NICE does not recommend lamotrigine for use in bipolar disorder.

Clinical considerations

Lamotrigine doses must be titrated slowly as it can cause serious skin reactions. Doses should not normally be increased more frequently than every two weeks to minimise the risk of developing this effect.

To revisit the key issues in this section, lithium is an effective mood stabiliser in mania and bipolar depression; however, it requires close monitoring due to its narrow therapeutic window and the potential for adverse effects on renal and thyroid functioning. Valproate is also an effective mood stabiliser in bipolar disorder, although it has such significant teratogenicity that it should normally be avoided in all women of child-bearing age for any indication (including epilepsy). Carbamazepine can be useful, particularly if lithium is not tolerated; however, it has a number of significant drug interactions which arise from its enzyme-inducing effects which make it less desirable for use. Lamotrigine may be effective for bipolar depression; however, its use is not currently recommended in NICE guidance.

Anxiolytics and hypnotics

Anxiety disorders are the most common psychiatric disorders to be diagnosed. Approximately 25% of adults will experience an anxiety disorder at some point in their life and although it can develop at any point, age of diagnosis is most commonly in adults aged 35–55 years. In order to meet the threshold diagnosis of an anxiety disorder, a certain number of symptoms must be experienced beyond a minimum specified period and cause considerable personal distress, with an associated impairment in day-to-day functioning (Baldwin et al., 2014).

453

A number of different anxiety disorders exist including generalised anxiety disorder (GAD), panic disorder, post-traumatic stress disorder (PTSD) and obsessive–compulsive disorder (OCD).

Anxiety symptoms often co-exist with other psychological symptoms, particularly depressive symptoms and especially those with severe anxiety symptoms.

Symptoms often consist of uncontrollable, disproportionate and widespread worry and a range of physical, mental and behavioural symptoms which can range in severity. Symptoms may often arise without obvious warning and in some cases be lifelong without any significant remission. The development of anxiety disorders is often complex and may include a number of factors, such as environmental stressors, genetic factors, chronic illness and substance misuse.

Many patients can have reservations about drug treatment for anxiety disorders, not least due to the potential adverse effects which can be associated with these and the potential for dependence with drugs such as Benzodiazepines. Professionals have a large role to play to ensure patients can understand the benefits associated with drug treatments and support them to balance these with the associated risks.

SSRIs are currently the first-line treatment approach for most anxiety disorders as they appear to have a relatively quick onset of action but remain effective in the longer term and are generally well tolerated (Baldwin et al., 2014), as discussed earlier in the chapter. Where drug treatment has been effective, this should usually be continued for at least 12 months (Bazire, 2018).

Benzodiazepines

Benzodiazepines are effective at managing symptoms of anxiety in the short term. They are the most commonly used anxiolytics and hypnotics and act at Benzodiazepine receptors which are associated with γ-aminobutyric acid (GABA) receptors. Examples include diazepam and lorazepam.

Although Benzodiazepines are widely prescribed, they are associated with a risk of dependence and tolerance and this risk is increased where these agents are used for an extended period of time. Physiological dependence involves adaptation of Benzodiazepine target receptors in the body resulting in larger doses being required to achieve the same therapeutic effect. Once tolerance is established, it is extremely difficult, but not impossible to withdraw Benzodiazepine therapy.

Withdrawal

Where tolerance to Benzodiazepines has developed, withdrawal usually begins by converting existing treatment to an equivalent daily dose of diazepam. This is because diazepam is relatively long acting with a half-life of approximately one to two days. This allows for once or twice daily administration and also for smaller dose reductions to be made. The Ashton Manual (2013) is a useful source for supporting the design of Benzodiazepine reduction and withdrawal schedules.

Place in therapy

Due to the known risks associated with their use, there are specific indications where Benzodiazepines are usually considered (Joint Formulary Committee, 2019).

Benzodiazepines are indicated for short-term relief (two to four weeks only) of anxiety that is severe, disabling or causing the patient unacceptable distress, occurring alone or in association with insomnia or short-term psychosomatic, organic or psychotic illness. Benzodiazepines should be used to treat insomnia only when it is severe, disabling, or causing the patient extreme distress. The use of Benzodiazepines to treat short-term "mild" anxiety is inappropriate and alternative approaches such as psychological therapy should be utilised instead.

Different Benzodiazepines may be used on account of their pharmacokinetic profile; some have a short onset and duration of action, such as lorazepam, and so are useful in symptoms of acute anxiety. The therapeutic effects of diazepam persist (ABPI, 2018d) for a prolonged period following administration; it has a half-life of one to two days but its metabolite is also pharmacologically active and has a half-life of two to five days (ABPI, 2019i).

Pregabalin

Pregabalin is an analogue of GABA, a neurotransmitter which inhibits the release of glutamate and noradrenaline, among other substances. It is licensed in the UK for management of seizures, neuropathic pain and GAD. The usual maintenance dose is between 150 and 600 mg given in two to three divided doses; the lower initial and maximum doses should be used for older patients and those with renal impairment (ABPI, 2019j; Joint Formulary Committee, 2019). Pregabalin is usually considered where antidepressant drugs are unsuitable or not tolerated (NICE, 2017) and they have been shown to have similar efficacy on anxiety symptoms as Benzodiazepines and are often better tolerated than a number of antidepressants indicated for anxiety disorders.

Adverse effects

Common side effects of pregabalin include dizziness and drowsiness and so patients should be cautious of this if they are driving or using machinery. This is most prominent on initiation and titration, with effects reducing after a few weeks. Weight gain is associated with longer-term treatment and may be seen in up to one-fifth of patients treated with pregabalin (Baldwin et al., 2014). The use of pregabalin has also been linked with an increased risk of suicidal ideation and suicidal behaviour; therefore, professionals must carefully assess this risk and provide close monitoring, particularly during initiation and dose titration of pregabalin (NICE, 2017). The main risks associated with pregabalin dependence appear to be overdose, suicidality and impaired driving (Expert Committee on Drug Dependence, 2018).

Interactions

Pregabalin has very few pharmacokinetic interactions with other drugs and many appear to be of little clinical significance. Significant risks do exist, however, when pregabalin is used concurrently with alcohol or CNS depressant drugs, such as opioids, and may result in fatality. Pregabalin has an elimination half-life of 6.3 hours and excretion is directly proportional to creatinine clearance; as such, doses must be reduced in cases of renal impairment (ABPI, 2019j).

Risk of misuse and dependence

Since 2008, there have been a significant number of cases of pregabalin misuse reported. Pregabalin is not known to act in the same way as traditional drugs of abuse; however, evidence from pre-marketing clinical trials demonstrated that it can commonly produce a feeling of euphoria, particularly at higher doses. Over the last 10 years, prescriptions for pregabalin in the UK have increased more than 11-fold with over 5.5 million issued in 2016 (Expert Committee on Drug Dependence, 2018). In April 2019, due to growing concern about misuse, both pregabalin and gabapentin were reclassified under the Misuse of Drugs Act 1971 as Class C substances and scheduled under the Misuse of Drugs Regulations 2001 as Schedule 3 controlled drugs (MHRA, 2019).

The risk of dependence and misuse is much higher for patients who have current or previous substance misuse, psychiatric co-morbidities and current opioid dependence (Expert Committee on Drug Dependence, 2018). Prior to treating with pregabalin professionals have a responsibility to carefully assess patient risk for potential misuse and dependence. Patients taking pregabalin must be observed for possible signs of misuse and dependence such as seeking dose escalation, drug-seeking behaviour and development of tolerance (MHRA, 2019).

To recap on this section, anxiety disorders have a high prevalence and may persist for prolonged periods without significant remission between episodes. SSRIs are usually effective in treating anxiety disorders and should be used first line. Benzodiazepines, though effective, should not be routinely used to manage anxiety due to their side effect profile, risk of dependence and difficulty to discontinue once treatment is established. Pregabalin is a well-tolerated, effective alternative to SSRIs for treating anxiety, though it is increasingly being misused and has recently been reclassified in legislation to reflect this.

Hypnotics

Sleep disorders are somewhat common in the general population, yet are relatively poorly understood by professionals. Insomnia can be broadly considered to be the difficulty initiating or maintaining sleep and often arises as the result of one or more factors. There is a high correlation between psychiatric disorders and insomnia, and this is most often reported in patients with major depressive disorder. Insomnia can have a number of important consequences, not least a detrimental impact on quality of life. It is also linked with an increased incidence of depression, suicide, physical health conditions (e.g. type 2 diabetes and hypertension) and road accidents (Wilson et al., 2019). With this in mind, effective and timely treatment is imperative.

Non-pharmacological approaches should always be considered whether or not medication is considered to be appropriate. A sensible first step is to identify any potentially contributing factors, such as pain, and address these wherever possible. Although encouraging sleep hygiene may also be helpful, there is actually no evidence to suggest that such approaches are effective, though it is widely supported in current literature and guidance. Psychological therapies have also been shown to be effective in treating insomnia and should usually be considered as a first-line approach before medication. The principles of sleep hygiene are outlined in Table 17.8 below

Medication for sleep is referred to by a number of terms including hypnotics, sedatives and tranquilisers. They may be indicated where non-pharmacological approaches have been unsuccessful, where there is significant distress or impairment in daytime functioning, or where risks may be increased (e.g. manic episode). Use of hypnotics should usually be on an "as required" basis with the minimum effective dose being used for the shortest duration possible to avoid development of tolerance and adverse effects, with treatment normally limited to a maximum of two to four weeks.

Table 17.8　Principles of sleep hygiene.

- Establish a regular bedtime routine, particularly going to bed and rising at the same time each day.
- Avoid sleeping or long periods of inactivity through the day.
- Avoid back-lit screens for at least one hour prior to retiring to bed; the blue light emitted is known to inhibit the release of melatonin.
- A warm bath or exercise a few hours before going to bed may promote sleep, though intense exercise should be avoided shortly before retiring as this is likely to have the opposite effect.
- Avoid caffeine, nicotine and alcohol for 6 hours before retiring to bed.
- Maintain a comfortable sleeping environment which is dark, quiet and has an ambient temperature.
- Do not remain in bed for prolonged periods while awake; if there is difficulty sleeping, move to another room until the feeling of tiredness returns, without engaging in any stimulating activity.

Source: Bazire 2018, Wilson et al. 2019.

Benzodiazepines

In addition to their role in treating anxiety symptoms, Benzodiazepines can also be effective as hypnotics for improving sleep latency and duration, at least in the short term. Adverse effects are common, however, including dizziness and drowsiness lasting into the following day, the so-called "hangover effect" (ABPI, 2017c). Temazepam, Loprazolam and Loremetazepam are the Benzodiazepines recommended for treatment of insomnia due to their relatively short duration of action, minimising the risk of residual drowsiness on rising. They are, however, more commonly associated with discontinuation effects (Joint Formulary Committee, 2019).

Z-Drugs

These are so-called because of the agents in this class – zopiclone and zolpidem. A third agent, zaleplon, has now been withdrawn in the UK. Despite acting on Benzodiazepine receptors, they have many benefits over Benzodiazepines, including a reduced incidence of dependence. They are both relatively short acting and so are unlikely to cause a "hangover effect." Zopiclone is has a slightly longer duration of action, though zolpidem is rapid in its onset, often within 15 minutes.

Melatonin

Melatonin is a naturally occurring hormone produced by the pineal gland in the brain and plays an important role in regulating sleep–wake cycle. Older people with insomnia are known to secrete less endogenous melatonin than those with normal sleep, and so exogenous melatonin is licensed for insomnia in patients over 55 for up to 13 weeks (Joint Formulary Committee, 2019). This is used at a dose of 2 mg in a modified release form to allow gradual release over a number of hours in an attempt to reflect the normal endogenous melatonin profile (Bazire, 2018; Wilson et al., 2019). It has a half-life of 3.5–4 hours (ABPI, 2019k).

Cautions

Due to their sedative action, hypnotics are known to increase risk of falls. This should be carefully risk assessed when considering their use and in particular for older people who may be at increased risk of fracture.

Patients using hypnotics should be warned about the risk of hangover effects and advised to avoid driving or carrying out skilled tasks if they are affected. It is illegal in England and Wales to drive with certain level of prescription drugs in the body if it impairs driving. Many Benzodiazepines are included on this list and the penalty if caught is a driving ban for a minimum of 12 months, an unlimited fine, up to six months in prison and a criminal record (UK Government, n.d.). While melatonin and Z-drugs are not listed, patients must be advised to avoid driving if impaired as a result of taking these drugs.

To summarise this section: underlying causes of insomnia should be identified and addressed wherever possible in preference to use of hypnotic medication. Where hypnotics are indicated, their use should be limited to a maximum of two to four weeks in most cases due to the risk of dependence (particularly with Benzodiazepines). Implementation of sleep hygiene practices may help with insomnia despite a lack of evidence to support their efficacy. Melatonin may be considered for patients over 55 years but treatment courses are only licensed for a maximum of 13 weeks.

Drugs for dementia

Dementia is a chronic, progressive disease characterised by deterioration in cognitive function beyond that associated with normal aging. It affects memory, thinking, orientation, comprehension, calculation, learning capacity, language and judgment but does not affect consciousness (WHO, 2019).

Although there is no cure for dementia, there are drugs available which aim to slow the progression of cognitive impairment and preserve functional ability, and these fall into two groups.

Acetylcholinesterase inhibitors

Some dementias, such as Alzheimer's disease, are associated with a reduced amount of acetylcholine in the brain. Acetylcholinesterase inhibitors like donepezil, galantamine and rivastigmine work by blocking the enzyme which breaks down acetylcholine to reduce further loss. Acetycholine is found all over the body and these drugs are not specific for the type found in the brain. As a result, common side effects include nausea, vomiting and diarrhoea. Other side effects may include bradycardia, tiredness, headache, dizziness and, rarely, aggression (ABPI, 2016).

The risk of side effects (particularly GI upset) can be minimised by titrating doses slowly and doses should not normally be increased more frequently than every four weeks (Joint Formulary Committee, 2019). Donepezil, galantamine and rivastigmine all have similar efficacy and they are all licensed for use in mild–moderate Alzheimer's disease. Rivastigmine is also approved for use in Parkinson's disease dementia. Although not licensed, NICE recommends acetylcholinesterase inhibitors for people with dementia with Lewy bodies (DLB) (NICE, 2018b). Where people are unable to tolerate oral rivastigmine, this is also available in a transdermal patch to avoid the drug entering the systemic circulation and reducing the likelihood of GI upset.

Pulse monitoring should be carried out before starting an acetylcholinesterase inhibitor as they can cause bradycardia; this may pose an additional risk of falls in a patient group which may already have additional risks in this regard (ABPI, 2018e).

Glutamate inhibitors

Memantine is licensed for treatment of patients with moderate to severe Alzheimer's disease. NICE (2018b) suggests memantine can be considered for patients with DLB if they cannot tolerate acetylcholinesterase inhibitors. Memantine is usually introduced at a dose of 5 mg and increased on a weekly basis to 20 mg, or the maximum dose tolerated. Common side effects associated with memantine include dizziness, drowsiness, unsteady gait/falls and tiredness. They may rarely cause seizures and acute agitation. Memantine is renally excreted and the maximum daily dose should be reduced to 10 mg if the eGFR is less than 29 (ABPI 2019I; Joint Formulary Committee, 2019).

Due to the emerging evidence in this area, NICE now supports the addition of memantine treatment for people with advancing Alzheimer's disease who are already treated with an acetylcholinesterase inhibitor (ABPI, 2019I).

To recap on this section, acetylcholinesterase inhibitors are recommended for treatment of mild–moderate Alzheimer's disease, DLB and mixed Alzheimer's dementia syndromes.

457

Memantine should be reserved for treatment of moderate–severe disease. The aim of drug treatment is to slow the progression of cognitive symptoms and it is not a cure for the disease. As dementia progresses, consideration can be given to adding memantine to existing acetyl-cholinesterase inhibitor treatment.

References

ABPI Medicines Compendium (2014). *Summary of product characteristics for mirtazapine 15mg tablets (Arrow)*. https://www.medicines.org.uk/emc/product/3192/smpc (accessed 20 October 2019).

ABPI Medicines Compendium (2015). *Summary of product characteristics for Edronax 4mg tablets*. https://www.medicines.org.uk/emc/product/1578 (accessed 31 October 2019).

ABPI Medicines Compendium (2016). *Summary of product characteristics for Nimvastid 1.5mg hard capsules*. https://www.medicines.org.uk/emc/product/4911/smpc (accessed 29 October 2019).

ABPI Medicines Compendium (2017a). *Summary of product characteristics for Nardil tablets*. https://www.medicines.org.uk/emc/product/228Ltd (accessed 21 August 2019).

ABPI Medicines Compendium (2017b). *Summary of product characteristics for Agomelatine Accord 25mg Film-coated tablets*. https://www.medicines.org.uk/emc/product/9887/smpc (accessed 30 September 2019).

ABPI Medicines Compendium (2017c). *Summary of product characteristics for Temazepam 10mg tablets*. https://www.medicines.org.uk/emc/product/8792/smpc (accessed 23 October 2019).

ABPI Medicines Compendium (2018a). *Summary of product characteristics for Paroxetine 10mg tablets*. https://www.medicines.org.uk/emc/product/9582/smpc (accessed 21 August 2019).

ABPI Medicines Compendium (2018b). *Summary of product characteristics for Epilim 100mg crushable tablets*. https://www.medicines.org.uk/emc/product/518/smpc (accessed 26 October 2019).

ABPI Medicines Compendium (2018c). *Summary of product characteristics for Lamictal tablets*. https://www.medicines.org.uk/emc/product/8052/smpc (accessed 26 October 2019).

ABPI Medicines Compendium (2018d). *Summary of product characteristics for Lorazepam 1mg tablets*. https://www.medicines.org.uk/emc/product/6137/smpc (accessed 23 October 2019).

ABPI Medicines Compendium (2018e). *Summary of product characteristics for Aricept tablets*. https://www.medicines.org.uk/emc/product/3776/smpc (accessed 29 October 2019).

ABPI Medicines Compendium (2019a). *Summary of product characteristics for Lustral 50mg tablets*. https://www.medicines.org.uk/emc/product/1070/smpc (accessed 20 October 2019).

ABPI Medicines Compendium (2019b). *Summary of product characteristics for fluoxetine 20mg capsules*. https://www.medicines.org.uk/emc/product/6013/smpc (accessed 22 October 2019).

ABPI Medicines Compendium (2019c). *Summary of product characteristics for venlafaxine 37.5mg tablets*. https://www.medicines.org.uk/emc/product/773/smpc (accessed 20 October 2019).

ABPI Medicines Compendium (2019d). *Summary of product characteristics for Cymbalta 30mg hard gastro-resistant capsules*. https://www.medicines.org.uk/emc/product/3880/smpc (accessed 30 October 2019).

ABPI Medicines Compendium (2019e). *Summary of product characteristics for Brintellix 10mg film-coated tablets*. https://www.medicines.org.uk/emc/product/10441/smpc (accessed 20 October 2019).

ABPI Medicines Compendium (2019f). *Summary of product characteristics for Denzapine 100mg tablets*. https://www.medicines.org.uk/emc/product/6120/smpc (accessed 25 October 2019).

ABPI Medicines Compendium (2019g). *Summary of product characteristics for Quetiapine 100mg film-coated tablets*. https://www.medicines.org.uk/emc/product/8233/smpc (accessed 20 October 2019).

ABPI Medicines Compendium (2019h). *Summary of product characteristics for Tegretol 100mg tablets*. https://www.medicines.org.uk/emc/product/1040/smpc (accessed 27 October 2019).

ABPI Medicines Compendium (2019i) *Summary of product characteristics for Diazepam tablets BP 2mg*. https://www.medicines.org.uk/emc/product/4523/smpc (accessed 30 September 2019).

ABPI Medicines Compendium (2019j). *Summary of product characteristics for Alzain 100mg capsules, hard*. https://www.medicines.org.uk/emc/product/1761/smpc (accessed 24 October 2019).

ABPI Medicines Compendium (2019k). *Summary of product characteristics for Circadin 2mg prolonged-release tablets*. https://www.medicines.org.uk/emc/product/2809/smpc (accessed 20 October 2019).

ABPI Medicines Compendium (2019l). *Summary of product characteristics for Ebixa 20mg film-coated tablets*. https://www.medicines.org.uk/emc/product/8220/smpc (accessed 01 October 2019).

Ashton, H. (2013). *Benzodiazepines: How they work and how to withdraw*. https://www.benzo.org.uk/manual (accessed on 29 September 2019).

Author unknown (2002). The Complex Interrelationship of Lithium and the Thyroid. *Psychiatric Times* **19** (1) https://www.psychiatrictimes.com/bipolar-disorder/complex-interrelationship-lithium-and-thyroid (accessed 27 September 2019).

Baldwin, D.S., Anderson, I.M., Nutt, D.J. et al. (2014). Evidence-based pharmacological treatment of anxiety disorders, post-traumatic stress disorder and obsessive-compulsive disorder: A revision of the 2005 guidelines from the British Association for Psychopharmacology. *Journal of Psychopharmacology*: **28** (5): 403–439. https://doi.org/10.1177/0269881114525674.

Barnes, T.R.E. and Schizophrenia Consensus Group of the British Association for Psychopharmacology (2011). Evidence-based guidelines for the pharmacological treatment of schizophrenia: recommendations from the British Association for Psychopharmacology. *Journal of Psychopharmacology*: 1–54. doi: 10.1177/0269881110391123.

Baxter, K. and Preston, C.L. (eds.) (2019). *Stockley's Drug Interactions*, 12e. London: Pharmaceutical Press http://www.new.medicinescomplete.com (accessed 22 September 2019).

Bazire, S. (2018). *Psychotropic Drug Directory 2018*. Dorsington: Lloyd-Reinhold Communications LLP.

Bird, A.M., Smith, T.L. and Walton, A.E. (2011). Current treatment strategies for clozapine-induced sialorrhea. *Annals of Pharmacotherapy* **45** (5): 667–675.

Buckingham, R. (ed.) (2019). *Martindale: The Complete Drug Reference*. London: Pharmaceutical Press http://www.new.medicinescomplete.com (accessed 30 October 2019).

Cheng, F., Jones, P.B., and Talbot, P.S. (2016). Antipsychotics. In: *Fundamentals of Clinical Psychopharmacology*, 4e (eds. I.M. Anderson and R.H. McAllister-Williams), 47–76. Boca Raton: CRC Press.

Cleare, A., Pariante, C.M. and Young, A.H. (2015). Evidence-based guidelines for treating depressive disorders with antidepressants: a revision of the 2008 British Association for Psychopharmacology guidelines. *Journal of Psychopharmacology* **29** (5): 459–525. https://doi.org/10.1177/0269881115581093.

Davies, J., Read, J., Hengartner, M.P. et al. (2019). Clinical guidelines on antidepressant withdrawal urgently need updating. *British Medical Journal* **365**: l2238. https://doi.org/10.1136/bmj.l2238.

Expert Committee on Drug Dependence (2018). *Critical Review Report: Pregabalin*. https://www.who.int/medicines/access/controlled-substances/Pregabalin_FINAL.pdf?ua=1 (accessed 22 September 2019).

Gartlehner, G., Hansen, R.A., Morgan, L.C. et al. (2011). Comparative benefits and harms of second-generation antidepressants for treating major depressive disorder: an updated meta-analysis. *Annals of Internal Medicine* **155** (11): 772–785.

Goodwin, G.M., Haddad, P.M., Ferrier, I.N. et al. (2016). Evidence-based guidelines for treating bipolar disorder: Revised third edition recommendations from the British Association for Psychopharmacology. *Journal of Psychopharmacology* **30** (6): 495–553. https://doi.org/10.1177/0269881116636545.

Joint Formulary Committee (2019). *British National Formulary (BNF)*. London: British Medical Journal (BMJ) Group and Pharmaceutical Press. https://www.medicinescomplete.com (accessed 30 September 2019).

Lohr, J.B. and Flynn, K. (1992). Smoking and schizophrenia. *Schizophrenia Research* **8**: 93–102. https://doi.org/10.1016/0920-9964(92)90024-Y.

Meadows, T. (2019). *If antidepressant-induced hyponatraemia has been diagnosed, how should the depression be treated?* https://www.sps.nhs.uk/articles/if-antidepressant-induced-hyponatraemia-has-been-diagnosed-how-should-the-depression-be-treated-2 (accessed on 21 August 2019).

Medicines Healthcare Regulatory Authority (MHRA) (2017). *Clozapine: reminder of potentially fatal risk of intestinal obstruction, faecal impaction, and paralytic ileus*. https://www.gov.uk/drug-safety-update/clozapine-reminder-of-potentially-fatal-risk-of-intestinal-obstruction-faecal-impaction-and-paralytic-ileus (accessed 28 September 2019).

Medicines Healthcare Regulatory Authority (MHRA) (2018a). *Summary of product characteristics for Priadel 400mg prolonged release tablets*. https://www.mhra.gov.uk/home/groups/spcpil/documents/spcpil/con1542949679637.pdf (accessed 28 September 2019).

Medicines Healthcare Regulatory Authority (MHRA) (2018b). *Valproate use by women and girls*. https://www.gov.uk/guidance/valproate-use-by-women-and-girls (accessed on 28 September 2019).

Medicines Healthcare Regulatory Authority (MHRA) (2019). *Pregabalin (Lyrica), gabapentin (Neurontin) and risk of abuse and dependence: new scheduling requirements from 1 April*. https://www.gov.uk/drug-safety-update/pregabalin-lyrica-gabapentin-neurontin-and-risk-of-abuse-and-dependence-new-scheduling-requirements-from-1-april (accessed 22 September 2019).

Montgomery, S.A., Nielsen, R., Poulsen, L. et al. (2014). A randomised, double-blind study in adults with major depressive disorder with an inadequate response to a single course of selective serotonin reuptake inhibitor or serotonin–noradrenaline reuptake inhibitor treatment switched to vortioxetine or agomelatine. *Human Psychopharmacology: Clinical and Experimental* **29**: 470–482. https://doi.org/10.1002/hup.2424.

National Health Service (NHS) (2009). *Antidepressants and suicide risk*. https://www.nhs.uk/news/mental-health/antidepressants-and-suicide-risk (accessed 22 September 2019).

National Institute for Health and Care Excellence (NICE) (2009). *Depression in adults: recognition and management*. *CG90*. https://www.nice.org.uk/guidance/CG90 (accessed 15 August 2019).

National Institute for Health and Care Excellence (NICE) (2014). *Psychosis and schizophrenia in adults: prevention and management*. *CG178*. https://www.nice.org.uk/guidance/cg178 (accessed 28 August 2019).

National Institute for Health and Care Excellence (NICE) (2015). *Vortioxetine for treating major depressive episodes*. *TA 367*. https://www.nice.org.uk/guidance/ta367 (accessed on 29 September 2019).

National Institute for Health and Care Excellence (NICE) (2017). *Generalized anxiety disorder. Clinical knowledge summary*. https://cks.nice.org.uk/generalized-anxiety-disorder#!topicSummary (accessed 28 September 2019).

National Institute for Health and Care Excellence (NICE) (2018a). *Bipolar disorder: assessment and management*. *CG185*. https://www.nice.org.uk/guidance/cg185 (accessed on 28 September 2019).

National Institute for Health and Care Excellence (NICE) (2018b). *Dementia: assessment, management and support for people living with dementia and their carers*. *NG97*. https://www.nice.org.uk/guidance/ng97 (accessed 1 October 2019).

National Institute for Health and Care Excellence (NICE) (2019). Antidepressant treatment in adults. https://pathways.nice.org.uk/pathways/depression/antidepressant-treatment-in-adults (accessed on 29 September 2019).

National Patient Safety Agency (NPSA) (2009). *Lithium therapy*. https://www.sps.nhs.uk/wp-content/uploads/2018/02/2009-NRLS-0921-Lithium-patientet-2009.12.01-v1.pdf (accessed 1 September 2019).

National Poisons Information Service (NPIS) (2016). *Lithium*. https://www.toxbase.org/Poisons-Index-A-Z/L-Products/Lithium (accessed 28 September 2019).

National Poisons Information Service (NPIS) (2017). *Amitriptyline*. https://www.toxbase.org/poisons-index-a-z/a-products/amitriptyline---------------/ (accessed 28 September 2019).

Owen, S. (2017). *Drug-induced hypersalivation – what treatment options are available?* https://www.sps.nhs.uk/wp-content/uploads/2015/11/UKMi_QA_Hypersalivationdruginduced_update-May-2017.doc (accessed 20 September 2019).

Qurashi, I., Stephenson, P., Nagaraj, C. et al. (2019). Changes in smoking status, mental state and plasma clozapine concentration: retrospective cohort evaluation. *BJPsych Bulletin*: **43** (6): 271-274. https://doi.org/10.1192/bjb.2019.50 (accessed 24 September 2019).

Royal College of Psychiatrists (RCPsych) (2014a). *Consensus statement on high-dose antipsychotic Medication CR190*. www.rcpsych.ac.uk/docs/default-source/improving-care/better-mh-policy/college-reports/college-report-cr190.pdf?sfvrsn=54f5d9a2_2 (accessed on 21 September 2019).

Royal College of Psychiatrists (RCPsych) (2014b). *Report of the second round of the National Audit of Schizophrenia (NAS2)*. www.rcpsych.ac.uk/docs/default-source/improving-care/ccqi/national-clinical-audits/ncap-library/national-audit-of-schizophrenia-document-library/nas_round-2-report.pdf?sfvrsn=6356a4b0_2 (accessed 29 September 2019).

Royal College of Psychiatrists (RCPsych) (2019). *Position statement on antidepressants and depression*. www.rcpsych.ac.uk/docs/default-source/improving-care/better-mh-policy/position-statements/ps04_19---antidepressants-and-depression.pdf?sfvrsn=ddea9473_5 (accessed 9 November 2019).

Shepherd, E. (2018). Injection technique 1: administering drugs via the intramuscular route. *Nursing Times* **114** (8): 23–25.

Smart, C., Anderson, I.M. and McAllister-Williams, R.H. (2016). Antidepressants and ECT. In: *Fundamentals of Clinical Psychopharmacology*, 4e (eds. I.M. Anderson and R.H. McAllister-Williams), 77–102. Boca Raton: CRC Press.

Stahl, S.M. (2008). *Stahl's Essential Psychopharmacology*, 4e. Cambridge: Cambridge University Press https://stahlonline.cambridge.org/essential_4th_chapter.jsf (accessed 30 October 2019).

Taylor, D., Sparshatt, A., Varma, S. et al. (2014). Antidepressant efficacy of agomelatine: meta-analysis of published and unpublished studies. *British Medical Journal* **348**: g1888. https://doi.org/10.1136/bmj.g1888.

Taylor, D.M., Barnes, T.R.E., and Young, A.H. (2019). *The Maudsley Prescribing Guidelines in Psychiatry*, 13e. Hoboken: Wiley Blackwell.

UK Government (n.d.). *Drugs and driving: the law*. https://www.gov.uk/drug-driving-law (accessed on 30 September 2019).

Waddell, L. and Taylor, M. (2008). A new self-rating scale for detecting atypical or second-generation antipsychotic side effects. *Journal of Psychopharmacology* **22**: 238–243. https://doi.org/10.1177/0269881107087976.

Wilson, S., Anderson, K., Baldwin, D. et al. (2019). British Association for Psychopharmacology consensus statement on evidence-based treatment of insomnia, parasomnias and circadian rhythm disorders: An update. *Journal of Psychopharmacology* **33** (8): 923–947. https://doi.org/10.1177/0269881119855343 (accessed 27 September 2019).

World Health Organisation (WHO) (2019). *Dementia key facts*. https://www.who.int/news-room/fact-sheets/detail/dementia (accessed 01 October 2019).

Further reading

Find out more about the current advice on valproate use and the Pregnancy Prevention Programme (PPP) from the Medicines Healthcare Regulatory Authority at https://www.gov.uk/guidance/valproate-use-by-women-and-girls.

Joint National Formulary. *The BNF provides monographs for drugs with a UK marketing authorisation and clinical treatment summaries.*

Taylor, D.M., Barnes, T.R.E. and Young, A.H. (2019). *The Maudsley Prescribing Guidelines in Psychiatry*, 13e. Hoboken: Wiley Blackwell www.bnf.nice.org.uk.

Practically useful advice on the prescribing of psychotropic agents in clinical situations based on a combination of literature review, clinical experience and expert contribution.

National Institute for Health and Care Excellence. *Evidence-based recommendations developed by independent committees, including professionals and lay members and consulted on by stakeholders.* www.nice.org.uk/guidance.

Multiple choice questions

1. Which of these drugs is not an SSRI antidepressant?
    (a) Fluoxetine
    (b) Sertraline
    (c) Mirtazapine
    (d) Citalopram
    (e) Paroxetine
2. How long after the last dose should a blood sample for a lithium trough level be taken?
    (a) 2 hours
    (b) 4 hours
    (c) 8 hours
    (d) 12 hours
    (e) 18 hours
3. Which of these is not a side effect associated with clozapine?
    (a) Hypothyroidism
    (b) Sedation
    (c) Constipation
    (d) Hypersalivation
    (e) Weight gain
4. Which of these Benzodiazepines has the longest duration of action?
    (a) Lorazepam
    (b) Temazepam
    (c) Clonazepam
    (d) Lormetazepam
    (e) Diazepam

5. Which of these is not considered to be an extrapyramidal side effect?
   (a) Chilblains
   (b) Akathisia
   (c) Tardive dyskinesia
   (d) Parkinsonism
   (e) Dystonia

6. Which of these rating scales is used to assess antipsychotic related side effects?
   (a) ACE-III
   (b) PHQ-9
   (c) Cornell
   (d) GASS
   (e) HAM-D

7. What is the maximum licensed daily dose of clozapine?
   (a) 50 mg
   (b) 250 mg
   (c) 375 mg
   (d) 750 mg
   (e) 900 mg

8. Foods rich in what must be avoided whilst taking MAOIs?
   (a) Tyramine
   (b) Creatine
   (c) Tyrosine
   (d) Phenylalanine
   (e) Tryptophan

9. Which of these is not a recommended sleep hygiene action?
   (a) Changing bed linen every day
   (b) Going to bed and rising at the same time each day.
   (c) Avoid sleeping or long period of inactivity through the day.
   (d) Avoid caffeine, nicotine and alcohol for six hours before retiring to bed.
   (e) Do not remain in bed for prolonged periods whilst awake

10. Approximately what proportion of people will experience an anxiety disorder?
    (a) 4%
    (b) 10%
    (c) 25%
    (d) 41%
    (e) 68%

11. Following the initial dose of clozapine, for how many hours should hourly monitoring of pulse, blood pressure and temperature be conducted?
    (a) 1 hour
    (b) 2 hours
    (c) 4 hours
    (d) 6 hours
    (e) 12 hours

12. In 2019 which controlled drug schedule was pregabalin reclassified into?
    (a) Schedule 5
    (b) Schedule 4
    (c) Schedule 3
    (d) Schedule 2
    (e) Pregabalin is not a controlled drug

13. Which of these drug classes is known to have a clinically significant interaction with lithium?
    (a) Opioid analgesics
    (b) Oral hypoglycaemics
    (c) Oral contraceptives
    (d) Non-steroidal anti-inflammatory drugs
    (e) Macrolide antibiotics
14. Which of these drugs is licensed for the treatment of Alzheimer's dementia
    (a) Galantamine
    (b) Paliperidone
    (c) Lamotrigine
    (d) Allopurinol
    (e) Oxybutynin
15. What is the therapeutic range for lithium trough levels?
    (a) 1.0–4.0 mmol/L
    (b) 6–10 mg/L
    (c) 0.1–0.5 mg/L
    (d) 0.4–1.0 mmol/L
    (e) 10–20 mmol/L

Find out more

The following are a list of mental health conditions. Take some time and write notes about each of the conditions. Think about the medications that may be used in order to treat these conditions and be specific about the pharmacokinetics and pharmacodynamics. Remember to include aspects of patient care. If you are making notes about people you have offered care and support to, you must ensure that you have adhered to the rules of confidentiality.

The Condition	Your Notes
Depression	
Bipolar Affective Disorder	
Schizophrenia/Psychosis	
Generalised Anxiety Disorder	
Alzheimer's Disease	

Chapter 18

Immunisations

Aby Mitchell

Aim

The aim of this chapter is to provide an overview of vaccinations, the pharmacology of vaccinations and the immunisation schedule.

Learning outcomes

After reading this chapter, the reader will understand:

1. Immunity and how vaccines work
2. The national immunisation program and diseases
3. Consent, legal and ethical issues around vaccination
4. Administration and storage of vaccines

Test your knowledge

1. What are the different types of immunity?
2. How are vaccines administered?
3. What are vaccine-preventable diseases?
4. What is the biggest challenge to improving global vaccine coverage?

Fundamentals of Pharmacology: For Nursing and Healthcare Students, First Edition. Edited by Ian Peate and Barry Hill.
© 2021 John Wiley & Sons Ltd. Published 2021 by John Wiley & Sons Ltd.

Introduction

Immunisations, also referred to as vaccinations, are the single greatest health promotion and health sector intervention alongside clean water (Who.int., 2019). However, from early experimentation to the development of new vaccines, widening of global immunisation programs, to vaccine availability and current media headlines, vaccination is not without its controversy. Ethical dilemmas lie between the balance of personal autonomy and choice and the risk to the entire population.

The first record of vaccination development was in 1797 by Edward Jenner. Following the discovery that if a person suffered an attack of cowpox (a relatively harmless disease from cattle) the individual could not contract smallpox (an infectious disease caused by the variola virus with symptoms such as rash and fever that could lead to blindness, scarring and in as many as 3 out of 10 cases death), Jennifer concluded that not only did cowpox protect against smallpox but that it could be transmitted from one person to another as a mechanism of protection. In the first experiment to test this theory, Jenner took cowpox from a milkmaid's hand and inoculated a small boy (James Phipps) who had not had smallpox. Months following the inoculation, James was exposed to the variola virus but never contracted the disease. This discovery by Jenner marked a turning point in public health, the start of national immunisation programs, and the declaration by the World Health Organization (WHO) of eradication of smallpox globally in 1980 (WHO.int, 2010).

Following the success of vaccinations in the twenty-first century and vaccination campaigns, the incidences of diseases which were considered common a few generations ago, such as mumps, polio and pertussis, have been greatly reduced in numerous geographical regions (see Table 18.1 that discusses vaccine preventable diseases). When vaccine coverage is at a high enough level to induce herd immunity (indirect protection from infectious diseases created when a large proportion of the population has become immune), it is possible for infections to be eliminated from the country. However, if this coverage is not maintained, it is possible for the disease to return. Now the WHO is working on eradicating poliomyelitis, which is still a significant endemic in Nigeria, Afghanistan and Pakistan (WHO, 2019a). Despite the UK's national immunisation program, outbreaks of diseases still exist today; for example, the measles outbreak in England 2018, which was linked to a Europe-wide outbreak (GOV. UK, 2018b).

The controversy of immunisations could perhaps be a consequence of the success of immunisation programs at eradicating particular diseases (see Table 18.2 for an overview of the national immunisation programme); subsequent generations may have no concept of the dangers of these diseases both to physical health and long-term well-being of individuals, groups and communities. Unfounded scare stories continue to circulate about vaccination side effects, and the perception that vaccines are unsafe lives on. Debates are still gaining momentum on social media platforms with a barrage of testimonials from 'anti-vax' campaigners regarding the supposed dangers.

The legacy of the 'Wakefield study' (Wakefield et al., 1998) continues to have global consequences influencing the population, despite the article's retraction from the *Lancet* and Wakefield's removal from the Medical Register following evidence of misconduct and unethical behaviour. The published study claimed to have identified a link between the MMR (measles, mumps and rubella) vaccine and autism. A subsequently published investigation uncovered the study to be fraudulent and more than 13 well-designed studies have definitively disproven any association between the MMR vaccine and autism (Amin et al., 2012). Yet, the damage to public health continues to be fueled by unbalanced media reporting. In 2008, for the first time in 14 years, measles was declared an endemic in England and Wales. In 2019, the WHO declared that the UK has lost its measles free status based on several benchmarks, most significantly vaccine uptake, which is currently at its lowest rate and has reduced from 95% (the WHO recommended coverage rate) to 87% (Gov.UK, 2019a). In some areas of the country, vaccine rates were as low as 66.7% in 2017/2018 (Screening & Immunisations Team, NHS Digital, 2018). The battle continues to restore parents trust in the vaccine.

Table 18.1 Vaccine-preventable diseases.

Disease	Prevalence	Spread	Complications	Signs and Symptoms
Hepatitis B A viral infection that attacks the liver and can cause acute and chronic disease	Low in the UK with a carriage rate of 0.1–0.5% This may vary between communities	Transmitted through contact with blood or other bodily fluids The virus can survive outside the body for at least 7 days	Liver cirrhosis Liver cancer	Symptoms specific to complications
HPV Human papillomavirus	Estimated 266 000 deaths caused by the virus and 528 000 new cases in 2012 Accounts for 12% of all female cancers globally	Sexually transmitted	• Cervical cancer • Anogenital cancers • Head and neck cancers	Majority – asymptomatic Symptoms specific to complications
Influenza Also known as flu An acute viral infection that attacks the upper respiratory tract, nose, throat, bronchi and less frequently lungs	The disease occurs worldwide with the emergence of different strains In the northern hemisphere, annual epidemics occur in the autumn and winter affecting approx. 5–15% of the population	Airborne droplets Contaminated hands and surfaces	Severe cases can be fatal Individuals at risk of serious complications are: • Pregnant women • Older people • Young children • People who are immune compromised • People with long-term chronic conditions • People with no or non-functioning spleen • Secondary bacterial infections	• Pyrexia • Cough • Headache • Muscle and joint pain • Malaise • Runny nose
Measles Highly contagious viral disease	991 confirmed cases in the UK in 2018 Global Vaccine Action Plan targeted measles for elimination in 5 WHO regions by 2020 Global measles deaths have decreased by	Transmitted via droplets from the nose, mouth or throat of the infected person The virus survives on surfaces for several hours	Serious complications can be fatal • Blindness • Encephalitis (an infection that causes swelling of the brain) • Diarrhoea • Symptom related dehydration	10–12 days post-infection • Pyrexia • Cold-like symptoms • White spots inside the mouth • Rash starting on the face and spreading downwards

467

(Continued)

Table 18.1 (Continued)

Disease	Prevalence	Spread	Complications	Signs and Symptoms
			• Pneumonia • Other severe respiratory infections	
Meningitis Neisseria meningitides (meningococcus) Of the 12 N. meningitides serogroups identifies A, B, C, X, W and Y	84% in recent years. However, measles is still common in developing countries No reliable estimates of global meningococcal disease burden due to inadequate surveillance in several parts of the world	Direct human to human contact or airborne droplets or secretions	Serious complications can be fatal • Septicemia • Brain damage	Average incubation 4 days but can range from 2 to 10 • Pyrexia • Nausea • Vomiting • Confusion • Headaches • Sensitivity to light • Seizure • Drowsy or unresponsive
Pneumococcal disease Streptococcus pneumoniae bacterium Over 90 different serotypes Only a small minority cause most disease	More than 5000 cases of invasive pneumococcal disease diagnosed in England each year. Incidence rates peek in December and January Rates of death are higher in developing countries	Airborne – respiratory droplets	Most susceptible are the: • Very young • Older people • People with no or non-functioning spleen • People who are immune compromised Serious complications can be fatal • Pneumonia • Meningitis • Septicemia	Symptoms specific to complications
Rubella Also known as German measles Togavirus	3 reported incidences in the UK 2018 Targeted for elimination in 5 WHO regions by 2020	Airborne – coughs and sneezes Contact with surfaces where the droplets have settled	Mild viral disease Most susceptible children and young adults Contraction of the disease just before conception or in early pregnancy can result in miscarriage, fetal death or congenital defects (congenital rubella syndrome)	14–21 days post-infection • Maculopapular rash (a rash with bumps) • Cold-like symptoms • Abdominal pain • Joint pain • Pyrexia • Lethargy • Lymph-adenopathy (enlargement of the lymph nodes) • Loss of appetite

Tetanus A non-communicable disease contracted through exposure to the spores of the bacterium *Clostridium tetani* Exists worldwide in animal intestinal tracts and soil	7 total reported incidences in the UK 2018 Rare due to vaccine programs	Soil or manure getting into a wound Contaminated drug injections	Can be contracted by people of all ages Particularly serious in newborn babies (happens in newborns in unsanitary conditions where the umbilical cord stump becomes infected). Can be prevented by immunising women of reproductive age or during pregnancy	4–21 days post-infection: • Muscles spasms in the jaw (trismus) • Swallowing and stiffness or pain in the muscles or the neck, back or shoulders • Spread of muscles spasms to the abdomen, upper arms and thighs • Pyrexia • Tachycardia
Tuberculosis (TB) *Mycobacterium tuberculosis*	Estimated 10.4 million new cases in 2016 and 1.7 million deaths 90% of cases occur in low or middle-income countries	Airborne droplets – coughing, sneezing, spitting	Severe cases can be fatal • Meningitis • Pneumonia • Increased risk of heart attack or stroke • Vision impairment • Weakening of the bones and joints	Approximately 1/3 of the world's population carry the disease but don't have symptoms (latent infection) • Flu-like symptoms • Chest pain • Persistent cough • Poor appetite • Sore throat • Night sweats • Weight loss

469

Source: Modified from WHO (2019b).

Table 18.2 National immunisation programs.

Age due	Diseases protected against	Vaccine	Administration site
8 weeks old	Diphtheria, tetanus, pertussis, polio, Hib, hepatitis b	DTap/IPV/Hib/HepB	Thigh
	Pneumococcal (13 serotypes)	Pneumococcal conjugate vaccine (PCV)	Thigh
	Meningococcal group B (MenB)	Men B	Left thigh
	Rotavirus	Rotavirus	By mouth
Twelve weeks old	Diphtheria, tetanus, pertussis, polio, Hib and hepatitis B	DTap/IPV/Hib/HepB	Thigh
	Rotavirus	Rotavirus	By mouth
Sixteen weeks old	Diphtheria, tetanus, pertussis, polio, Hib and hepatitis B	DTap/IPV/Hib/HepB	Thigh
	Pneumococcal (13 serotypes)	Pneumococcal conjugate vaccine (PCV)	Thigh
One year old (one or after the child's first birthday)	MenB	MenB	Left thigh
	Hib and MenC	Hib/MenC	Upper arm/thigh
	Pneumococcal	PCV	Upper arm/thigh
	Measles, mumps and rubella (German measles)	MMR	Upper arm/thigh
	MenB	MenB booster	Left thigh
Eligible paediatric age groups	Influenza (each year from September)	Live attenuated influenza vaccine	Both nostrils
	Diphtheria, tetanus, pertussis and polio	DTap/IPV	Upper arm
	Measles, mumps and rubella	MMR (check the first dose given)	Upper arm

Three years four months old or soon after	Diphtheria, tetanus, pertussis and polio	DTap/IPV	Upper arm
Boys and girls aged 12 to 13 years	Cancers caused by human papillomavirus (HPV) types 16 and 18 (and genital warts caused by types 6 and 11)	HPV (two doses 6–24 months apart)	Upper arm
	Measles, mumps and rubella	MMR (check the first dose given)	Upper arm
Fourteen years old (school year 9)	Tetanus, diphtheria and polio	Td/IPV (check MMR status)	Upper arm
	Meningococcal groups A, C, W and Y disease	MenACWY	Upper arm
65 years old	Pneumococcal (23 serotypes)	Pneumococcal Polysaccharide Vaccine (PPV)	Upper arm
65 years of age and older	Influenza (each year from September)	Inactivated influenza vaccine	Upper arm
70 years old	Shingles	Shingles	Upper arm

Source: GOV.UK (2019b).

While the media shares some responsibility, often so too must the language used in the health sector. Vaccine controversy extends beyond the MMR vaccine, and the 1970s and 1980s saw a major scare around the pertussis vaccine and neurological complications. Anti-vaccine movements focused on side effects of the HPV vaccine and recent tabloid reports have linked autism and fears over a link to multiple sclerosis. Current uptake of the flu vaccine across the UK falls short of the 75% and above WHO target, and the UK has the lowest uptake of flu vaccine in at-risk groups (Royal Society for Public Health, 2019). Survey results suggest that the main reason for poor flu vaccine uptake were: concerns about side effects, effectiveness of vaccine and perceived risk of getting the flu (RSPH, 2018). Other issues around vaccine uptake, particularly in working-age adults, centre around timing of appointments, availability and location of appointments, and forgetting appointments (RSPH, 2018).

Ethics

Mandatory vaccination was tried in the UK in the late 1800s with smallpox but was abandoned following hostility and considerable resistance from certain community groups. To this day there has been no reintroduction of compulsory childhood vaccines in the UK. Other parts of the globe have tried different approaches to mandatory vaccination. Since 2017, the Italian government has changed its law on compulsory vaccination following measles outbreaks and a drop in the vaccine uptake to below 80%. Other countries, such as Australia, have incentivised vaccination by linking it to social-welfare payments and in some US states mandatory vaccination is a requirement for school and daycare entry. The question remains: should vaccination be mandatory and what are the implications for this?

Over the last two decades, much consideration has been given to defining ethical principles relevant to public health. There is some suggestion that the most relevant principles (labelled moral considerations) are:

- producing benefits;
- avoiding, preventing and removing harm;
- producing the maximum balance of benefits over harm and cost;
- fair distribution of benefits and burdens and ensuring public participation;
- respect of autonomous choices and actions;
- protection of privacy and confidentiality;
- keeping promises and commitments;
- transparency, disclosing information, honesty;
- building and maintaining trust.

(Source: Childress et al., 2002; Amin et al., 2012).

Amin et al. (2012) consider a change in practical approaches to improve vaccine uptake is required. To contribute to a 'vaccine friendly environment', healthcare professionals should focus on: addressing patent/guardian vaccine safety concerns; enhancing population awareness of vaccine-preventable disease risks; and promoting a better public understanding of herd immunity. With increasing concerns around antibiotic resistance, health promotion and patient education to improve vaccine uptake and prevent the spread of infectious diseases would reduce the number of people acquiring harmful infections and limit the spread of antibiotic resistance.

It is acknowledged that vaccination programs have a positive economic impact (RSPH, 2018). Vaccination can lead to long-term societal savings across the health sector and workforces, including reduction in economic inequality, improved school attendance and fertility decline (RSPH, 2018).

Immunity

Immunity is the body's ability to protect itself from infectious disease. There are three main types of immunity:

1. Innate or non-specific immunity.
2. Acquired immunity.
3. Active and passive immunity.

Innate or non-specific immunity is present from birth. It is the body's natural resistance to pathogens and antigens; for example, intact skin, salivary enzymes and neutrophils which provide an initial response to infection. Acquired immunity is gained by the body over time; for example, the antibodies developed after an infection passed through the placenta at birth or by vaccination. Active and passive immunity are the two basic mechanisms for acquiring immunity. See Figure 18.1 for the types of immunity.

Active immunity is protection produced by an individual's immune system when exposed to an antigen; it is usually long-lasting and can be acquired by natural disease or vaccination. For example, recovery from Hepatitis-A virus gives a natural active immune response which usually provides life-long protection. Therefore, the purpose of a vaccination is to provide immunity similar to that elicited from natural infection. Passive immunity is the transfer of antibodies from immune individuals, commonly across the placenta or less often from the transfusion of blood or blood products including immunoglobulin. The protection which occurs in the uterus by cross-placental transfer of antibodies from mother to child is more effective against certain infections (e.g. tetanus and measles) than for others (e.g. polio and whooping cough). This protection is temporary and only lasts for a few weeks or months until the antibody is degraded and lost.

473

The primary aim of vaccination is to promote immunity in the vaccinated individual. This reduces the risk of unvaccinated members of the population or those who cannot be vaccinated being exposed to infection. This is known as population (or 'herd') immunity. The level of vaccination needed to achieve herd immunity varies by disease.

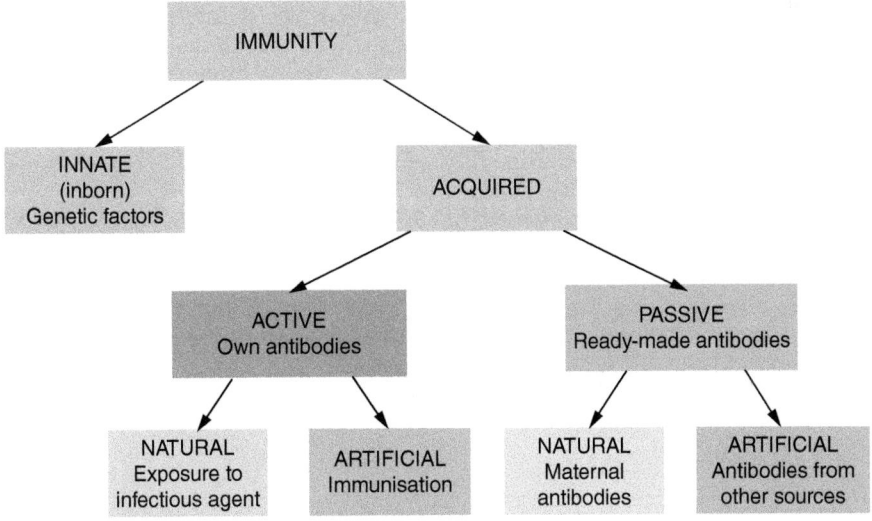

Figure 18.1 Types of immunity.

How vaccines work

Vaccines induce active immunity and provide immunological memory which enables the immune system to recognise and rapidly respond when exposed to the natural infection in the future. Vaccines are made from inactivated (killed) or live-attenuated organisms, secreted products, recombinant components or the constituents of cell walls. There is no evidence to suggest that vaccines increase susceptibility to serious infections and infection rates are generally lower in a vaccinated child (GOV.UK, 2018a).

Inactivated vaccines that are administered to an individual who has not had prior exposure to the disease elicit a primary antibody response (two or more injections may be required in infants to elicit such a response). This is called the primary course. Depending on the time and potency of the vaccination, further injections lead to an accelerated response, which is known as a secondary response. Even if the levels of detectable antibodies fall, the immune system has been primed and an individual may be still be protected. Further reinforcement of the vaccine, for example, the flu vaccine, are used to boost immunity and provide a longer-term protection. A common myth with these vaccines is that they cause the disease/virus they are trying to prevent. This is unfounded as the component of the disease/virus in these vaccines is killed and therefore cannot create the disease pathogens.

Live vaccines, for example, the MMR, usually elicit a full, long-lasting antibody response after one or two doses. To promote an immune response, the live organism needs to replicate (grow) in the vaccinated host over a period of days or weeks. The live vaccine promotes the same response in the body as it does to a natural infection. It does this without causing the actual disease. However, some responses may cause a mild form of the disease, for example, a localised rash, although this is very rare. See Table 18.3 for the pharmacodynamics and pharmacokinetics of vaccines.

Despite a plethora of evidence identifying the impact of the vaccination program in the UK, no vaccine offers 100% protection and a small proportion of the population get infected despite vaccination (Who.int., 2019). Vaccine failure can occur in two main ways. Primary failure occurs when an individual fails to make an initial immunological response to the vaccine. This leaves the individual susceptible to infection, for example, the 5–10% of children (GOV.UK, 2018a) who do not respond to the measles component of the first MMR dose. However, the risk of measles is reduced by offering an additional dose before the child starts school. Secondary failure is when an individual responds well initially to the vaccine but protection wanes over time. Consequently, the incidence rate of failure increases over time. Those individuals who do acquire the infection despite vaccination may have a milder form of the disease and are less likely to experience serious complications, such as hospitalisation or death, compared to those who have not been vaccinated at all. The pertussis vaccine, for example, provides high protection against whooping cough after three doses but declines as the child gets older. A fourth booster is given to improve protection during school years.

The complete routine immunisation schedule is regularly updated and must be checked online line before giving immunisations. Public Health England (PHE) (2016) provides an algorithm for individuals with incomplete or uncertain vaccine history. This helps healthcare professionals to bring individuals living in the UK in line with the national schedule. Leaflets about childhood vaccines in different languages can be accessed online (NHS Scotland, 2013).

The Green Book

For the latest up-to-date information on vaccines and vaccination procedures for vaccine preventable infectious diseases in the UK, nurses should consult the online Green Book https://www.gov.uk/government/collections/immunisation-against-infectious-disease-the-green-book. Chapters are regularly reviewed and updated as guidance changes. As a result, nurses are advised not to print copies of the Green Book.

Clinical considerations

Consent

Consent to vaccination must be given freely following relevant, properly explained information about the vaccination with an opportunity for the individual to ask questions. Nurses and other healthcare professionals should explain the benefits and risks of immunisation and how data on immunisation is stored in line with data protection and Caldicott guidance (principles to protect patient information). The information provided should be easy to understand by the individual in a written or verbal format. Consent is only valid if the individual providing consent is offered as much information as reasonably possible to make a decision. Case law on this area is currently evolving and more information can be found in a Department of Health publication 'Reference guide to consent for examination or treatment, Second edition' (Department of Health, 2009). Giving an immunisation without consent could lead to legal action against the nurse by the Nursing and Midwifery Council (NMC). Accountability always lies with the nurse who is accountable for any actions and omissions, regardless of advice or directions from another healthcare professional (NMC, 2018).

Storage

The correct storage of vaccinations is important to ensure safe, effective vaccination. Vaccine effectiveness may be compromised if vaccines become too hot or too cold at any time. Vaccines deteriorate over time and any changes to the recommended temperature – including during transportation – may speed up irreversible loss of potency. This can result in a failed immune response and poor protection. Additionally, inappropriate or inadequate storage can result in wastage and unnecessary costs to the healthcare economy. Vaccination storage should ensure that:

475

- only vaccines or other drugs are stored in the refrigerator;
- different shelves are designated for different vaccines to reduce error (a list on the outside of the door to highlight this is useful);
- the temperature of the fridge is recorded daily;
- stock is rotated (oldest at the front);
- vaccines are stored in the original packaging (many vaccines are sensitive to the light and efficacy can deteriorate if left out of the box for any length of time);
- correct stocks are ordered (avoid over-ordering).

Clinical considerations

Vaccines should be stored:

- in original packages retaining batch numbers and expiry dates according to manufacturer's guidelines;
- usually at 2 °C to 8 °C;
- in a place that protects from light.

The cold chain

The 'cold chain' is the term used to describe maintaining cold conditions for vaccines throughout storage and transportation according to the manufacturer's recommended temperature range until administration. See Figure 18.2 for an example of a cold chain system.

Table 18.3   Pharmacodynamics and pharmacokinetics of vaccines.

	Vaccine type	How vaccines are absorbed	How the body responds to the vaccine	Precautions/side effects
Influenza vaccine	The injectable vaccine contains an inactivated (killed component of the virus). The live attenuated nasal vaccine LAIV contains a 'live' (a weakened component of the virus that has been altered to make it non-infectious) virus. Live attenuated vaccines create a longer-lasting immunity but are not suitable for all members of the population.	Intramuscular injections are given straight into the muscle at a 90-degree angle. The fluid from the injection remains in the muscle tissue and is slowly absorbed into the muscle capillaries.	Up to 2 weeks following vaccination the body develops antibodies. These are known as B-cells and T-cells. These cells fight the infection and remember what the vaccine looks like. Immunological memory enables the immune system to recognise and respond to natural infection. When an individual comes into contact with the virus again the B-cells and T-cells trigger an immune response.	Vaccines should not be given if individuals who have a known life-threatening allergic reaction to vaccines or any ingredient in the vaccine. LAIV should not be given to children or adolescents who are clinically severely immunocompromised due to conditions or immunosuppressive therapy such as acute and chronic leukaemias; lymphoma; HIV infection not on highly active antiretroviral therapy (HAART); cellular immune deficiencies; and high dose corticosteroids Side effects: Pain, swelling or redness at the injection site, low-grade fever, malaise, shivering, fatigue, headache, myalgia and arthralgia. A small painless nodule (induration) at the injection site.
Pneumovax	Pneumococcal polysaccharide vaccine PSV23 (protects against 23 types of pneumococcal bacteria) and Pneumococcal conjugate vaccine PCV13 or Prevnar 13 (protects against 13 kinds of pneumococcal bacteria that cause serious infections like pneumonia). The polysaccharide is a type of vaccine that is created to look like the surface of certain bacteria to help the body build protection against that germ. The conjugate is a type of vaccine that joins a protein to part of the bacteria which improves vaccine protection and elicits a greater immune response.	This vaccine can be given IM or subcutaneously. IM vaccines are known to produce less localised reactions. In a subcutaneous vaccine, the fluid is absorbed slowly into the body through the layer of fat under the skin.	See above for response to the vaccine	Nasal congestion/rhinorrhea, reduced appetite, weakness and headache are common adverse reaction following administration of LAIV. Confirmed life-threating allergic reaction as above. Precautions: If an individual is acutely unwell. Side effects: Children 6 weeks to 5 years of age – fever, irritability, decreased appetite and increased and/or decreased sleep. Adults – Mild soreness and induration at the site of injection lasting one to three days and, less commonly, a low-grade fever may occur.

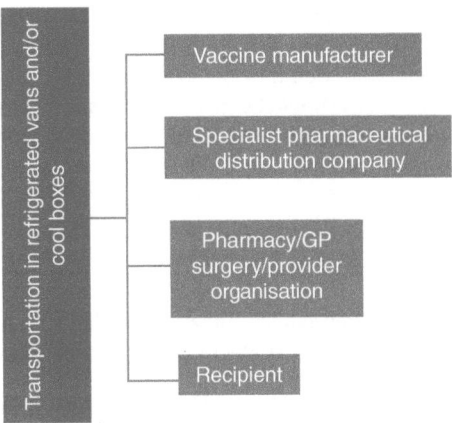

Figure 18.2   A typical cold chain system. Source: Modified from the Department of Health (2013).

Clinical considerations

For guidance around disruptions to the cold chain, see 'Refrigerator failure or disruption of the cold chain' Green Book. Guidance on incorrect storage of vaccines, breaches, incorrect diluent used, etc., can be found at: www.hpa.org.uk/webc/HPAwebfile/HPAweb_C/1267551139589.

Any out-of-date stock should be removed from the refrigerator and disposed of according to local policies. Vaccines should never be used past their expiry date. If an expired vaccine has been administered, this must be reported using the local untoward incident reporting procedure. Additional advice should be sought. It is often necessary to re-administer the vaccine dose.

If the vial or syringe containing the vaccine is damaged or not intact, the vaccine should not be used. These should be labelled as damaged and either disposed of according to local policy or reported as a defect.

Contraindications

Although almost all individuals can be vaccinated safely, there are a few exceptions where vaccination is contraindicated or should be deferred. GOV.UK (2018a) suggest that consideration on whether to avoid specific vaccinations should be taken when:

- The individual has a confirmed history of an anaphylactic reaction to either a component of the vaccine or to a previous vaccination.
- The individual has a primary or acquired immunodeficiency, is on current or recent immunosuppressive or immunosuppressive biological therapy.
- An infant is born to a mother who received immunosuppressive biological therapy during pregnancy.
- The women is pregnant.

Confirmed anaphylactic reaction to a previous vaccination is extremely rare (Gov. UK, 2013a). Individuals who do have a confirmed anaphylactic reaction to a vaccination or a component of the vaccination should be given an alternative vaccine. Individuals who have confirmed anaphylaxis to eggs should be given vaccines that are egg-free or have a very low ovalbumin content; for example, Flucelax or Fluad (Gov.UK, 2013a). Recent data suggests that there is no association between the MMR vaccine and hypersensitivity to egg antigens. For further information, the Green Book, Chapter 6, lists some of the most common allergens and vaccines.

Anaphylaxis

Anaphylaxis is a severe, generalised, life-threatening allergic reaction (National Institute for Clinical Excellence [NICE], 2011). It is characterised by several signs and rapidly deteriorating symptoms:

- swallowing and breathing difficulties;
- swollen mouth, throat or tongue;
- rapid breathing rate (tachypnea);
- rapid heart rate (tachycardia);
- urticaria (rash and itching);
- drop in blood pressure (hypotension).

Treatment of an anaphylactic reaction should be based on life support principles:

- Use the Airway, Breathing, Circulation, Disability, Exposure (ABCDE) to recognise and treat problems.
- Call early for help.
- Treat the greatest threat to life first.

Source: Resuscitation Council (2016).

Patient group direction/patient specific direction

Nurses administering vaccinations must be aware of their legal position if the vaccine has not been individually prescribed by a doctor. The Medicines Act 1968 does not permit nurses or healthcare practitioners who are not qualified prescribers to administer prescription-only medicines (POMS) unless one of these three types of instruction are in place.

- signed prescription;
- signed Patient Specific Direction (PSD);
- Patient Group Direction (PGD).

A PSD is a written instruction from a doctor or independent prescriber for a medicine to be supplied or administered to a named patient. See Figure 18.3 for an example of a PSD.

To be completed by Practice Nurse/Healthcare professional upon administration of the vaccine

Name of Vaccine administered	Zostavax
Batch Number	12345678
Expiry Date	09/9/2020
Strength of Vaccination	19 4000 PFU
Dose	0.65 mL
Site of injection/method of administration	IM right deltoid
Date vaccine administered	12/11/2019
Notes	Immunisation explained to the patient Informed consent obtained

Signed   A Nurse_____

Print Name   Anne Nurse_____

Qualifications_____ RN _____

Date_____12/11/2019_____

   PGDs are written agreements for the supply and administration of medicines to a group of patients who have not been individually identified before presentation for treatment. PGDs allow a range of healthcare professionals to supply or administer a medicine directly to a patient with an identified clinical condition without them seeing a prescriber. It is the responsibility of the healthcare professional working with the PGD to assess that the patient fits the criteria set out in the PGD. The PGD should include certain particulars:

- The period the direction has effect.
- The description or class of POM.
- Any restrictions on the quantity of medicine.
- The clinical situations which the POMS of that description may treat.
- The clinical criteria under which a person is eligible for the treatment.
- Whether any class of person is excluded.
- Whether there are any circumstances in which further advice should be sought.
- The applicable dosage and maximum dosage.
- The route of administration.
- Frequency of administration.
- Any relevant warnings to note.
- Whether there is any follow-up action to be taken in any circumstances.
- Details of records to be kept of the supply, or the administration, of medicines under the direction.

Source: Gov.UK (2018a).

   For further information, the National Prescribing Centre has produced a practical guide and competency framework for the use of PGDs available at https://www.guidelinesinpractice.co.uk/searchresults?qkeyword=pGD.

Example of a PSD

Patient Specific Direction (PSD)

Name of Patient   _Brenda Brown _____

DOB   ____01/01/1948_____

Address   __1 Rainbow Cottage _____

                    ___Windsor_____ _____

                    ___SL4 9GN

_____

I authorise for the above-named patient to receive the following vaccination:

Name of Vaccination:	Zostavax
Strength of Vaccination	19,400 PFU
Dose	0.65 mL
Frequency	Once
Site of injection/method of administration	IM or SC deltoid region of the upper arm

and that this can be administrated by the Practice Nurse/Health Care Professional who is suitably qualified to do so and is employed by this practice

Signed A Doctor_____

Print Name   Alan Doctor_____

Position/role   General Practitioner_____

Date _____   11/11/2019 _____

Expiry date of this PSD _____11/12/2019 _____

Figure 18.3   An example of a patient specific direction.

Skills in practice

Immunisation procedures

Those nurses administering vaccinations are professionally accountable for their actions and omissions (NMC, 2018). All healthcare professionals advising on immunisation or administering vaccines must be deemed competent with regards to preparation and storage, cold chain, administration before, during, and after, and recognition and treatment of anaphylaxis.

Nurses administering vaccines must be trained in the management of anaphylaxis and must have immediate access to epinephrine (adrenaline).

How to administer an immunisation

- Prior to administration ensure that:
- consent is obtained;
- there are no contraindications to the vaccine being given;
- the individual or carer has been fully informed about the vaccine and understands the procedure;
- the individual/carer is aware of any possible adverse reactions and how to treat these.

Most vaccines are given by intramuscular (IM) injection. Injections given IM, rather than deep subcutaneously (SC), are found to be less likely to cause local reactions (Diggle et al., 2006). The Bacillus Calmetter-Guerin (BCG) vaccine is given by intradermal injection and varicella vaccines are given SC. No vaccines are given intravenously. Before administration, locate a site on the patient which avoids all major nerves and blood vessels.

The preferred sites for IM and SC immunisations are the anterolateral aspect of the thigh and deltoid area of the upper arm (see Figures 18.4 and 18.5).

If two or more injections need to be given at the same time, these should be administered in a different limb. However, if it is only possible to use one limb (for example, in cases of lymphedema) the vaccines can be administered in the same limb 2.5 cm apart. All sites of administration should be documented. Nurses should avoid giving immunisations into the buttock, due to the risk of sciatic nerve damage (Piggot, 1988; Villarejo and Pascaul, 1993).

The following good practice should be followed:
- ensure that the expiry date has not passed;
- store vaccines under appropriate cold chain conditions;
- wash hands;
- wear protective clothing and follow universal precautions if infection risk;
- use a sterile syringe and needle when withdrawing from a vial;
- prepare vaccines only when you are ready to administer them;

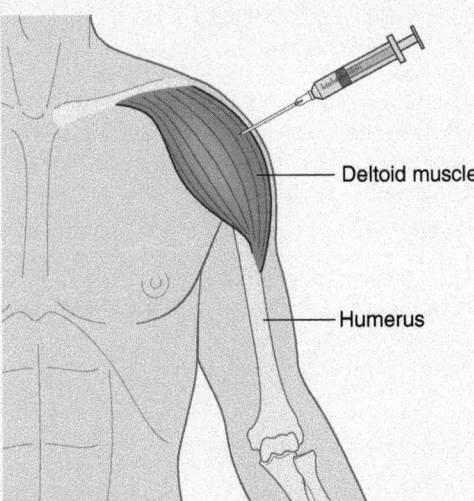

Deltoid muscle

Humerus

Figure 18.4   Location of the deltoid muscle. Source: From Peate and Wild 2nd Ed Nursing Practice Knowledge and Care Fig 19.12 page 391.

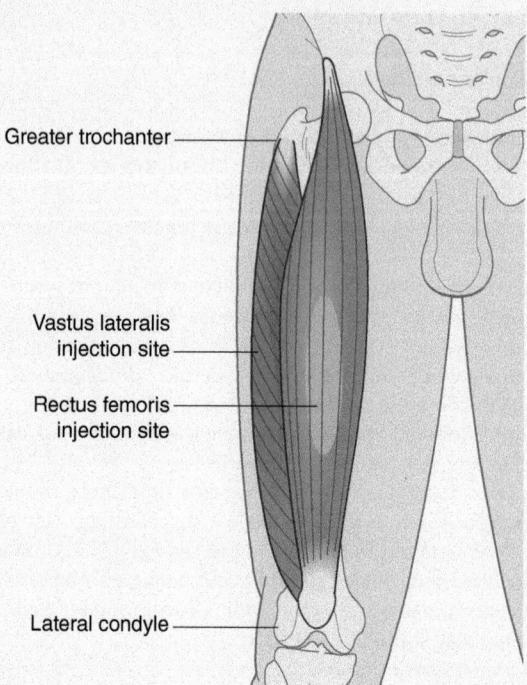

Greater trochanter

Vastus lateralis
injection site

Rectus femoris
injection site

Lateral condyle

Figure 18.5   Location of the rectus femoris and vastus lateralis muscles of the thigh. Source: From Peate and Wild 2nd Ed Nursing Practice Knowledge and Care Fig 19.13 page 391.

- the needle should not be left in the vial for multiple withdrawals;
- the vial is marked with:
  o date and time of reconstruction or first use;
  o initials of the person who reconstituted or first used the vial;
  o the period of time the vaccine can be used for;
- ensure patient dignity at all times;
- wash hands again before administration.

IM injection should be given with the needle at a 90° angle to stretched not bunched skin (Gov.UK, 2013b). The skin does not need to be disinfected before administration. Only if the skin is visibly ocedure must be adhered to. The following information should be recorded accurately:

Recipients of any vaccine should be observed for immediate side effects. Equipment used for vaccination, including vials and ampules, must be disposed of in a puncture-resistant 'sharps box' and local policy and procedure must be adhered to. The following information should be recorded accurately

- vaccine name, product, batch number, expiry date;
- dose administered;
- site;
- date given;
- name and signature of vaccinator.

Episode of care

Mrs. Oban arrives at the immunisation clinic to see the practice nurse Grace Brown. Mrs. Oban is 42 years old. She has had asthma since childhood, which is uncontrolled (she does not like taking her inhalers) and has a previous history of breast cancer resulting in a left-sided mastectomy. Mrs. Oban has been advised to attend the clinic for her annual flu vaccination. She fits the criteria with her chronic respiratory disease and immunosuppression following chemotherapy for her breast cancer.

Mrs. Oban has not had a flu vaccine for the last two years and explains that last time she had the vaccination it gave her the flu. Grace is aware that this is a common misconception, and explains that in some cases the vaccine can cause flu-like symptoms such as fever, headaches and muscle pains for a few days but it is not possible to get the flu. Grace is confident with her knowledge of the flu vaccine and explains that the influenza vaccine is an inactivated vaccine which means there are no active viruses in the vaccine. Grace advises Mrs. Oban that patients with sub-optimal immune function as a result of disease or treatment are recognised to be at increased risk of flu-related complications, such as pneumonia, and other serious complications. Mrs. Oban is in the high-risk category and although she may not make a full antibody response to the vaccine, it is highly recommended. Grace also recommends that anyone living in the same household where close contact is unavoidable should also be given the vaccine. This will provide further protection for Mrs. Oban against the flu. For further information, Grace suggests that Mrs. Oban looks at the NHS UK website with her family
https://www.nhs.uk/conditions/vaccinations/who-should-have-flu-vaccine/.

Mrs. Oban states that she read somewhere on the internet that a side effect to immunisation is Guillain-Barré syndrome (GBS). Guillan-Barré syndrome is an acute disorder where the body attacks the peripheral nervous system causing weakness and paralysis of the limbs. Grace is aware of GBS and knows that it is a rare vaccine side effect. She refers to the information given in Chapter 19 of the Green Book. Grace explains to Mrs. Oban that the risk of GBS following this vaccination is extremely low and incidence is reported to be less than two cases in one million vaccinated people (NHS Online, 2020). Grace is aware that Mrs. Oban is extremely anxious regarding the vaccination and advises her that the vaccine may give a localised reaction of pain, tenderness, swelling and redness or a small nodule at the injection site but these symptoms will disappear in a few days.

After a long discussion, Mrs. Oban consents to the vaccine. Grace checks if she has had her pneumococcal vaccine as there is no record of this at the surgery. Mrs. Oban confirms that she has not had the vaccine. She would be happy to have the vaccine today with the flu vaccine but explains that she has mild lymphedema in her left arm following her mastectomy. Grace is happy that there are no contraindications to Mrs. Oban having this vaccine. She knows that she can give both vaccines in the right arm 2.5 cm apart. Grace is aware that she can give both these vaccines under the practice PGD. If Mrs. Oban did not meet the criteria for both of these, for example, an egg allergy, Grace would need to give the vaccines under a PSD.

When Grace goes to the fridge to collect the vaccine she checks the temperature of the fridge and the last time that this was recorded. She takes the vaccine from the front of the fridge as she knows that new stock is added to the back. Grace checks the batch number and expiry date of each vaccine before administration and administers the influenza vaccine IM and the pneumo-coccal vaccine subcutaneously into Mrs. Oban's upper right arm.

Grace observes Mrs. Oban for 15 minutes following the vaccinations and has the adrenaline box close by in case of an anaphylactic reaction. Grace has recently had a basic life support update and knows that she will need to contact the emergency services in the event of an ana-phylaxis. She has ensured that there is plenty of space in the clinic room if she should need to lie Mrs. Oban flat and has already checked that she is not pregnant. If Mrs. Oban was pregnant, Grace would lie her on her life side when placing Mrs. Oban in the recovery position to prevent the baby from compressing one of the main blood vessels in the abdomen (Resus Council, 2016).

Grace knows that to confirm an anaphylaxis following a vaccination she must look for three rapidly deteriorating symptoms. Grace is aware that in the event of anaphylaxis Mrs. Oban should receive 0.5 mL of adrenaline deep IM, in the middle of the outer thigh (through clothing if necessary), with a second dose five minutes later if the symptoms persist (Resus Council, 2016). Following recovery from anaphylaxis, Grace knows that Mrs. Oban must be referred to the allergy clinic for testing.

Grace records the name of the vaccine, batch number, expiry date, site of both injections, dose, date and all information given about the vaccine in Mrs. Oban's notes. Mrs. Oban appears to be fine following the vaccination and is looking forward to going home for a cup of tea. Grace reminds her about the potential of a localised reaction to the vaccines and advises Mrs. Oban to make an appointment with the practice nurse for an asthma review.

Episode of care

Madelaine is 14 years old, she attends the HPV vaccine clinic at school for her first HPV vaccine. Dorothy Green is the school nurse administering the vaccines and askes Madelaine for her signed parental consent form. Madelaine explains that her parents have not signed the form because they are anti vaccines. They believe that the body creates its own defences for infectious diseases. Dorothy knows that there are common myths around vaccinations and asks Madelaine about her perception of vaccines. Madelaine informs Dorothy that she has read the leaflet provided by the school and information about the vaccine on the internet and would still like to have it despite the lack of parental consent.

Dorothy knows that children under the age of 16 are able to consent to medical treatment without parental permission or knowledge under the UK common law known as Gillick competence. Dorothy checks the guidance in the Green Book, Chapter 2 (GOV.UK, 2017) regarding Gillick competence. She asks Madelaine questions about the proposed procedure to ensure that Madelaine has a full understanding. Dorothy is happy that Madelaine is fully aware of the reason for the vaccine, understands about the Human Papilloma Virus, the number of doses, route of vaccination and any possible side effects. During this discussion, Madelaine mentions that she has read somewhere on social media that a girl died following a HPV vaccine. Dorothy explains to Madeline that full regulated research has been carried out on the HPV vaccine and there were found to be no evidence of side effects or risks associated with the vaccine (Arbyn et al., 2018). Dorothy confirms with Madelaine that there are two doses of the vaccine which are usually given 6 to 24 months apart. Dorothy knows that if Madelaine does not have the vaccine until after her 15th birthday she will require three doses of the vaccine.

Following the initial consultation, Dorothy acknowledges that although ideally parents should be involved in the decision-making process, she is confident that Madelaine can consent to treatment. Dorothy is aware that there is no requirement for this consent to be in writing but completes full documentation of her conversation with Madelaine for her records. During the consultation, Dorothy asks Madelaine of her current vaccination status. Madelaine is unsure if she has ever had any vaccines and her parents have always referred to them as unnecessary. Dorothy refers to the government's uncertain or incomplete vaccine status documents: https://www.gov.uk/government/publications/vaccination-of-individuals-with-uncertain-or-incomplete-immunisation-status.

According to the schedule, Madelaine could have her Tetanus, diptheria and polio (Td/IPV), meningitis ACWY (MenACWY) and MMR vaccines at the same time as the HPV vaccine. These vaccines would need to be given preferably in a different limb or at least 2.5 cm apart in the same limb. Dorothy decides that is this a sensitive issue that may require more discussion and time for Madelaine to think. She gives Madelaine some information leaflets and online links about these vaccines and asks her to read the literature before her second dose of the HPV vaccine. Dorothy encourages Madelaine to speak with her parents about this and see if they can reach a decision together.

Dorothy decides that it is best to just give the HPV vaccine today. Dorothy administers that HPV vaccine intramuscularly in Madelaine's left upper arm to reduce the risk of localised reaction. She records the name of the vaccine, batch number, expiry date, site of the injection, dose, date and all information given about the vaccine the HPV vaccine and other vaccines in Madelaine's notes. Dorothy reminds Madelaine that she will need a further dose of the vaccine and to read all the information leaflets on other vaccinations she has provided.

Conclusion

This chapter has discussed immunity, how vaccines work, diseases and vaccination schedules. The controversy surrounding vaccination and consideration to ethical principles have been described. The chapter has outlined immunisation procedures and the nurse's role in vaccination. Nurses administering vaccinations need to ensure that they keep up to date on, and know where to find information on, national and local policies. It is the nurse's responsibility to ensure patients are provided with the right information to assist with decision-making and to discuss vaccination status with those in specific target groups or with an uncertain or incomplete vaccination status.

References

Amin, A., Parra, M., Kim-Farley, R., and Fielding, J. (2012). Ethical issues concerning vaccination requirements. *Public Health Reviews* 34 (1): 1–20.

Arbyn, M., Simoens, C., Xu, L., and Martin-Hirsch, P. (2018). Prophylactic vaccination against human papillomaviruses to prevent cervical cancer and its precursors. *Cochrane Database of Systematic Reviews* (5).

Childress, J.F., Faden, R.R., Garre, R.D. et al. (2002). Public health ethics: mapping the terrain. *The Journal of Law, Medicine & Ethics* 30: 170–178.

Department of Health (2013). Immunisation against infectious disease (Green book. London: Department of Health (https://www.gov.uk/government/collections/immunisation-against-infectious-disease-the-green-book).

Department of Health (2009). *Reference guide to consent for examination or treatment*, 2e. London: Department of Health https://assets.publishing.service.gov.uk/government/uploads/system/uploads/attachment_data/file/138296/dh_103653__1_.pdf (accessed 4 August 2020).

Diggle, L., Deeks, J.J., and Pollard, A.J. (2006). Effect of needle size on immunogenicity and reactogenicity of vaccines in infants: randomised controlled trial. *BMJ* 333: 571–574.

GOV.UK (2013a). Contraindications and special considerations: the green book, chapter 6. https://www.gov.uk/government/publications/contraindications-and-special-considerations-the-green-book-chapter-6 (accessed 1 September 2019).

GOV.UK (2013b). Immunisation by nurses and other health professionals: the green book, chapter 5. https://www.gov.uk/government/publications/immunisation-by-nurses-and-other-health-professionals-the-green-book-chapter-5 (accessed 27 August 2019).

GOV.UK (2017). Consent: the green book, chapter 2. https://www.gov.uk/government/publications/consent-the-green-book-chapter-2 (accessed 5 September 2019).

GOV.UK (2018a). Immunity and how vaccines work: the green book chapter 1. https://www.gov.uk/government/publications/immunity-and-how-vaccines-work-the-green-book-chapter-1 (accessed 21 August 2019).

GOV.UK (2018b). Measles outbreaks across England. https://www.gov.uk/government/news/measles-outbreaks-across-england (accessed 2 October 2019).

GOV.UK (2019a). Measles in England - Public health matters. https://publichealthmatters.blog.gov.uk/2019/08/19/measles-in-england (accessed 1 September 2019).

GOV.UK (2019b). Complete routine immunisation schedule. https://www.gov.uk/government/publications/the-complete-routine-immunisation-schedule (accessed 5 September 2019).

NHS Online (2020). Guillain-Barré syndrome. https://www.nhs.uk/conditions/guillain-barre-syndrome/causes/ (accessed 15 September 2020).

NHS Scotland (2013). A guide to childhood immunisations up to 5 years of age. http://library.nhsggc.org.uk/media/224977/6016-GuideToChildhoodImmunisationsToFiveYearsOfAge.pdf (accessed 5 September 2019).

NICE (2011). Anaphylaxis: Assessment to confirm an anaphylactic episode and the decision to refer after emergency treatment for a suspected anaphylactic episode. www.nice.org.uk/guidance/CG134 (accessed 18 August 2019).

Nursing and Midwifery Council (NMC) (2018). The Code: Professional standards of practice and behaviour for nurse, midwives and nursing associates. www.nmc.org.uk/standards/code/read-the-code-online (accessed 5 September 2019).

Piggot, J. (1988). Needling doubts about where to vaccinate. *British Medical Journal* 297 (6656): 1130.

Plotkin, S.A. and Orenstein, W.A. (eds.) (2008). *Vaccines*, 5e. Philadelphia: WB Saunders Company.

Public Health England (PHE) (2016). Vaccination of individuals with uncertain or incomplete immunisation status algorithm. https://assets.publishing.service.gov.uk/government/uploads/system/uploads/attachment_data/file/852475/Algorithm_immunisation_status_Jan2020.pdf (accessed 4 August 2020).

Resuscitation Council (2016). Emergency treatment of anaphylactic reactions. https://www.resus.org.uk/sites/default/files/2020-06/EmergencyTreatmentOfAnaphylacticReactions%20%281%29.pdf (accessed 26 August 2019).

Royal Society for Public Health (2019). Moving the needle. Promoting vaccination uptake across the life course. https://www.rsph.org.uk/our-work/policy/vaccinations/moving-the-needle-promoting-vaccination-uptake-across-the-life-course.html (accessed 25 September 2019).

Screening & Immunisations Team, NHS Digital (2018). Childhood vaccination coverage statistics England, 2017–18. https://files.digital.nhs.uk/55/D9C4C2/child-vacc-stat-eng-2017-18-report.pdf (accessed August 2020).

Villarejo, F.J. and Pascaul, A.M. (1993). Injection injury of the sciatic nerve (370 cases). *Child's Nervous System* 9: 229–232.

Wakefield, A., Murch, S., Anthony, A. et al. (1998). RETRACTED: Ileal-lymphoid-nodular hyperplasia, non-specific colitis, and pervasive developmental disorder in children. *The Lancet* 351 (9103): 637–641.

Who.int (2010). The Smallpox Eradication Programme – SEP (1966–1980). https://www.who.int/features/2010/smallpox/en (accessed 20 August 2019).

Who.int (2019). Immunization. https://www.who.int/topics/immunization/about/en (accessed 30 August 2019).

World Health Organization (WHO) (2004). *Immunization in Practice: A Guide for Health Workers*. WHO.

World Health Organization (2019a). GPEI – endemic countries. http://polioeradication.org/where-we-work/polio-endemic-countries (accessed 20 September 2019).

World Health Organization (2019b). Vaccines and diseases. https://www.who.int/immunization/diseases/en (accessed 30 August 2019).

Further reading

Public Health England (2013, updated September 2014). The Green Book. https://www.gov.uk/government/collections/immunisation-against-infectious-disease-the-green-book (accessed 15 September 2020).

Royal Society for Public Health (2019). Moving the needle: Promoting vaccination uptake across the life course. https://www.rsph.org.uk/static/uploaded/3b82db00-a7ef-494c-85451e78ce18a779.pdf (accessed 15 September 2020).

Multiple choice questions

1. What disease mainly affects children under five and remains endemic in two countries?
   (a) Measles
   (b) TB
   (c) Polio
   (d) Smallpox

2. Which vaccine preventable diseases are airborne?
   (a) Diptheria
   (b) Influenza
   (c) Pertussis
   (d) All of the above
3. What is an attenuated vaccine?
   (a) A weakened form of the bacteria that causes disease
   (b) A killed form of the bacteria that causes the disease
   (c) A replicate form of the bacteria that causes the disease
   (d) All of the above
4. What is herd immunity?
   (a) Immunity from diseases in cattle
   (b) Short-term immunity following vaccination
   (c) Resistance to the spread of a contagious disease if a sufficiently high proportion of individuals are immune
   (d) Immunity which results from the production of antibodies by the immune system in response to an antigen
5. How can you administer a vaccine?
   (a) IM, SC or orally
   (b) SC or IV
   (c) IV or IM
   (d) Orally or SC
6. What would you do if you are unsure of someone's immunisation history?
   (a) Leave it until the can confirm what vaccines they have had
   (b) Assume they have had them all
   (c) Check the PHE algorithm
   (d) Assume to be unimmunised and give a full course of immunisations
7. What are the contraindications to vaccination?
   (a) The individual has a confirmed history of an anaphylactic reaction to either a component of the vaccine or to a previous vaccination
   (b) The individual has a primary or acquired immunodeficiency, is on current or recent immunosuppressive or immunosuppressive biological therapy
   (c) An infant is born to a mother who received immunosuppressive biological therapy during pregnancy
   (d) All of the above
8. What are the signs of an anaphylactic reaction?
   (a) Pain at the injection site
   (b) Itchy rash
   (c) Raised temperature
   (d) Swollen lips
9. What temperature should a vaccine be stored at?
   (a) 4–6 °C
   (b) 2–6 °C
   (c) 2–8 °C
   (d) 1–5 °C

487

10. What is informed consent?
    (a) Consent given by a patient for a procedure
    (b) Consent given after the patient has received and understood the full information before the procedure
    (c) Consent given by a parent for a child
    (d) Consent in the presence of a witness

11. How old do you have to be by law to be able to consent to medical treatment?
    (a) 16 or over
    (b) 15 or over
    (c) 18
    (d) under 16 when the child demonstrates full understanding

12. When might a PSD be used?
    (a) For a named patient
    (b) For a group of patients
    (c) For a group of patients identified with a clinical condition
    (d) All of the above

13. What is a common localised reaction to a vaccine?
    (a) Pain at the injection site
    (b) Tenderness and swelling at the injection
    (c) Urticaria
    (d) Drop in blood pressure

14. What would you do if a patient refuses vaccination?
    (a) Tell them they have no choice this is a legal requirement
    (b) Provide all the information you can and help the patient make an informed decision
    (c) Write on the notes that the patient refused
    (d) Advise them to come back another day

15. What should you record in the patients notes following administration of a vaccination?
    (a) Vaccine name, product, batch number, expiry date
    (b) Dose and site administered
    (c) Date given, name and signature of vaccinator
    (d) All of the above

Find out more

The following are a list of conditions that are associated with immunisations. Take some time and write notes about each of the conditions. Think about the medications that may be used in order to treat these conditions and be specific about the pharmacokinetics and pharmacodynamics. Remember to include aspects of patient care. If you are making notes about people you have offered care and support to, you must ensure that you have adhered to the rules of confidentiality.

The condition	Your notes

The condition	Your notes

Normal Values

There are a variety of techniques that those who analyze blood use in the laboratory to identify the various components. These techniques can differ from laboratory to laboratory, it is essential that when assessment of blood results is undertaken, referral to the local laboratory's normal values is made. Variation occurs across the UK, Europe, and globally.

Hematology
Full blood count
Hemoglobin (males) 13.0–18.0 g/dl
Hemoglobin (females) 11.5–16.5 g/dl
Hematocrit (males) 0.40–0.52
Hematocrit (females) 0.36–0.47
MCV 80–96 fl
MCH 28–32 pg
MCHC 32–35 g/dl
White cell count $(4–11) \times 10^9$ l

White cell differential
Neutrophils $1.5–7 \times 10^9$ l
Lymphocytes $1.5–4 \times 10^9$ l
Monocytes $0–0.8 \times 10^9$ l
Eosinophils $0.04–0.4 \times 10^9$ l
Basophils $0–0.1 \times 10^9$ l
Platelet count $150–400 \times 10^9$ l
Reticulocyte count $(25–85) \times 10^9$ l or 0.5–2.4%

Erythrocyte sedimentation rate
Westergren
Under 50 years:
    Males 0–15 mm/1st hour
    Females 0–20 mm/1st hour
Over 50 years:
    Males 0–20 mm/1st hour
    Females 0–30 mm/1st hour

Plasma viscosity 1.50–1.72 mPa s^1 (at 25 °C)

Coagulation screen
Prothrombin time 11.5–15.5 seconds
International normalized ratio < 1.4
Activated partial thromboplastin time 30–40 seconds
Fibrinogen 1.8–5.4 g/l
Bleeding time 3–8 minutes

Coagulation factors
Factors II, V, VII, VIII, IX, X, XI, XII 50–150 IU/dl

Fundamentals of Pharmacology: For Nursing and Healthcare Students, First Edition. Edited by Ian Peate and Barry Hill.
© 2021 John Wiley & Sons Ltd. Published 2021 by John Wiley & Sons Ltd.

Factor V Leiden Present or not
Von Willebrand factor 45–150 IU/dl
Von Willebrand factor antigen 50–150 IU/dl
Protein C 80–135 IU/dl
Protein S 80–120 IU/dl
Antithrombin III 80–120 IU/dl
Activated protein C resistance 2.12–4.0
Fibrin degradation products <100 mg/l
D-dimer screen <0.5 mg/l

Hematinics
Serum iron 12–30 μmol/l
Serum iron-binding capacity 45–75 μmol/l
Serum ferritin 15–300 μg/l
Serum transferrin 2.0–4.0 g/l
Serum B_{12} 160–760 ng/l
Serum folate 2.0–11.0 μg/l
Red cell folate 160–640 μg/l
Serum haptoglobin 0.13–1.63 g/l

Hemoglobin electrophoresis
Hemoglobin A > 95%
Hemoglobin A2 2–3%
Hemoglobin F < 2%

Chemistry
Serum sodium 137–144 mmol/l
Serum potassium 3.5–4.9 mmol/l
Serum chloride 95–107 mmol/l
Serum bicarbonate 20–28 mmol/l
Anion gap 12–16 mmol/l
Serum urea 2.5–7.5 mmol/l
Serum creatinine 60–110 μmol/l
Serum corrected calcium 2.2–2.6 mmol/l
Serum phosphate 0.8–1.4 mmol/l
Serum total protein 61–76 g/l
Serum albumin 37–49 g/l
Serum total bilirubin 1–22 μmol/l
Serum conjugated bilirubin 0–3.4 μmol/l
Serum alanine aminotransferase 5–35 U/l
Serum aspartate aminotransferase 1–31 U/l
Serum alkaline phosphatase 45–105 U/l (over 14 years)
Serum gamma glutamyl transferase 4–35 U/l (<50 U/l in males)
Serum lactate dehydrogenase 10–250 U/l
Serum creatine kinase (males) 24–195 U/l
Serum creatine kinase (females) 24–170 U/l
Creatine kinase MB fraction <5%
Serum troponin I 0–0.4 μg/l
Serum troponin T 0–0.1 μg/l
Serum copper 12–26 μmol/l
Serum caeruloplasmin 200–350 mg/l
Serum aluminum 0–10 μg/l
Serum magnesium 0.75–1.05 mmol/l
Serum zinc 6–25 μmol/l
Serum urate (males) 0.23–0.46 mmol/l

Serum urate (females) 0.19–0.36 mmol/l
Plasma lactate 0.6–1.8 mmol/l
Plasma ammonia 12–55 µmol/l
Serum angiotensin-converting enzyme 25–82 U/l
Fasting plasma glucose 3.0–6.0 mmol/L
Hemoglobin A1 C 3.8–6.4%
Fructosamine <285 µmo/l
Serum amylase 60–180 U/l
Plasma osmolality 278–305 mosmol/kg

Lipids and lipoproteins
Target levels will vary depending on the patient's overall cardiovascular risk assessment
Serum cholesterol <5.2 mmol/l
Serum LDL cholesterol <3.36 mmol/l
Serum HDL cholesterol >1.55 mmol/l
Fasting serum triglyceride 0.45–1.69 mmol/l

Blood gases (breathing air at sea level)
Blood H$^+$ 35–45 nmol/l
pH 7.36–7.44
PaO$_2$ 11.3–12.6 kPa
PaCO$_2$ 4.7–6.0 kPa
Base excess ±2 mmol/l

Carboxyhemoglobin
Non-smoker <2%
Smoker 3–15%

Immunology/rheumatology
Complement C3 65–190 mg/dl
Complement C4 15–50 mg/dl
Total hemolytic (CH50) 150–250 U/l
Serum C-reactive protein <10 mg/l

Serum immunoglobulins
IgG 6.0–13.0 g/l
IgA 0.8–3.0 g/l
IgM 0.4–2.5 g/l
IgE <120 kU/l
Serum β_2-microglobulin <3 mg/l

Cerebrospinal fluid
Opening pressure 50–180 mmH$_2$O
Total protein 0.15–0.45 g/l
Albumin 0.066–0.442 g/l
Chloride 116–122 mmol/l
Glucose 3.3–4.4 mmol/l
Lactate 1–2 mmol/l
Cell count ≤5 mL^{-1}

Differential
Lymphocytes 60–70%
Monocytes 30–50%
Neutrophils None
IgG/ALB ≤0.26
IgG index ≤0.88

Urine

Albumin/creatinine ratio (untimed specimen) <3.5 mg/mmol (males)
<2.5 mg/mmol (females)
Glomerular filtration rate 70–140 ml/min
Total protein <0.2 g/24 hours
Albumin <30 mg/24 hours
Calcium 2.5–7.5 mmol/24 hours
Urobilinogen 1.7–5.9 µmol/24 hours
Coproporphyrin <300 nmol/24 hours
Uroporphyrin 6–24 nmol/24 hours
δ-Aminolevulinate 8–53 µmol/24 hours
5-Hydroxyindoleacetic acid 10–47 µmol/24 hours
Osmolality 350–1000 mosmol/kg

Feces

Nitrogen 70–140 mmol/24 hours
Urobilinogen 50–500 µmol/24 hours
Fat (on normal diet) <7 g/24 hours

Answers

Chapter 1
1. (a); **2.** (c); **3.** (c); **4.** (c); **5.** (d); **6.** (b); **7.** (c); **8.** (c); **9.** (b); **10.** (a); **11.** (b); **12.** (d); **13.** (b); **14.** (a); **15.** (b)

Chapter 2
1. (c); **2.** (a); **3.** (b); **4.** (b); **5.** (c); **6.** (b); **7.** (d); **8.** (c); **9.** (b); **10.** (a); **11.** (c); **12.** (c); **13.** (c); **14.** (b); **15.** (c)

Chapter 3
1. (b); **2.** (c); **3.** (c); **4.** (a); **5.** (d); **6.** (d); **7.** (a); **8.** (c); **9.** (c); **10.** (a); **11.** (d); **12.** (d); **13.** (d); **14.** (d); **15.** (d)

Chapter 4
1. (a); **2.** (c); **3.** (c); **4.** (b); **5.** (b); **6.** (a); **7.** (a); **8.** (b); **9.** (c); **10.** (b); **11.** (b); **12.** (a); **13.** (c); **14.** (a); **15.** (b)

Chapter 5
1. (a); **2.** (a); **3.** (e); **4.** (b); **5.** (a); **6.** (d); **7.** (b); **8.** (d); **9.** (a); **10.** (a); **11.** (c); **12.** (a); **13.** (a); **14.** (c); **15.** (a)

Chapter 6
1. (b); **2.** (c); **3.** (b); **4.** (c); **5.** (b); **6.** (a); **7.** (c); **8.** (b, c); **9.** (b); **10.** (d); **11.** (c); **12.** (c); **13.** (d); **14.** (c); **15.** (d)

Chapter 7
1. (c); **2.** (c); **3.** (c); **4.** (a); **5.** (b); **6.** (a); **7.** (c); **8.** (b); **9.** (b); **10.** (c); **11.** (b); **12.** (a); **13.** (c); **14.** (c); **15.** (c)

Chapter 8
1. (c); **2.** (a); **3.** (c); **4.** (b); **5.** (c); **6.** (a); **7.** (c); **8.** (b); **9.** (a); **10.** (d); **11.** (c); **12.** (d); **13.** (d); **14.** (b); **15.** (a)

Fundamentals of Pharmacology: For Nursing and Healthcare Students, First Edition. Edited by Ian Peate and Barry Hill.
© 2021 John Wiley & Sons Ltd. Published 2021 by John Wiley & Sons Ltd.

Chapter 9

1. (b); 2. (d); 3. (b); 4. (c); 5. (a); 6. (d); 7. (d); 8. (d); 9. (a); 10. (a); 11. (a); 12. (b); 13. (d); 14. (d); 15. (b)

Chapter 10

1. (c); 2. (b); 3. (b); 4. (d); 5. (b); 6. (b); 7. (c); 8. (b); 9. (a); 10. (a, b); 11. (b, c); 12. (b, c, d); 13. (e); 14. (a, d); 15. (a, c)

Chapter 11

1. (a); 2. (c); 3. (c); 4. (a); 5. (b); 6. (d); 7. (a); 8. (c); 9. (b); 10. (d); 11. (b); 12. (c); 13. (c); 14. (a); 15. (b)

Chapter 12

1. (c); 2. (d); 3. (c); 4. (c); 5. (b); 6. (b); 7. (d); 8. (a); 9. (d); 10. (a); 11. (a); 12. (c); 13. (c); 14. (b); 15. (d)

Chapter 13

1. (a); 2. (c); 3. (b); 4. (c); 5. (a); 6. (c); 7. (d); 8. (d); 9. (b); 10. (a); 11. (d); 12. (c); 13. (c); 14. (c); 15. (c)

Chapter 14

1. (b); 2. (a); 3. (b); 4. (d); 5. (c); 6. (b); 7. (d); 8. (a); 9. (d); 10. (c); 11. (b); 12. (a); 13. (b); 14. (d); 15. (d)

Chapter 15

1. (c); 2. (a); 3. (a); 4. (d); 5. (c); 6. (b); 7. (a); 8. (c); 9. (b); 10. (d); 11. (a); 12. (c); 13. (d); 14. (a); 15. (c)

Chapter 16

1. (d); 2. (b); 3. (d); 4. (d); 5. (a); 6. (c); 7. (c); 8. (b); 9. (c); 10. (c); 11. (c); 12. (c); 13. (b); 14. (d); 15. (a)

Chapter 17

1. (c); 2. (d); 3. (a); 4. (e); 5. (a); 6. (d); 7. (e); 8. (a); 9. (a); 10. (c); 11. (d); 12. (c); 13. (d); 14. (d); 15. (d)

Chapter 18

1. (c); 2. (d); 3. (a); 4. (c); 5. (a); 6. (c); 7. (d); 8. (b); 9. (c); 10. (b); 11. (d); 12. (c); 13. (b); 14. (b); 15. (d)

Index

Note: Page numbers in *italic* refer to figures.
Page numbers in **bold** refer to tables.

Fundamentals of Pharmacology: For Nursing and Healthcare Students, First Edition. Edited by Ian Peate and Barry Hill.
© 2021 John Wiley & Sons Ltd. Published 2021 by John Wiley & Sons Ltd.